Postgraduate Manual of
OBSTETRICS & GYNECOLOGY
for Practical Examination

AF096828

Postgraduate Manual of
OBSTETRICS & GYNECOLOGY
for Practical Examination

Third Edition

Editors

Sumita Mehta
DGO DNB FICOG MAMS
Senior Specialist and Head
Department of Obstetrics and Gynecology
Babu Jagjivan Ram Memorial Hospital
New Delhi, India

Sandhya Jain
MD DNB FICOG MRCOG (UK)
Director-Professor
Department of Obstetrics and Gynecology
University College of Medical Sciences and
Guru Teg Bahadur Hospital
New Delhi, India

Shalini Rajaram
MD FAMS FICOG
Professor and Program Lead
Department of Obstetrics and Gynecology
All India Institute of Medical Sciences
Rishikesh, Uttarakhand, India

Neerja Goel
MD FAMS FIMSA FICOG FFGSI
Senior Consultant
Department of Obstetrics and Gynecology
School of Medical Sciences and Research and
Sharda Hospital, Sharda University
Greater Noida, Uttar Pradesh, India

Foreword
Amita Suneja

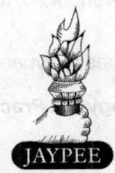

JAYPEE BROTHERS MEDICAL PUBLISHERS
The Health Sciences Publisher
New Delhi | London

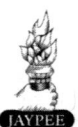 **Jaypee Brothers Medical Publishers (P) Ltd**

Headquarters
Jaypee Brothers Medical Publishers (P) Ltd
EMCA House, 23/23-B
Ansari Road, Daryaganj
New Delhi 110 002, India
Landline: +91-11-23272143, +91-11-23272703
+91-11-23282021, +91-11-23245672
Email: jaypee@jaypeebrothers.com

Corporate Office
Jaypee Brothers Medical Publishers (P) Ltd
4838/24, Ansari Road, Daryaganj
New Delhi 110 002, India
Phone: +91-11-43574357
Fax: +91-11-43574314
Email: jaypee@jaypeebrothers.com

Overseas Office
JP Medical Ltd
83 Victoria Street, London
SW1H 0HW (UK)
Phone: +44 20 3170 8910
Fax: +44 (0)20 3008 6180
Email: info@jpmedpub.com

Website: www.jaypeebrothers.com
Website: www.jaypeedigital.com

© 2024, Jaypee Brothers Medical Publishers

The views and opinions expressed in this book are solely those of the original contributor(s)/author(s) and do not necessarily represent those of editor(s) or publisher of the book.

All rights reserved. No part of this publication may be reproduced, stored or transmitted in any form or by any means, electronic, mechanical, photocopying, recording or otherwise, without the prior permission in writing of the publishers.

All brand names and product names used in this book are trade names, service marks, trademarks or registered trademarks of their respective owners. The publisher is not associated with any product or vendor mentioned in this book.

Medical knowledge and practice change constantly. This book is designed to provide accurate, authoritative information about the subject matter in question. However, readers are advised to check the most current information available on procedures included and check information from the manufacturer of each product to be administered, to verify the recommended dose, formula, method and duration of administration, adverse effects and contraindications. It is the responsibility of the practitioner to take all appropriate safety precautions. Neither the publisher nor the author(s)/editor(s) assume any liability for any injury and/or damage to persons or property arising from or related to use of material in this book.

This book is sold on the understanding that the publisher is not engaged in providing professional medical services. If such advice or services are required, the services of a competent medical professional should be sought.

Every effort has been made where necessary to contact holders of copyright to obtain permission to reproduce copyright material. If any have been inadvertently overlooked, the publisher will be pleased to make the necessary arrangements at the first opportunity.

Inquiries for bulk sales may be solicited at: jaypee@jaypeebrothers.com

Postgraduate Manual of Obstetrics & Gynecology for Practical Examination

First Edition: 2009

Second Edition: 2018

Third Edition: **2024**

ISBN: 978-93-5696-891-2

Printed in India

Contributors

Astha Srivastava MD DNB MRCOG
Senior Consultant
Department of Obstetrics and Gynecology
Sarvodaya Hospital
Greater Noida, Uttar Pradesh, India

Abha Sharma MD
Senior Specialist
Department of Obstetrics and Gynecology
University College of Medical Sciences and
Guru Teg Bahadur Hospital
New Delhi, India

Amita Suneja MD FAMS FIMCH FICOG
Director-Professor and Head
Department of Obstetrics and Gynecology
University College of Medical Sciences and
Guru Teg Bahadur Hospital
New Delhi, India

Anita Matai MD FICOG MAMS FIMSA FICMCH
Consultant
Department of Obstetrics and Gynecology
Max Super Specialty Hospital
New Delhi, India

Ankita Jain MS
Senior Resident
Department of Obstetrics and Gynecology
University College of Medical Sciences and
Guru Teg Bahadur Hospital
New Delhi, India

Annu Kumari MD DNB
Senior Resident
Department of Obstetrics and Gynecology
University College of Medical Sciences and
Guru Teg Bahadur Hospital
New Delhi, India

Anshuja Singla MD
Professor
Department of Obstetrics and Gynecology
University College of Medical Sciences and
Guru Teg Bahadur Hospital
New Delhi, India

Archana Mehta MD MAMS FICOG
Professor and Head
Department of Obstetrics and Gynecology
School of Medical Sciences and Research and
Sharda Hospital, Sharda University
Greater Noida, Uttar Pradesh, India

Archana Mishra MD
Professor
Department of Obstetrics and Gynecology
Vardhman Mahavir Medical College and
Safdarjung Hospital
New Delhi, India

Bindiya Gupta MS
Professor
Department of Obstetrics and Gynecology
University College of Medical Sciences and
Guru Teg Bahadur Hospital
New Delhi, India

Himsweta Srivastava MD
Director-Professor
Department of Obstetrics and Gynecology
University College of Medical Sciences and
Guru Teg Bahadur Hospital
New Delhi, India

Latika Chawla
MD DNB Fellow Maternal and Fetal Medicine
Additional Professor
Department of Obstetrics and Gynecology
All India Institute of Medical Sciences
Rishikesh, Uttarakhand, India

Contributors

Manpreet Singh
MD FCCP FIMSA FACEE FCCS MAMS FICA
Professor
Department of Anesthesiology and
Intensive Care
Government Medical College and Hospital
Chandigarh, India

Mayuri Ahuja DGO DNB
Assistant Professor
Department of Obstetrics and Gynecology
School of Medical Sciences and Research and
Sharda Hospital, Sharda University
Greater Noida, Uttar Pradesh, India

Namita Grover MD
Consultant
Department of Obstetrics and Gynecology
Shalby Hospital
Mohali, Punjab, India

Nazia Parveen MS
Assistant Professor
Department of Obstetrics and Gynecology
University College of Medical Sciences and
Guru Teg Bahadur Hospital
New Delhi, India

Neerja Goel MD FAMS FIMSA FICOG FFGSI
Senior Consultant
Department of Obstetrics and Gynecology
School of Medical Sciences and Research and
Sharda Hospital, Sharda University
Greater Noida, Uttar Pradesh, India

Neha Kumar MS MCh (Gynecological Oncology)
Senior Consultant
Department of Gynecologic Oncology
Amrita Hospital
Faridabad, Haryana, India

Om Kumari
DGO MS PDCC (Maternal & Fetal Medicine)
Associate Professor
Department of Obstetrics and Gynecology
All India Institute of Medical Sciences
Rishikesh, Uttarakhand, India

Pakhee Aggarwal MS FICOG MRCOG MIPHA
Senior Consultant
Department of Gynecologic Oncology and
Robotic Surgery
Indraprastha Apollo Hospital
New Delhi, India

Penzy Goyal MS MRCOG
Senior Resident
Department of Obstetrics and Gynecology
University College of Medical Sciences and
Guru Teg Bahadur Hospital
New Delhi, India

Pikee Saxena MD FICOG MNAMS PGCC PGDCR
Director-Professor
Department of Obstetrics and Gynecology
Lady Hardinge Medical College and
Smt Sucheta Kriplani Hospital
New Delhi, India

Priyanka Mathe MS FICMCH
Associate Professor
Department of Obstetrics and Gynecology
University College of Medical Sciences and
Guru Teg Bahadur Hospital
New Delhi, India

Rachna Agarwal MD
Director-Professor and Unit Head
Department of Obstetrics and Gynecology
University College of Medical Sciences and
Guru Teg Bahadur Hospital
New Delhi, India

Rajeev Kumar Thapar MD DIT MAMS
Professor and Head
Department of Pediatrics
School of Medical Sciences and Research and
Sharda Hospital, Sharda University
Greater Noida, Uttar Pradesh, India

Rashmi Gupta MBBS Mphil (HHSM)
CMO, In-charge Family Planning
Department of Obstetrics and Gynecology
University College of Medical Sciences and
Guru Teg Bahadur Hospital
New Delhi, India

Rashmi Malik MD
Professor
Department of Obstetrics and Gynecology
University College of Medical Sciences and
Guru Teg Bahadur Hospital
New Delhi, India

Rashmi Salhotra MD MAMS
Professor
Department of Anesthesiology
University College of Medical Sciences and
Guru Teg Bahadur Hospital
New Delhi, India

Richa Aggarwal MD
Professor
Department of Obstetrics and Gynecology
University College of Medical Sciences and
Guru Teg Bahadur Hospital
New Delhi, India

Richa Sharma MS MNAMS FICOG FICMCH FMAS
Director-Professor
Department of Obstetrics and Gynecology
University College of Medical Sciences and
Guru Teg Bahadur Hospital
New Delhi, India

Ruchi Narayan MD (Radiology)
Senior Resident
Department of Radiology
School of Medical Sciences and Research and
Sharda Hospital, Sharda University
Greater Noida, Uttar Pradesh, India

Ruchi Srivastava MS MAMS FICOG
Professor and Unit Head
Department of Obstetrics and Gynecology
School of Medical Sciences and Research and
Sharda Hospital, Sharda University
Greater Noida, Uttar Pradesh, India

Rupali Bhatia MS
Ex-Senior Resident
Department of Obstetrics and Gynecology
Babu Jagjivan Ram Memorial Hospital
New Delhi, India

Saloni Chadha DrNB (Gyne Oncology) MS
Resident
Department of Obstetrics and Gynecology
Vardhman Mahavir Medical College and
Safdarjung Hospital
New Delhi, India

Samta Gupta MS MAMS FICOG
Professor and Unit Head
Department of Obstetrics and Gynecology
School of Medical Sciences and Research and
Sharda Hospital, Sharda University
Greater Noida, Uttar Pradesh, India

Sandhya Jain MD DNB FICOG MRCOG (UK)
Director-Professor
Department of Obstetrics and Gynecology
University College of Medical Sciences and
Guru Teg Bahadur Hospital
New Delhi, India

Shailza Vardhan MS
Assistant Professor
Department of Obstetrics and Gynecology
School of Medical Sciences and Research and
Sharda Hospital, Sharda University
Greater Noida, Uttar Pradesh, India

Shalini Rajaram
MD FAMS FICOG
Professor and Program Lead
Department of Obstetrics and Gynecology
All India Institute of Medical Sciences
Rishikesh, Uttarakhand, India

Shelly Agarwal MS FICOG
Professor and Unit Head
Department of Obstetrics and Gynecology
School of Medical Sciences and Research and
Sharda Hospital, Sharda University
Greater Noida, Uttar Pradesh, India

Shivangini Sahay MS
Senior Resident
Department of Obstetrics and Gynecology
School of Medical Sciences and Research and
Sharda Hospital, Sharda University
Greater Noida, Uttar Pradesh, India

Smiti Jain DGO DNB MRCOG
Consultant
Department of Obstetrics and Gynecology
Greater Noida, Uttar Pradesh, India

Sonam Singh MS
Ex-Senior Resident
Department of Obstetrics and Gynecology
Babu Jagjivan Ram Memorial Hospital
New Delhi, India

Sonia Chawla MS
Senior Consultant and Gyne Laparoscopic Surgeon
Department of Obstetrics and Gynecology
Shanti Gopal Hospital
New Delhi, India

Sruthi Bhaskaran MS
Professor
Department of Obstetrics and Gynecology
University College of Medical Sciences and
Guru Teg Bahadur Hospital
New Delhi, India

Sumeet Singla MD DNB MNAMS
Professor
Department of Medicine
Maulana Azad Medical College
New Delhi, India

Sumita Mehta DGO DNB FICOG MAMS
Senior Specialist and Head
Department of Obstetrics and Gynecology
Babu Jagjivan Ram Memorial Hospital
New Delhi, India

Surinder Singh Gulati MD
Senior Consultant
Department of Obstetrics and Gynecology
School of Medical Sciences and Research and
Sharda Hospital, Sharda University
Greater Noida, Uttar Pradesh, India

Upasana Verma MS DNB
Associate Professor
Department of Obstetrics and Gynecology
University College of Medical Sciences and
Guru Teg Bahadur Hospital
New Delhi, India

Vashudha Gupta MS
Associate Professor
Department of Obstetrics and Gynecology
All India Institute of Medical Sciences
Rishikesh, Uttarakhand, India

Vikas Yadav DNB MD FAGE FICMCH D ART FMAS
Associate Professor and IVF Head
School of Medical Sciences and Research and
Sharda Hospital, Sharda University
Greater Noida, Uttar Pradesh, India

Vineeta Rathi MD
Director-Professor
Department of Radiodiagnosis
University College of Medical Sciences and
Guru Teg Bahadur Hospital
New Delhi, India

Vishal Gupta MD (Radiology)
Professor and Head
Department of Radiology
School of Medical Sciences and Research and
Sharda Hospital, Sharda University
Greater Noida, Uttar Pradesh, India

Foreword

It is with great pleasure and a sense of profound professional privilege that I write the foreword for the book titled *Postgraduate Manual of Obstetrics & Gynecology for Practical Examination*. In an era where medical knowledge is expanding at an unprecedented rate, the importance of a comprehensive, yet focused, educational resource cannot be overstated. This textbook, meticulously crafted by esteemed authors in the field, provides a detailed yet concise overview of obstetrics and gynecology, tailored specifically to the needs of students preparing for crucial examinations.

What sets this book apart is its unique approach to combining essential theoretical knowledge with practical clinical insights in a question-answer format. The chapters are structured to facilitate easy understanding, covering a wide range of topics from fundamental concepts to the latest advancements in the field. The authors have done an admirable job in distilling complex concepts into understandable segments without losing the depth and rigor required at this level of study.

The learned editors are passionate teachers with vast experience and are known for their in-depth knowledge of the subject and perfection. They have done an admirable job and deserve high appreciation for their devoted efforts. It is their vision which is being materialized into a very practical and useful book.

This book is not just a tool for exam preparation; it is a gateway to becoming a competent and compassionate healthcare professional in the field of obstetrics and gynecology. I strongly recommend this book to all students who are embarking on this challenging yet immensely rewarding journey.

Amita Suneja
MD FAMS FIMCH FICOG
Director-Professor and Head
Department of Obstetrics and Gynecology
University College of Medical Sciences and
Guru Teg Bahadur Hospital
New Delhi, India
President
Association of Obstetricians and
Gynaecologists of Delhi (AOGD) (2022–23)

Preface to the Third Edition

Our journey in creating this textbook began with a clear vision: To bridge the gap between theoretical knowledge and its practical application in obstetrics and gynecology. We recognized the need for a resource that not only prepares students for their examinations but also equips them with a robust understanding of real-world clinical scenarios they will encounter in their medical careers.

In crafting this book, we have meticulously curated content that encompasses the entire spectrum of obstetrics and gynecology. The book will serve as a reference manual to students for the practical examination. The book will serve as a reference manual to students for the practical examination as it discusses all topics relevant to viva voce in detail with ample illustrations. Furthermore, the question/answer format which is a unique feature of the book will help students learn the art of good presentation.

In response to the rapid advancements in the medical field, we have brought out the third edition of the book with a purpose of updating the chapters in the previous edition and adding new chapters on emerging trends and technologies in obstetrics and gynecology. The new edition includes chapters like Robotic Surgery in Gynecology, Medical Termination of Pregnancy Act with Amendments, Assisted Reproductive Technologies and Surrogacy, and Principles of Counseling in Obstetrics and Gynecology, thereby ensuring that our readers are up-to-date with the latest developments. The manual will be immensely beneficial to the students and will add to their armamentarium of knowledge regarding recent advances in the field of obstetrics and gynecology which will subsequently help them to perform better in examinations.

Collaboration has been at the heart of this endeavor. We have had the privilege of working with a team of distinguished authors whose contributions have been instrumental in bringing depth and diversity to the content. We extend our heartfelt gratitude to all contributors for their invaluable insights and dedication to this project.

In closing, we sincerely hope that this book not only serves as a comprehensive manual for students preparing for their examinations but also lays a foundation for lifelong learning in a constantly evolving medical landscape. We are honored to be a part of your educational journey and wish you the very best in your endeavors.

Sumita Mehta
Sandhya Jain
Shalini Rajaram
Neerja Goel

Preface to the First Edition

Over the years, we have felt the need for a comprehensive manual to aid the postgraduate students in their practical examinations. Though the students are well prepared for the theory examination, there is always a want for a book which will help them in answering the Viva-Voce questions completely and confidently.

Keeping this in mind, we have written the manual which will serve as companion to the students in reparation for the practical examination. The contents are divided into various sections which cover in detail with ample illustrations of all the topics relevant to Viva-Voce. It also includes the question/answer format which will help the students to learn the art of presenting answers during examination.

We hope this book will help our exam-going students to perform better in their exams and a feedback to this book would be welcomed.

Neerja Goel
Sumita Mehta
Shalini Rajaram
Himsweta Srivastava

Acknowledgments

We wish to acknowledge the support and encouragement we received from our respective institutions for allowing and encouraging us to pursue our academic venture.

No work of excellence can be done in isolation. We would like to thank all the authors for their unconditional support in bringing out the third edition and for providing excellent updated chapters on various subjects. Their invaluable input, meticulous attention to detail, and commitment to excellence have significantly enriched the quality of this textbook. We are honored to have worked alongside such esteemed professionals.

We also express our sincere thanks to the entire publishing team at M/s Jaypee Brothers Medical Publishers (P) Ltd, New Delhi, India, for their expertise and dedication in bringing this project to fruition.

We are profoundly grateful to our families for their unwavering support and encouragement throughout this process. Their patience, understanding, and belief in our work have been our pillars of strength.

Lastly, we thank the students, our readers, for whom this book is written. Your endless quest for knowledge has motivated us to create resources that support your academic and professional growth.

Contents

1. **History Taking and Examination of Long/Short Cases** 1
   Shalini Rajaram, Om Kumari, Namita Grover, Neerja Goel

2. **Immunization in Pregnancy** 17
   Pakhee Aggarwal, Sandhya Jain

3. **First- and Second-trimester Aneuploidy Screening** 23
   Astha Srivastava, Sandhya Jain

4. **Fetal Monitoring** 29
   Sruthi Bhaskaran, Himsweta Srivastava, Shalini Rajaram

5. **Maternal Pelvis and Fetal Skull** 44
   Himsweta Srivastava

6. **Normal Labor** 50
   Rashmi Malik, Annu Kumari

7. **Abnormal Presentations** 67
   Smiti Jain, Amita Suneja, Anita Matai

8. **Instrumental Delivery** 86
   Sumita Mehta, Sonam Singh

9. **Obstetric Procedures** 96
   Abha Sharma, Sruthi Bhaskaran

10. **Obstetric Drills** 108
    Upasana Verma, Sumita Mehta

11. **Maternal Resuscitation** 120
    Rashmi Salhotra

12. **Neonatal Resuscitation** 126
    Rajeev Kumar Thapar

13. **Instruments** 149
    Shalini Rajaram, Sandhya Jain, Om Kumari, Vashudha Gupta

14. **Endoscopy: Laparoscopy and Hysteroscopy** 172
    Sumita Mehta, Shalini Rajaram, Latika Chawla

15. **Robotic Surgery in Gynecology** 187
    Latika Chawla, Shalini Rajaram

16. **Incisions** 194
    Sonia Chawla, Bindiya Gupta

17. **Sutures, Needles, and Meshes** 203
    Rachna Agarwal, Penzy Goyal

18. **Disease-specific Investigations in Obstetrics and Gynecology** 218
    Sumita Mehta, Rupali Bhatia

19. **Obstetric Specimens** 233
    Pikee Saxena, Archana Mishra, Saloni Chadha

20. **Gynecology Specimens** 249
    Ruchi Srivastava, Shailza Vardhan, Neerja Goel

21. **Imaging: Hysterosalpingogram, X-ray, and CT Scan** 280
    Himsweta Srivastava, Richa Aggarwal, Vineeta Rathi

22. **Ultrasonography in Obstetrics** 298
    Vishal Gupta, Ruchi Narayan

23. **Drugs in Obstetrics and Gynecology** 310
    Sandhya Jain, Nazia Parveen, Astha Srivastava, Sumeet Singla

24. **Prescription Writing** 334
    Neerja Goel, Anshuja Singla, Ankita Jain

25. **Contraception** 348
    Rashmi Malik, Annu Kumari

26. **Medical Termination of Pregnancy Act with Amendments** 371
    Richa Sharma

27. **Consent in Family Planning: Medicolegal Aspects** 377
    Rashmi Gupta

28. **Definitions** 394
    Archana Mehta, Shivangini Sahay, Neerja Goel, Anshuja Singla

29. **Anesthetic Techniques** 406
    Manpreet Singh, Namita Grover

30. **Fluids and Electrolytes** 415
    Manpreet Singh, Namita Grover

31. **Assisted Reproductive Technologies and Surrogacy** 428
    Vikas Yadav, Neerja Goel

32. **Principles of Counseling in Obstetrics and Gynecology** 438
    Surinder Singh Gulati

33. **Normal Values of Investigations Related to Obstetrics and Gynecology** 455
    Samta Gupta

34. **Classification in Obstetrics and Gynecology** 459
    Priyanka Mathe, Neha Kumar

35. **New FIGO Classification of Gynecological Cancers** 471
    Shelly Agarwal, Mayuri Ahuja

Index *483*

Plate 1

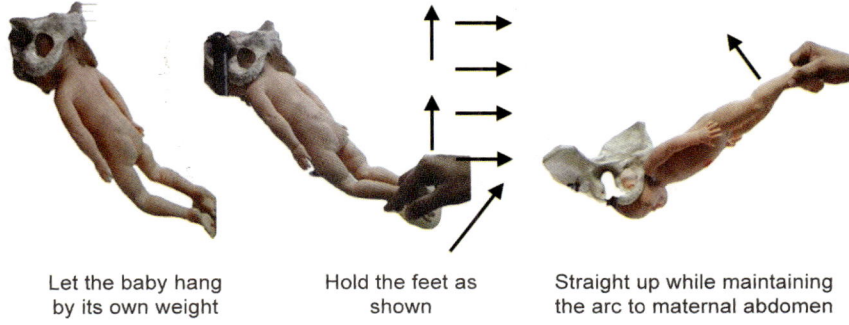

Let the baby hang by its own weight

Hold the feet as shown

Straight up while maintaining the arc to maternal abdomen

Fig. 1: Burns–Marshall technique. *(Chapter 7)*

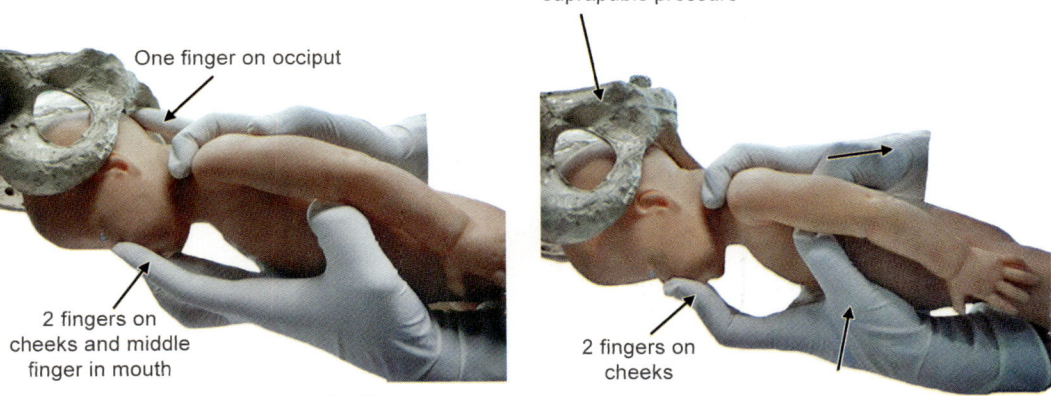

One finger on occiput

2 fingers on cheeks and middle finger in mouth

Fig. 2: Original Mauriceau–Smellie–Veit method. *(Chapter 7)*

Assistant gives the suprapubic pressure

2 fingers on cheeks

Fig. 3: Modified Mauriceau–Smellie–Veit method. *(Chapter 7)*

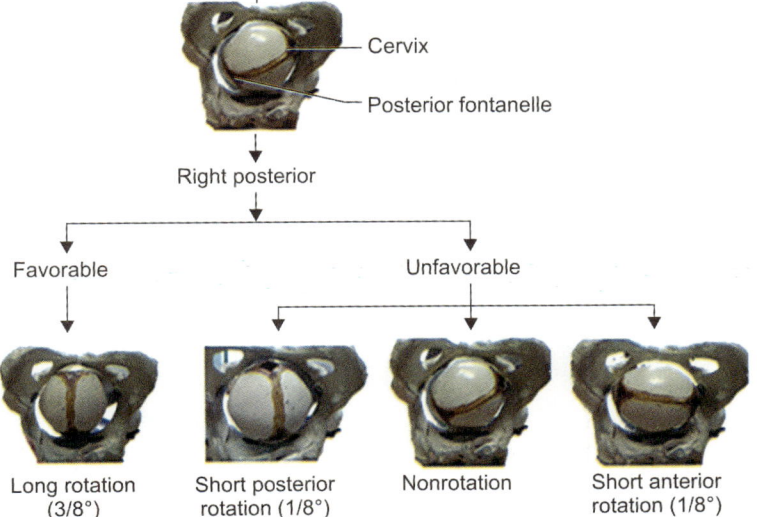

Symphysis pubis

Cervix

Posterior fontanelle

Right posterior

Favorable

Unfavorable

Long rotation (3/8°)

Short posterior rotation (1/8°)

Nonrotation

Short anterior rotation (1/8°)

Fig. 7: Diagrammatic representations showing favorable and unfavorable rotation of occipitoposterior position. *(Chapter 7)*

Plate 2

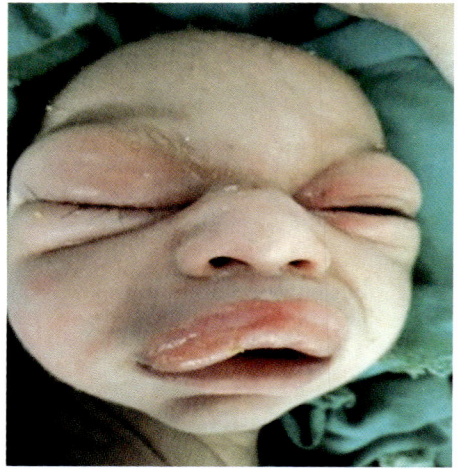

Fig. 8: Edema in face presentation. *(Chapter 7)*

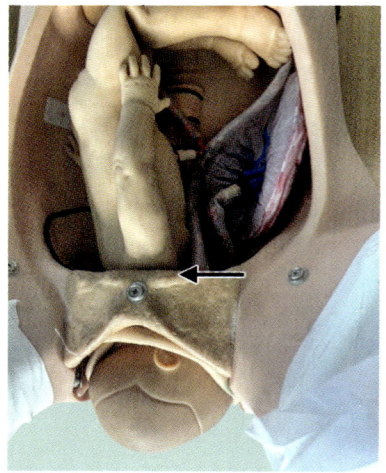

Fig. 1: Shoulder dystocia. *(Chapter 10)*

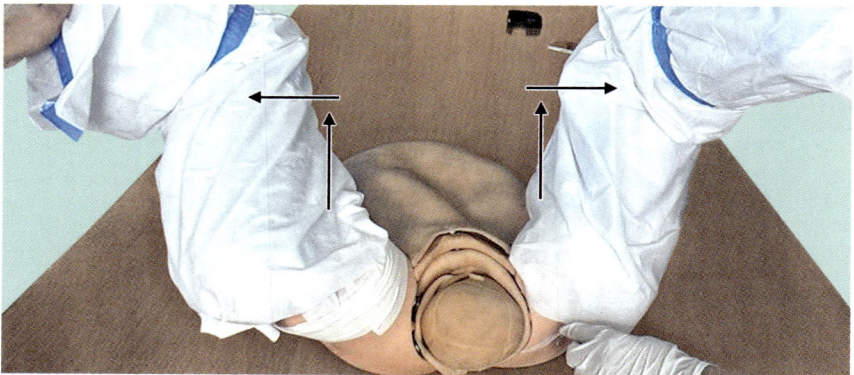

Fig. 2: McRoberts maneuver. *(Chapter 10)*

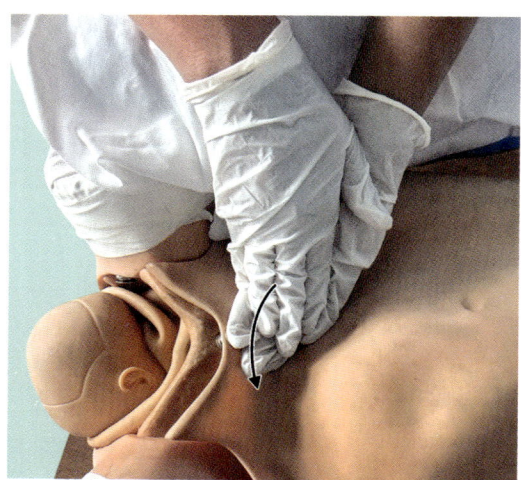

Fig. 3: Suprapubic pressure. *(Chapter 10)*

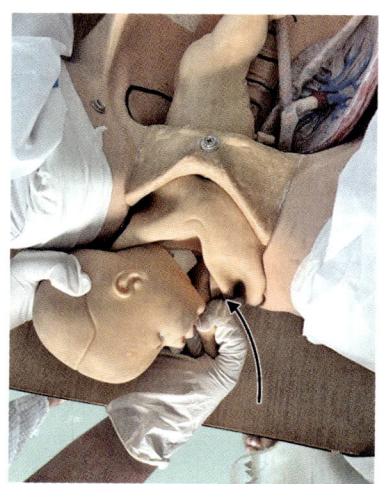

Fig. 4: Posterior arm extraction. *(Chapter 10)*

Plate 3

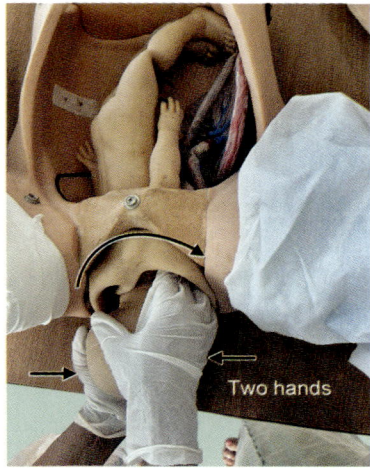

Fig. 5: Woods corkscrew maneuver. *(Chapter 10)*

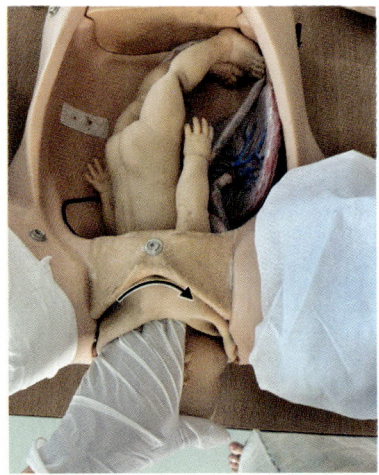

Fig. 6: Rubin's maneuver. *(Chapter 10)*

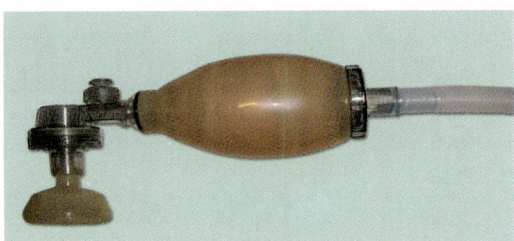

Fig. 3: Self-inflating bag and mask. *(Chapter 12)*

Plate 4

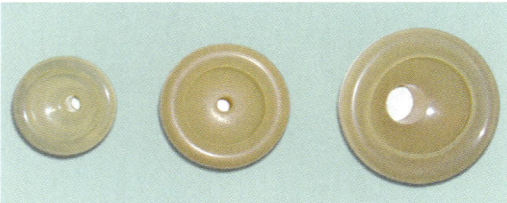

Fig. 6: Various sizes of face cushioned and rounded masks: 00, 0, and 1. *(Chapter 12)*

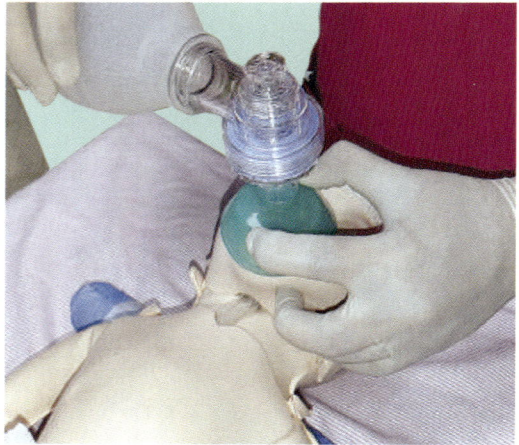

Fig. 8: PPV with "C" and "E" clamp to provide tight seal. (PPV: positive-pressure ventilation). *(Chapter 12)*

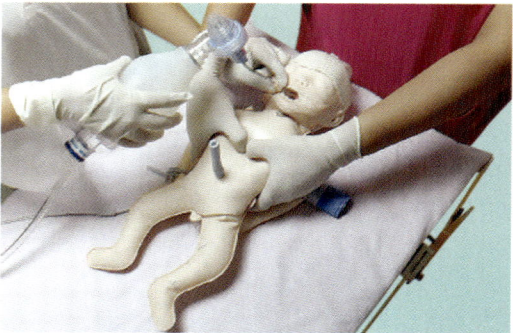

Fig. 9: Chest compression from the head end and PPV from the side of the baby. *(Chapter 12)*

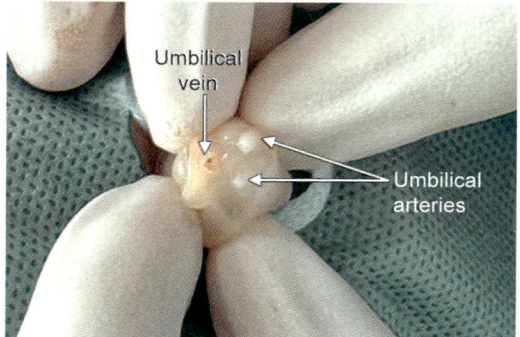

Fig. 10: Umbilical cord showing umbilical two arteries and one vein. *(Chapter 12)*

Plate 5

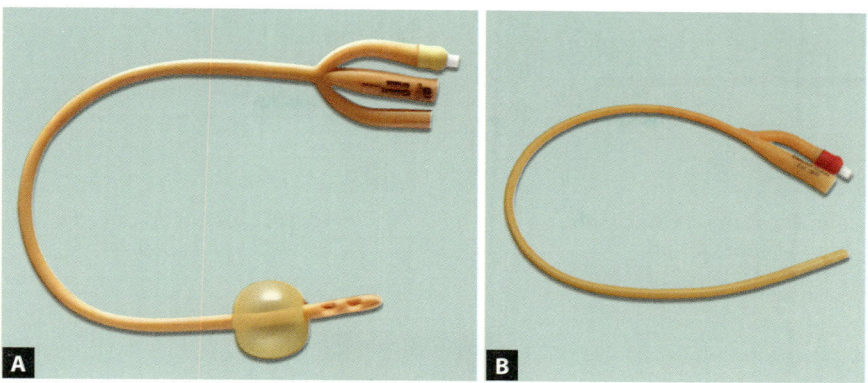

Figs. 28A and B: Foley's catheter image. *(Chapter 13)*

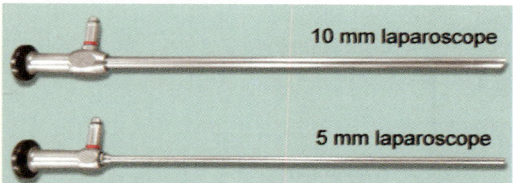

Fig. 1: Laparoscope (10 mm, 5 mm). *(Chapter 14)*

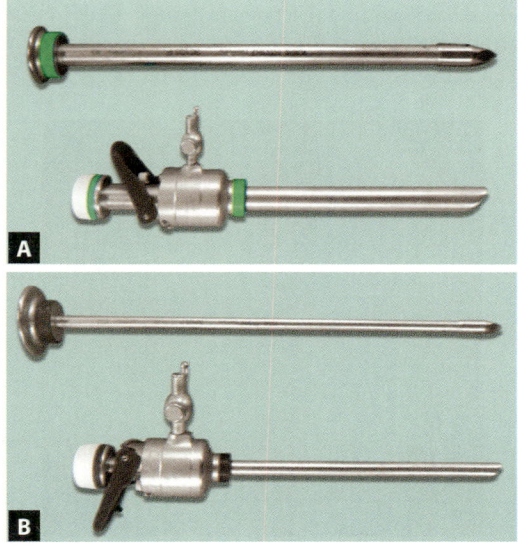

Figs. 2A and B: (A) 10 mm trocar and cannula; (B) 5 mm trocar and cannula. *(Chapter 14)*

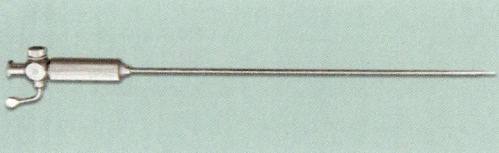

Fig. 3: Veress needle. *(Chapter 14)*

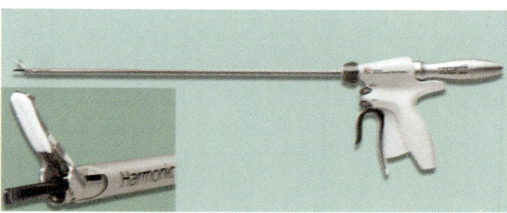

Fig. 5: Harmonic ace. *(Chapter 14)*

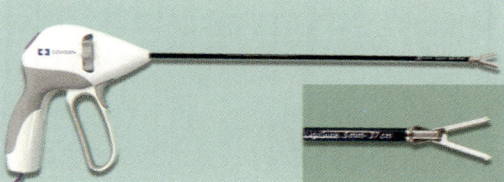

Fig. 6: LigaSure. *(Chapter 14)*

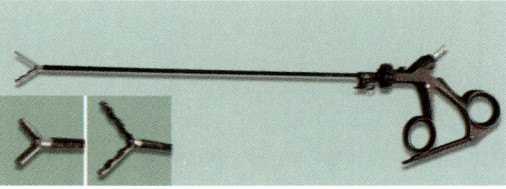

Fig. 8: Laparoscopic tooth and nontooth graspers. *(Chapter 14)*

Plate 6

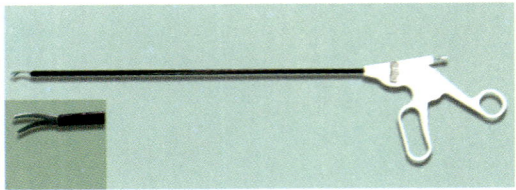

Fig. 9: Laparoscopic scissors.
(Chapter 14)

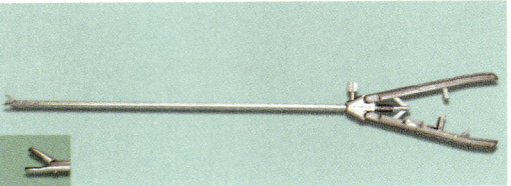

Fig. 10: Laparoscopic needle holder.
(Chapter 14)

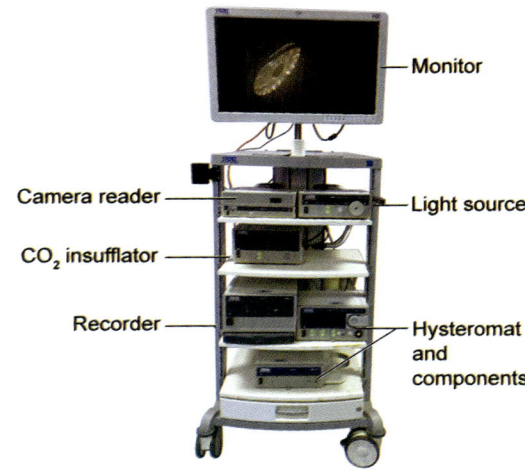

Fig. 11: Overview of a laparoscopy cart, consisting of a monitor, a camera reader, light source, CO_2 insufflator, recorder, and hysteromat. *(Chapter 14)*

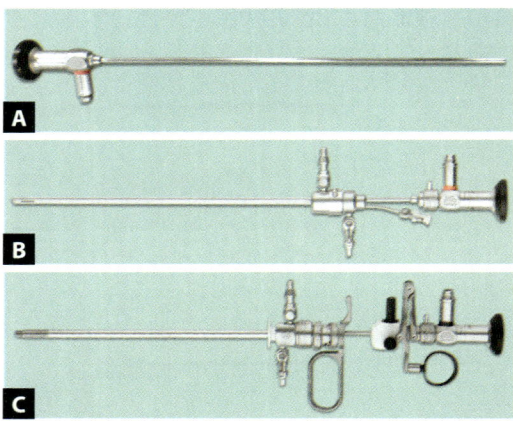

Figs. 12A to C: (A) 5-mm Hysteroscope; (B) Hysteroscope with working side channel; (C) Hysteroscope with working element for operative intervention. *(Chapter 14)*

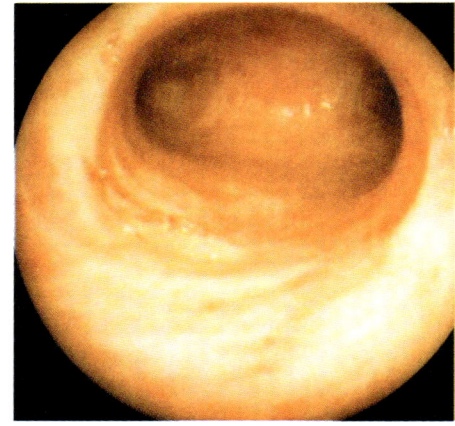

Fig. 13: Panoramic view of uterine cavity with a hysteroscope. Tubal ostium is seen on either side *(Chapter 14)*

Plate 7

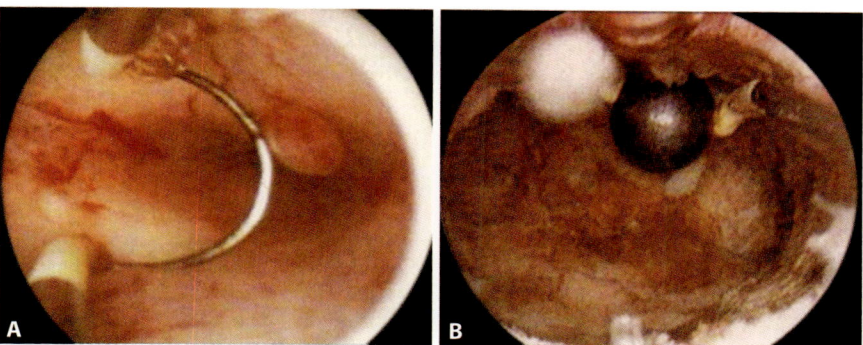

Figs. 14A and B: (A) Endometrial resection with cutting loop; (B) Rollerball endometrial ablation. *(Chapter 14)*

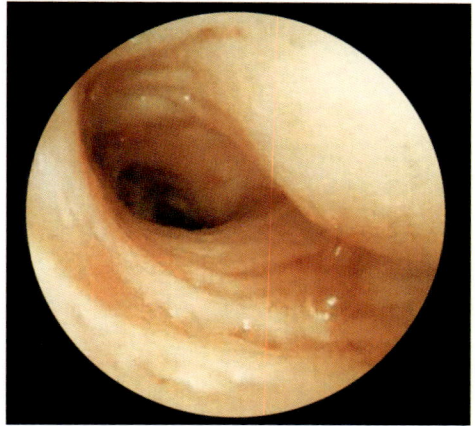

Fig. 15: Submucous fibroid covered by homogeneous endometrium. *(Chapter 14)*

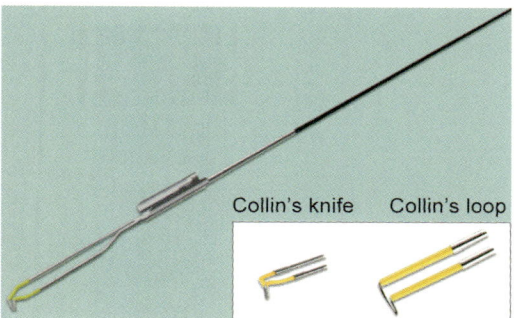

Fig. 16: Collin's knife and loop. *(Chapter 14)*

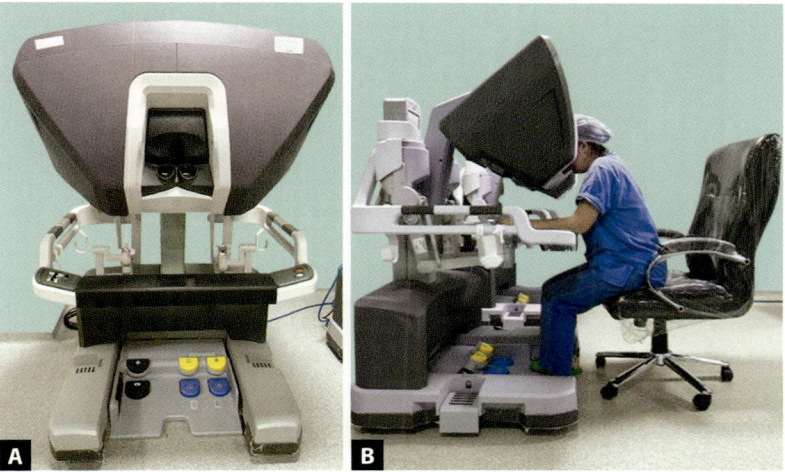

Figs. 1A and B: (A) Surgeon console; (B) Surgeon sitting comfortably at console while operating. *(Chapter 15)*

Plate 8

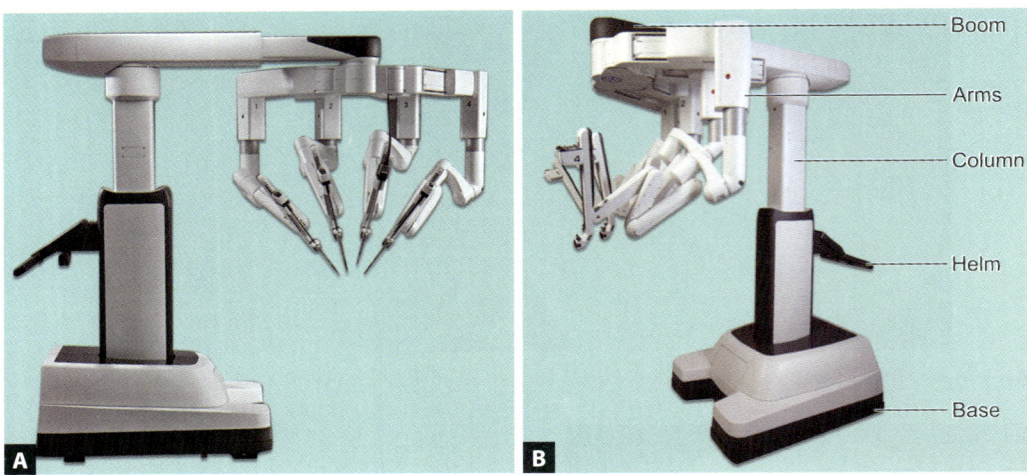

Figs. 2A and B: (A) Patient cart; (B) Components of patient cart. *(Chapter 15)*

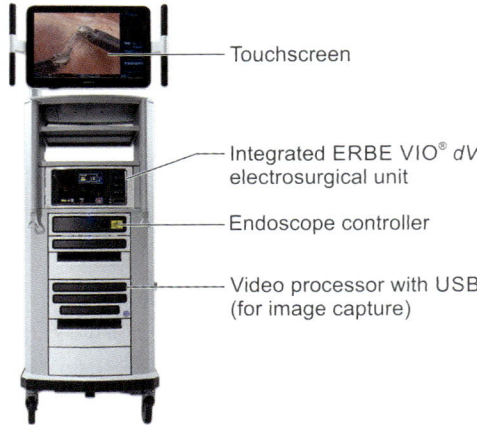

Fig. 3: Components of vision cart. *(Chapter 15)*

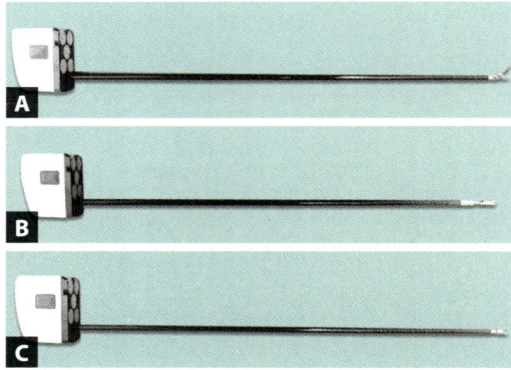

Figs. 4A to C: (A) Fenestrated bipolar forceps; (B) Monopolar scissors; (C) Needle driver. *(Chapter 15)*

Plate 9

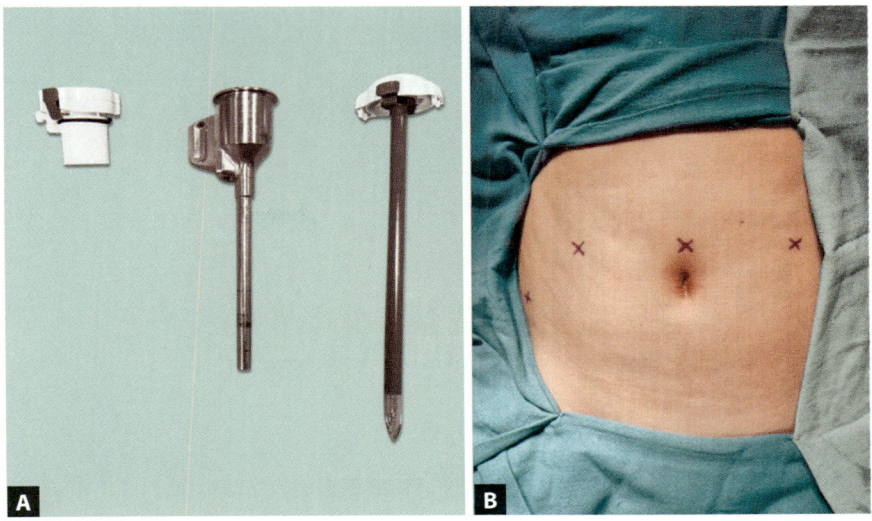

Figs. 5A and B: (A) Robotic trocar and cannula 8 mm; (B) Port placement in robotic gynecological surgery. *(Chapter 15)*

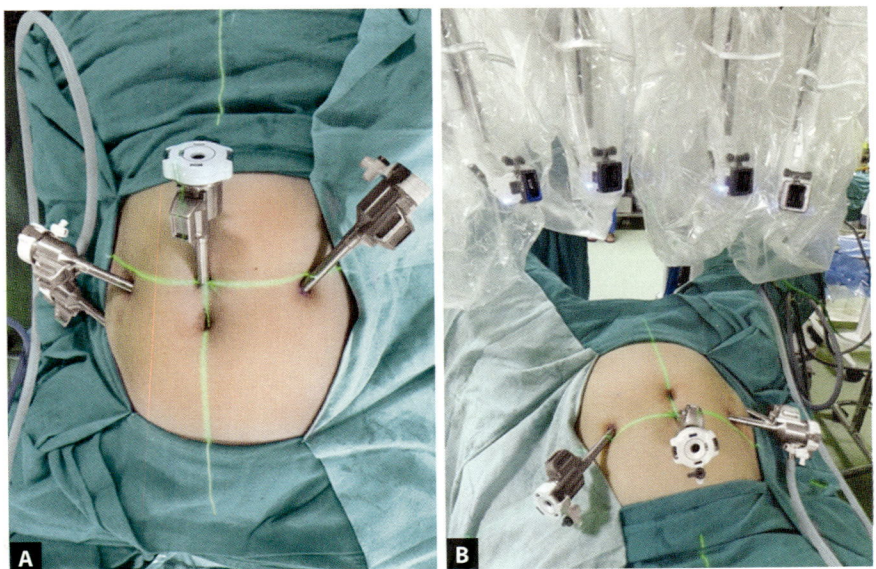

Figs. 6A and B: (A) External targeting using laser line; (B) Robotic arms draped and ready for docking. *(Chapter 15)*

Plate 10

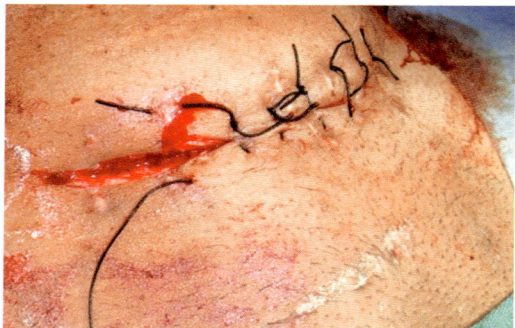

Fig. 1: Far–far suture placement. *(Chapter 17)*

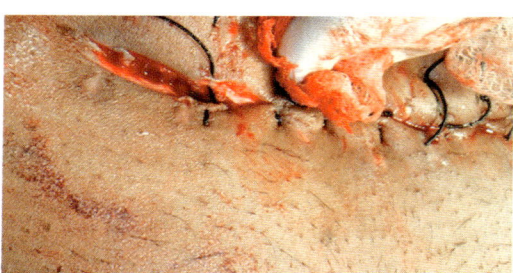

Fig. 2: Near–near suture placement. *(Chapter 17)*

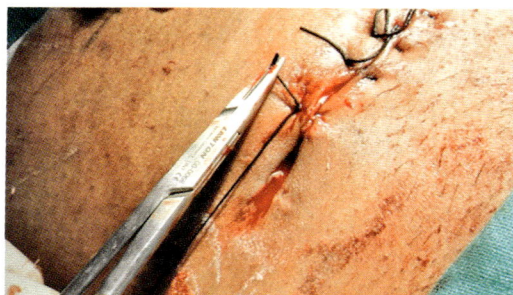

Fig. 3: Final knot is on the side where the suture began. *(Chapter 17)*

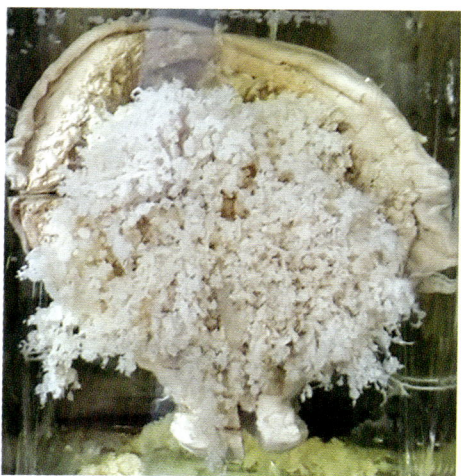

Fig. 1: Hydatidiform mole. *(Chapter 19)*

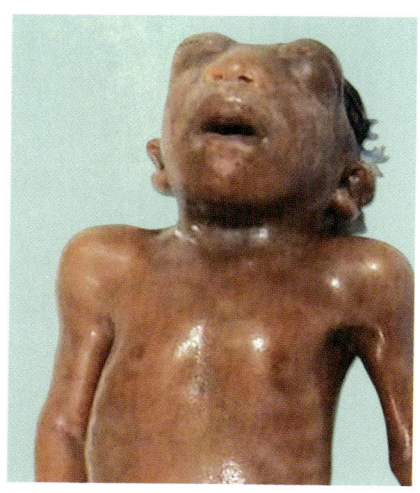

Fig. 2: Anencephaly. *(Chapter 19)*

Plate 11

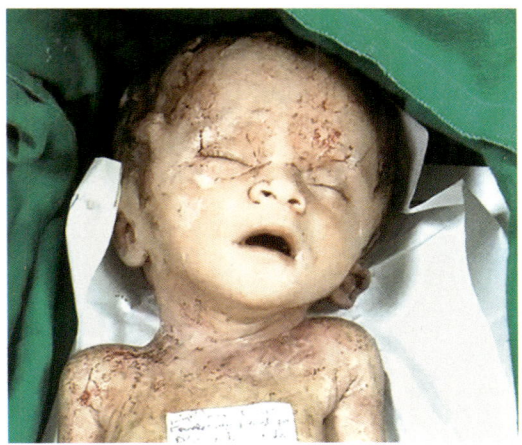

Fig. 3: Hydrocephalus. *(Chapter 19)*

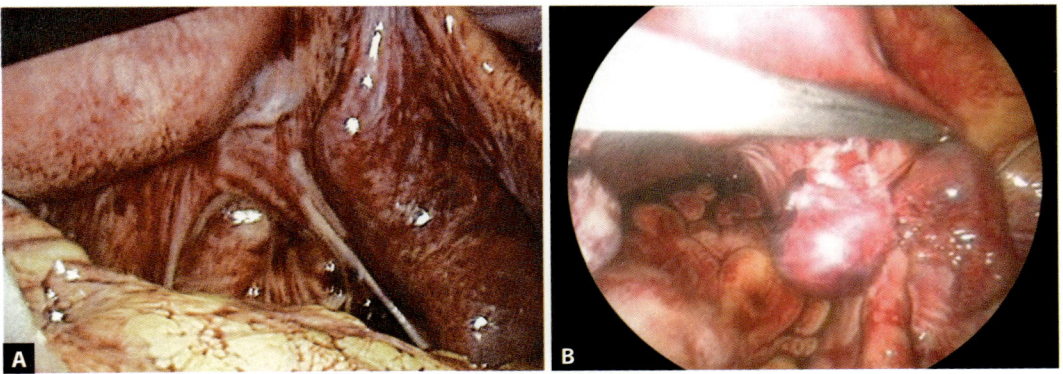

Figs. 5A and B: Ectopic tubal gestation. *(Chapter 19)*

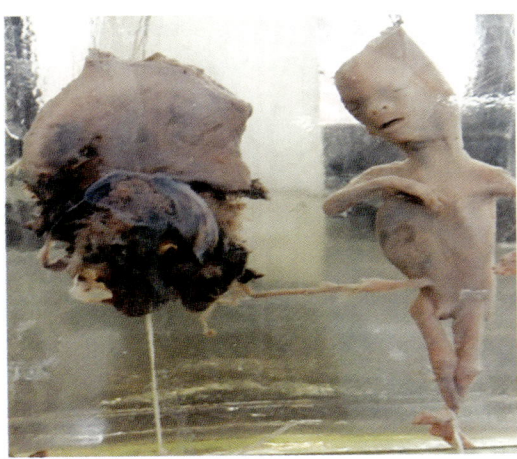

Fig. 6: Ectopic pregnancy in a ruptured rudimentary horn with fetus. *(Chapter 19)*

Plate 12

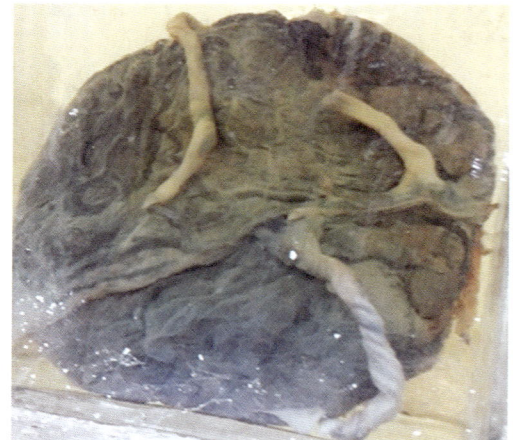

Fig. 8: Placenta of triplet delivery. *(Chapter 19)*

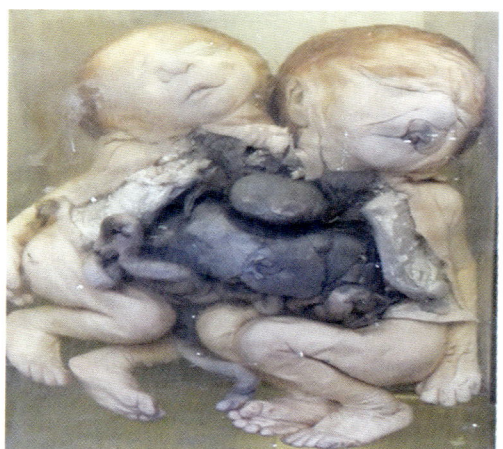

Fig. 9: Conjoint twins. *(Chapter 19)*

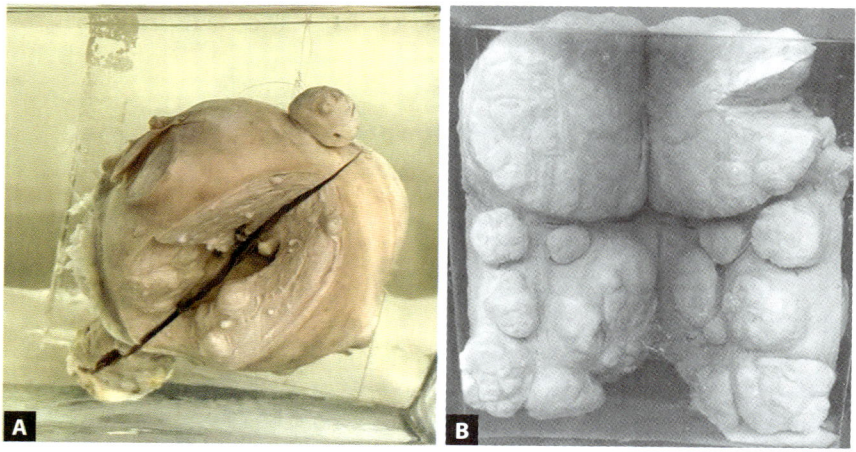

Figs. 3A and B: Multiple leiomyoma. *(Chapter 20)*

Plate 13

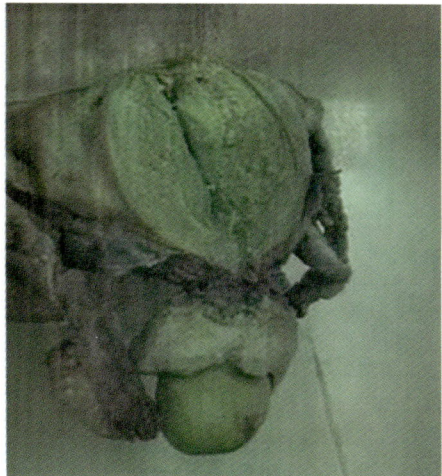

Fig. 4: Cervical fibroid. *(Chapter 20)*

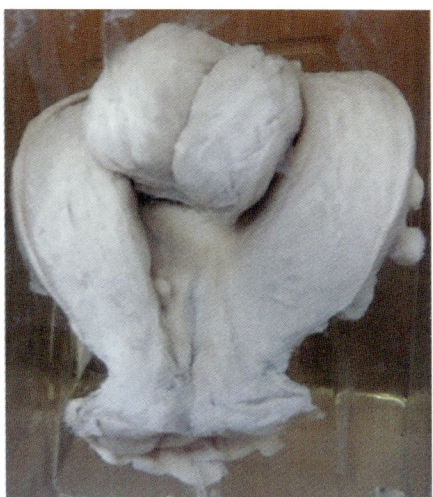

Fig. 5: Submucosal fibroid. *(Chapter 20)*

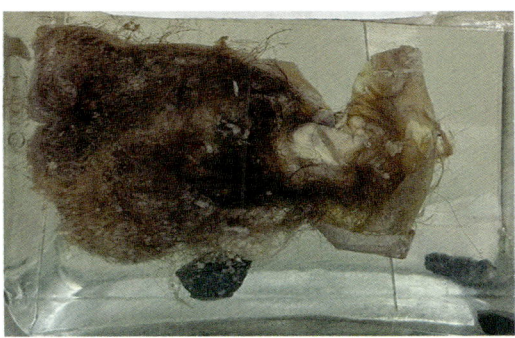

Fig. 8: Dermoid cyst. *(Chapter 20)*

Plate 14

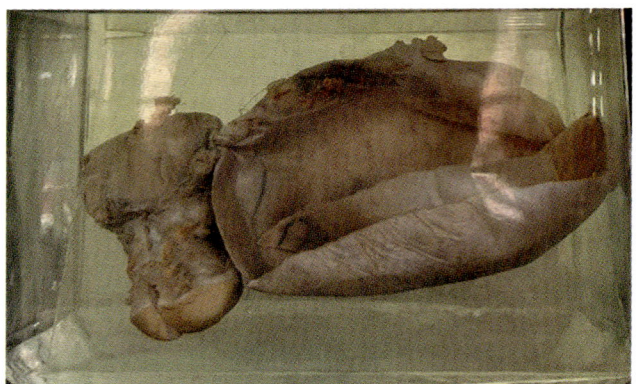

Fig. 10: Serous cystadenoma of ovary. *(Chapter 20)*

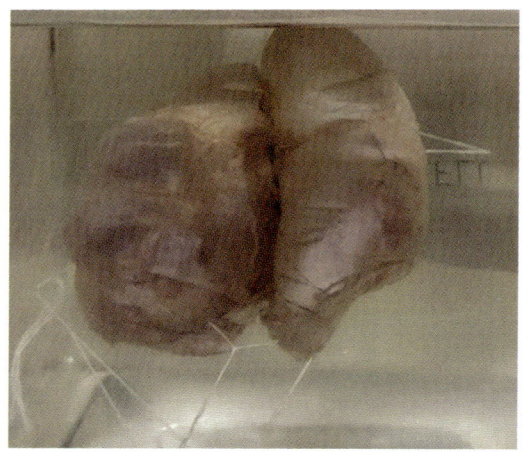

Fig. 11: Mucinous cystadenoma of ovary. *(Chapter 20)*

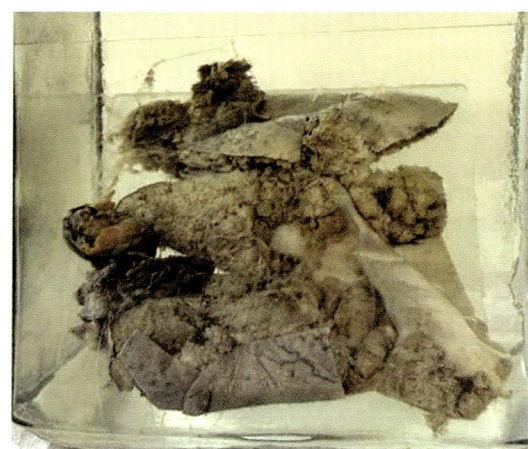

Fig. 12: Papillary serous cystadenocarcinoma of ovary. *(Chapter 20)*

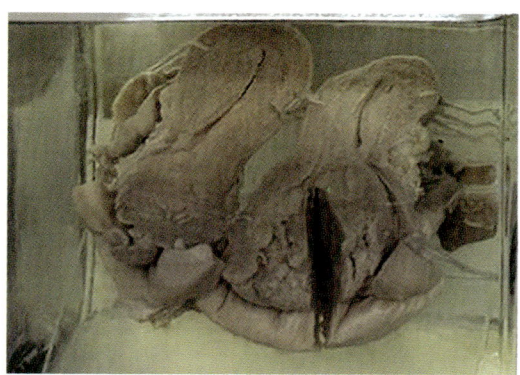

Fig. 17: Cervical carcinoma. *(Chapter 20)*

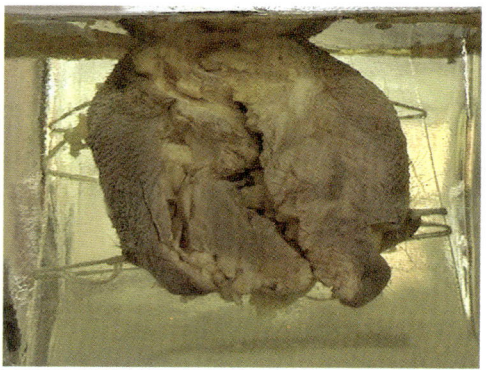

Fig. 18: Vulval carcinoma. *(Chapter 20)*

Plate 15

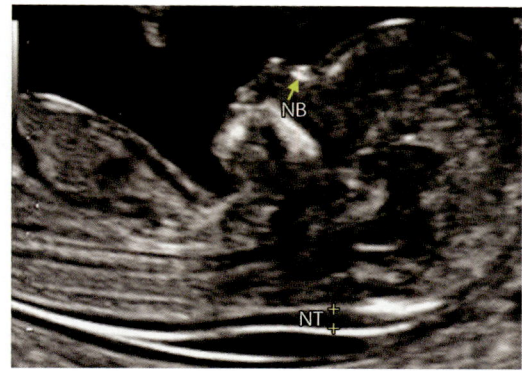

Fig. 1: Nuchal translucency (NT) and nasal bone (NB). *(Chapter 22)*
Courtesy: The Fetal Medicine Foundation.

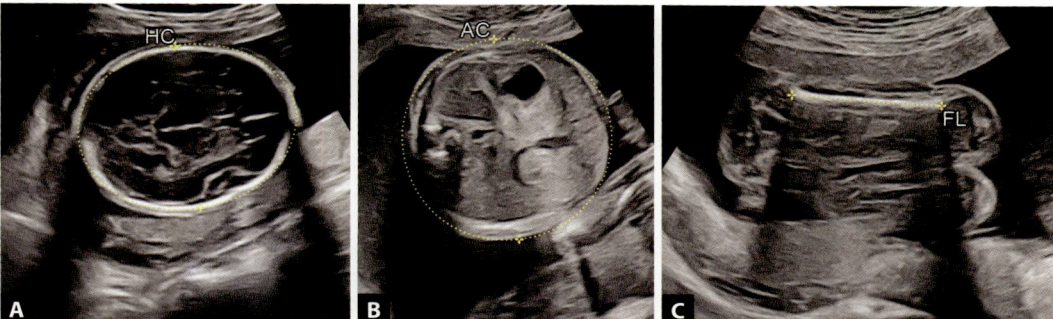

Figs. 2A to C: Standard fetal biometry. Sonographic measurements of (A) head circumference (HC), (B) abdominal circumference (AC), and (C) femur length (FL). *(Chapter 22)*
Source: ISUOG Practice Guidelines (updated): performance of the routine mid-trimester fetal ultrasound scan.

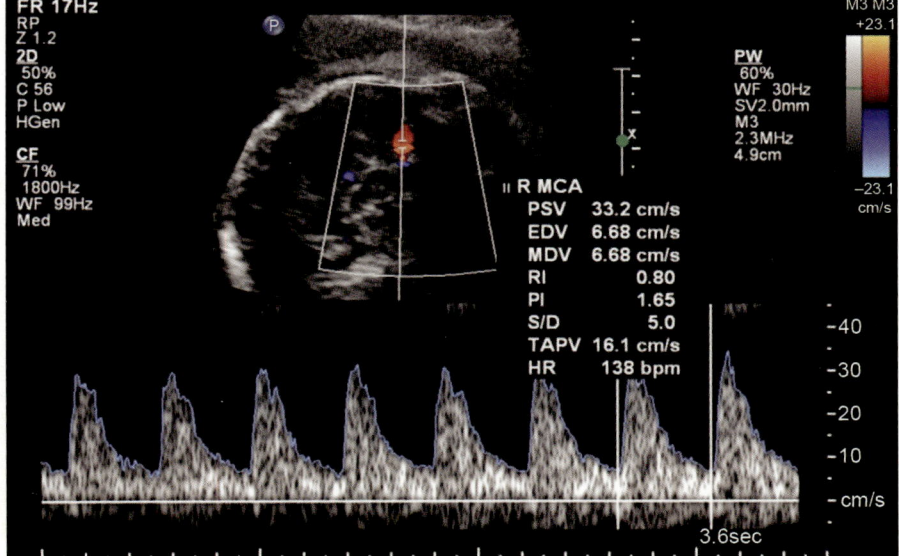

Fig. 3: Normal middle cerebral artery Doppler. *(Chapter 22)*
Courtesy: Radiopedia.

Plate 16

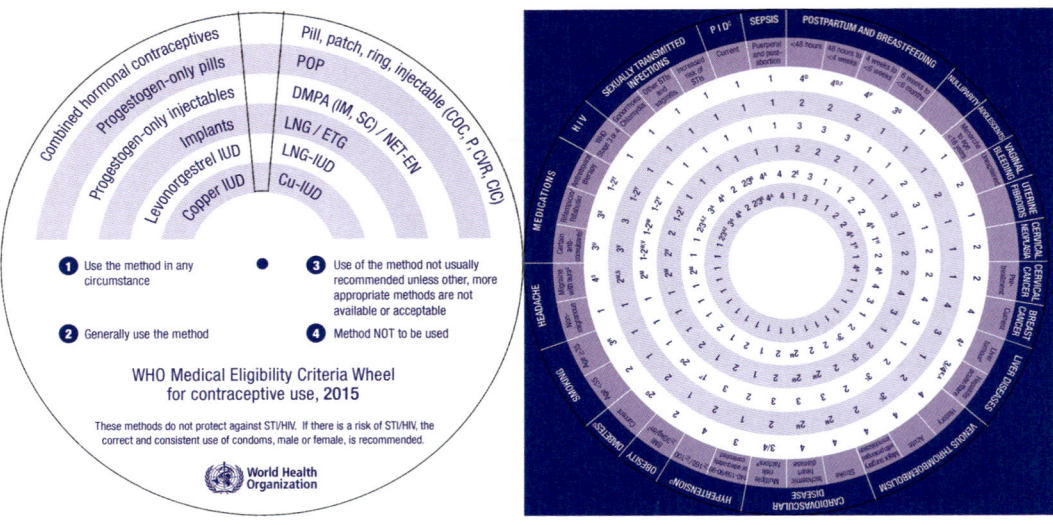

Fig. 1: Medical Eligibility Categories (MEC) wheel. *(Chapter 25)*

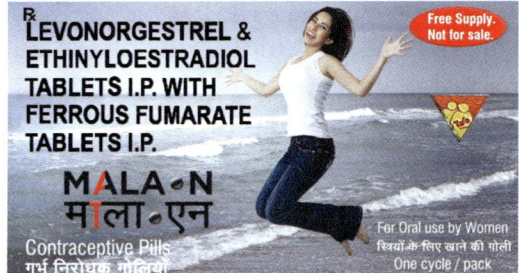

Fig. 7: Mala N. *(Chapter 25)*

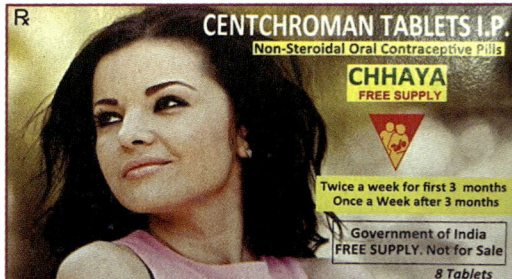

Fig. 8: Centchroman. *(Chapter 25)*

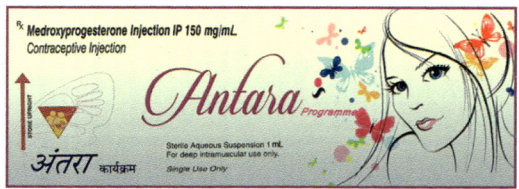

Fig. 12: Progestin-only contraceptive. *(Chapter 25)*

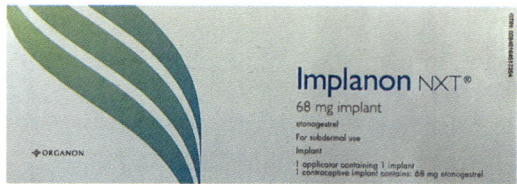

Fig. 13: Implanon NXT. *(Chapter 25)*

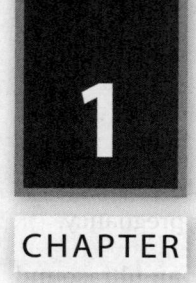

CHAPTER 1

History Taking and Examination of Long/Short Cases

Shalini Rajaram, Om Kumari, Namita Grover, Neerja Goel

■ OBSTETRIC HISTORY TAKING

The headings under which history is taken are as follows:
- Name
- Age
- Occupation
- Religion
- Education status
- Socioeconomic status
- Booked/registered/unbooked
- Gestational age—last menstrual period (LMP), period of gestation (POG), expected date of delivery (EDD)
- Presenting complaints
- History of present pregnancy
- Obstetric history—obstetric score (gravida, para, abortions, preterm labor), history of previous pregnancies
- Menstrual history—LMP, previous cycles; normal, frequent (<21 days), infrequent (>35 days), amount of flow; normal, heavy, scanty
- Past medical/surgical history
- Immunization history
- Family history—hypertension (HTN), diabetes mellitus (DM), tuberculosis (TB), allergies, genetic disorders, multiple births, blood dyscrasias
- Personal history
- Dietary history
- General/systemic/obstetric examination.

What is the importance of age?

There is an increased risk of obstetric complications and adverse pregnancy outcome at both ends (young gravida <19 years and elderly gravida >35 years) of age spectrum.

What are the problems associated with a teenage pregnancy?

- *Medical problems:* Anemia, malnutrition, preeclampsia
- *Obstetric problems:* Miscarriage, fetal growth restriction, fetal malpresentation, cephalopelvic disproportion (CPD), preterm delivery, and psychological stress.

What are the problems associated with pregnancy in women more than 35 years of age?

- Increased risk of chromosomal anomalies and miscarriages
- Increased incidence of medical diseases in pregnancy like chronic and gestational HTN, preeclampsia, gestational DM, and obesity
- Increased risk of pregnancy complications like abruptio placentae, fetal growth restriction, postdatism, cervical dystocia, incoordinate uterine contractions, malpositions (occipitoposterior), malpresentations, and prolonged labor due to reduced elasticity of the soft tissues
- Due to impaired mobility of joints, there is an increased risk of operative vaginal delivery and its accompanying maternal and fetal complications
- Fetal macrosomia
- Higher incidence of lactation failure in puerperium.

When is the patient said to be booked?
Women with at least three antenatal visits are said to be booked.

What is a registered pregnancy?
Registered pregnancy is when a woman has visited a health facility the first time and is registered but subsequently does not attend the antenatal clinics for checkups.

How are the antenatal visits scheduled?
First visit/booking visit: Ideally, the first visit should be before 10 weeks of gestation. A thorough medical, obstetric, and family history along with physical examination must be carried out. Gestational age assessment and assignment of EDD is done. Also, risk categorization for subsequent pregnancy management is done.

Number of antenatal visits: 10 routine antenatal visits for nulliparous women and 7 for parous women.

In low-risk pregnancy, once every 4 weeks till 28 weeks after 20 weeks, every 2 weeks from 28 to 36 weeks, and weekly till delivery. In high-risk pregnancy, antenatal visits are to be individualized as per need.

First antenatal visit: Measure woman's height and weight and calculate body mass index.
- Offer blood test to check for full blood count, blood group, and rhesus D status.
- Screen for infectious disease in pregnancy; HIV, syphilis, and hepatitis B.
- Assess a woman's risk factor for pre-eclampsia, and those at risk should be advised aspirin 150 mg once a day.
- Assess risk for gestational diabetes and offer oral glucose tolerance test at 24–28 weeks POG.
- Assess risk for venous thromboembolism and refer for further management if required.
- Screen for thalassemia and sickle cell anemia.
- Discuss and share information about fetal anomaly screening during pregnancy.

Second antenatal visit: Offer an ultrasound scan between 11 and 13 + 6 weeks for determining gestational age, detect multiple pregnancy, and if opted for, screen for common aneuploidies and pre-eclampsia.

Third antenatal visit: Offer an ultrasound scan between 18 and 20 + 6 weeks to screen for fetal anomalies and determine placental location.

Antenatal visits between 24 and 28 weeks: Hemoglobin and hematocrit are retested to assess anemia and to modify iron supplementation. Screening for gestational DM and antibody screening for Rh-negative women.

Subsequent visits: Surveillance for maternal–fetal well-being is done.
- At each antenatal visit, enquire the woman about her general health and well-being; measure blood pressure (BP), weight, urine dipstick test for proteinuria, and fetal movements after 24 weeks; and review and reassess the plan of care.
- Offer symphysis fundal height (SFH) measurement at each antenatal appointment after 24 weeks but no more frequently than every 2 weeks. In case of SFH large or small for gestational age, offer an ultrasound for fetal growth and fetal well-being.
- Do not routinely offer ultrasound scans after 28 weeks for uncomplicated singleton pregnancies.
- After 28 weeks, apart from fetomaternal surveillance, discuss and give information regarding preparation for labor, birth, and postnatal self and baby care. Contraceptive

counseling should be initiated during the antenatal period.
- Identify women who need additional care. High-risk pregnancy may require weekly antenatal visits for fetomaternal surveillance.

How do you screen for aneuploidies?
- All antenatal women should be offered prenatal genetic screening for aneuploidies in the first-trimester (11–13 + 6 weeks POG) and/or second-trimester screening.
- First-trimester combined screening for aneuploidy includes risk assessment by maternal age, ultrasound for nuchal translucency (NT), nasal bone, maternal serum measurement of free β-human chorionic gonadotropin (β-hCG) and pregnancy-associated plasma protein A (PAPP-A) glycoprotein at 11 to 13 + 6 weeks gestation.
- *Second trimester:* Serum quadruple marker (β-hCG, PAPP-A, inhibin-A, estradiol) and mid-trimester anomaly scan at 18–22 weeks for structural abnormalities.

Women with screen positive for aneuploidies are categorized as low, intermediate, and high risk:

Low-risk women: No further test for aneuploidies is required and routine antenatal care for pregnancy is continued.

Intermediate risk: Additional screening test [ultrasound markers, noninvasive prenatal screening test (NIPT)]/diagnostic test is advisable.

High risk: Diagnostic test (chorionic villous sampling or amniocentesis) for fetal karyotype or chromosomal microarray is required.

What is noninvasive prenatal screening test?
Noninvasive prenatal screening test screens for an abnormal number of chromosomes. The test has a high sensitivity and specificity for trisomies 21, 18, and 13. It does not screen for all types of chromosomal disorders.

The test is performed on fetal-derived cell-free fetal DNA fragments (<200 bp) present in maternal plasma. 5–20% of cell-free DNA (cf-DNA) in maternal plasma is of fetal origin as the product of placental apoptosis. The test can be done as early as 10 weeks of pregnancy and up until delivery.

What are the advantages of noninvasive prenatal screening test over other screening tests?
Screening with cf-DNA has high sensitivity, specificity, and low false-positive rate for common trisomies. Detection rates for trisomies 21, 18, and 13 are 99%, 96.3%, and 91%, respectively. It can detect sex chromosome abnormalities too.

What are the disadvantages of cell-free DNA screening test?
- Testing with cf-DNA is of high cost.
- Although NIPS has a better detection rate, it is still not diagnostic. A positive screen test necessitates a diagnostic test for further confirmation.
- It cannot detect other rare autosomal trisomies.
- Do not assess risk for fetal structural anomalies like neural tube defects.
- Sometimes results are not reported, indeterminate, or uninterpretable (a "no call" test result) which require further genetic counseling, comprehensive ultrasound evaluation, and diagnostic testing.

What does gravida/parity denote?
- *Gravida*—denotes a present pregnancy irrespective of gestational maturity.
- *Parity*—denotes a previous pregnancy that has progressed beyond the period of viability (28 weeks) and the woman has delivered, irrespective of the ultimate outcome.

Who is a grand multipara and what are the problems associated with grand multipara?
Grand multipara is a woman who has given birth to at least four viable neonates, i.e., after 28 weeks of pregnancy.

The associated complications are:
- Pendulous abdomen, which leads to malpresentation
- Pronounced lordosis, which leads to increase in pelvic inclination and nonengagement of fetal head at term
- Medical problems, e.g., anemia, HTN, and gestational DM
- Multiple pregnancy
- Placenta previa
- Contracted pelvis due to osteomalacic changes in pelvis due to repeated childbirth
- Rupture uterus
- Postpartum hemorrhage (PPH).

How do you write the obstetric score?
If a woman is pregnant now for the fourth time and has had previous three normal full term pregnancies and all are alive, her formula is G4P3L3 or GTPAL system can be used, gravida term preterm abortion live issues, so this will be written as G4 30 0 3.

How is gestational age calculated?
As per Naegele's formula, add 9 calendar months and 7 days to the 1st day of LMP, e.g., woman with LMP as 05-05-2023; her EDD will be calculated as 12-02-2024. So count forward 9 months and add 7 days.

Another method is to count the remaining days from a known EDD, divide by 7 (for weeks), and minus from 40 weeks (total duration of pregnancy). For example, if a woman's EDD is 28-12-2023 and you have examined her on 01-11-2023, her gestational age is 31 weeks + 1 day as 57 days are remaining.

How do you determine the reliability of gestational age?
The reliability of gestational age is excellent, if the following conditions are met:
- Patient was not using oral contraceptives (OCP).
- Had three or more regular periods before the last one and the last period was normal in duration and amount of flow.
- An ultrasound measurement of crown–rump length (CRL) obtained at 6–11 weeks supports current gestational age most accurately (±5 days).
- Clinical history and physical or ultrasound examination performed between 12 and 20 weeks support current gestational age (±10 days).
- Gestational age corresponds to 36 weeks since the patient had a positive serum or urine pregnancy test soon after she misses her period.
- Fetal heart tones were documented 20 weeks before EDD by a nonelectronic fetoscope.
- Pregnancies achieved during infertility treatment following administration of clomiphene, gonadotropins, and hCG have a known date of conception.

How is estimated date of delivery calculated in women with irregular cycles?
For longer cycles—add the extra days to get EDD; e.g., for a woman with a 45-day cycle and LMP 3-1-20, EDD as calculated would be 25-10-202.3

For shorter cycles—subtract the shorter days to get EDD; e.g., for a woman with a 20-day cycle and LMP 3-1-2023, EDD could be 30-9-2023.

What is the best method for dating of pregnancy in women with irregular cycles?
First-trimester ultrasound with measurement of CRL is the best method for accurate estimation of gestational age.

What are the important questions to be asked in history of present pregnancy?
First trimester
- Spontaneous conception or with assisted reproductive technique
- History of periconceptional intake of folic acid
- Confirmation of pregnancy by urine pregnancy test and/or first-trimester ultrasound
- History of hyperemesis, fever with rash, drug intake, radiation exposure, urinary tract infection (UTI), and threatened abortion.

Second trimester
- History of immunization with tetanus toxoid, COVID vaccine, anti-D in nonisoimmunized Rh-negative woman, MMR (measles, mumps, and rubella) vaccination, HPV (human papillomavirus) vaccination
- Date of quickening
- Iron and calcium supplementation
- Mid-trimester anomaly scan done or not
- History of swelling over body, excessive weight gain, decreased urine output, blurring of vision, epigastric discomfort, right hypochondriac pain, easy fatigability, dyspnea, and orthopnea
- High BP records
- History of abnormal blood sugar reports after oral glucose tolerance test.

Third trimester
- History of any bleeding per vaginum (painless/preceded by trauma), amount of bleed, and color of bleed
- Leaking per vaginum
- High BP records
- Perceiving fetal movements or not
- History of any medical or surgical event in any trimester.

What is the importance of fever with rash in the first trimester?
Viral infections during pregnancy in the first trimester may be associated with congenital anomalies in a fetus. Hence, a high index of suspicion and screening for infection is important.

Rubella infection: This is the most worrisome viral infection during pregnancy. It is a mild febrile illness with a generalized maculopapular rash, arthralgias or arthritis, lymphadenopathy (usually suboccipital, postauricular, and cervical), and conjunctivitis. 20–50% of infections may be asymptomatic. It may lead to congenital rubella syndrome.

Parvovirus B19 infection: It is a respiratory illness that may vary from mild asymptomatic illness to severe febrile illness with rash, arthralgia, viral myocarditis, and rarely an aplastic crisis. Approximately 30–50% of pregnant women are immune to infection due to prior exposure to the infection. Effects on pregnancy include risk of fetal loss and fetal pleural or pericardial effusion. It causes severe fetal anemia and may lead to hydrops fetalis.

Cytomegalovirus (CMV) infection: It is the most common congenital viral infection in newborn. This is the leading infectious cause of mental disability and sensorineural deafness. CMV infection is transmitted by contact with infected nasopharyngeal secretion, urine, saliva, semen, and cervical and vaginal secretions. Primary infection during pregnancy is associated with a 40% risk of fetal infection. Ultrasound may detect cerebral ventriculomegaly, intracranial calcification, and microcephaly in case of fetal affection.

What is the significance of urinary tract infection in pregnancy?
Urinary tract infection in pregnancy has been associated with adverse pregnancy outcomes, including preterm delivery, low-birth-weight infants, preeclampsia, and anemia. The spectrum of UTI includes asymptomatic bacteriuria, symptomatic acute cystitis, and acute pyelonephritis.

Asymptomatic bacteriuria: Presence of significant bacterial counts in the urine without symptoms. The incidence in pregnancy is around 2–10%. Identification and treatment of asymptomatic bacteriuria reduce the risk of adverse pregnancy outcome. The screening is done with a culture of a clean-catch urine sample. If culture shows bacteriuria, women should be treated by appropriate antibiotics.

When should the tetanus immunization be given?
- TT is replaced by Td (tetanus toxoid and reduced diphtheria toxin).
- Pregnant women who have not received three doses of Td should undertake a series of vaccinations at 0, 4 weeks, and 6–12 months after the initial dose.
- First dose Td as early as possible (first contact).
- At least one of these doses to be Tdap.
- Tdap (tetanus toxoid, reduced diphtheria, and acellular pertussis component).
- Tdap vaccine is safe in pregnancy.
- All pregnant women should receive a single dose of Tdap during pregnancy (27–36 weeks' window) who are immunized with Td vaccine previously.

What is Rh isoimmunization in pregnancy?
When a Rh-negative woman is exposed to a red cell antigen that is not present in her blood, the immune response results in the production of immunoglobulin G (IgG) antibodies. The transplacental passage of these antibodies attacks the fetal red blood cells (RBCs) that are positive for these surface antigens, resulting in hemolytic disease in fetus and newborn.

What are the predisposing conditions for Rh alloimmunization during pregnancy?
Antepartum and intrapartum events that commonly cause transplacental leakage of fetal blood and red cell alloimmunization are:
- Abortion
- Ectopic pregnancy
- Placental abruption
- Hemorrhage due to placenta previa
- Obstetric procedures such as chorionic villous sampling, amniocentesis, and fetal blood sampling
- Manual removal of placenta.

How can alloimmunization be prevented during pregnancy?
Prophylactic administration of anti-D immunoglobulin during antenatal and postnatal periods can reduce the incidence of alloimmunization from 1 to 0.1%.

What is anti-D immunoglobulin?
Anti-D immunoglobulin is a polyclonal antibody derived from human plasma. The dose of 300 µg, administered deep intramuscular, can neutralize 15 mL of Rh-positive RBCs.

What is routine antenatal anti-D prophylaxis?
Routine antenatal anti-D prophylaxis (RAADP) (300 µg) is recommended for all Rh-negative women with no evidence of alloimmunization [indirect Coombs test (ICT) negative] at 28 weeks. The second dose is given after delivery, preferably within 72 hours, if the newborn is D-positive.

What is quickening?
Quickening is perception of active fetal movements by a pregnant woman. It is usually felt around 18–20 weeks in primipara and 2 weeks earlier in multipara.

What are the recommendations for iron supplementation?
The World Health Organization (WHO) recommends 60 mg elemental iron and 400 µg of folic acid once or twice daily for 6 months in pregnancy in countries with a prevalence of anemia >40% and for an additional 3 months postpartum.

The Ministry of Health, Government of India, has now recommended intake of 100 mg of elemental iron with 500 µg of folic acid in the second half of pregnancy for a period of at least 100 days.

What are the recommendations for folic acid supplementation?
Prophylactic dose of 500 µg of folic acid supplementation is recommended and to be started preconceptionally.

In women with previously affected children with neural tube defects, history of anticonvulsant therapy, or pregestational DM, 4 mg/day is recommended.

As 4 mg tablets are not available, 5 mg is prescribed for at least 12 weeks before planning pregnancy and continued in the first trimester.

What is normal weight gain in pregnancy?
Recommendations for weight gain in pregnancy for singleton gestation **(Table 1)**:
- The range of weight gain for women carrying twins is 16–20 kg.
- *Young adolescents:* Weight gain at the upper end of range.
- *Short women:* Weight gain at the lower end of range.
- The rate of weight gain in the second half of pregnancy is 500 g/week.

What are the important points to be asked in obstetric history?
- Duration of marriage
- *Number of pregnancies:* Full term/preterm/abortion (induced or spontaneous)/ectopic pregnancy/living children/multiple gestation
- Consanguinity
- Contraceptive history in the interpregnancy period.

Was this a spontaneous pregnancy or after ovulation induction?
Take a detailed history for each pregnancy beginning with an obstetric formula; e.g., if a

TABLE 1: Recommendations for weight gain in pregnancy.

	BMI (prepregnancy) (kg/m²)	Recommended weight gain (kg)
Low	<18.5	13–18
Normal	18.5–24.9	11–16
High (overweight)	25–29.9	7–11
Obese	≥30	5–9
(BMI: body mass index)		

woman is pregnant now for the fourth time and has had previous three normal full-term pregnancies and all are alive, her formula is G4P3L3 or the GTPAL system can be used, gravida-term-preterm-abortion-live issues, so this will be written as G4-3-0-0-3.

- *Antepartum*—whether booked or not, iron/calcium intake, any history of high BP records, abnormal blood sugar reports, bleeding/leaking per vaginum, any history of surgery in the past, any associated medical disorder.
- *Intrapartum*—term or preterm, duration of labor pains, spontaneous or induced labor, mode of delivery, place of delivery, conduct of delivery by trained personnel, instrumentation, increased blood loss, blood transfusion, lower segment cesarean section (LSCS)—emergency/elective, indication for cesarean section, and perioperative complications, if any.
- *Postpartum*
  - *For women with a normal delivery:* History of PPH, fever, foul-smelling discharge, return to normal activity (in days/weeks), when did she start lactating, and duration of lactation
  - *For women who have undergone cesarean section:* Period of catheterization, suture removal, status of stitch line, any postoperative fever, establishment of successful lactation, duration of lactation, congestion of breasts, inverted nipples, and secondary PPH
- Baby (weight/sex), congenital anomaly, breastfeeding; immunization of newborn, and milestones.

How much spacing is required between pregnancies?
A minimum spacing of 3 years is required to replenish the iron and calcium stores and for the woman to lactate successfully for at least 2 years and to recover physically and psychologically before another pregnancy.

What are the dietary recommendations in a normal pregnant woman?
- Pregnancy—2,200–2,500 kcal/day and protein 1.5 g/kg/day body weight.
- Caloric intake should increase by approximately 300 kcal/day during pregnancy.
- Lactation—extra 600 kcal/day and 20 g protein/day.
- Calcium—1,000 to 1,200 mg/day for development of fetal bones.

What are the recommendations for rest in pregnancy?
An average of 10 hour/day (8 hours at night and 2 hours at noon) rest is required in pregnancy, especially in the last 6 weeks.

GENERAL AND SYSTEMIC EXAMINATION

- General condition (consciousness and orientation)
- Built, height, and weight
- BMI = Weight (kg)/height (m^2) (prepregnancy)
- Nutritional status—skin (any lesion, bruising, edema, rashes), hair (coarse, sparse, thin suggestive of protein deficiency), glossitis (ulceration of tongue and swelling may suggest vitamin B_{12} deficiency), cheilitis (dry and cracked lips), angular stomatitis (riboflavin deficiency), bleeding gums (vitamin C/riboflavin deficiency)
- Pallor—mild, moderate, severe
- Hydration—good/dehydrated
- Icterus—yellowish discoloration of sclera and skin (hyperbilirubinemia)
- Cyanosis-bluish discoloration of skin due to poor circulation
- Clubbing

- Edema—pedal edema/abdominal edema/on dependent body parts like sacrum/vulva
- *Generalized lymphadenopathy:* It is defined as involvement of three or more noncontiguous lymph node areas. (Any palpable inguinal lymph node >2 cm and any other lymph node >1 cm is significant.) Look for lymph nodes in inguinal and supraclavicular regions.
- Pulse rate, rhythm, volume, character, radiofemoral delay, peripheral pulsations, and any specific characters (e.g., slow rising pulse, water hammer pulse).
- Jugular venous pulse is seen in good light with the patient reclining at an angle of 45°; the neck should be well supported so that neck muscles, especially sternocleidomastoid, are relaxed. In normal health, it is 6–8 cm from mid right atrium and corresponds to sternal angle and therefore not seen (normal pressure—6–8 cm water).
- BP—sitting position and right upper arm.
- Respiratory rate (RR)—normal is 14–16 beats/min.
- Temperature—mean oral temperature is 36.8° ± 0.4°C or 98.2° ± 0.7°F and rectal temperature 0.4°C (0.7°F) higher than oral temperature.
- Fever—elevation in body temperature with an increase in hypothalamic set point, and hyperpyrexia—>41.5°C (106.7°F)
- *Orodental hygiene*
- *Thyroid* examination
- Pedal edema (first appears at the ankle, dorsum of foot, and then extends upward to the legs).

Breast examination: See for normal pregnancy changes—increase in size, Montgomery tubercles (enlarged sebaceous glands around the areola and the secretions of which helps to keep the areola and nipple moist), secondary areola, nipples become large erectile and deeply pigmented, secretions from nipple from 12 to 16 weeks, any nodule, and secretion from nipple should be noted. It is important to note whether nipples are everted or inverted.

OBSTETRIC EXAMINATION

Obstetrical examination aims at diagnosing lie, presentation, position, and attitude of the fetus.

Preliminaries
- Verbal consent
- Ensure privacy
- Ask woman to evacuate bladder
- Thighs should be semi-flexed
- Abdomen fully exposed from xiphisternum to mid-thigh (use a sheet to cover lower limbs)
- Examiner to stand on the right side of the patient.

Inspection
- Uterine ovoid is longitudinal, transverse, or oblique
- Undue enlargement of uterus
- Skin—striae, scar marks, scratch marks, shining skin (may be suggestive of polyhydramnios or ascites)
- Umbilicus—normal/everted
- Hernial orifices.

Palpation
Correct dextrorotation

Fundal height: The ulnar border of the left hand is placed over the uppermost level of fundus and approximate duration of pregnancy is ascertained in terms of weeks of gestation as fundal height.

Fundus of uterus is just palpable above the symphysis pubis at 12 weeks. It is midway between umbilicus and symphysis pubis at 16 weeks and at the level of umbilicus at 24 weeks. Below level of umbilicus is 20 weeks and above is 26 weeks. The distance between umbilicus and xiphisternum is divided into three parts: (1) Fundus of uterus corresponds to the upper border of lower third at 28 weeks, (2) upper border of lower two-thirds at 32 weeks, and (3) at xiphisternum at 36 weeks. At term, uterine fundus corresponds to 32 weeks but flanks are full.

Conditions where the height of uterus is more than the period of amenorrhea: Full bladder, mistaken dates, twins, polyhydramnios, big baby, pelvic tumors (ovarian/fibroid), hydatidiform mole, and concealed abruptio placenta.

Conditions where the height of uterus is less than the period of amenorrhea: Mistaken dates, scanty liquor, preterm premature rupture of membranes (PPROM), fetal growth restriction, and intrauterine death.

Obstetric grips:
- *Fundal grip:* The whole of the fundal area is palpated using both hands laid flat on it to ascertain which pole of fetus is lying at fundus (irregular, broad, and soft mass suggestive of breech whereas smooth, hard, globular mass is suggestive of head).

  In transverse lie, neither of fetal poles is palpated at the fundal area. Head is felt in either lumbar region.
- *Lateral or umbilical grip:* The hands are to be placed flat on either side of umbilicus to palpate the back, limbs, and anterior shoulder.
- *First pelvic grip (Leopold's fourth maneuver):* To ascertain the presenting part, attitude, and engagement (done facing the patient's feet).

  Four fingers of both the hands are placed on either side of the midline in the lower pole of uterus and parallel to inguinal ligament. The fingers are pressed downward and backward in a manner of approximation of fingertips to palpate the part occupying the lower pole of the uterus (presentation).
- *Second pelvic grip (Pawlik's grip or Leopold's third maneuver):* It is done facing toward the patient's face. The overstretched thumb and four fingers of the right hand are placed over the lower pole of the uterus, keeping the ulnar border of the palm over the symphysis pubis to ascertain the presenting part and engagement. In an unengaged head, it can be moved freely from side to side and both the poles (occiput and sinciput) remain at the same level.
- *Engagement of head:* Head is engaged when the greatest horizontal plane, the biparietal diameter, has passed the plane of pelvic brim. Both the poles are not felt per abdomen. However, sinciput can be felt with difficulty in engaged head.

  There is divergence of examining fingers while trying to push downward (convergence of fingers—unengaged head).

Causes of unengaged head at term in primigravida:
- Deflexed head
- CPD due to contracted pelvis
- Big head or combination of both
- Polyhydramnios
- Hydrocephalus
- Placenta previa
- Pelvic tumors—ovarian or fibroid
- High-pelvic inclination.

Importance of palpating anterior shoulder:
- It helps in ascertaining rotation of the head and helps in diagnosing occipitoposterior position.

- In labor, it helps to know the progress of labor where it rotates medially and descends downward.

Auscultation:
- Fetal heart sounds
- Heard best through the back in the spinoumbilical line with the bell of the stethoscope
- In breech presentation—around umbilicus
- In occipitoposterior position—near the mother's flank.

Pelvic assessment: In the inlet, only the anteroposterior (AP) diameter is measured, which is the diagonal conjugate (DC). It is clinically estimated by measuring the distance from sacral promontory (SP) to the lower margin of symphysis pubis. Two fingers of the dominant hand are introduced into the vagina and SP is felt. The obstetric conjugate is computed by subtracting 1.5–2 cm (depending on height and inclination of pubic symphysis) from DC. If the DC is >11.5 cm, it is assumed that the pelvic inlet is of adequate size for vaginal delivery of a normal-sized fetus.

In the mid-cavity, feel for the concavity of the sacrum from above downward and side to side. Assess for the side walls, sacrosciatic notch (SSN) (it is adequate when two fingers can be easily placed over the sacrospinous ligament covering the notch), and ischial spines (IS) (their prominence and distance between them by pronated first and middle finger). In normal cases, they should not touch both the spines simultaneously.

Pelvic assessment is completed by measuring the distance between ischial tuberosities (ISD), which is adequate, if it easily accommodates a closed fist (or four knuckles) and subpubic angle (SPA) is >90°.

To summarize the above, findings may be written as follows in the case sheets: SP not tipped, side walls parallel (II), SSN 2F, IS-NP (not palpable), ISD-N (normal), SPA >90°, TDO (transverse diameter of outlet or intertuberous diameter) 4K, and DC 11.5 cm.

GYNECOLOGICAL HISTORY TAKING

What are the important points to be noted in history?
- Chief complaints—in chronological order
- History of present illness
- Menstrual history
- Treatment history
- *Past medical history:* DM, TB, HTN, cardiac disease, asthma, or thyroid disorders. Presence of these requires care during an operative procedure.
- *Past surgical history:* Includes general, obstetrical, or any gynecological surgery. Enquiry should be done for the nature of surgery, any operative complications, postoperative course, and histopathological report if available.
- *Obstetric history:* Detailed obstetric history.
- *Family history:* HTN, DM, allergies, TB, genetic disorders. Malignancy of ovary, endometrium, breast, and colon in relatives must be documented.
- *Personal history:* Occupation, marital status, allergy to certain drugs, or any drug intake for long time.

What are the important points to be noted in menstrual history?
- Age of onset of the first period (menarche)
- Regularity of cycle
- Duration of cycle (*normal range:* 2–7 days)
- Length of cycle (*normal range:* 21–35 days)
- *Amount of bleeding:* Excess is indicated by the number of pads used/day or passage of clots (30–80 mL menstrual blood flow per cycle is normal).

- **LMP:** First day of LMP
- Association with dysmenorrhea

What is abnormal uterine bleeding?
Abnormal uterine bleeding (AUB) is bleeding from the uterine cavity that is abnormal in volume, frequency, regularity, and duration and occurs in absence of pregnancy.

What is heavy menstrual bleeding?
Excessive menstrual blood loss which interferes with a women's physical, social, and/or material quality of life is heavy menstrual bleeding (HMB). Bleeding is excessive either in amount or in duration or both.

What are the causes of heavy menstrual bleeding?
Pelvic causes
- Fibroid uterus
- Adenomyosis
- Pelvic inflammatory disease (PID)
- Early stages of pelvic TB (tubercular endometritis)
- Pelvic endometriosis
- Granulosa cell tumor of ovary
- Chronic tubo-ovarian mass
- Endometrial hyperplasia and/or endometrial carcinoma
- Intrauterine contraceptive device (IUCD) in utero.

Systemic causes
- Hypothyroidism or hyperthyroidism
- Liver dysfunction
- Idiopathic thrombocytopenic purpura (ITP), leukemia, Von Willebrand's disease
- Congestive cardiac failure.

What is PALM-COEIN classification (FIGO 2011) for categorization of causes of abnormal uterine bleeding?
Structural causes (PALM): Polyp, Adenomyosis, Leiomyoma, Malignancy, and hyperplasia.

Nonstructural systemic causes (COEIN): Coagulopathy, Ovulatory dysfunction, Endometrial, Iatrogenic, Not yet identified

What are the causes of frequent cycles?
- Ovarian congestion as in fibroid, PID, and endometriosis
- Pelvic congestion syndrome
- Abnormality of pituitary–ovarian axis as in perimenarchal and premenopausal states.

What are the causes of intermenstrual bleeding?
- Endometrial polyps
- Submucous fibroid
- Endometrial carcinoma
- Cervical ectropion
- Cervical polyps
- Carcinoma cervix
- Any lesion in vagina or vulva
- Ovulatory mid-cycle bleed
- IUCD use
- Breakthrough bleeding with OCP use.

Enumerate causes of infrequent cycles.
- Perimenarchal and premenopausal
- Hypothyroidism
- Hyperprolactinemia
- Familial
- Polycystic ovary syndrome (PCOS) and other causes of hyperandrogenism.

What are the causes of scanty periods?
- Tuberculous endometritis
- Uterine synechiae
- Chronic OCP use causing endometrial atrophy
- Thyroid dysfunction
- Premenopausal
- Constitutional (malnutrition).

What is dysmenorrhea?
Painful menstruation of sufficient magnitude so as to incapacitate day-to-day activities is dysmenorrhea.

What are the types of dysmenorrhea?
Dysmenorrhea is of two types:
1. Primary
2. Secondary

Primary dysmenorrhea: No identifiable pathology, mostly confined to ovulatory cycle. Pain starts with the onset or just before menses.

Secondary dysmenorrhea: Secondary to pelvic pathologies which include:
- *Intrauterine:* Fibroid, adenomyosis (usually late onset), and IUCD
- *Extrauterine:* PID, endometriosis, and adhesions due to previous surgery
- *Obstructive abnormality:* Cervical stenosis and Müllerian abnormality
- *Triple dysmenorrhea:* It is characteristic of endometriosis. Pain begins before the onset of menstruation and persists during and for a few days after cessation of menstruation.

What are the causes of acute pelvic pain?
- *Pregnancy related:* Ectopic gestation, abortion, and red degeneration of leiomyoma during pregnancy
- *Infection related:* Acute PID, tubo-ovarian abscess, and endometritis
- *Adnexa related:* Ovarian torsion, hemorrhage, and rupture of ovarian cyst or corpus luteum
- *Visceral distention related:* Ovarian hyperstimulation syndrome, hematometra, or pyometra
- *Gastrointestinal (GI) causes:* Diverticulitis, appendicitis, inflammatory bowel disease, bowel obstruction, and gastroenteritis, pancreatitis
- *Genitourinary causes:* Cystitis, pyelonephritis, and ureteric colic.

What are the causes of chronic pelvic pain?
Chronic pelvic pain is defined as intermittent or constant pain in the lower abdomen or pelvis of at least 6 months' duration, not occurring exclusively with menstruation or intercourse and not associated with pregnancy.
- *Gynecologic causes:* Endometriosis, chronic PID, adhesions, pelvic congestion, fibroid, PID, and ovarian masses—remnant ovary and residual ovary
- *GI:* Irritable bowel syndrome and ulcerative colitis
- *Genitourinary:* Cystourethritis and interstitial cystitis
- *Neurologic:* Nerve entrapment syndrome
- *Musculoskeletal:* Scoliosis and spondylosis
- *Myofascial:* Acute intermittent porphyria, abdominal migraine, and psoas spasm.

GYNECOLOGIC EXAMINATION
- *General and systemic examination (see Obstetric section)*
- *Breast examination:* See and palpate for any lump, abnormal discharge, or any other abnormality in nipple areola complex.
- *Thyroid:* Look for abnormal enlargement, contour, asymmetry, and mass for thyroid abnormality
- Cardiovascular and respiratory system examination.

Enumerate important points in abdominal examination.

Prerequisite: Bladder should be empty.

Inspection:
- Distension (due to any lump and ascites)
- *Eversion of umbilicus:* Due to raised intra-abdominal pressure and is seen in large tumor, ascites, and pregnancy
- *Striae:* Pregnancy, parous women, obese subjects, and women having large tumors
- *Scar marks:* Indicate previous surgery and whether healed by primary or secondary intention

- *Mobility of the abdominal wall with breathing:* In case of pelvic peritonitis, movement of lower abdomen below umbilicus is restricted.
- *Hernial orifices:* For any evidence of hernia
- Any visible pulsations (in case of any aneurysm)
- Distended veins (e.g., in case of portal HTN).

Palpation: The clinician should stand to the right side of the patient. It is desirable to palpate the liver and spleen with the right hand and use the sensitive ulnar border of the left hand from above downward to palpate masses arising from pelvis and growing into the abdomen. The upper and lateral margins of such tumors can be felt, but the lower border cannot be reached.

On palpation, look for size, site, mobility from side to side and from above to down, surface, margins, consistency (myomas—firm, ovarian neoplasm feels cystic/fluctuant, pregnant uterus is soft, full bladder feels tense, and tender), tenderness—extreme tenderness below umbilicus suggestive of pelvic irritation seen in women with ectopic pregnancy, PID, torsion of ovarian cyst, a ruptured corpus luteal hematoma, red differentiation of fibroid, and sarcoma. When describing a pelvic mass, the size is described according to the size of a gravid uterus. For example, if the mass is just below umbilicus, it is described as a mass of "20 weeks gravid uterus size" and so on.

Percussion:
- Uterine fibroids and ovarian masses are dull on percussion, but flanks are resonant as the bowel is pushed laterally.
- Dullness at flanks and presence of shifting dullness suggest presence of free fluid.

Auscultation:
- Peristaltic bowel sounds
- Hyperperistalsis indicates bowel obstruction.
- Feeble or absent bowel sounds are suggestive of paralytic ileus.
- Fetal heart sounds.
- Soufflé in vascular neoplasm and pregnancy.

What are the causes of abdominopelvic masses or pelvic masses?
- Uterine—fibroid, adenomyosis, and pregnancy
- Ovarian—functional cyst, neoplastic cyst, chocolate cyst, and inflammatory tubo-ovarian masses
- Tubal—hydrosalpinx, pyosalpinx, and ectopic gestation
- Others—paraovarian cyst, appendicular mass, GI malignancy, retroperitoneal mass, and pelvic kidney.

Pelvic Examination

Prerequisites
- Patient's bladder must be empty—exception being a case of stress urinary incontinence
- Presence of third party, preferably female staff nurse, if the examiner is a male
- Consent of the patient or consent of her parents or *guardian* (if she is minor or insane)
- A light source should be available.
- Sterile gloves, antiseptic solution, instruments for examination.

How is a pelvic examination conducted?
Local examination of external genitalia
Inspect the vulva comprising mons pubis, labia majora, labia minora, and clitoris. Look for any abnormality of clitoris, labia, perineum, and pubic hair. If normal looking, say "external

genitalia healthy". In postmenopausal women, external genitalia are described as atrophic and occasionally genital prolapse can be seen. In hyperandrogenic states, look for clitoral hypertrophy and in cases of primary amenorrhea, look for gonads in the inguinal region and labia majora. Retract the labia and look for discharge and hematocolpos.

In case of stress urinary incontinence, urine comes out through urethral meatus during coughing or straining.

Per speculum examination
- Examine the vagina for rugosities, vascularization, atrophy, keratinization, laceration, nodules, and any discharge or prolapse.
- Examine cervix for discharge, ectropion, nabothian cyst, polyp, and growth.

Per vaginum examination
- *Anteverted uterus:* Cervix pointing downward and backward and uterus felt between the abdominal hand and fingers placed in anterior fornix.
- *Retroverted uterus:* Cervix pointing upward and uterus felt between the abdominal hand and fingers placed in posterior fornix.
- *Anteflexion:* There is anterior flexion of uterine body over cervix of 90° and vice versa in retroflexion. There could be various combinations of version and flexion as retroversion with retroflexion and vice versa.

The points to be determined with regard to the cervix and the uterus are the size, shape, position, mobility, consistency, and tenderness caused by pressure or movement.

Palpate any adnexal mass and its size, position, consistency, mobility, and tenderness.

Rectal examination
- It is useful when vaginal examination is not possible (e.g., unmarried female)
- It is a useful adjunct to vaginal examination and is the best approach for feeling the uterosacral ligaments, POD, and other parts of the broad ligament and is therefore used for assessing growth arising from cervix.
- It is useful to diagnose enterocoele, hematocolpos, hematometra, pelvic abscess, chronic ectopic, ovarian metastasis, and endometriosis.

Combined Rectal and Vaginal Examination (P/V/R)
This is done by inserting the index finger into vagina and middle finger into rectum. This combined method has a special value in determining whether a lesion is situated within the bowel or between the bowel and the genital tract and in staging of carcinoma cervix.

What are the steps to be taken by a medical officer while examining a case of sexual assault?
Take a detailed history and perform a thorough examination maintaining the victim's privacy. A valid consent is mandatory. Sexual Assault Care and Forensic Evidence (SAFE) kits launched by the center for enquiry into health and allied themes (CEHAT) are available in hospitals at the national level. It comprises five forms, which need to be filled. They are: (1) consent form, (2) medical history form, (3) sexual assault history, (4) forensic evidence and general examination form, and (5) discharge/summary slip.

It also consists of a manual to guide examination, which contains the following items:
- Bulb for blood grouping and DNA analysis
- Swabs for collecting evidence from mouth/body/and genital area

- Catchment paper for nail clippings/body scraping/comb/scissors
- Distilled water ampule to moisten swabs
- Paper bags to collect evidence and a white sheet of paper on which a woman stands and undresses so that debris is collected
- Photographs of injuries
- Body maps showing in detail the size, color, and body location of injuries (also contusions, ecchymoses, snatches, abrasions, laceration, grip marks, and bite marks)
- Colposcopic examination of the female genitalia after staining the vagina with toluidine blue and washing with 1% acetic acid and photographing the injuries sustained in the vagina
- Emergency contraception.

All samples should be preserved properly and quickly forwarded to concerned laboratories for examination. If there is oral or rectal penetration, proper samples should be collected from these sites. Breast development in young victims should especially be recorded because young girls who are assaulted may mature to adult appearing females during the interim between the assault and trial. Other signs of fondling or sadistic trauma, i.e., ecchymosis, bite marks, and hickeys, should be noted on breast.

Simultaneously, an accused should be examined at the earliest possible. Samples of blood, blood stains, semen, sputum, sweat, hair, and nail clippings should be obtained and sent for DNA profiling and other necessary investigations.

CHAPTER 2: Immunization in Pregnancy

Pakhee Aggarwal, Sandhya Jain

INTRODUCTION

Infants can be protected from many infections by passive immunization if mothers are immunized in pregnancy. Maternal immunization can protect both mother and fetus in their high-risk period of life. This chapter deals with various vaccines and their safety profiles **(Box 1)**.

BOX 1: Summary of vaccines in pregnancy.

Vaccines recommended in pregnancy:
- Tetanus toxoid (TT) vaccine
- Tetanus toxoid, acellular pertussis, and reduced diphtheria toxoid (Tdap) vaccine
- Influenza vaccine

Vaccines contraindicated in pregnancy:
- Measles, mumps, rubella (MMR) vaccine
- Varicella vaccine
- Live influenza vaccine
- Typhoid oral vaccine
- BCG vaccine
- Zoster vaccine (both live and recombinant)
- HPV vaccine

Vaccines which are safe and can be given in special circumstances:
- Hepatitis A vaccine
- Hepatitis B vaccine
- Typhoid intramuscular vaccine
- Antirabies vaccine
- Respiratory syncytial virus (RSV)
- COVID-19 vaccine
- Polio vaccine (live and inactivated)
- Yellow fever vaccine (live)
- Meningococcal vaccine
- Pneumococcal vaccine
- *Haemophilus influenzae* vaccine

What is the concept of maternal immunization?

Maternal immunization against vaccine-preventable infections protects the mother from developing that infection during pregnancy, thereby preventing perinatal transmission to the baby. The ideal time to vaccinate is prepregnancy, but some vaccinations are given during pregnancy to protect the newborn by providing passive immunity against neonatal infections. In addition, even though immune adaptations occur in pregnancy, vaccine efficacy is similar in pregnant and nonpregnant patients.

What are the vaccines routinely recommended in pregnancy?

Routinely recommended vaccines in pregnancy are safe, provide passive immunity to the newborn, and are not associated with miscarriage. These are mainly three:
1. Tetanus toxoid (TT)
2. Tetanus, reduced diphtheria toxoid, acellular pertussis (Tdap) vaccine
3. Influenza vaccine

What are the general guidelines for immunization in pregnancy?

- Pregnancy should always be ruled out before immunizing women of the reproductive age group. This can be ascertained with reasonable certainty if the woman does not have any signs and symptoms of pregnancy and either of the following—abstained since last periods/on a regular contraceptive/within 4 weeks

> **BOX 2:** Live and nonlive vaccines.
>
> *Live vaccines:*
> - Measles, mumps, rubella (MMR)
> - Varicella
> - Live influenza vaccine
> - Typhoid oral vaccine
> - BCG
> - Zoster vaccine
> - MMR-V vaccine
> - Rubella vaccine
> - Oral polio vaccine
> - Yellow fever vaccine
>
> *Nonlive (inactivated/recombinant vaccines):*
> - Hepatitis A
> - Hepatitis B
> - Typhoid injectable vaccine
> - Antirabies vaccine
> - Respiratory syncytial virus (RSV)
> - COVID-19 vaccine
> - Polio injectable vaccine
> - Inactivated zoster vaccine
> - Tetanus toxoid (TT)
> - Tdap
> - Influenza vaccine
> - Meningococcal vaccine
> - Pneumococcal vaccine
> - *Hemophilus influenzae* vaccine
> - Human papillomavirus (HPV) vaccine

- Toxoids, inactivated viral or bacterial vaccines, and immune globulins are considered safe in pregnancy; there is no risk to the fetus or teratogenicity or miscarriage.
- Following delivery, even while breastfeeding, women should be immunized with the vaccines which could not be administered in pregnancy [measles, mumps, and rubella (MMR), varicella, human papillomavirus (HPV)] or those which were recommended but missed (Tdap, TT, Influenza).
- Maternal antibodies crossing the placenta are of immunoglobulin G (IgG) type. The levels of antibody peak at 4 weeks after vaccination; hence, the timing of vaccination is important for passive immunity of fetus (e.g., pertussis vaccine given between 28 and 32 weeks). Vaccines which are given for both maternal and fetal production can be given irrespective of the gestational age (e.g., influenza vaccine given as per the flu season).

postpartum/within a week of abortion or last menstrual period/fitting within the criteria of lactational amenorrhea
- Live or live-attenuated viral and bacterial vaccines are contraindicated in pregnancy **(Box 2)**.
- If a pregnant woman is given live or live-attenuated vaccine by mistake, she should be counseled regarding the risks of teratogenicity, but it should not be considered as a reason for medical termination of pregnancy.
- If a patient is given live or live-attenuated vaccine in the preconception period, she should be counseled to plan pregnancy after a gap of 4 weeks. For varicella, the manufacturer recommendation is 3 months.

What is tetanus prophylaxis?

Active immunization: Two doses of 0.5 mL TT intramuscular (IM) in deltoid region 4–6 weeks apart are administered. The first dose is given as soon as a patient visits a healthcare facility. Vaccine efficacy is 90%.

Only one booster dose is required, if the previous pregnancy was within 3 years and the mother received complete prophylaxis in previous pregnancy. If there is doubt, two doses are to be given.

In disaster situations, give blanket cover to all pregnant women with a single dose of TT.

Passive immunization: Single dose of tetanus immunoglobulin (TIG) 250–500 IU IM is recommended.

What do you mean by neonatal tetanus high risk, control area, and neonatal tetanus elimination?

Neonatal tetanus high-risk areas
- Incidence of neonatal tetanus (NNT) more than 1/1,000 live births
- TT second dose coverage <70%
- Attended deliveries <50%

Neonatal tetanus control areas
- Incidence of NNT <1/1,000 live births
- Tetanus toxoid second dose coverage >70%
- Attended deliveries >50%

Neonatal tetanus elimination
- Incidence of NNT <0.1/1,000 live births
- Tetanus toxoid second dose coverage >90%
- Attended deliveries >75%.

Target: Tetanus prophylaxis to 100% of pregnant women to achieve NNT elimination.

What is Tdap vaccination?

Vaccination with tetanus toxoid, acellular pertussis, and reduced diphtheria toxoid is recommended in pregnancy, between 27 and 36 weeks of pregnancy. This is to be given in each pregnancy, irrespective of previous vaccination, even if pregnancy occurs within 3 years, as it is also to transmit passive immunity to the fetus. Its main role is in prevention of neonatal pertussis, especially for the first 6 weeks of life, as infant immunization starts at 6 weeks. Giving at the recommended gestation has the benefits of transplacental transfer of antibodies as well as through the breast milk, maximizing neonatal protection though passive immunity. Vaccinating too early (before 27 weeks) and too late (beyond 36 weeks) gives suboptimal protection compared to between 27 and 36 weeks as per the Advisory Committee on Immunization Practices (ACIP).

If it is not administered in pregnancy, it should be given while breastfeeding to protect the infant through passive transfer of antibodies in breast milk, but it may take at least 2 weeks for antibody levels to be sufficient. If Tdap is given prior to 27 weeks, due to any reason, it does not need to be repeated after 27 weeks.

Household contacts, looking after infants, who have not been immunized previously, should be vaccinated with single-dose Tdap to prevent neonatal infection. It does not need to be repeated, unlike for pregnant patients.

How is influenza vaccination given in pregnancy?

The ACIP and American College of Obstetricians and Gynecologists (ACOG) recommend influenza vaccination for all pregnant women or likely to be pregnant or postpartum during the flu season. Flu season occurs in September–October in the northern hemisphere and March–April in the southern hemisphere. Hence, vaccination is given based on the flu season and the prevalent strains of influenza and is independent of pregnancy trimesters. As is it an inactivated vaccine, it can be safely administered without any fetal complications or risk of miscarriage. Live-attenuated influenza vaccine (LAIV) is not recommended during pregnancy. It is not necessary for pregnant women to avoid contact with individuals who have received live virus vaccine.

Pregnant and postpartum women have more complications due to influenza infection compared to nonpregnant women. There is a higher risk of intensive care unit (ICU) admission, stillbirth, and preterm birth with maternal influenza infection. Vaccination reduces the risk of influenza-like illness and influenza-related hospitalizations, in addition to providing passive immunity to the fetus (IgA through breast milk and IgG through transplacental transfer). The adjuvant in the vaccine (thiomersal) is generally thought to be safe. Inactivated influenza vaccine is not associated with any adverse maternal or fetal events.

What are the consequences of varicella infection in pregnancy and its management?

Varicella (chickenpox) is a highly infectious and contagious disease caused by varicella zoster virus. The primary infection caused by varicella zoster is chickenpox, while reactivation due to an immunocompromised state causes herpes zoster. This infection can be transmitted by direct contact, droplets by coughing or sneezing, and transplacentally from mother to baby.

Varicella infection, if occurs in first and second trimesters, causes congenital varicella syndrome in fetus, and neonatal varicella zoster, if infection occurs in late third trimester or close to term. Congenital varicella syndrome typically presents as skin scarring, limb reduction deformities, and eye and central nervous system (CNS) defects.

Varicella infection in adults is more severe, and associated with complications like pneumonia, encephalopathy, and death. Thus, women of child-bearing age who are not immune and not planning pregnancy in the near future and are at risk of exposure (e.g., school health nurses, daycare center staff, hospital workers) should be vaccinated with varicella vaccine (2 doses, 4-8 weeks apart). Pregnancy should be deferred for a month following vaccination. This is active immunization. It provides 100% seroconversion and immunity against chickenpox infection. There is a theoretical risk of varicella infection to the fetus, if a pregnant lady is given varicella vaccine. Therefore, when a woman of reproductive age group is given varicella injection, she should be counseled to plan pregnancy after 4 weeks. If injection is given by mistake to a pregnant woman, then risks should be explained, although it is not an indication for termination of pregnancy.

Passive immunization: Specific immunoglobulins are available and can be given safely as postexposure prophylaxis (exposure to varicella or herpes zoster) in pregnant women. *Dose*—12U/10 kg body weight (maximum of 625U) IM preferably within 72 hours and not later than 96 hours of exposure. Individuals receiving varicella immunoglobulin and babies born to mothers with varicella should be isolated for 21-28 days as immunoglobulins may prolong the incubation period.

Varicella zoster immunoglobulins (VZIG) should be given to the babies whose mother developed chickenpox 7 days before delivery and 2 days following delivery.

Varicella virus vaccine is recommended for children 12 months to 12 years of age who did not have chickenpox in earlier age.

What are the risks of herpes zoster infection in pregnancy and what is the treatment?

Reactivation of herpes zoster infection in mother causes viremia, but it does not cause clinical disease. Therefore, the risk of intrauterine varicella zoster virus infection is remote. The immunoglobulins transferred to fetus by the transplacental route are also protective for the fetus. Postexposure prophylaxis is not required. Zoster vaccine (Zostavax®) should not be administered to pregnant women. Pregnancy should not be terminated, if the patient is vaccinated during pregnancy by mistake.

What are indications for measles, mumps, and rubella?

Measles, mumps, and rubella vaccine is live-attenuated vaccine and therefore is contraindicated in pregnancy. MMR vaccine is usually given in childhood when the immunization schedule is followed. Immunity to rubella and measles (IgG positivity) is part of preconception screening, and so if someone has missed childhood vaccination or immunity cannot be demonstrated with certainty, the MMR vaccine should be administered, before pregnancy planning. Similar to varicella vaccine, if the MMR vaccine is given to women of reproductive age group, pregnancy should be planned after 4 weeks. There is a theoretical risk of congenital rubella syndrome, if the vaccine is inadvertently given during pregnancy but it is not evidence based, so patients should not be counseled for medical termination of pregnancy. If a woman is not immunized in childhood with MMR vaccine and she becomes pregnant without immunization, she can be immunized in the postpartum period.

Can hepatitis A vaccine be given in pregnancy?

Hepatitis A vaccine is an inactivated virus vaccine. It can be given in pregnancy, if the benefits are more than risks. In high-risk populations (such as planned travel to endemic area, drug abusers, occupational risk for infection, etc.), vaccination is recommended in pregnancy as acute hepatitis in pregnancy can cause significant morbidity. Vaccination is not associated with adverse effects to the pregnancy or fetus (although data is limited).

Can hepatitis B vaccine be given in pregnancy, if the patient has not been previously immunized?

Available vaccines contain noninfectious Australia antigen (HBsAg) Hepatitis B surface antigen, as they are recombinant vaccines. Therefore, the vaccine does not pose risks to the developing fetus. So, it can be given when postexposure prophylaxis is recommended in pregnant women. It can also be given to patients to complete the immunization schedule started before pregnancy (0, 1, 6 months) and if someone is at high risk for acquiring hepatitis B (e.g., health care workers).

What are the risks if the mother is Australia antigen positive, and how do you manage such a case?

Australia antigen positivity in pregnant females in India ranges from 0.6% to 12.3% (average 2–3%). Acute infection with hepatitis B causes antigenemia in 7% of fetuses with the incidence increasing to 40–67%, if infection occurs in the third trimester. The mother, if immune, passes antibodies by the transplacental route to the fetus.

The dose of hepatitis B vaccine in an adult is 20 µg at 0, 1, and 6 months. The protective efficacy with a three-dose schedule is as high as 95%. Neonates born to HBsAg-positive mothers should receive:

- Hepatitis B vaccine 10 µg IM at 0, 6, 10, and 14 weeks
- Specific immunoglobulin [hepatitis B immunoglobulin (HBIG)] should be given preferably within 12 hours to 7 days of birth. 0.5 mL IM at 0, 3, and 6 months should be administered.
- Interferon alpha-2 therapy is successful but has a lot of side effects.

Women, who are at risk for hepatitis B vaccine infection during pregnancy (e.g., multiple sexual partners, drug abusers, HbsAg-positive partner), should be vaccinated.

What is to be done if a pregnant woman is exposed to measles?

If a pregnant woman comes into contact with measles, certain precautions should be taken. Specific immunoglobulin is not available but standard immunoglobulin has a definite role.

Dose—0.25 mL/kg body weight in healthy persons and 0.5 mL/kg in immunocompromised person up to maximum of 15 mL,

IM, preferably within 72 hours to 6 days of exposure.

What is the treatment if a pregnant woman is exposed to dog/mammalian bite?
Antirabies postexposure prophylaxis regimen (vaccine and immunoglobulin both) is followed as per standard recommendations. Pregnancy is not a contraindication for postexposure prophylaxis of rabies, as it is an inactivated vaccine. Pre-exposure prophylaxis may be considered if the risk of exposure is high. There are no increased risks of abortion, premature births, or fetal abnormalities associated with rabies vaccination.

Is human papillomavirus vaccine safe in pregnancy?
Human papillomavirus vaccines are not recommended in pregnant women. However, as they do not contain active virus, if a woman is inadvertently vaccinated without knowing that she is pregnant, medical termination of pregnancy is not recommended. The schedule of HPV vaccine is 0, 2, and 6 months; if any of the doses fall during pregnancy, they can be deferred to post-partum without any loss in efficacy. Breastfeeding is not a contraindication to vaccination.

Can typhoid vaccine be given in pregnancy?
Data on the use of either typhoid vaccine in pregnant women are limited. In general, live vaccines like Ty21a (live-attenuated oral vaccine) are contraindicated in pregnancy. Inactive capsular polysaccharide vaccine (Typhim Vi) should be given to pregnant women only if it is clearly needed, e.g., travel to endemic area. More importantly, as typhoid is acquired from contaminated food or water, avoiding such substances affords better protection as vaccination is only partially protective.

What about COVID-19 vaccination?
After the COVID pandemic, vaccination has developed rapidly and the indications for vaccination remain the same for pregnant and nonpregnant women. The vaccines approved by the World Health Organization (WHO) are either protein-based subunit vaccines or inactivated virus or mRNA based and are considered safe in pregnancy based on available data, as they are not live vaccines and benefits outweigh the risks. These are given IM in the deltoid region.

■ SUGGESTED READING

1. American College of Obstetricians and Gynecologists. (2018). Influenza Vaccination During Pregnancy: Committee Opinion No 732, 2018. [online] Available from https://www.acog.org/clinical/clinical-guidance/committee-opinion/articles/2018/04/influenza-vaccination-during-pregnancy [Last accessed April, 2024].
2. American College of Obstetricians and Gynecologists. (2022). Maternal immunization. Practice advisory October 2022. [online] Available from https://www.acog.org/clinical/clinical-guidance/practice-advisory/articles/2022/10/maternal-immunization [Last accessed April, 2024].
3. United States Centers for Disease Control and Prevention. (2022). Pregnancy and Vaccination: Guidelines for Vaccinating Pregnant Women, 2022. [online] Available from https://www.cdc.gov/vaccines/pregnancy/hcp-toolkit/guidelines.html [Last accessed April, 2024].
4. United States Centers for Disease Control and Prevention. (2022). Pregnancy and vaccination: Guidelines for Vaccinating Pregnant Women. [online] Available from https://www.cdc.gov/vaccines/pregnancy/hcp-toolkit/guidelines.html [Last accessed April, 2024].
5. World Health Organization. (2023). Draft landscape of COVID-19 candidate vaccines. [online] Available from https://www.who.int/publications/m/item/draft-landscape-of-covid-19-candidate-vaccines [Last accessed April, 2024].

CHAPTER 3

First- and Second-trimester Aneuploidy Screening

Astha Srivastava, Sandhya Jain

■ INTRODUCTION

The most common autosomal trisomy among live births is trisomy 21 (Down syndrome). The primary target of prenatal aneuploidy screening is early detection of pregnancies at high risk for Down syndrome. First-trimester combined and integrated tests are available for screening of trisomy 21 (Down syndrome), trisomy 18 (Edwards syndrome, the second most common autosomal trisomy among live births), and trisomy 13 (Patau syndrome). Prenatal screening can also be performed using cell-free DNA in maternal circulation. Cell-free DNA can diagnose 98–99% of pregnancies affected by Down syndrome.

■ ANEUPLOIDY SCREENING

Who are the candidates for screening?

As per American College of Obstetricians and Gynecologists, every pregnant female should be offered aneuploidy screening before 20 weeks of period of gestation and they have the option of invasive testing irrespective of maternal age.

Who are the candidates for diagnostic tests?

A diagnostic rather than screening test is a reasonable choice for women irrespective of age who are at high risk of Down syndrome or other aneuploidies, i.e.:
- Woman with history of fetal trisomy in previous pregnancy.
- Current pregnancy has at least one major or two minor structural anomalies in the fetus.
- Pregnant woman or her partner having chromosomal translocation, inversion, or aneuploidy.

What do you mean by first-trimester screening test? Enumerate the timings of biochemical screening and ultrasound.

First-trimester screening for aneuploidies is done between 9 and 13 weeks of gestation (in the late first trimester). The screening test consists of biochemical markers plus NT measurement on ultrasound. Biochemical markers tested are—maternal serum beta human chorionic gonadotropin (beta-hCG) and maternal serum pregnancy-associated plasma protein (PAPP-A).

These three together comprise the *"combined test"*.

Combined tests together with maternal age provide a patient-specific risk. Detection rate (DR) of combined test for Down syndrome is approximately 85% (DR or sensitivity = 85%) with a false-positive rate (FPR) of 5%. The combined test performs slightly better than the second-trimester quadruple test (i.e., the DR is higher and/other FPR is lower).

Timing: The blood tests and ultrasound examination for the combined test are most commonly performed at the same time between 11 and 13 weeks of gestation. Some protocols opt for blood collection at around

9 weeks of gestation, so that the results are available for immediate reporting when the ultrasound is performed later.

Beta-human chorionic gonadotropin: The levels are usually twice as high in pregnancies affected with fetal Down syndrome than in normal pregnancy. It can be assayed in free or total form. Free beta-hCG is effective at 9–13 weeks and the performance improves as gestational age advances within this interval. Total beta-hCG is effective at 11–13 weeks.

Pregnancy-associated plasma protein: It is a complex, high-molecular-weight glycoprotein, and levels are lower in affected pregnancies. In contrast to beta-hCG, PAPP-A performance as a screening marker decreases with increasing gestational age between 9 and 13 weeks.

Nuchal translucency: Fetal NT thickness measured between 10 and 13 gestational weeks is increased in fetuses with Down syndrome. NT performance as a screening marker decreases with advancing gestation between 10 and 13 weeks. NT is the translucent nuchal space at the posterior fetal neck observed sonographically in the midsagittal plane **(Fig. 1)**. The most commonly used cutoffs to classify NT as abnormal are the 95th and 99th percentiles for gestational age. The normal NT is 3.0–4.0 mm. Various calculators are available online that enable a clinician to enter the fetal crown rump length and NT measurement to obtain the estimated gestational age and percentile for NT. Measurement of NT should be combined with serum marker results for screening. One exception to this recommendation is for fetuses with a cystic hygroma or significantly enlarged NT. These pregnancies are at particularly high risk of aneuploidy. Enlarged

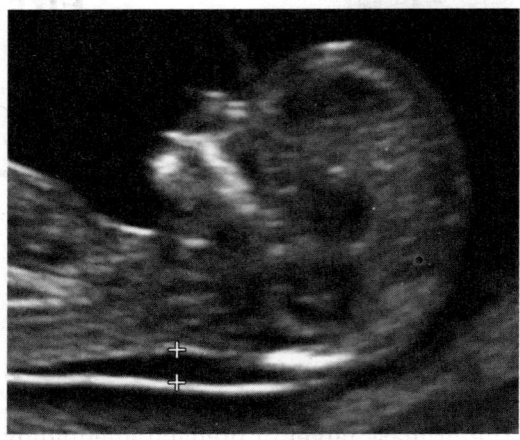

Fig. 1: Nuchal translucency.

NT has also been associated with other structural malformations.

What is quadruple test?

Second-trimester quadruple test: It measures the level of the biochemical markers alpha fetoprotein (AFP), unconjugated estriol (uE3), hCG, and inhibin A in maternal serum.

Maternal serum AFP and uE3 levels are, on average, reduced by 25–30% in pregnancies affected by Down syndrome and hCG and inhibin A levels are, on average, twice as high as those in unaffected pregnancies. Ideal timing for quadruple test is between 15 and 18 weeks of gestation, but it can be done till 22 weeks.

For women, who first present for prenatal care in the second trimester, the quadruple test is the best available biochemical marker for Down syndrome screening. Since it involves measurement of AFP, it also serves as a screening test for open neural tube defects. An elevated risk of trisomy 18, when present, is also reported. Some screening programs include reporting of elevated risk of Smith–Lemli–Opitz syndrome (SLOS), when present. Trisomy 13 is not detected by the quadruple test.

What do you mean by integrated test?

Integrated screening tests measure biochemical markers of Down syndrome in both the first and second trimesters and may or may not include ultrasound measurement for NT. Since, the second-trimester portion of the integrated test includes measurement of maternal serum AFP levels, these tests also screen for open neural tube defects.

There are three types of integrated test:
1. The *full integrated test* measures serum PAPP-A at 10–13 weeks and sonographic NT at 11–13 weeks, as the first step. These results are integrated with results of the quadruple test performed on a second serum sample collected at 15–18 weeks to determine the risk of trisomy 21.
2. The *serum integrated test* differs from the full integrated test by not including ultrasound measurement of NT, especially in areas where ultrasound expertise is not there.
3. *Stepwise sequential testing* is a modified version of the full integrated test that provides risk estimates after the first step. In most protocols, the sequential screening process involves performing the first-trimester portion of the full integrated test; reporting risks of Down syndrome to the patient and offering chorionic villus sampling (CVS) to high-risk women. Women whose screen does not place them at very high risk go on to complete the second-trimester portion of the test. The benefit of *stepwise sequential testing* is that pregnant women at highest risk of aneuploidy benefit from early detection of affected fetuses, whereas women at lower risk benefit from the high DR and low false-positive rates of second-trimester screening.

What is noninvasive prenatal test?

Noninvasive prenatal testing (NIPT) means testing maternal blood for cell-free DNA. It is used for Down syndrome screening and also for screening of trisomy 18, 13, and sex chromosomal aneuploidies. It is more accurate than combined test or quadruple test, as it can detect >99% of pregnancies complicated by Down syndrome. However, inconclusive result can be obtained in 1–5% of samples. Inconclusive result is obtained, if the proportion of fetal DNA present in the sample is not high enough to give an accurate result. High cost of cell-free DNA limits its use for screening women at low risk for Down syndrome, but it is widely accepted for those at high risk.

High-risk groups in which cell-free DNA testing can be used as primary testing comprise the following:
- Pregnant female 35 years or older at delivery
- Soft marker associated with an increased risk of aneuploidy (trisomy 13, 18, or 21) on fetal ultrasound
- History of trisomy detectable by cell-free DNA screening (trisomy 13, 18, or 21) in prior pregnancy
- Balanced Robertsonian translocation with increased risk of fetal trisomy 13 or 21 in pregnant woman or her partner.

Enumerate the management of screening results.

Screen-negative test result: A screen-negative result means the fetus is at low risk as defined by the specific laboratory cutoffs (e.g., <1 in 250), but does not rule out the possibility of Down syndrome or trisomy 18. It is not appropriate to tell women with a screen-negative result that their test was "normal" or "negative", as they may interpret these terms to mean the fetus definitely has a normal karyotype. After a low-risk result, further testing is not recommended.

Screen-positive test result: A screen-positive test result means the fetus is at increased risk of Down syndrome as defined by the specific laboratory cutoff (e.g., ≥1 in 250). Women, who screen positive on a biochemical marker-based test, may undergo secondary screening or a diagnostic procedure. A secondary screening test aims to collect additional information about risk that screen-positive women can use in deciding whether to proceed to diagnostic testing. Secondary screening is performed with a cell-free DNA test. Because of the high sensitivity and specificity of cell-free DNA tests, many patients with falsepositive biochemical marker tests will be reclassified as screen negative with minimal risk of misclassification of true positives. Women who choose secondary screening with a cell-free DNA test and are secondary screen positive should be offered an invasive test for definitive diagnosis because false-positive results are possible (<0.1%). Patient may also go for diagnostic test (CVS or amniocentesis) directly without going for secondary screening.

Diagnostic testing: In the first trimester, diagnostic test performed is CVS; the results of which can be obtained within 2 days, if a direct preparation is performed; and final results from cultured cells take 7–10 days. Amniocentesis is performed in second trimester to obtain fetal cells for chromosomal analysis. Result of amniocentesis from cultured cells takes approximately 8–14 days.

Fluorescent in situ hybridization targets chromosomes 13, 18, 21, X, and Y. It is used for rapid aneuploidy screening after amniocentesis and can also be performed on interphase cytotrophoblasts from CVS, if the direct preparation fails to yield sufficient useable metaphases for a complete karyotype. Analysis of the full karyotype is generally performed to allow detection of any aneuploidy (not just Down syndrome and trisomy 18) as well as detection of major structural chromosomal abnormalities (e.g., translocations, inversions, and marker chromosomes).

Ultrasound Markers

Soft markers are ultrasound findings of uncertain significance. They are often associated with normal fetuses (i.e., normal variants), usually have no clinical sequelae, and are transient, resolving with advancing gestation or after birth. They do carry an increased risk for fetal aneuploidy, however, correlation with the patient's biochemical risk status should be done. Isolated soft markers are identified in 11–17% of normal fetuses. The prevalence is higher in aneuploid fetuses and the likelihood of aneuploidy is significantly increased when more than one marker is present.

First-trimester Ultrasound Markers

These include:
- Nuchal translucency
- Nasal bone (NB)
- Ductus venosus (DV)
- Tricuspid regurgitation (TR)
- Frontomaxillary angle (FMA)
- Intracranial translucency
- Structural anomalies

Nuchal translucency has been already discussed above.

Nasal bone hypoplasia: The frequency of absent nasal bone in euploid, trisomy 13, trisomy 18, and trisomy 21 is 2.5%, 45%, 53%, and 60%, respectively. Individuals with trisomy 21 often have short nasal root depth. Based on this observation, absence of visualization of the fetal nasal bone ossification has been investigated as a possible fetal marker of Down syndrome. When the fetal profile is viewed in the midsagittal plane, the nasal bone synostosis appears as a thin echogenic line within the bridge of the nose. The nasal bone is considered present, if this line is more echogenic than the overlying skin, and absent, if it is not visualized or less echogenic than the overlying skin. The optimum time for nasal bone assessment is at crown rump length of 65–74 mm (13–13.5 weeks of gestation). Absent nasal bone ossification earlier in gestation could reflect delayed maturation in a euploid fetus, rather than actual absence of the structure.

Ductus venosus Doppler: Abnormal ductal blood flow in 3.7% of euploid fetuses and 69.1%, 71.3%, 64.5%, and 76.2% of fetuses with trisomies 21, 18, and 13, and Turner syndrome, respectively.

Tricuspid valve Doppler and fetal aneuploidy: Assessment of tricuspid flow in the first trimester can also be used to detect aneuploid fetuses. Prevalence of TR varies with gestational age and increases as the NT measurement increases. The prevalence of TR in euploid fetuses is 1%, whereas in fetuses with trisomies 21, 18, 13, and monosomy X, the prevalence is 56%, 33%, 30%, and 38%, respectively.

Fetal heart rate, maxillary length, ear length, femur length, and humeral length are other fetal measurements affected in chromosomally abnormal fetuses in first-trimester ultrasound.

Ultrasound in Second Trimester

Nuchal fold: The nuchal fold is measured in the second trimester. The nuchal fold is the measurement between the outer edges of the occipital bone to the outer margin of the skin and is taken in the axial plane. An increase in this measurement is also associated with aneuploidy. An increased nuchal fold is detected in 20–33% of fetuses with Down syndrome and 0.5–2% of euploid fetuses.

Echogenic bowel: Fetal echogenic bowel refers to increased echogenicity (brightness) of the fetal bowel noted on second-trimester sonographic examination. It may be first identified in the first trimester but is more commonly identified in the second trimester. It has been found in 1–2% of normal fetuses and 13–21% of fetuses with Down syndrome.

Pyelectasis: Pyelectasis or mild hydronephrosis is a common finding in fetuses. Studies that defined pyelectasis as renal pelvic diameter of ≥4 mm at 15–19 weeks of gestation demonstrated pyelectasis in 10–25% of fetuses with Down syndrome and 1–3% of euploid fetuses. Aneuploidy is present in 0.3–0.9% of fetuses with isolated pyelectasis.

Ventriculomegaly: Mild ventriculomegaly is detected in 4–13% of fetuses with Down syndrome and 0.1–0.4% of euploid fetuses.

Shortened long bones: Fetuses with Down syndrome have slightly shorter long bones than their normal counterparts. A shortened humerus appears to be a better predictor of Down syndrome than a shortened femur.

Echogenic intracardiac focus: The sonographic criteria for echogenic intracardiac foci are brightness equivalent to that of bone. Echogenic intracardiac foci usually occur as a single focus in the left ventricle, but multiple foci, biventricular foci, or a right ventricular location can also occur. Echogenic intracardiac foci may be first identified in the first trimester, but identification of this early in pregnancy is rare. In the second trimester, 21–28% of fetuses with Down syndrome have an echogenic intracardiac focus, while this is seen in 3–5% of normal.

Choroid plexus cysts: These are most common in the second trimester. They usually disappear by the third trimester; and those that persist are usually asymptomatic and benign. Choroid plexus cysts are present in 30–50% of fetuses with trisomy 18 compared with 0.6–3% of all second-trimester fetuses.

Others: Although more prevalent in patients with Down syndrome, sandal gap toe, short ear length, and a hypoplastic wedge-shaped middle phalanx of the fifth digit that causes it to curve toward the fourth finger (clinodactyly) are also common normal variants.

The frequency of chromosomal abnormalities is increased in fetuses with sonographic evidence of structural anomalies, i.e., cystic hygroma, fetal growth restriction, single umbilical artery, etc.

Genetic Sonogram

A "genetic sonogram" uses ultrasound to assess the fetus for both structural anomalies and soft markers suggestive of Down syndrome. It is typically performed in the second trimester but may be useful in first-trimester screening as well. Ultrasound findings are incorporated into a mathematical formula that refines a priori Down syndrome risk estimates. It is not useful as a follow-up screening test for women who have undergone a highly sensitive Down syndrome screening test, such as cell-free DNA testing.

■ SUGGESTED READING

1. ACOG Committee on Practice Bulletins. ACOG Practice Bulletin No. 77: screening for fetal chromosomal abnormalities. Obstet Gynecol. 2007;109(1):217-27.
2. Gil MM, Quezada MS, Revello R, Akolekar R, Nicolaides KH. Analysis of cell free DNA in maternal blood in screening for fetal aneuploidies: updated meta-analysis. Ultrasound Obstet Gynecol. 2015;45(3):249-66.
3. Hurt L, Wright M, Dunstan F, Thomas S, Brook F, Morris S, et al. Prevalence of defined ultrasound findings of unknown significance at the second trimester fetal anomaly scan and their association with adverse pregnancy outcomes: the Welsh study of mothers and babies population-based cohort. Prenat Diagn. 2016;36(1):40-8.

CHAPTER 4

Fetal Monitoring

Sruthi Bhaskaran, Himsweta Srivastava, Shalini Rajaram

What are the indications for antepartum fetal testing?
Antepartum fetal testing is used in pregnancies with increased risk of intrauterine fetal demise. Some indications are mentioned in Box 1.

What are the recommendations for antepartum fetal testing?
Initiation of antepartum fetal surveillance depends on the neonatal survival, risk of fetal demise, risk of iatrogenic prematurity (due to false-positive test result), and severity of maternal medical condition.

When to initiate?
For high-risk cases, testing should start after 32 0/7 weeks.

Testing may be required to be started as early as 26–28 weeks in pregnancies with multiple risk factors or complications.

Frequency of testing:
- *Weekly:* If maternal medical condition is stable and test result is reassuring
- *Biweekly:* High-risk pregnancies
- *Daily:* Fetal growth restriction with abnormal Doppler

What are the various antepartum fetal surveillance techniques?
The various techniques in clinical use are daily fetal movement count, nonstress test (NST), contraction stress test (CST), biophysical profile (BPP), modified BPP, and umbilical artery Doppler velocimetry.

How reassuring is a normal antepartum fetal surveillance result?
In most of the cases, a normal antepartum fetal test result is highly reassuring (low false-negative rate—incidence of stillbirth occurring within 1 week of a normal test result). The negative predictive value is 99.8% for the NST and is >99.9% for the CST, BPP, and modified BPP.

BOX 1: Indications for antepartum fetal testing.

Maternal conditions:
- Overt diabetes mellitus
- Hypertension
- Systemic lupus erythematosus
- Chronic renal disease
- Antiphospholipid syndrome
- Hyperthyroidism (poorly controlled)
- Hemoglobinopathies (sickle cell, sickle cell-hemoglobin C, or sickle cell-thalassemia disease)
- Cyanotic heart disease

Pregnancy-related conditions:
- Gestational hypertension
- Preeclampsia
- Decreased fetal movement
- Gestational diabetes mellitus (poorly controlled or medically treated)
- Oligohydramnios
- Fetal growth restriction
- Late-term or post-term pregnancy
- Isoimmunization
- Previous fetal demise (unexplained or recurrent risk)
- Monochorionic multiple gestation (with significant growth discrepancy)

How is a contraction stress test performed and interpreted?
The basis of CST is that fetal oxygenation will be transiently worsened by uterine contractions. In an already hypoxic fetus, the resultant intermittent decreased oxygenation will, in turn, lead to the fetal heart rate (FHR) pattern of late decelerations.

Procedure: Contractions are induced with either nipple stimulation or intravenous (IV) oxytocin. The patient is placed in the lateral recumbent position and FHR and uterine contractions are recorded simultaneously with an external fetal monitor. An adequate uterine contraction is indicated when at least three contractions persist for at least 40 seconds each in a 10-minute period.

Interpretation: The results of the CST are categorized as follows:
- *Negative:* When there are no late or significant variable decelerations
- *Positive:* When late decelerations occur with 50% or more of contractions (even if frequency is less than three contractions in 10 minutes)
- *Equivocal-suspicious:* When there are intermittent late decelerations or significant variable decelerations
- *Equivocal:* When FHR decelerations occur in the presence of contractions more frequent than every 2 minutes or lasting longer than 90 seconds
- *Unsatisfactory:* When there are less than three contractions in 10 minutes or an uninterpretable tracing

Relative contraindications to the CST include conditions that are also contraindications to labor or vaginal delivery.

What is the basic principle of nonstress test?
The basis of NST is that the heart rate of a fetus that is not acidotic or neurologically depressed will temporarily accelerate with fetal movement. Heart rate reactivity is considered to be a good indicator of normal fetal autonomic function.

What is a reactive nonstress test?
- *At or beyond 32 weeks:* When there are two or more FHR accelerations that peak at least 15 bpm above the baseline and last 15 seconds or more but less than 2 minutes, within 20 minutes, it is reactive.
- *Before 32 weeks:* Acceleration of 10 bpm or more above the baseline for 10 seconds or longer. Accelerations with or without fetal movement can be accepted.

The NST should be conducted for at least 20 minutes, which may be extended to 40 minutes or longer to take into account the variations of the fetal sleep–wake cycle.

What is nonreactive nonstress test?
The test is considered nonreactive, if there are no accelerations with spontaneous or repeated external stimulation during a 20-minute period, which may be extended to 40 minutes.

What is the difference between nonstress test and contraction stress test?
The rationale behind NST is that the presence of spontaneous FHR accelerations associated with fetal movements (fetal reactivity) is an indicator of fetal well-being. Whereas, CST is a test of uteroplacental function and relies on evidence that uteroplacental blood flow decreases markedly during uterine contractions which a normal healthy fetus can tolerate. But a fetus with chronic or acute problems will not be able to tolerate this hypoxic stress and will demonstrate this

by decelerations of the FHR following the contractions.

What is the difference between nonstress test and cardiotocography?
Nonstress test is done when the patient is not in labor, whereas cardiotocography (CTG) is done for fetal heart evaluation in labor.

What is baseline fetal heart rate?
- The normal baseline FHR is between 110 and 160 bpm.
- The mean FHR during a 10-minute segment rounded to 5 bpm excluding the following:
  - Periodic or episodic changes
  - Periods of marked FHR variability
  - Segments of the baseline that differ by at least 25 bpm

What is the above nonstress test showing (Fig. 1)?
The above NST is showing periods of fetal bradycardia with FHR <110 bpm.

What is fetal heart rate bradycardia and its causes?
Fetal heart rate below 110 bpm is termed as bradycardia, but a rate between 100 and 119 bpm with normal variability is not indicative of fetal compromise. It may be seen with head compression in second stage of labor. Causes of fetal bradycardia:
- Severe fetal hypoxia with or without acidemia
- Congenital heart block
- Maternal hypothermia (as seen in cardiopulmonary bypass for open heart surgery)

What is fetal tachycardia and what are its causes?
Fetal heart rate above 160 bpm is called tachycardia.

The most common cause of fetal tachycardia is maternal fever due to chorioamnionitis or any other cause. Fetal tachycardia due to maternal infection is not associated with fetal compromise.
- Maternal administration of parasympatholytic drugs (atropine) or sympathomimetic drugs (isoxsuprine, ritodrine, and terbutaline)
- Cardiac arrhythmias
- Epidural analgesia causing maternal hypotension and fetal hypoxia

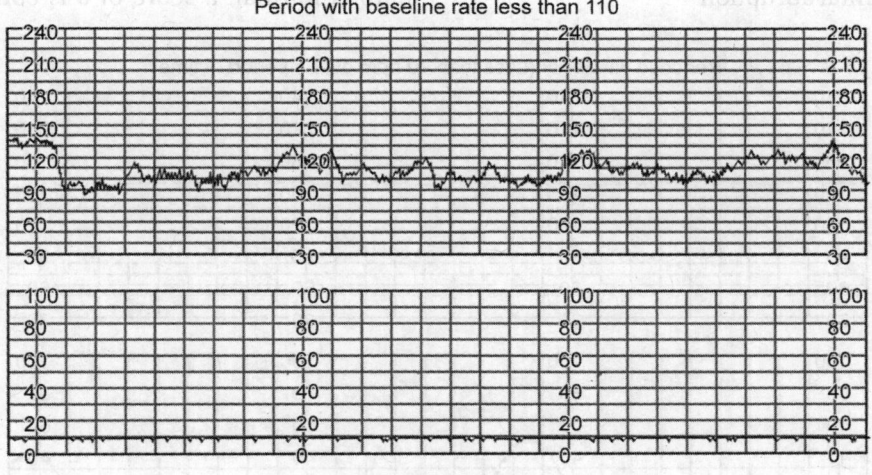

Fig. 1: Fetal heart tracing.

- Presence of decelerations associated with fetal tachycardia is indicative of fetal compromise.

What is baseline variability in fetal heart rate?

The baseline fluctuation in baseline fetal heart rate occurring at 3–5 cycles per minute, measured by estimating the difference between the highest peak and lowest trough of fluctuation in a 1-minute segment of the trace, is called baseline variability. Normal baseline variability is 5–25 bpm.

- Baseline variability is an important index of cardiovascular function.
- Baseline variability is said to be reduced if it is <5 bpm **(Fig. 2)**.

Enumerate few causes of fetal death within 7 days of normal nonstress test.

- Postmaturity
- Meconium aspiration
- Acute asphyxial insult
- Intrauterine infection
- Abnormal cord position
- Malformations
- Placental abruption

What are the components of biophysical profile and how is it scored?

Biophysical profile comprises five components:

1. *NST:* More than or equal to two accelerations of ≥15 bmp for ≥15 seconds within 20–40 minutes (may be omitted if all four sonographic features are normal)
2. *Fetal breathing movements:* One or more episodes of rhythmic fetal breathing movements of 30 seconds or more within 30 minutes
3. *Fetal movement:* Three or more discrete body or limb movements within 30 minutes
4. *Fetal tone:* One or more episodes of extension of a fetal extremity with return to flexion, or opening or closing of a hand
5. *Determination of the amniotic fluid volume:* A single deepest vertical pocket >2 cm in two planes perpendicular to each other is considered evidence of adequate amniotic fluid.

Each of the five components is assigned a score of either 2 (present, as previously defined) or 0 (not present). A score of 8 or 10 is normal, a score of 6 is considered

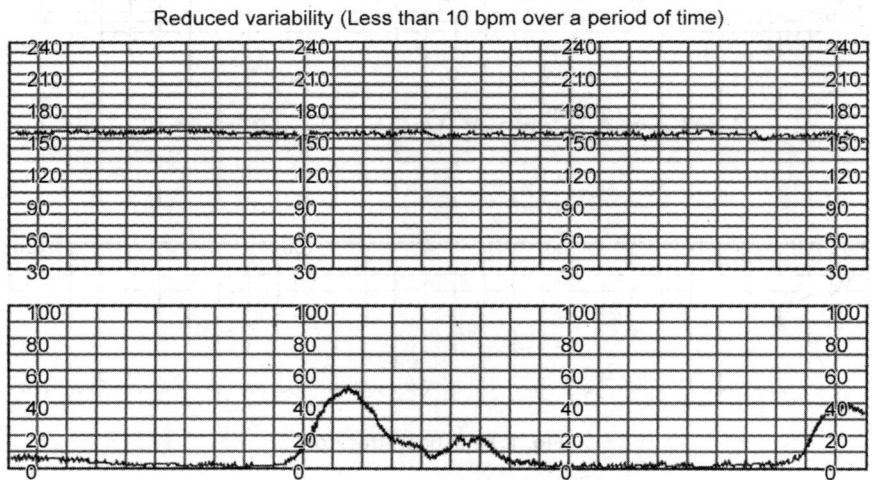

Fig. 2: Reduced baseline variability.

equivocal, and a score of 4 or less is abnormal. Further evaluation should be done in case of oligohydramnios (defined as an amniotic fluid volume of 2 cm or less in the single deepest vertical pocket) regardless of the composite score.

What is modified biophysical profile?
The modified BPP combines the NST with amniotic fluid assessment. NST is a short-term indicator of fetal acid–base status, whereas amniotic fluid volume assessment is an indicator of long-term placental function.

What is the recommended management of abnormal antepartum fetal test?
- Antepartum fetal surveillance tests have high false-positive rates and low positive-predictive values; hence, abnormal tests are usually followed by another test or delivery depending on test results, maternal and fetal condition, and gestational age.
- Decreased fetal movement reported by mother should be evaluated by an NST, CST, BPP, or modified BPP.
- Abnormal NST or a modified BPP should be followed by testing with either a CST or a BPP. A BPP score of 6 out of 10 is considered equivocal and should prompt further evaluation or delivery based on gestational age. If gestational age is at or beyond 37 0/7 weeks, consider delivery. If gestational age is less than 37 0/7 weeks, a repeat BPP in 24 hours.
- A BPP score of 4, delivery is warranted (in pregnancies at less than 32 0/7 weeks of gestation, management should be individualized with extended monitoring). In most circumstances, a BPP score of less than 4 should result in delivery.

How should a finding of oligohydramnios affect the decision for delivery?
In case of uncomplicated isolated and persistent oligohydramnios (deepest vertical pocket measurement <2 cm), delivery at 36–37 weeks of gestation is recommended. If pregnancy is <36 0/7 weeks of gestation with intact membranes and oligohydramnios, the decision for expectant management or delivery should be individualized based on gestational age and the maternal and fetal condition.

What is the role of umbilical artery and other Doppler velocimetry studies?
The main role of Doppler studies is in assessment of growth-restricted fetuses, and currently there is no evidence of its role in fetuses with normal growth.

What are the various methods of intrapartum fetal surveillance?
Intermittent auscultation (IA), CTG, fetal scalp blood sampling—routinely practiced fetal lactate measurement, continuous fetal blood pH monitoring fetal pulse oximetry, and ST waveform analysis are various methods of intrapartum fetal surveillance.

What are the current recommendations for intermittent auscultation?
- Intermittent auscultation is recommended in both low-risk and high-risk pregnancies where the facility for continuous CTG monitoring is not available.
- Intermittent auscultation of the FHR should be offered to low-risk women in established first stage of labor by either stethoscope or Doppler ultrasound. It should be carried out immediately after a contraction for at least 1 minute, at least every 15 minutes in active phase of first stage, and every 5 minutes in second stage of labor. Accelerations and decelerations are recorded, if heard.

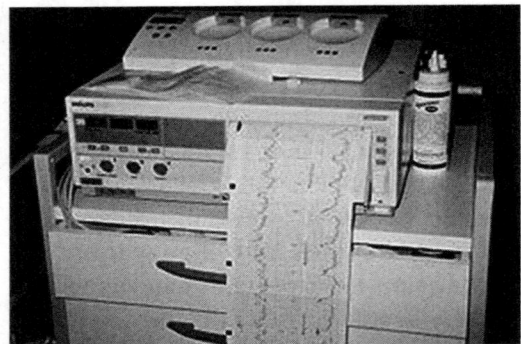

Fig. 3: Cardiotocograph machine.

- Maternal pulse can also be palpated, if a FHR abnormality is suspected, to differentiate between the two heart rates.
- In high-risk pregnancy, continuous CTG monitoring is recommended **(Fig. 3)**.

What are abnormal findings on intermittent auscultation?
- *Baseline FHR:* Below 110 bpm or above 160 bpm
- *Decelerations:* Presence of repetitive or prolonged (>3 minutes) decelerations
- *Contractions:* More than five contractions in a 10-minute period

What should be done if on intermittent auscultation, an increase in the FHR (as plotted on the partogram) of ≥20 bpm from the start of labor, or a deceleration is heard?
- More frequent auscultation (e.g., after 3 consecutive contractions)
- Reassess antepartum, intrapartum risk factors (new and existing), contraction frequency, progress of labor

What should be done if abnormal findings are detected and persist on intermittent auscultation?
Patient should be put on continuous CTG and if there are no nonreassuring or abnormal features on the trace after 20 minutes, remove the CTG and return to IA.

What are the indications for use of cardiotocography?
High-risk pregnancy:
- Postmaturity, suspected fetal growth restriction or macrosomia, oligohydramnios/polyhydramnios, multiple pregnancy, maternal vascular disease, severe hypertension/preeclampsia, antepartum hemorrhage (APH), uterine scar, epidural analgesia, preexisting diabetes mellitus, gestational diabetes requiring medication, hypertensive disorder requiring medication
- Temperature of 38°C or above on a single reading, or 37.5°C or above on two consecutive readings 1 hour apart
- Vaginal blood loss other than a show
- Rupture of membranes >24 hours before the onset of established labor
- Reduced fetal movements in the last 24 hours

Low-risk pregnancy: If any of the following risk factors are present or arise during labor:
- Suspected chorioamnionitis or sepsis, or a temperature of 38°C or above
- Contractions lasting >2 minutes, or ≥5 contractions in 10 minutes
- Fresh vaginal bleeding, blood-stained liquor
- Maternal pulse >120 beats per minute on 2 occasions 30 minutes apart
- Severe hypertension (160/110 mm Hg or above)
- Hypertension [either systolic blood pressure (SBP) of ≥140 mm Hg or diastolic blood pressure (DBP) ≥90 mm Hg on 2 consecutive readings taken 30 minutes apart, measured between contractions] with or without +2 proteinuria
- Oxytocin use
- Delay in first or second stage of labor
- Significant meconium-stained liquor
- Fetal heart rate deceleration on IA

What is the speed of cardiotocography trace?

Recommended scaling factors are 30 bpm per vertical centimeter (30–240 bpm) and at 3 cm/min paper speed. NICE (2022) recommends a speed of 1 cm/min.

What are the features documented while interpreting cardiotocography trace?

- Baseline FHR, baseline variability, presence or absence of decelerations, and presence of accelerations
- To classify the CTG trace, categorize the four features (contractions, baseline FHR, variability, decelerations) as *white, amber, or red* (indicating increasing levels of concern) and use alongside the presence of accelerations.
- *Categorization of contractions:* White—<5 contractions in 10 minutes, *amber*—≥5 contractions in 10 minutes, or hypertonus (contraction lasting for ≥2 minutes)

What is the normal baseline fetal heart rate, tachycardia, and bradycardia?

- *Normal baseline FHR*: White—110–160 bpm
- *Amber*—FHR—100 and 109 bpm with normal baseline variability and no variable or late decelerations [maternal heart rate, postdated pregnancy, hypothermia, beta-blockers, and fetal arrhythmias—atrioventricular (AV) block should be ruled out] or increase in baseline FHR of ≥20 bpm from the start of labor or since the last review an hour ago.
- *Red—tachycardia:* A baseline FHR >160 bpm minutes [*causes*—maternal pyrexia, epidural analgesia, initial stages of nonacute fetal hypoxemia, beta-agonist drugs (salbutamol, ritodrine, terbutaline, etc.), parasympathetic blockers (atropine), fetal arrhythmias (supraventricular tachycardia and atrial fibrillation)]
- *Red—bradycardia:* A baseline FHR <100 bpm

What is variability?

Oscillations in FHR evaluated as average amplitude of signal over 1-minute segment calculated by the difference in beats per minute between the highest FHR and the lowest FHR in a 1-minute segment of the trace between contractions, excluding decelerations and accelerations.

- *White:* 5–25 bpm
- *Amber:* <5 bpm for 30–50 minutes in baseline segment *or* increased variability of >25 bpm for up to 10 minutes
- *Red:* <5 bpm for >50 minutes, or >25 bpm for >10 minutes, or sinusoidal.

How to interpret variability findings on CTG?

- Variability between 5 and 25 bpm is normal.
- Intermittent periods of decreased variability are normal, especially during periods of quiescence ("sleep") or due to opioids
- *Reduced variability:* Assess for intrapartum risk factors and check other CTG findings like baseline FHR
- *Increased variability:* Shorter episodes lasting few minutes may indicate worsening fetal condition.

Define decelerations in fetal heart rate.

Transient episode of slowing of FHR below the baseline of more than 15 bpm for more than 15 seconds is called deceleration.

In a trace with reduced variability, decelerations may be 'shallow', so the above criteria need to be interpreted accordingly.

What is the type of deceleration in Figure 4?
Early deceleration: It is uniform, repetitive, and periodic slowing of FHR with onset early in the contraction and return to baseline at the end of the contraction with normal variability. It is usually benign and caused by head compression.

What is the type of deceleration in the cardiotocography shown in Figure 5?
This CTG shows late decelerations (U-shaped and/or with reduced variability). It is defined as one in which deceleration is gradual with onset to nadir taking 30 seconds and the nadir occurring after the peak of contraction. These are rarely below 30–40 bpm and are not accompanied by accelerations. They indicate chemoreceptor-mediated response to fetal hypoxemia. Late deceleration is associated with low-umbilical artery pH and pO_2 levels. It signifies uteroplacental insufficiency.

What is the cardiotocography in Figure 6 depicting?
It shows variable decelerations—decelerations that exhibit rapid drop (onset to nadir <30 seconds), good variability within decelerations, rapid recovery to baseline, and varying relationship to contractions. They constitute the majority of decelerations during labor. They indicate a baroreceptor-mediated response to increased arterial pressure as seen in umbilical cord compression.

Concerning characteristics in variable decelerations include—lasting more than 60 seconds, reduced variability within the deceleration, failure or slow return to baseline fetal heart rate, and loss of previously present shouldering.

When is variable deceleration nonreassuring?
When variable decelerations drop from baseline by 60 bpm or less and take 60 seconds or less to recover and are present for over

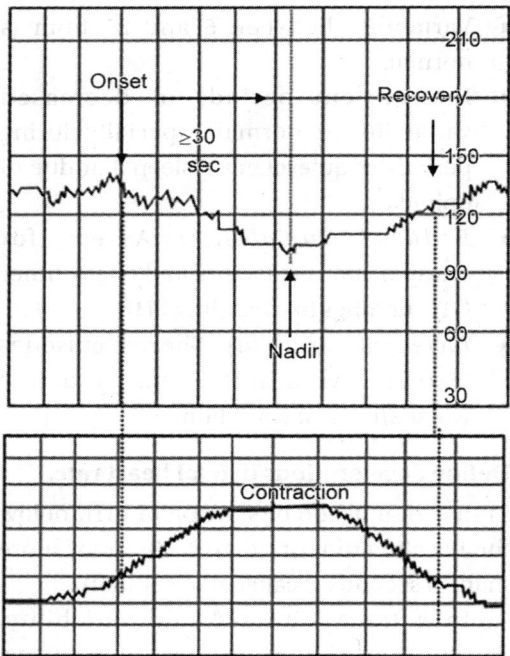

Fig. 4: Fetal heart deceleration (early).

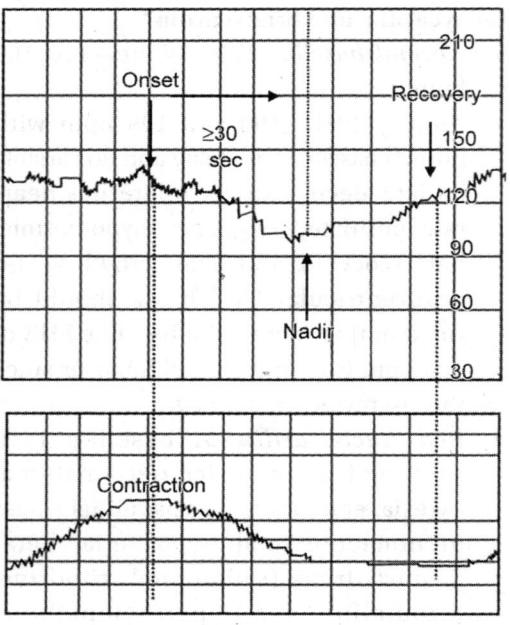

Fig. 5: Fetal heart deceleration (late).

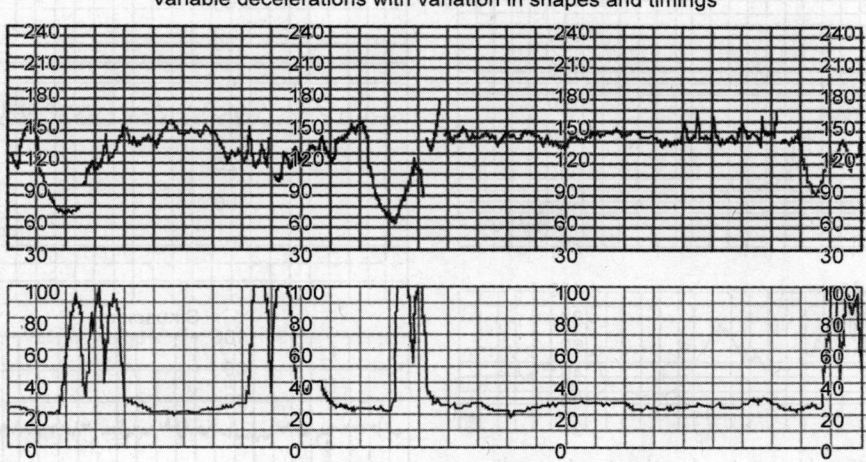

Fig. 6: Fetal heart deceleration (variable).

90 minutes, occurring with over 50% of contractions.

Or

When variable decelerations drop from baseline by more than 60 bpm or take over 60 seconds to recover and are present for up to 30 minutes, occurring with over 50% of contractions.

When is variable deceleration indicative of fetal hypoxia/acidosis?

When nonreassuring variable decelerations are observed even after 30 minutes of starting conservative measures or accompanied by tachycardia (baseline FHR more than 160 bpm) and/or reduced baseline variability (less than 5 bpm).

How do you categorize decelerations according to color?

- *White:* No decelerations, or early decelerations, or variable decelerations that are not evolving to have concerning characteristics.
- *Amber:* Repetitive variable decelerations with any concerning characteristics for <30 minutes, or variable decelerations with any concerning characteristics for >30 minutes, or repetitive late decelerations for <30 minutes.
- *Red:* Repetitive variable decelerations with any concerning characteristics for >30 minutes, or repetitive late decelerations for >30 minutes, or acute bradycardia, or a single prolonged deceleration lasting 3 minutes or more.

Describe the graph given in Figure 7.

This is showing a *prolonged deceleration*, which is an abrupt decrease in FHR to levels below the baseline that lasts 3-minute or longer but less than 10 minutes from onset to return to baseline.

Causes of such a deceleration include:
- Cervical examination
- Uterine hyperactivity
- Cord entanglement
- Maternal supine hypotension
- Maternal hypoxia
- Placental abruption
- Umbilical cord knots or prolapse
- Eclampsia
- Maternal epilepsy
- Application of fetal scalp electrode
- Epidural analgesia

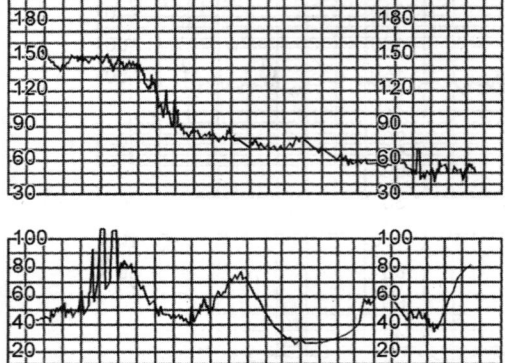

Fig. 7: Fetal heart deceleration (prolonged).

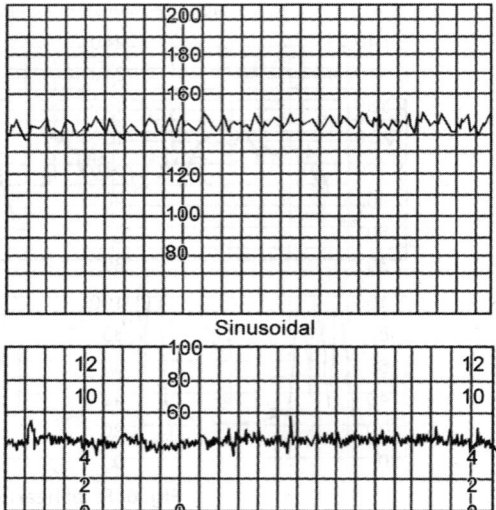

Fig. 8: Sinusoidal fetal heart.

Decelerations lasting more than 5 minutes with FHR maintained at less than 80 bpm with reduced variability indicate acute fetal hypoxia/acidosis and require emergent intervention.

How do you categorize cardiotocography trace based on all characteristics?
- CTG categorization is a tool which quickly communicates the current state of the CTG and should be used together with antenatal and intrapartum risk factors.
- CTG categorization (contractions, baseline, variability, and decelerations)

Normal: No amber or red features (all 4 features are white)

Suspicious: Any 1 feature is amber

Pathological: Any 1 feature is red, or 2 or more features are amber.

How does the interpretation change during second stage of labor?
- Ensure the fetal heart rate is differentiated from the maternal heart rate at least once every 5 minutes.
- If fetal heart rate decelerations are present look for other signs of hypoxia (rise in the baseline FHR or a reduction in variability)
- Onset of hypoxia is both more common and more rapid in the active second stage of labor—an increase in the baseline FHR of ≥20 bpm from the start of labor or since the last review an hour ago is a *red feature in active second stage labor*.
- Consider discouraging pushing and stopping any oxytocin infusion to allow the baby to recover, unless birth is imminent and review.

What is sinusoidal pattern (Fig. 8)?
It is a regular oscillation of the baseline long-term variability resembling a sine wave. This smooth and undulating pattern lasts at least 10 minutes and has a relatively fixed period of 3–5 cycles per minute with an amplitude of 5–15 bpm above and below the baseline. Baseline variability is absent.

What are the causes of sinusoidal pattern?
- Fetal anemia due to Rh-isoimmunization
- Ruptured vasa previa
- Twin-to-twin transfusion syndrome
- Massive fetal hemorrhage from anti-coagulant therapy
- Cordocentesis

- Maternal administration of sedatives and analgesics such as meperidine, pethidine, and butorphanol.

What is pseudosinusoidal pattern?

The intrapartum sine wave-like baseline variation with periods of acceleration is called pseudosinusoidal pattern. In this, the baseline variability is preserved—not flattened. This type of sinusoidal pattern, which alternates with normal fetal heart pattern, does not carry ominous prognosis.

What is the management of nonreassuring cardiotocography (Tables 1 and 2)?

Conservative management of abnormal cardiotocography:
- Check, if the mother had any CNS depressant drug
- Check fetal maturity—baseline tachycardia, reduced baseline variability; poor or absent FM accelerations are sometimes normally exhibited by the fetus under 34 weeks of pregnancy
- Reposition the mother
- Reposition transducer
- Discontinue oxytocin, subcutaneous terbutaline 0.25 mg if hyperstimulation/hypertonus
- Start oxygen inhalation—if maternal hypoxia
- Check maternal pulse—maternal tachycardia may be associated with fetal tachycardia
- Check BP, if hypotensive episode has occurred then tracing abnormality due to this is possible
- Start IV fluids, if patient is hypotensive or dehydrated
- Continue continuous CTG monitoring and analyze the tracing every 10 minutes

TABLE 1: Cardiotocography—classification criteria, interpretation, and recommended management.

	Normal	Suspicious	Pathological
Baseline	110–160 bpm	Lacking at least one characteristic of normality, but with no pathological features	<100 bpm
Variability	5–25 bpm	Same	Variability of <5 beats/min for >50 minutes or variability of >25 beats/min for >10 minutes or sinusoidal pattern
Decelerations	No repetitive decelerations	Same	Repetitive variable decelerations with any concerning characteristics for >30 minutes, repetitive late decelerations for >30 minutes or 1 prolonged deceleration >3 minutes
Interpretation	Fetus with no hypoxia/acidosis	Fetus with a low probability of having hypoxia/acidosis	Fetus with high probability of hypoxia/acidosis
Clinical Mx	No intervention	Action to correct reversible causes. if identified, close monitoring or additional methods to evaluate fetal oxygenation	Immediate action to correct reversible causes, additional methods to evaluate fetal oxygenation, or if this is not possible—expedite delivery

TABLE 2: Recommended management according to NICE, 2022.

Normal	Suspicious	Pathological
• Continue CTG • Continue to perform a full risk assessment at least hourly and document	*No additional intrapartum risk factors* • Perform a full risk assessment • If accelerations are present then fetal acidosis is unlikely • Undertake conservative measures as described *Additional intrapartum risk factors (slow progress, sepsis or meconium)* • Perform a full risk assessment • Look for possible underlying causes • Conservative measures as described • Consider—fetal scalp stimulation or expediting birth	• Exclude acute events (for example, cord prolapse, placental abruption, or uterine rupture) • Perform a full risk assessment • Look for possible underlying causes • Undertake conservative measures as described *If still pathological despite conservative measures* • Evaluate the whole clinical picture and expedite birth *If acute bradycardia, or a single prolonged deceleration for 3 minutes or more:* • Expedite birth simultaneously undertaking conservative measures

(CTG: cardiotocography)

Obstetric reassessment of the case to be done: Whether patient is elderly, diabetic, hypertensive, nephrotic, an assisted reproductive technology (ART) pregnancy, or whether fetus is premature, postdated or growth restricted.

Per-vaginal examination is done to assess progress of labor and prepare for immediate delivery.

How should the recordkeeping of cardiotocography trace be done?

- Date and time clocks on the cardiotocograph monitor are set correctly.
- Label traces with the woman's name, date of birth, hospital number, maternal pulse at the start of CTG, and date of CTG.
- Keep cardiotocograph traces for 25 years and, if possible, store them electronically.
- In cases where there is concern of possible brain injury to baby, photocopy of cardiotocograph traces should be stored indefinitely in case of possible adverse outcomes.

What are the other methods of revalidation in intrapartum situation?

- Vibroacoustic stimulation test (VAST)
- Scalp-stimulation test
- Combining CTG and ST change in fetal electrocardiogram (ECG)
- Pulse oximetry
- Fetal blood sampling (FBS) and instant lactate assay

What is vibroacoustic stimulation test (Fig. 9)?

In this test, an acoustic stimulation to the fetus is given by the use of an artificial larynx placed over maternal abdomen. A normal response is a FHR acceleration of at least 15 bpm for at least 15 seconds occurring within 15 seconds after the stimulation. This test is based on the following observation that: (1) fetal cochlear apparatus gets mature enough to appreciate acoustic stimulation from 28 weeks of gestation and (2) the auditory sensation is one of the first to get affected by hypoxia. The graph in **Figure 9** depicts a reactive VAST test.

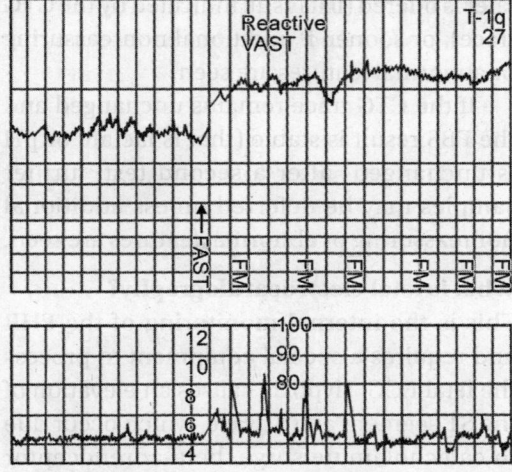

Fig. 9: Fetal acceleration after vibroacoustic stimulation testing.

What is the auditory frequency of acoustic stimulation used in vibroacoustic stimulation test?

The auditory frequency used is 75–85 Hz. It has been found that more fetuses respond to lower frequency acoustic stimulation, for example, 82 Hz than higher frequency of stimulation, for example, 1,000 Hz or more. This is because abdominal wall and uterine wall attenuate significant degrees of external noises of frequencies higher than 1,000 Hz, hence it appears that fetuses do not perceive noises of high frequency and if such quality of stimulus is used, VAST may be negative.

What is the duration of stimulus in vibroacoustic stimulation test?

Acoustic stimulus to be used for a period of 1–3 seconds only. More mature the fetus lesser the duration of stimulus required to elicit qualifying response because of the greater maturity of its cochlear apparatus.

What is a reactive vibroacoustic stimulation test?

Vibroacoustic stimulation test is said to be reactive, if any of the following response is seen:

- Two or more fetal heart acceleration of at least 15 bpm lasting for at least 15 seconds in 10-minute period
- If there occurs at least one acceleration lasting for 60 seconds
- If there occurs sustained acceleration by at least 15 bpm and lasting for at least 3 minutes or more
- If there occurs a series of 2–5 accelerations lasting for 20–60 seconds each

A maternal perception of fetal movement soon after giving the stimulus makes the test even more worthy of labeling as reactive.

Vibroacoustic stimulation is used as a method to exclude fetal sleep in the cases of flat CTG.

What are the factors influencing vibroacoustic stimulation test?

- Thickness of the abdominal wall
- The amount of amniotic fluid
- Pressure exerted by the examiner in holding the stimulator against the abdomen
- The state of the battery of the stimulator

Can vibroacoustic stimulation test be used in preterm fetuses?

In pregnancies less than 36 weeks, VAST gives unusual FHR pattern, which is difficult to interpret, hence this test is not very useful in these cases.

How is fetal blood sampling for pH and lactate done and how are the results interpreted?

In cases of suspicious or pathological CTG, FBS may be used. However, when pathological CTGs indicate a severe and acute event, FBS is not recommended and immediate action should be taken.

The NICE 2022 states that recommendation could not be made due to insufficient evidence. They noted that limited evidence showed that fetal blood sampling does not improve outcomes for women and babies compared with CTG alone, or compared with CTG in combination with fetal scalp stimulation and it may delay expediting birth.

Procedure: Cervical dilation should be at least 3 cm and membranes should be ruptured. The nature and position of the presenting part should be ascertained. An amnioscope (the diameter of which can vary according to cervical dilation) is inserted into the vagina and the lighting equipment is attached. With the amnioscope held tightly in place, the presenting part is dried using small swabs and a thin layer of paraffin is applied to the presenting part, so that blood will form in a large drop and not spread over the skin, thus causing loss of carbon dioxide by diffusion. The incision on the fetal skin should not exceed 2 mm. After a blood drop has formed, it is collected in a heparin-coated capillary and analyzed.

Contraindications: Active genital herpes infection hepatitis B, C, D, E, or to human immunodeficiency virus (HIV) seropositive, suspected fetal blood disorders, uncertainty about the presenting part, or when artificial rupture of membranes is inappropriate.

Results:
Lactate (mmol/L) pH interpretation:

Less than or equal to 4.1	More than or equal to 7.25	Normal
4.2–4.8	7.21–7.24	Intermediate
More than or equal to 4.9	Less than or equal to 7.20	Abnormal

If the fetal blood sample result is normal, repeat sampling no more than 1 hour later is offered (if it is still indicated by the CTG trace), or sooner, if additional nonreassuring or abnormal features are seen.

If the fetal blood sample result is borderline, repeat sampling no more than 30 minutes later is offered (if it is still indicated by the CTG trace), or sooner, if additional nonreassuring or abnormal features are seen.

If the CTG trace remains unchanged and the FBS result is stable (that is lactate or pH is unchanged) after a second test, further samples may be deferred unless additional nonreassuring or abnormal features are seen.

What is fetal electrocardiography?
This is the internal monitoring of the FHR and requires a special equipment to process the fetal ECG. Hypoxia causes an elevation of the ST segment and T wave, which occur due to catecholamine surge, beta-adrenoceptor activation, and myocardial glycogenolysis.

Combined CTG and ST changes are a more specific sign of hypoxia than CTG changes alone and, therefore, this combined modality can significantly reduce cesarean section rates.

What is near-infrared spectroscopy?
It is a noninvasive technique to measure changes in the concentration of oxy-/deoxyhemoglobin in real time. Biologic tissue is relatively transparent to light in the near-infrared region of the spectrum (700–1,000 nm) and this is the basis of spectroscopy. It is possible to transmit near-infrared light through less than 8 cm of tissue and hence spectroscopic information can be obtained.

The changes in fetal cerebral oxygenation during labor have been studied using this technique.

■ SUGGESTED READING
1. Campos D, Arulkumaran S. FIGO consensus guidelines on intrapartum fetal monitoring: Introduction. Int J Gynecol Obstet. 2015;131:3-4.
2. Campos D, Spong C, Chandraharan E; FIGO Intrapartum Fetal Monitoring Expert Consensus Panel. FIGO consensus guidelines on intrapartum fetal monitoring:

Cardiotocography. Int J Gynecol Obstet. 2015;131:13-24.
3. Cunningham F, Leveno K, Bloom S, Hauth J, Rouse D, Spong C. Williams Obstetrics, 23rd edition. New York: The McGraw Hill companies. Inc.; 2010.
4. Lewis D, Downe S. FIGO consensus guidelines on intrapartum fetal monitoring: Intermittent auscultation. Int J Gynecol Obstet. 2015;131:9-12.
5. NICE Guidelines. (2022). Fetal monitoring in Labour (NG 229). [online] Available from https://www.nice.org.uk/guidance/ng229/resources/fetal-monitoring-in-labour-pdf-66143844065221. [Last accessed April, 2024]
6. The American College of Obstetricians and Gynecologists. Practice bulletin no. 145: antepartum fetal surveillance. Obstet Gynecol. 2014;124:182-92.
7. Visser G, Campos D. FIGO consensus guidelines on intrapartum fetal monitoring: adjunctive technologies. Int J Gynecol Obstet. 2015;131:25-9.

5
CHAPTER

Maternal Pelvis and Fetal Skull

Himsweta Srivastava

■ MATERNAL PELVIS

Mention bony landmarks of the pelvic brim.
From anterior to posterior—upper border of symphysis pubis, pubic crest, pubic tubercle, pectineal line, iliopubic eminence, iliopectineal line, sacroiliac articulation, anterior border of the ala of sacrum, and sacral promontory **(Fig. 1)**.

Pelvic brim is the plane of division between the false and true pelvis.

What is inclination of pelvis?
In the erect posture, the pelvis is tilted forward such that the plane of inlet makes an angle of 55° with the horizontal and is called angle of inclination of pelvis.

What is high inclination?
High inclination is said to occur when the angle of inclination is increased due to sacralization of 5th lumbar vertebra. It is obstetrically significant because (1) it causes delay in engagement as the uterine axis fails to coincide with that of inlet, (2) it favors occipitoposterior position, and (3) there is delay in descent of head due to long birth canal and flat sacrum.

What is axis of pelvic brim?
The axis of the brim is represented by an imaginary straight line drawn perpendicular to the plane of the brim at its center. This line when extrapolated upward will pass from umbilicus and downward, it will reach up to the coccyx **(Fig. 1)**.

What are the various diameters of the pelvic inlet?
The true conjugate or anteroposterior diameter is measured from the center of the sacral promontory behind to the inner margin of the upper border of the symphysis pubis in front. It measures 11.0 cm.

The two oblique diameters are measured from the sacroiliac articulation behind to the iliopectineal eminence on the opposite side

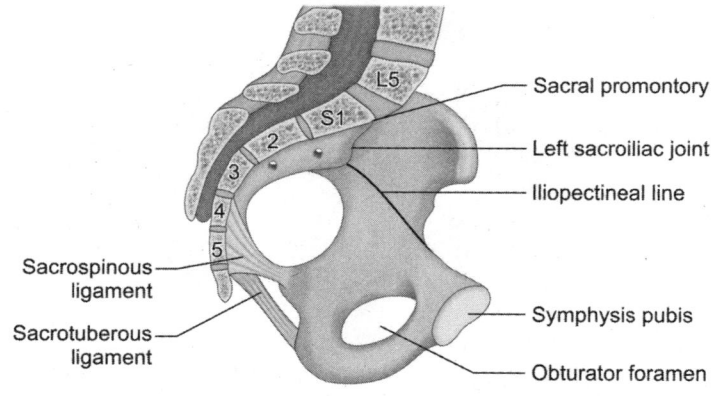

Fig. 1: Pelvic brim.

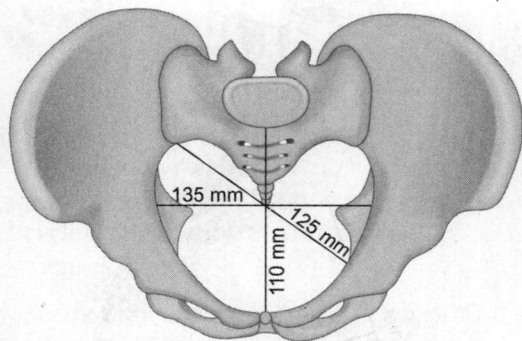

Fig. 2: Diameters of pelvic inlet.

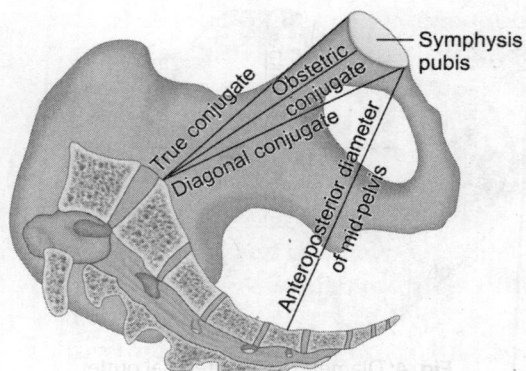

Fig. 3: Diagonal conjugate.

in front, the right oblique diameter being measured from the right sacroiliac joint. It measures 11.8 cm.

Transverse diameter is the distance between the two furthest points on the pelvic brim. It is 12.8 cm **(Fig. 2)**.

What is obstetric conjugate?
Obstetric conjugate is the distance between the midpoints of the sacral promontory and prominent bony projection in the midline on the inner surface of the pubic symphysis. It is the shortest anteroposterior diameter in the anteroposterior plane of inlet. It measures 10 cm.

What is diagonal conjugate and its significance?
Diagonal conjugate is measured clinically during pelvic assessment. It is the distance between the lower border of symphysis pubis and the midpoint on the sacral promontory; it measures 12 cm. Obstetric conjugate is computed by subtracting 1.5–2.0 cm from the diagonal conjugate depending on the width and inclination of pubic symphysis **(Fig. 3)**.

What is obstetrical outlet?
Obstetrical outlet is a segment of the pelvis bounded above by the plane of the least pelvic dimensions and below by the anatomical outlet.

Describe the boundaries of plane of least pelvic dimension or narrow pelvic plane.
This plane is bounded anteriorly by the lower border of the symphysis pubis, laterally by the tip of ischial spines, and posteriorly by the lower border of the last sacral vertebra. It is the narrowest plane in the pelvis, and the distance between the ischial spines is the shortest diameter of the normal pelvis and measures 10.7 cm. This narrow pelvic plane represents the plane of the outlet.

What is the anatomic significance of narrow pelvic plane in obstetrics?
- It marks the beginning of the forward curve of the pelvic axis.
- It corresponds to the origin of the levator ani muscles.
- It is the level where the completion of internal rotation of the head occurs (or the level of arrest when rotation does not occur).
- The ischial spines are easily felt on vaginal examination, and the interischial diameter (IID) is useful for determining the degree of descent of the fetal head into the pelvis. (If the head reaches IID, it is certain that it has engaged except in excessive molding or face presentation.)
- It is a landmark for pudendal nerve block analgesia.

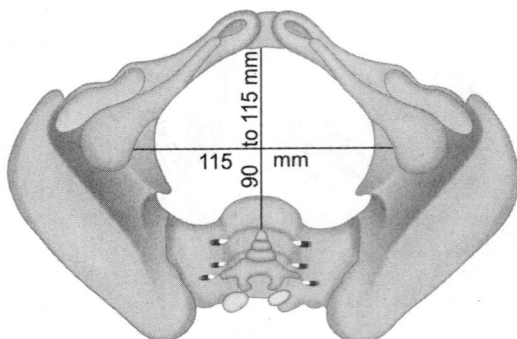

Fig. 4: Diameters of obstetrical outlet.

Describe anatomical outlet.
Anatomical outlet is bounded in front by the lower border of the symphysis pubis; laterally by the ischiopubic rami, ischial tuberosity, and sacrotuberous ligament; and posteriorly by the tip of coccyx. Hence, it consists of two triangular planes with a common base formed by a line joining the ischial tuberosities.

What are the various diameters of obstetrical outlet?
- *Bispinous diameter:* 10.7 cm
- *Intertuberous diameter:* 12.5 cm
- *Anteroposterior diameter:* 11 cm **(Fig. 4)**.

Describe cavity of the pelvis. What is its diameter?
Cavity of the pelvis is the segment of the pelvis bounded above by the inlet and below by the plane of least pelvic dimensions. It forms a curved canal with a shallow anterior (3.75 cm) and a deep posterior wall (11.25 cm), the lateral wall of the cavity being 7.5 cm deep.

Diameters of cavity
Anteroposterior diameter: 12 cm
Transverse diameter: 12 cm approximately (due to the presence of soft tissues over sacrosciatic notch).

What is the plane of the cavity?
Plane of the cavity is bounded in front by the center of the symphysis pubis and behind

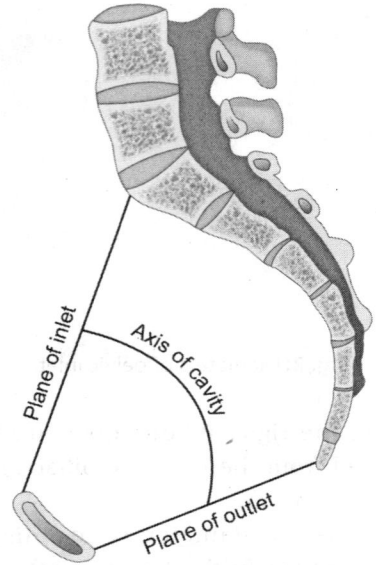

Fig. 5: Curve of Carus

by the junction of the sacral 2nd and 3rd vertebrae. It is the plane of the widest pelvic dimension.

What is the difference between anatomical pelvic axis (curve of Carus) and obstetrical pelvic axis (Fig. 5)?
Anatomical pelvic axis is formed by joining the axes of inlet, cavity, and outlet. It is uniformly curved with the convexity fitting with the concavity of the sacrum.

But as the pelvic cavity is almost cylindrical in shape in its upper 3/4th, the head descends in the axis of the pelvic inlet until near the level of the ischial spines and then it begins to curve forward near the plane of the pelvic outlet. The axis through which the fetus negotiates the pelvis is called the obstetrical axis of pelvis. So the obstetrical axis is directed first downward and backward up to the level of ischial spines and then directed abruptly forward.

What is Caldwell–Moloy classification?
Caldwell–Moloy developed a classification of the anatomical variation of pelvis.

This classification is based on measurement of the greatest transverse diameter of the inlet and its division into anterior and posterior segments, thus determining the shape of the inlet. Besides this, the classification is also based on the width of the sacrosciatic notch and the size of the subpubic angle. According to this classification, pelvis is divided into four types, namely *gynecoid, anthropoid, android,* and *platypelloid*.

Describe the four types of pelvis depending upon the shape of inlet.
1. *Gynecoid:* The posterior segment and anterior segment are almost equal and spacious, and the inlet is almost round. This type is seen in 50% of females.
2. *Android:* The posterior sagittal segment is much shorter than the anterior sagittal diameter limiting the use of the posterior space by the fetal head. Also, the anterior segment is narrow and triangular. This type carries poor prognosis for vaginal delivery.
3. *Anthropoid:* The anteroposterior diameter is greater than the transverse. This results in an oval anteroposterior pelvis with a narrow and pointed anterior segment. It is found in 1/3rd of women. It is also referred to as *transversely contracted pelvis*. Direct occipitoanterior or occipitoposterior positions of the head are common.
4. *Platypelloid:* It has a flattened gynecoid shape with short anteroposterior and wide transverse diameter. It also corresponds to the *flat pelvis*. It favors engagement of the fetal head in transverse diameter (Fig. 6).

Does change in maternal position during labor from supine to squatting or chest-knee position have any effect on pelvic outlet?
Based on magnetic resonance examinations, it has been seen that chest-knee or squatting position causes significant increase of interspinal and intertuberous diameters compared to the supine position during labor.

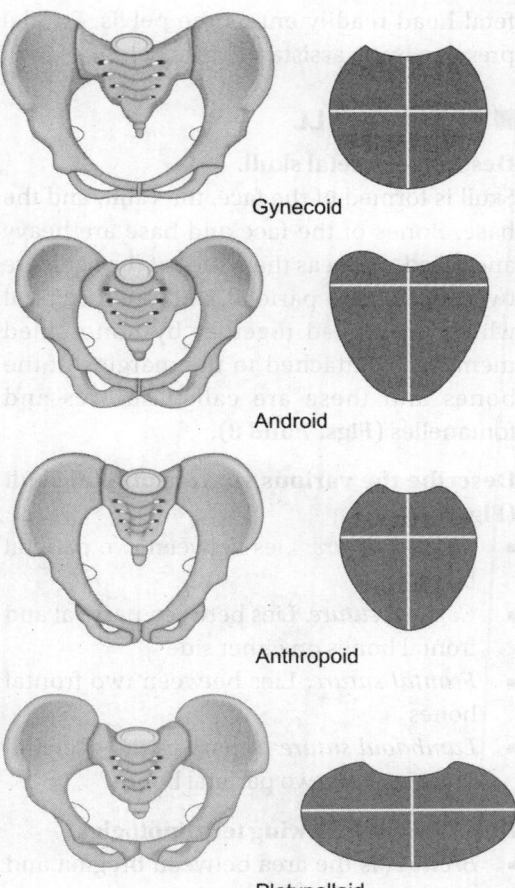

Fig. 6: Types of pelvis.

Describe Mueller–Hillis maneuver.
Mueller–Hillis maneuver is a clinical maneuver to predict disproportion. In an occiput presentation, the fetal brow and the suboccipital region are grasped through the abdominal wall with the fingers and firm pressure is directed downward in the axis of the inlet. During concomitant vaginal examination, a flexed fetal head that overrides the symphysis pubis is clear evidence of disproportion. If no disproportion exists, the

fetal head readily enters the pelvis. Fundal pressure by an assistant is also helpful.

FETAL SKULL

Describe the fetal skull.

Skull is formed of the face, the vault, and the base. Bones of the face and base are heavy and fused, whereas the bones of the vault are two frontal, two parietal, and one occipital which are united together by nonossified membranes attached to the margins of the bones and these are called sutures and fontanelles **(Figs. 7 and 8)**.

Describe the various sutures of fetal skull (Fig. 9).
- *Sagittal suture:* Lies between two parietal bones
- *Coronal suture:* Lies between parietal and frontal bones on either side
- *Frontal suture:* Lies between two frontal bones
- *Lambdoid suture:* Separates the occipital bone and the two parietal bones.

Describe the following terminologies.
- *Brow:* It is the area between bregma and root of the nose.
- *Face:* It is the area between the root of the nose and supraorbital ridge on one side and by the junction of the floor of the mouth with neck on the other side.
- *Vertex:* It is a quadrangular area bounded anteriorly by the bregma and coronal sutures, behind by the lambda and lambdoid sutures, and laterally by a line passing through the parietal eminences.
- *Sinciput:* It is the area lying in front of the anterior fontanelle and corresponds to the area of the brow.
- *Occiput:* It is the area limited to the occipital bone.

Describe the two fontanelles.

Fontanelle is a wide gap in the suture line.

Anterior fontanelle (bregma): It is formed by joining of the four sutures: Frontal (anteriorly), sagittal (posteriorly), and coronal on either side. It is diamond shaped and measures 3 cm × 2 cm. It gets ossified 18 months after birth.

Posterior fontanelle (lambda): It is formed by junction of three suture lines: Sagittal suture anteriorly and lambdoid suture on either side. It is triangular in shape and measures 1.2 cm × 1.2 cm. It becomes bony at term.

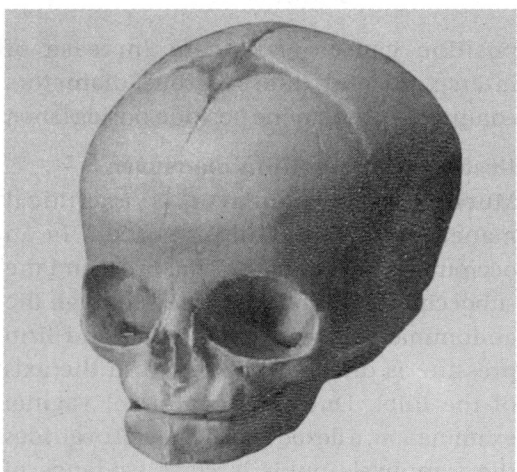

Fig. 7: Fetal skull.

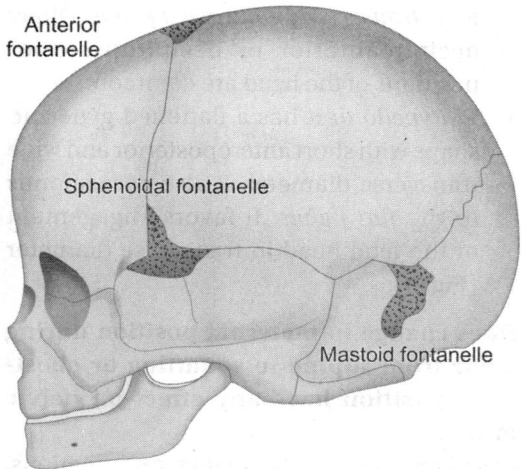

Fig. 8: Fontanelles.

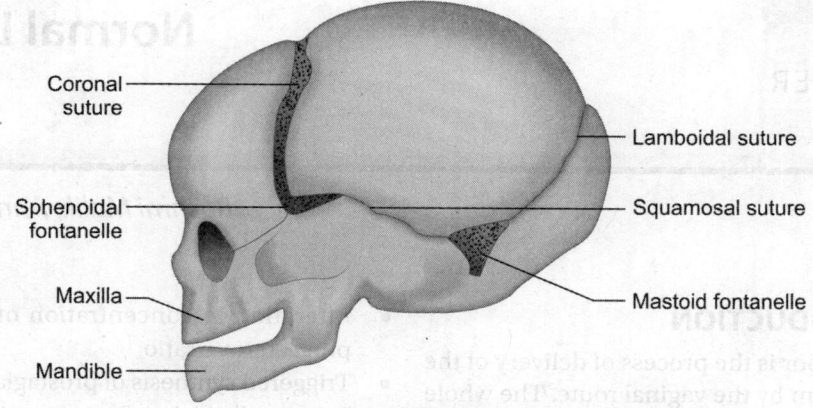

Fig. 9: Sutures of fetal skull.

TABLE 1: Various diameters of the fetal skull.		
Diameter		*Presentation*
Suboccipitobregmatic—extends from the nape of the neck to the centers of the bregma	9.4 cm (3¾″)	Vertex (complete flexion)
Suboccipitofrontal—from the nape of neck to the anterior end of the anterior fontanelle or center of the sinciput	10.0 cm (4″)	Vertex (incomplete flexion)
Occipitofrontal—extends from the occipital eminence to the root of the nose (glabella)	11.3 cm (4½″)	Vertex (marked deflexion)
Mentovertical—extends from the midpoint of the chin to the highest point on the sagittal suture	13.8 cm (5½″)	Brow (partial extension)
Submentovertical—extends from junction of floor of the mouth and neck to the highest point on the sagittal suture	11.3 cm (4½″)	Face (incomplete extension)
Submentobregmatic—extends from junction of floor of the mouth and neck to the center of the bregma	9.4 cm (3¾″)	Face (complete extension)

What is the obstetric importance of anterior fontanelle?
- If it is palpated during internal examination, it denotes deflexion of head.
- It facilitates molding of the head.
- Since it ossifies long after birth, it helps in accommodating brain growth.

What are the various diameters of the fetal skull?
The various diameters of the fetal skull are shown in **Table 1**.

What is molding of the head?
Molding of the head is alteration of the shape of the forecoming head while passing through the resistant birth passage during labor.

It is of three grades:
- *Grade 1:* Suture lines touch but do not overlap.
- *Grade 2:* Suture lines overlap but are easily separated by examining fingers.
- *Grade 3:* Fixed overlapping of suture lines

CHAPTER 6

Normal Labor

Rashmi Malik, Annu Kumari

■ INTRODUCTION

Normal labor is the process of delivery of the fetus at term by the vaginal route. The whole process consists of four stages and involves cervical changes (dilatation and effacement), descent of fetal head, and rotation resulting in final delivery of the baby followed by delivery of the placenta and membranes. It is important to have complete knowledge of the mechanism and conduct of normal labor as complications can arise at any stage and normal labor may become abnormal.

■ NORMAL LABOR

What is normal labor?

Normal labor is defined as:
- Spontaneous in onset
- With vertex presentation
- Unaided (without the help of forceps/ventouse)
- Completed within a period of 24 hours
- With vaginal delivery of full-term live births (37–40 weeks)
- Without any complication to the mother and fetus

What percentage of patients delivers on expected date of delivery?

Only 4% of pregnant women deliver on the given expected date of delivery (EDD). 80% deliver 2 weeks earlier or 1 week later.

What are the theories of initiation of labor?

Proposed theories are:
- Fetoplacental contribution—accelerated production of estrogen and prostaglandin
- Alteration in concentration of estrogen: progesterone ratio
- Triggered synthesis of prostaglandins
- Increased activity of receptors in uterus

How will you differentiate between true and false labor pains?

Differentiation between true and false labor pains has been described in **Table 1**.

TABLE 1: True and false labor pains.	
False labor	**True labor**
Discomfort especially in lower abdomen and groin	Discomfort starting in the back and sweeping around the abdomen
Contractions occur at irregular intervals	Contractions occur at regular intervals
No increase in frequency and intensity or duration of contractions	Progressive increase in frequency, intensity, and duration of contractions
Interval between contractions remains long	Interval between contractions gradually shortens
No or little change in cervix	Progressive cervical dilatation and effacement
Pain does not coincide with uterine contractions	Pain coincides with uterine contractions
Emptying of bowel may lead to relief of symptoms	Emptying of bowel does not lead to relief of symptoms but contractions may be augmented

What are the stages of labor?

Labor is conventionally divided into four stages of labor:

First stage: The first stage of labor is the stage of cervical dilatation. With the establishment of true labor pains, the first stage of labor starts and during this stage the cervix progressively dilates to 10 cm, i.e., full dilatation (end of first stage). It is further divided into latent phase and active phase. During latent phase, there is some effacement and slow cervical dilatation. The contractions are weak (<2 per 10 minutes). The active phase is characterized by painful contractions of increasing frequency, intensity, and duration accompanied by a rapid rate of cervical change (usually >1 cm/hour). During this phase, the descent of the presenting part also occurs. The earlier active phase was presumed to begin when the cervix has reached 3–4 cm dilatation. But evidence suggests that actually labor progresses at a much slower pace in many women, and the World Health Organization (WHO) has now recommended that active labor starts at 5 cm and the progression may be slower than 1 cm/hour in many cases. New definitions have been given so as to avoid unnecessary interventions (Labour Care Guide, WHO 2020). There is no defined limit of latent phase, and it may vary between women. The active phase generally does not exceed 12 hours in primigravidas and 10 hours in multigravidas.

Second stage: The second stage begins with full dilatation of cervix till delivery of baby. The onset of second stage is characterized by:
- Full cervical dilatation
- Bulging thinned-out perineum
- Gaping anus and vagina
- Head visible at the perineum

Third stage: The third stage starts after delivery of the baby till delivery of the placenta and membranes.

Fourth stage: The fourth stage is the period of observation for 1–2 hours after delivery. During this period, complications like postpartum hemorrhage (PPH) can occur. During this period, the parturient should be closely observed every 15 minutes for pulse, blood pressure (BP), size of the uterus and tone, and perineum for bleeding or swelling.

Define fetal lie.

Fetal lie is the relation between the longitudinal axis of the fetal ovoid and the longitudinal axis of the uterus.
- Longitudinal—95.5%
- Transverse
- Oblique—0.5%
- Unstable

What is meant by fetal presentation?

Fetal presentation is the part of the fetus that lies in the lower pole of the uterus. The presenting part enters first in the pelvis when labor begins **(Table 2)**.

Define fetal position.

Fetal position is the relation of an arbitrarily chosen point of the fetal presenting part in relation to the four quadrants of the maternal pelvis.
- Left occipitotransverse (LOT)—40%
- Right occipitotransverse (ROT)—24%
- Left occipitoanterior (LOA)—13%
- Right occipitoanterior (ROA)—10%
- Right occipitoposterior (ROP)—7.1%

TABLE 2: Fetal presentation.

Presentation	Percentage (%)	Incidence
Cephalic	96.8	–
Breech	2.7	1 in 36
Transverse	0.3	1 in 335
Compound	0.1	1 in 1,000
Face	0.05	1 in 2,000
Brow	0.01	1 in 10,000

What is meant by engagement?
Engagement is the mechanism by which the greatest transverse diameter of the fetal head and biparietal diameter (9.4 cm) is at or has passed the pelvic inlet (brim). In a vertex presentation, when engagement occurs, the lower-most portion of the vertex would be at the level of ischial spines.

How does descent occur in normal labor?
The mechanisms causing descent are:
- Intrauterine fluid pressure
- Uterine contractions and downward pressure of the fundus on the breech (fetal axis pressure)
- Bearing-down efforts of the abdominal muscles
- Extension and straightening of the fetal body

How do you assess the descent of head during labor?
Descent of the head can be assessed by both abdominal and vaginal examinations.

Abdominal examination (fifth's formula): In this method, the number of fifths of fetal head above the pelvic brim is estimated. And this is done by the number of fingers that can be placed over the fetal head palpable above pubic symphysis. A free-floating head will be completely above the pelvic brim and will be 5/5 palpable. When the head engages in the pelvis, i.e., biparietal diameter enters the pelvic brim, 2/5th of the head is palpable abdominally (**Figs. 1A to D**).

Vaginal examination: To determine descent vaginally, the position of the leading-most part is assessed in relation to the plane of ischial spines (**Figs. 2A and B**).

When the leading-most part is at the level of ischial spines, this is zero station and if it is above it, it is represented in minus values and if it is below the level of ischial spines, it is labeled as plus value varying from 0 to –5 and 0 to +5, respectively. The numerical value is the distance from the level of ischial spines in centimeters.

What are the prerequisites for adequate rotation?
- Well-flexed head
- Efficient uterine contraction
- Favorable shape at the midpelvis

How do you assess normal pelvis on pelvic assessment?
Pelvic assessment is done with the patient lying in dorsal position with buttocks on the edge of the examination table. The bladder should be emptied before examination. With sterile precautions, vaginal examination is done. First, we try to reach the sacral promontory. In a normal gynecoid pelvis, it

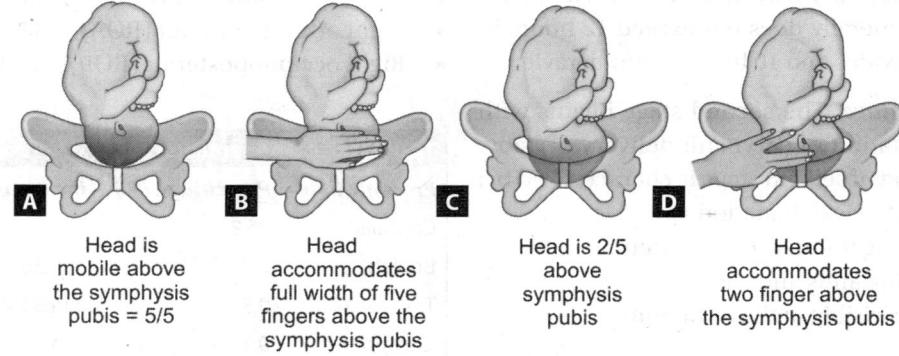

A	B	C	D
Head is mobile above the symphysis pubis = 5/5	Head accommodates full width of five fingers above the symphysis pubis	Head is 2/5 above symphysis pubis	Head accommodates two finger above the symphysis pubis

Figs. 1A to D: Fifth's method of assessing descent of fetal head.

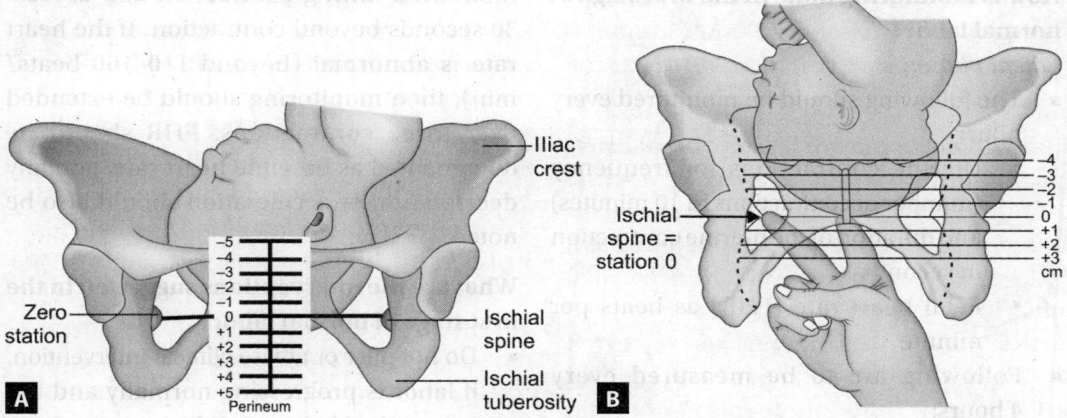

Figs. 2A and B: Assessment of fetal descent on vaginal examination.

is not reachable with the middle finger. If it is reached, then a point is marked on the gloved hand at the entry in pubic arch. This will later help in measuring the diagonal conjugate and later calculating the true conjugate from it.

Then fingers are moved down and sideways on the sacrum. The normal pelvis has well-curved sacrum and coccyx is movable. Then moving laterally side walls are checked, which are well curved. Ischial spines are not very prominent or long in normal pelvis and the interischial diameter is determined by spreading the two fingers sideways and positioning one each on each ischial spine. In normal situations, it is not possible to feel both ischial spines at the same time. Sacrosciatic notches are wide and accommodate two fingers. Then the posterior surface of the pubic symphysis is palpated to see if it is well curved and smooth or not. Now, the subpubic angle is checked, and it should accommodate two fingers easily. Lastly, the outlet is checked by keeping the fist between ischial tuberosities (transverse diameter of the outlet). It easily accommodates four knuckles in a normal pelvis.

Routine pelvimetry at admission is not recommended in healthy pregnant women.

What is the role of admission test?
Admission test is a short cardiotocography record taken on admission in labor. It mimics contraction stress test utilizing the spontaneous contractions and acting as a screening test to predict the increased risk of intrapartum hypoxia. The evidence does not support the policy of admission test in low-risk cases as the sensitivity of test is low and false positives are high.

What is respectful maternity care as recommended by WHO?
The World Health Organization (WHO) recommends that all women should receive respectful maternity care during labor and delivery. The services should be provided maintaining their respect, dignity, and confidentiality. There should not be any harm or mistreatment. Continuous support should be provided during labor and women should be involved in all decisions by the process of informed choices.

How is monitoring done in the first stage of normal labor?

Latent phase:
- The following should be monitored every hour:
  - Uterine contractions for frequency (number of contractions in 10 minutes) and duration of the uterine contraction in seconds
  - Fetal heart rate (FHR) as beats per minute
- Following are to be measured every 4 hours:
  - Pulse, BP, and temperature.
- If membranes rupture during the latent phase, the time of rupture should be recorded and color of the liquor should be checked to rule out any abnormality like meconium or blood staining. At the time of rupture of membranes, fetal heart should be auscultated and pelvic examinations should also be done to rule out any cord prolapse.

Active phase
- Monitor the following every 30 minutes:
  - Maternal pulse, uterine contractions, and FHR
  - Look for presence of meconium or blood-stained liquor or cord prolapse.
- Monitor the following every 4 hours:
  - Temperature and BP
  - *Vaginal examination:* Cervical dilatation (in cm) and descent of fetal head

How is fetal heart rate monitoring done in the active phase of labor?

Fetal heart rate should be monitored by intermittent auscultation every 15–30 minutes in active labor and every 5 minutes in the second stage. The heart rate should be counted for at least 1 minute. It should be monitored during contraction and at least 30 seconds beyond contraction. If the heart rate is abnormal (beyond 110–160 beats/min), then monitoring should be extended over three contractions. FHR should be documented as baseline heart rate, and any deceleration or acceleration should also be noted.

What are the interventions suggested in the first stage of normal labor?

- Do not offer or advise clinical intervention, if labor is progressing normally and the woman and baby are well.
- Inform women about the length of first stage (*primi*: average 8 hours and rarely beyond 18 hours; *multi*: average 5 hours and rarely beyond 12 hours). Also inform that the exact limits of latent phase have not been established and may vary widely.
- No need for active management routinely
- No need for routine amniotomy
- Early amniotomy with oxytocin augmentation should not be routinely used.

What supportive care is recommended during labor?

An important component of respectful maternity care is providing supportive care during labor. There are four components:
1. *Birth companion:* Ideally, a companion of woman's choice should be with her during labor.
2. *Pain relief:* Pain relief of her choice including medical and nonpharmacological measures should be given.
3. *Oral fluids and food intake* is recommended in low-risk women during labor.
4. *Position:* She should be encouraged to be mobile or be in upright position as per her choice during the first stage.

What pain relief choices a woman can be given during labor?
A woman during labor can opt for any of the following for pain relief methods:
- Epidural analgesia
- *Parenteral opioids:* Fentanyl, pethidine, or diamorphine
- Nonpharmacological measures including relaxation techniques focusing on guided muscle relaxation, breathing exercises, music therapy, mindfulness, etc.
- Manual methods like massage or warm packs application

How is prelabor rupture of membranes (PROM) managed at term pregnancy?
Prelabor rupture of membranes (PROM) is defined as rupture of membranes more than 1 hour before the onset of labor. If a woman at term presents with PROM, the following should be done:
- Sterile per speculum examination for confirmation
- No digital examination in absence of contractions
- Assess fetal movements and FHR
- *Counseling:*
  - The risk of serious neonatal infection is 1%, rather than 0.5% for women with intact membranes.
  - 60% of women with PROM will go into labor within 24 hours.
- Induction of labor, if spontaneous contractions do not start in 24 hours
- Temperature charting 4 hourly
- No need of C-reactive protein (CRP) and vaginal swab culture

What is a partograph?
A partograph is a tool for the management of labor. It is a printed graph representing the stages of labor on which a record of all observations and interventions is plotted. The normal progress in active labor is assessed by the descent of the fetus, the dilatation of the cervix, FHR, the color of the amniotic fluid, the presence of molding, the pattern of uterine contractions, the general condition of the mother, and the medications that have been given to the mother (**Fig. 3**).

What is alert line?
Alert line is a predrawn line on the partograph, starting at 3 cm dilatation with a slope of 1 cm dilatation/hour. This is the minimum rate of cervical dilatation in normal labor. If the cervical dilatation graph shifts to the right of alert line, one has to become alert and re-evaluate the patient for the possible causes of slow dilatation like cephalopelvic disproportion (CPD), hypotonic uterine contractions, etc. This line is mainly for the smaller peripheral health centers, where emergency obstetric services like cesarean section facilities are not available. If the graph shifts to the right of alert line at such centers, laboring woman should be shifted to the higher center.

What is action line?
The action line is a predrawn line on the partograph, drawn parallel and 4 hours to the right of alert line. When the graph shifts to the right of the action line, some action has to be taken like augmentation with oxytocin or cesarean section.

What are the principles of a WHO partograph?
Principles on which a WHO partograph is based are as follows:
- The duration of the latent phase should not be more than 8 hours. If after 8 hours the patient is still in labor but has not entered the active phase, assessment and interventions are required.
- After 3 cm dilatation, labor enters into active phase.

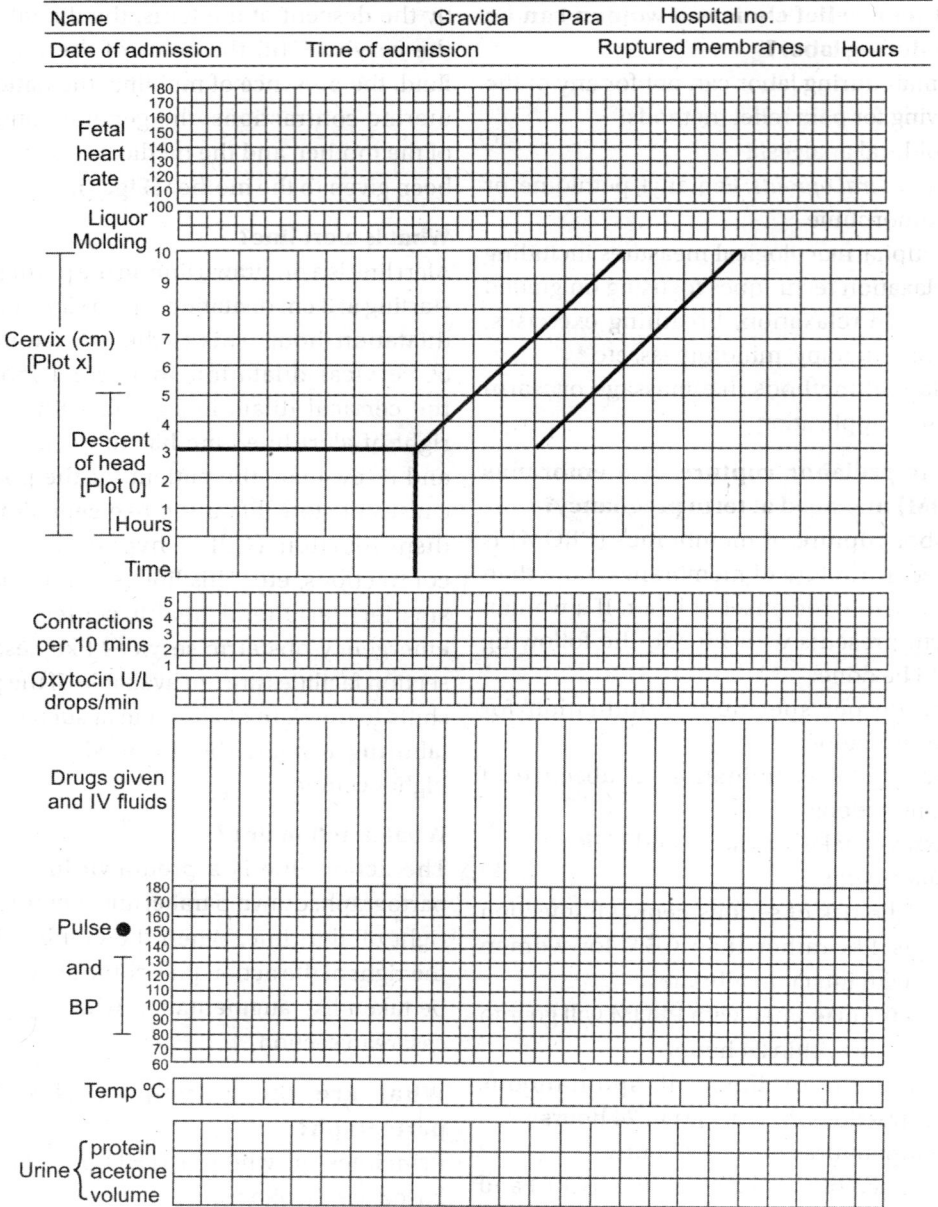

Fig. 3: Partograph.

- During active phase, the minimum dilatation rate should be 1 cm/hour. If there is lag, one should become alert. That is why an alert line is drawn as a slope of 1 cm/hour.
- The action line is 4 hours on the right of the alert line. This is based on the observation that a lag period of 4 hours between intervention and slowing of labor (alert) does not compromise the outcome.

This gives time for shifting of patient at the periphery also and avoids unnecessary intervention.

There is no need to perform vaginal examination more frequently than every 4 hours, unless indicated otherwise.
- Using a partograph with preset alert and action lines is more useful.

What is a modified WHO partograph?
The WHO partograph has been modified to make it simple and easy to be used by skilled birth attendants **(Fig. 4)**. In this modification, latent phase recording has been removed. Recording on a partograph is started when a laboring woman has a cervical dilatation of 4 cm.

What abnormal labor patterns can you diagnose with the help of a partograph?
Three main labor patterns can be seen:
1. Prolonged disorders
2. Protraction disorders
3. Arrest disorders

What is the labor diagnosis in partograph given in Figure 5?
This partograph shows *normal labor* as documented by:
- Normal FHR
- Clear liquor
- Cervical dilatation line has remained toward left of alert line
- Progressive descent of fetal head
- No augmentation
- Maternal condition as documented by pulse rate, BP, urine output, and temperature remained normal.
- Hypotonic uterine contractions

What is the cause of prolonged active phase in partograph given in Figure 6?

What is the labor abnormality in the partograph given in Figure 7?
This partograph shows features suggestive of *obstructed labor* **(Fig. 7)**.
- Cervical dilatation line shifting to the right
- No descent of fetal head in active phase
- Good uterine contractions
- Increasing molding of head
- Progressive deterioration of fetal condition as suggested by meconium-stained liquor and fetal bradycardia

What is Labor Care Guide (Fig. 8)?
The WHO has now recommended Labor Care Guide (LCG) for care of women in labor. It includes all assessment and documentation related to maternal and fetal monitoring during labor. Though primarily designed for low-risk labors, it is now recommended for all women irrespective of risk status. Documentation on LCG is to be initiated when cervical dilatation is 5 cm or more (as per definition of active phase, WHO 2020). It has seven sections:
1. Patient identification and general information including labor information
2. Supportive care
3. Care of the baby
4. Care of the woman
5. Labor progress
6. Medication
7. Shared decision-making

For sections 2–7, observations are documented after monitoring.

There is an alert column in which thresholds for abnormal values are given. If observations fall in that, further assessment and actions are to be taken by the healthcare provider.

What are similarities between Labor Care Guide and partograph?
Both are graphic representation of progress of labor, i.e., cervical dilatation and descent of head with time during the active phase of labor.

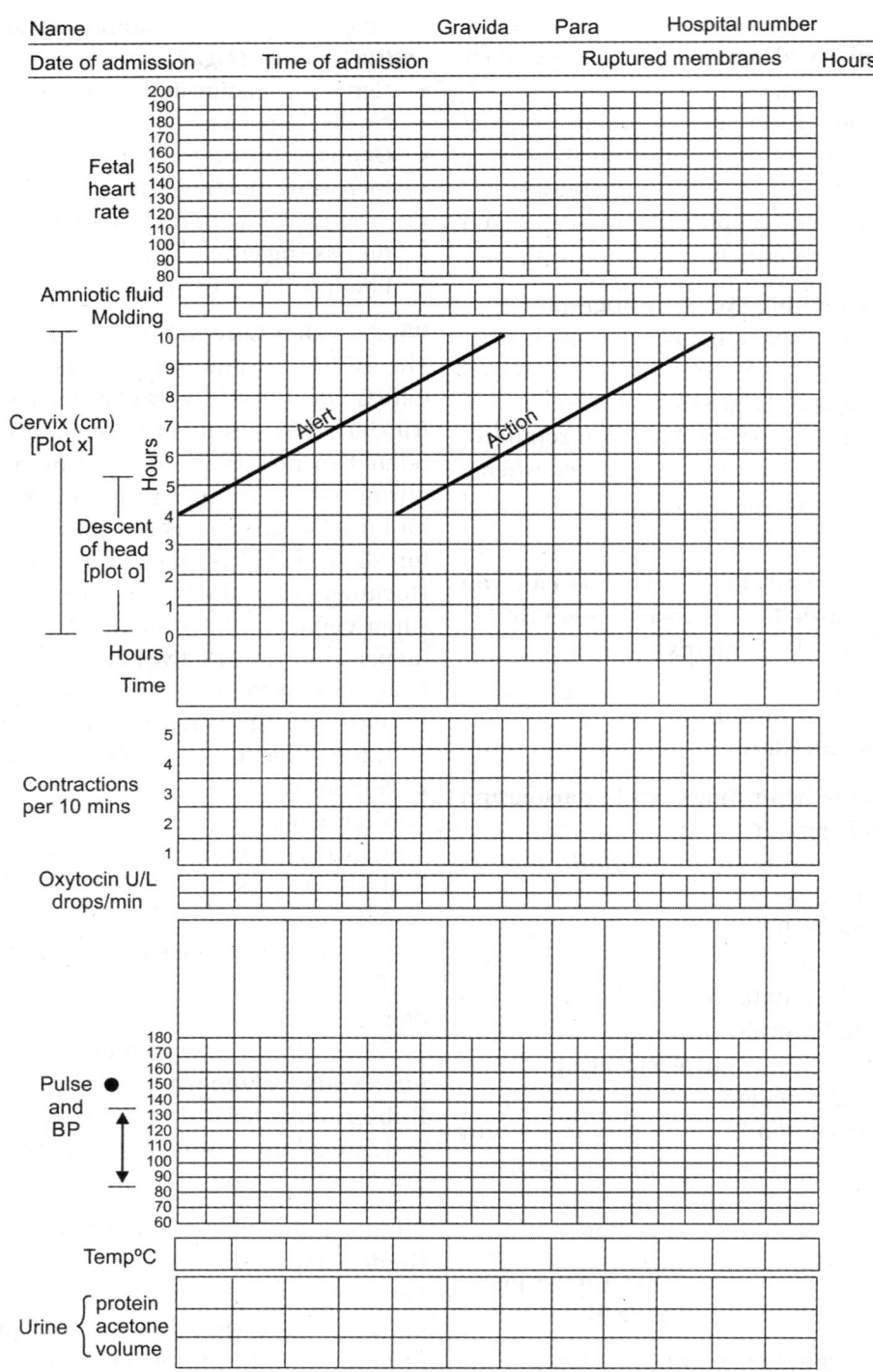

Fig. 4: Modified World Health Organization partograph.

Fig. 5: Partograph depicting normal labor.

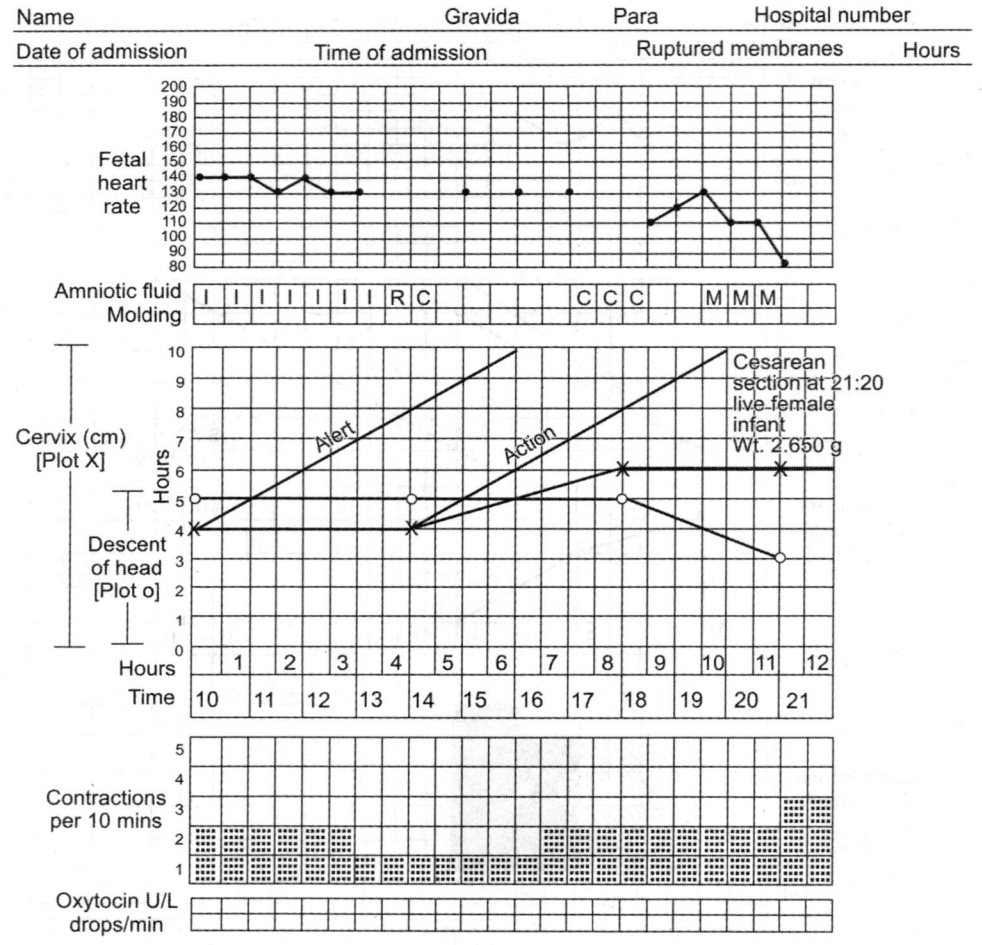

Fig. 6: Partograph showing prolonged active phase of labor.

Both provide for documentation of parameters for maternal and fetal well-being during labor.

How does Labor Care Guide differ from a (modified) partograph?

Both are the documentation of observations during labor, but LCG has certain differences and added few sections which were not there in the partograph **(Table 3)**:

- The second section is supportive care including companion, pain relief, oral intake, and position.
- There is a section for monitoring and documentation during the second stage also.
- Active stage is taken as 5 cm onward; therefore, documentation is started after a cervical dilatation of 5 cm or more, while in the partograph it was taken as 4 cm.
- There is no alert and action line. Normal labor in many women progresses at rates slower than 1 cm/hour. As per LCG if all other observations are normal, labor progression is considered abnormal if cervical dilatation remains at 5 cm for

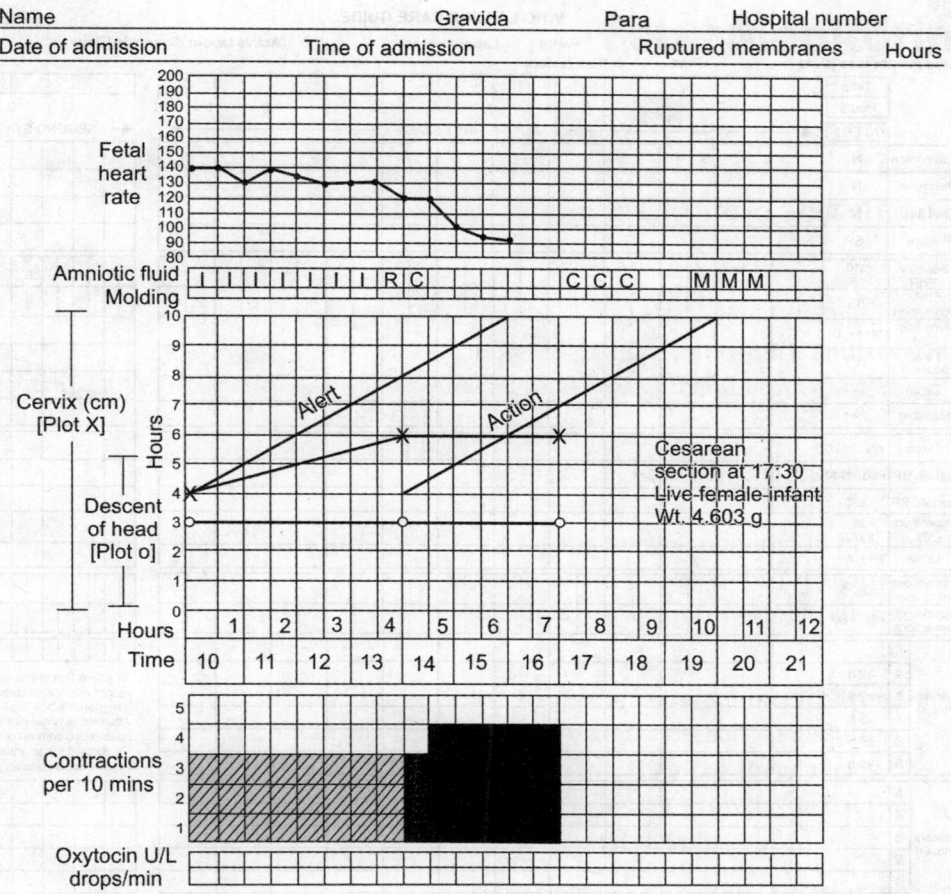

Fig. 7: Partograph showing obstructed labor.

≥6 hours, 6 cm for ≥5 hours, 7 cm for ≥3 hours, 8 cm for ≥2.5 hours, and 9 cm for ≥2 hours.
- There is an alert column wherein thresholds for abnormal values are given for all observations.
- The last section is for shared decision-making including overall assessment and further plan.
- The approach to be followed is Assess → Record → Check → Plan.

What is the mechanism of normal labor?
Normal labor is defined as the manner in which the fetus adjusts itself to pass through the parturient canal with minimal difficulty.

The cardinal movements are:
- Engagement
- Descent
- Flexion
- Internal rotation
- Extension
- Restitution
- External rotation
- Expulsion

What are the different phases of the second stage of labor?
The second stage of labor has two distinct phases:

WHO LABOUR CARE GUIDE

Name					Parity		Labour onset				Active labour diagnosis [Date			]
Ruptured membranes [Date			] Time		] Risk factors									

			Time	:	:	:	:	:	:	:	:	:	:	:	:	:	:	:
			Hours	1	2	3	4	5	6	7	8	9	10	11	12	1	2	3
			ALERT	←				ACTIVE FIRST STAGE							→	← SECOND STAGE →		
SUPPORTIVE CARE		Companion	N															
		Pain relief	N															
		Oral fluid	N															
		Posture	SP															
BABY		Baseline FHR	<110, ≥160															
		FHR deceleration	L															
		Amniotic fluid	M+++, B															
		Fetal position	P, T															
		Caput	+++															
		Moulding	+++															
WOMAN		Pulse	<60, ≥120															
		Systolic BP	<80, ≥140															
		Diastolic BP	≥90															
		Temperature (°C)	<35.0, ≥37.5															
		Urine	P++, A++															
LABOUR PROGRESS		Contractions per 10 min	≤2, >5															
		Duration of contractions	<20, >60															
	Cervix [Plot X]	10																	
		9	≥2 h															
		8	≥2.5 h															
		7	≥3 h															
		6	≥5 h															
		5	≥6 h															
	Descent [Plot O]	5																	
		4																	
		3																	
		2																	
		1																	
		0																	
MEDICATION		Oxytocin (U/L, drops/min)																	
		Medicine																	
		IV fluids																	
SHARED DECISION-MAKING		ASSESSMENT																	
		PLAN																	
		INITIALS																	

In active first stage, plot 'X' to record cervical dilatation. Alert triggered when lag time for current cervical dilatation is exceeded with no progress. In second stage, insert 'P' to indicate when pushing begins.

INSTRUCTIONS: CIRCLE ANY OBSERVATION MEETING THE CRITERIA IN THE 'ALERT' COLUMN, ALERT THE SENIOR MIDWIFE OR DOCTOR AND RECORD THE ASSESSMENT AND ACTION TAKEN. IF LABOUR EXTENDS BEYOND 12H, PLEASE CONTINUE ON A NEW LABOUR CARE GUIDE.

Abbreviations: Y – Yes, N – No, D – Declined, U – Unknown, SP – Supine, MO – Mobile, E – Early, L – Late, V – Variable, I – Intact, C – Clear, M – Meconium, B – Blood, A – Anterior, P – Posterior, T – Transverse, P+ – Protein, A+ – Acetone

Fig. 8: WHO Labor Care Guide.

Source: who-labour-care-guide.pdf available at https://www.who.int/docs/default-source/reproductive-health/maternal-health/who-labour-care-guide.pdf?sfvrsn=bd7fe865_10. [Last accessed April, 2024].

TABLE 3: Differences between partograph and labor care guide.

Partograph	Labor care guide
Active phase defined as starting from 4 cm of cervical dilatation	Active phase defined as starting from 5 cm of cervical dilatation
Fixed 1 cm/hour "alert" line and "action" lines 4 hours on right of alert line	Evidence-based time limits at each centimeter of cervical dilatation
No second-stage section	Documentation of monitoring in second stage
No recording of supportive care interventions	Separate section giving recording of labor companionship, pain relief, oral fluid intake, and posture
Records strength, duration, and frequency of uterine contractions	Records duration and frequency of uterine contractions
There is no explicit directive to address deviations from the expected observations of any labor parameter, except for the alert and action lines related to cervical dilatation	Recordings need to be compared with alert thresholds for each parameter and deviations need to be highlighted
No section to record the actions taken	A section for documentation of final assessment and plan of action is there

1. *Latent/passive/descent phase:* In this phase, descent of presenting part and rotation occurs.
2. *Active or pelvic floor phase:* During this phase, delivery of the baby occurs by expulsion.

What are the fetal and maternal risks during the second stage of labor?

Fetal risk:
- Fetal descent may precipitate cord compression.
- Intense uterine activity and expulsive efforts reduce placental blood flow.

Maternal risk: Injury to pelvic floor muscles (active phase)

When do you suspect abnormality in second stage (dystocia) and when is it termed prolonged?

Suspect second-stage labor abnormalities (dystocia), if:
- No urge to push after 1 hour of full-cervical dilatation
- Inadequate progress in terms of rotation and/or descent of the presenting part after 1 hour of active phase in nullipara or 30 minutes in multipara
- Delivery not imminent within 2 hours of active phase in nulliparous and 1 hour in multipara

Prolonged second stage:
- Arbitrary limits of the second stage of labor are not necessary and should be guided by fetal, maternal status, and observation of continuous process of descent and rotation of presenting part.
- Can be safely extended, if maternal and fetal assessments are normal and there is continuous progress. If these conditions are met, then the second stage is considered prolonged, if it exceeds:
  - *Nulliparas with epidural:* 4 hours
  - *Nulliparas without epidural:* 3 hours
  - *Multiparas with epidural:* 3 hours
  - *Multiparas without epidural:* 2 hours

How is the second stage of labor managed?
Monitoring in the second stage of labor:
- Check uterine contractions, FHR, mood, and behavior.
- Continue recording in the partograph.
- Intermittent FHR auscultation every 5 minutes and BP hourly
- Emotional support, hydration, and pain relief
- Encourage any position that a woman feels comfortable
- She should be guided by her own desire to push
- If pushing is ineffective, supportive care: Encouragement, emptying bladder, and change of position
- Oxytocin, if contractions are inadequate
- *Reminder:*
  - Massaging or stretching the perineum has not been shown to be beneficial.
  - Do not apply fundal pressure to help deliver the baby—it may harm mother and baby.

What is the evidence regarding episiotomy?
Evidence does not support routine episiotomy in all labors. A Cochrane review on the restricted use of episiotomy was published and the results found were as follows:
- With restricted use of episiotomy, the incidence of severe vaginal and perineal lacerations, postdelivery perineal pain, dyspareunia, or urinary symptoms like incontinency were not increased and were similar to the routine use of episiotomy group.
- With restricted use episiotomy, there was less risk of posterior perineal trauma and the subsequent need of perineal suturing while there was little increase in the anterior perineal trauma.

Therefore, it was concluded that restricted use of episiotomy should be done as per evidence.

What are the techniques recommended to avoid perineal trauma?
The various approaches recommended for avoiding perineal trauma during delivery are perineal massage, warm perineal compresses, and "hands on" perineal guarding. These have been shown to reduce perineal trauma. Evidence on Ritgen's maneuver being uncertain, it is not recommended.

What are the ways of separation of placenta?
- *Schulze method:* It is a more common method (80%). In this, the central part of the placenta separates first, blood collects behind it, and then margins separate and the gush of blood comes out.
- *Matthew Duncan method:* It is less common (20%). In this, the placenta starts separating from the margins.

What are the signs of placental separation?
The signs of placental separation occur within 5 minutes of placental separation:
- The patient complains of pains associated with uterine contractions.
- There will be a slight amount of vaginal hemorrhage.
- The extravulval portion of the cord lengthens.
- The fundus of the uterus rises above the umbilicus.
- There will be a soft elevation above the symphysis with a depression immediately above and indicating that the placenta has separated from the fundus and is lying in the lower uterine segment.
- If the fundus of the uterus is gently grasped and raised, the cord will not recede if the placenta has separated, whereas if the placenta is still adherent to the uterus, the portion of the cord just outside the vulva will be drawn into the vagina.

What are the physiological mechanisms to control bleeding in the third stage of labor?
Control of hemorrhage is due to three factors:
1. The contraction and retraction of the uterus constricting the vessels passing through the uterine wall to the placental site.
2. The occlusion of the torn vessels themselves
3. The formation of the blood clots, which favor the closure of the lumen of the vessels.

What are the components of active management of third stage of labor?
- Use of uterotonic for prevention of PPH (within 1 minute of delivery):
  - Oxytocin 10 IU intravenous (IV) or intramuscular (IM) is the most preferred.
  - Alternative choices are Injection Methergine/fixed-dose combinations of oxytocin and methergin or oral misoprostol 600 µg.
- Late cord clamping (after 1–3 minutes) while simultaneous essential newborn care is being done.
  - Clamp the cord within 5 minutes in order to perform controlled cord traction (CCT)
  - Early cord clamping (<1 minutes), if a neonate is asphyxiated and needs resuscitation.
- Controlled cord traction
- Sustained uterine massage not recommended
- Postpartum abdominal uterine tonus assessment

Give names and dosages of different oxytocic drugs that can be used for active management of third stage.
- Oxytocin 5U IV or 10U IM
- Methergine 0.2 mg IV or IM
- Misoprostol 600 µg oral/sublingual/rectal
- Injection Prostodin (15-methyl-PGF2α) 250 µg IM

Enumerate steps of controlled cord traction.
Steps of controlled cord traction are **(Fig. 9)**:
1. Apply clamp on the umbilical cord as close to the perineum as possible.
2. This clamp is held with one hand to apply traction.
3. Place the other hand on the patient's abdomen just above symphysis pubis.
4. When the uterus contracts, the cord is pulled gently downward, so as to deliver the separated placenta.
5. Simultaneously with the abdominal hand, countertraction is applied by pushing the uterus upward.
6. The traction should not be applied when the uterus is relaxed or without countertraction, as this will result in inversion of the uterus.
7. If with one traction placenta does not deliver in 30–40 seconds, release traction and wait for the next contraction.

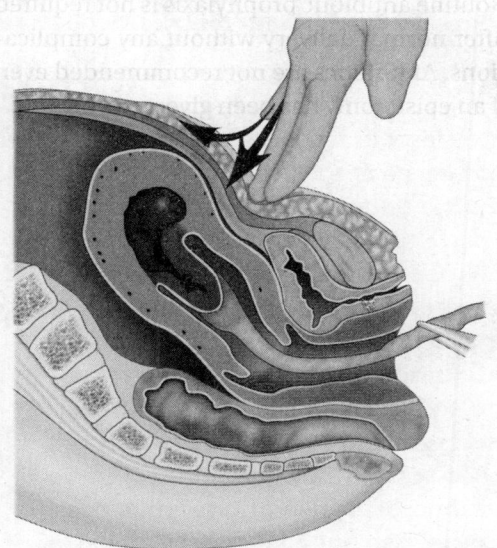

Fig. 9: Controlled cord traction.

8. Repeat the steps when the uterus contracts again.

What is prolonged third stage?
Prolonged third stage is more than 30 minutes in active management and 60 minutes in physiological management.

What is immediate care given to a newborn baby?
- Routine oral/nasal suctioning is not recommended as babies start breathing on their own if amniotic fluid is clear.
- The baby should be kept on the mother's abdomen for skin-to-skin contact with the mother for the first hour. This prevents neonatal hypothermia and also promotes breastfeeding.
- Breastfeeding should be encouraged and established as early as possible within the first hour of birth.

The baby should be adequately clothed, and bathing of neonate should be delayed for 24 hours.

Should antibiotic prophylaxis be given after normal delivery?
Routine antibiotic prophylaxis is not required after normal delivery without any complications. Antibiotics are not recommended even if an episiotomy has been given.

SUGGESTED READING

1. Approaches to limit intervention during labor and birth. ACOG Committee Opinion No.766 2019.
2. Preboth M. ACOG guidelines on antepartum fetal surveillance. American College of Obstetricians and Gynecologists. Am Fam Physician. 2000;62(5):1184, 1187-8. PMID: 10997537.
3. Rosen H, Yogev Y. Assessment of uterine contractions in labor and delivery. Am J Obstet Gynecol. 2023;228(5S):S1209-S1221.
4. Ross-Davie M, Brodrick A, Randall W, Kerrigan A, McSherry M. 2. Labour and birth. Best Pract Res Clin Obstet Gynaecol. 2021;73:91-103.
5. Vogel JP, Pingray V, Althabe F. Gibbons L, Berrueta M, Pujar Y, et al. Implementing the WHO Labour Care Guide to reduce the use of Caesarean section in four hospitals in India: protocol and statistical analysis plan for a pragmatic, stepped-wedge, cluster-randomized pilot trial. Reprod Health. 2023;20(1):18.
6. World Health Organization. WHO labour care guide: user's manual. 2020. https://www.who.int/publications/i/item/9789240017566.
7. World Health Organization. WHO recommendations: Intrapartum care for a positive childbirth experience Geneva: World Health Organization; 2018.

CHAPTER 7

Abnormal Presentations

Smiti Jain, Amita Suneja, Anita Matai

■ BREECH PRESENTATION

What is breech presentation?
Breech presentation is when the fetus is in longitudinal lie and podalic pole (fetal buttocks or legs or feet) occupies the lower uterine segment.

What is the most common form of malpresentation?
Breech is the most common malpresentation. The incidence is about 25–33% at 28 weeks and drops to 5% at 34 weeks and to 3% at term.

Enumerate the etiology of breech presentation.

Fetal factors
- Prematurity—smaller size of fetus and comparatively larger volume of amniotic fluid facilitate any pole occupying lower segment, so breech is commonly seen.
- Fetal anomaly—e.g., anencephaly, hydrocephaly, sacrococcygeal teratoma.
- Multiple gestation—causes crowding.
- Abnormalities in limb strength of fetus due to hypotonia in lower limbs causing extended fetal legs.
- Fetal neurological impairment affecting general fetal movements may contribute to some neuromuscular dysfunction and consequent breech presentation, e.g., meningomyelocele.
- Fetal growth restriction.

Maternal factors
- Older maternal age
- Multiparity
- Uterine anomalies (e.g., unicornuate or septate uterus)
- Contracted pelvis
- Polyhydramnios and oligohydramnios
- Maternal diabetes (increased risk of fetal anomalies)
- *Prior breech delivery:* Recurrence risk is 10% with previous one breech birth and 27% with previous two breech deliveries
- Uterine fibroid

Placental factors
- Placenta previa
- Cornual-fundal implantation of placenta
- Short umbilical cord

What are the varieties of breech presentation?

Complete breech: Usually seen in multiparas. Here, bilateral hip and knee joints are flexed.

Incomplete breech:
- *With extended legs (frank):* Bilateral hip joints are flexed and bilateral knee joints are extended. It is the most common type of breech presentation at term. It is usually seen in primiparas and accounts for more than 50% of breech fetuses in labor.
- *With extended thighs (presence of one or both feet or knees below the breech):*
  - Knee—lower limbs extended at hip joint but flexed at knee joint
  - Footling—lower limbs extended at both hip and knee joints.

How is breech presentation diagnosed?
Abdominal examination
- *Fundal grip:* Head is felt as a hard, round, mobile, and ballotable structure (usually felt lateral to midline).
- *Pelvic grip:* Breech or podalic pole-occupying lower segment is softer, irregular, less defined in outline, and usually lies above the brim. However, with extended legs (frank breech), the presenting part feels quite firm and is mostly deeply engaged. It can be mistaken for a vertex presentation, if both poles are not simultaneously felt.
- The fetal heart sounds are heard at or a little above the umbilicus.

Vaginal examination: In flexed breech, vaginal examination in early labor reveals a presenting part that is high up and ill-defined. The cervix dilates slowly and there is an elongated sausage-shaped bag of membranes owing to the irregular shape of the presenting part, allowing a large amount of liquor amnii to descend below it. At times, a small foot may be felt through the membranes. With cervix, well-dilated, and ruptured membranes, the diagnosis can be almost certainly made when soft buttocks, small spinous processes, and anal opening are felt. In flexed breech, one or both feet may be felt. Foot may be mistaken for hand before rupture of membranes. But afterward, foot may be distinguished by the heel and the toes, which are very characteristic. At times, scrotum is also felt.

Breech presentation could be easily mistaken with face presentation. Differentiation is possible as the mouth and malar eminences form a triangular shape while in breech presentation, ischial tuberosities and anus lie in a straight line. Alveolar margins are felt during examination when the finger enters the mouth in face presentation, while in breech presentation, a gripping sensation of anal sphincter is felt and no bony margins are felt.

What is the antenatal management of breech presentation?
When breech presentation is documented beginning 36 weeks of gestation, the following should be done:
- Counseling and discussion regarding the mode of delivery.
- Antenatal ultrasonography (USG) should be done to rule out congenital anomalies and placenta previa.

There are three management options:
1. *External cephalic version (ECV):* All women near term (36 weeks) with breech presentation should be offered ECV after the contraindications to ECV have been ruled out [American College of Obstetricians and Gynecologists (ACOG) 2016]. Details of ECV are discussed in later chapters.
2. *Vaginal delivery:* Patients with breech presentation can be left for vaginal delivery, if:
   - Fetopelvic disproportion (FPD) is ruled out.
   - No maternal complicating factors are present, e.g., heart disease, severe preeclampsia, precious pregnancy, abruption.
   - Estimated fetal weight is between 2 and 3.5 kg.
   - *Favorable fetal attitude:* Frank breech and no hyperextension of fetal head.
   - Fetus is dead or has gross congenital malformations incompatible with life.
   - Availability of an experienced obstetrician and pediatrician at the time of delivery is assured.

Primigravida with breech presentation can also be offered vaginal delivery, if she fulfills the above-mentioned criteria.

In an attempt to select the mode of delivery, various scoring systems have been made, e.g., Westin scoring and Zatuchni-Andros scoring (see Chapter 35).

3. *Lower segment cesarean section (LSCS):* Cesarean section is advocated, if:
- Fetal weight >3.8–4 kg
- Suspected FPD-associated maternal complications, precious pregnancy, bad obstetric history (BOH), and prior perinatal or neonatal birth trauma
- Hyperextended fetal head
- Footling presentation
- Severe fetal growth restriction
- Previous LSCS with breech presentation.

What is the management of breech in labor?

Management of breech presentation in first stage of labor:
- Informed consent explaining both fetal and maternal risks of breech vaginal delivery
- Part preparation and enema
- A per vaginam (pv) examination for pelvic assessment by a senior obstetrician in labor room
- Maintenance of adequate maternal hydration and nutrition
- Continuous epidural analgesia
- Maintain a partogram with careful fetal heart monitoring
- Patient is counseled not to bear down prematurely
- A pv examination at rupture of membranes should always be done to rule out cord prolapse.

Management of breech vaginal delivery in second stage of labor:

There are three methods of breech vaginal delivery:
1. *Spontaneous breech delivery:* It usually occurs in a multigravida with a small baby who may deliver unsupervised; it is not encouraged.
2. *Assisted breech delivery:* The fetus is delivered with assistance of the obstetrician supervising labor. It should be encouraged in all cases.
3. *Breech extraction:* When the entire body of the fetus is extracted by the obstetrician with minimal aid from the mother. It is carried out under anesthesia in case of fully dilated cervix with maternal or fetal distress, cord prolapse, or following internal podalic version. It is done very infrequently in modern obstetrics for a live baby. The only indication for breech extraction in a live baby is delivery of second twin after internal podalic version of transverse lie.

What is the mechanism of labor in spontaneous breech delivery?

Bitrochanteric diameter (10 cm) is the engaging diameter with left sacroanterior, the most common position. Engagement occurs in one of the oblique diameters of pelvis, descent occurs, and once anterior buttock strikes the pelvic floor, it rotates 1/8th of a circle. After rotation, descent continues until the perineum is distended by the advancing breech, and the anterior hip appears at the vulva. By lateral flexion of the fetal body, the posterior hip is delivered followed by the anterior hip. After delivery of buttocks, legs, and feet may be born spontaneously or require assistance. There is slight external rotation, with the back turning anteriorly and the shoulders (bisacromial diameter) come to lie in one of the oblique diameters (same as oblique diameter as occupied by buttocks). The shoulders then descend rapidly and undergo internal rotation to occupy the anteroposterior plane. Immediately following the shoulders, the well-flexed head enters the pelvis in the oblique diameter and descends and rotates to bring the posterior portion of the neck under the symphysis pubis. The head is then born by flexion (chin, face, and brow are born first followed by the occiput).

How is an assisted breech delivery conducted?

In addition to the requirements for the conduct of normal labor, the following are the prerequisites when planning an assisted breech delivery:
- Skilled obstetrician
- One assistant
- Anesthetist and availability of operation theater (OT)
- Availability of cross-matched blood
- Pudendal block and infiltration of perineum with local anesthetic
- Instruments for giving episiotomy
- Breech towel
- Piper's or long forceps for the aftercoming head of breech, if needed
- Trolley for neonatal resuscitation
- Pediatrician
- Staff nurse
- Watch/clock—to note the time taken for delivering the baby after the baby is born up to the umbilicus. *This should not be more than 3–5 minutes.*

Patient is put into lithotomy position in the second stage of labor and brought to the edge of the table, once the fetal anus is visible and anterior buttock distends the perineum.

Parts are cleaned and draped and bladder emptied. Local anesthesia (pudendal block with infiltration of the perineum) is given. Pudendal block allows manipulations, if necessary, at a higher level in the vagina and relaxes the pelvic floor facilitating delivery.

With each contraction, breech characteristically "climbs the perineum" at which time a wide generous episiotomy is given. "Climbing the perineum" is synonymous to "crowning" in vertex presentation.

Masterly inactivity is the rule of thumb and delivery is allowed by maternal efforts alone up to the umbilicus. Thereafter, disengage the extended legs and pull down a loop of cord, which may be on quite a stretch. If the cord is short, it is divided between artery forceps and time noted (average safe interval is 5 minutes). Further, descent is allowed by maternal efforts.

The trunk is held with breech towel and the buttocks grasped using pelvifemoral grip encouraging the sacrum to turn anteriorly. Look for the presence of arms folded across the chest with the visibility of the lower angle of the anterior scapula of the baby. If they fail to deliver spontaneously, they are hooked out. If extended, they are brought down by Lovset's maneuver.

The fetus hangs by its own weight at the vulva encouraging flexion of the head. When the nape of neck is visible under the pubic arch, the baby is grasped by both the ankles with the fingers in-between the two. Maintaining a steady traction and forming a wide arch of circle, the trunk is swung in upward and forward direction over the maternal pubes. The fetal head is finally delivered by movement of flexion. Simultaneously, the perineum is guarded, which prevents the head from emerging too quickly. This is the *Burns–Marshall method* (Fig. 1). It has few failures and a fetal mortality of under 3%.

If this maneuver fails, either *Mauriceau–Smellie-Veit (MSV) maneuver* or preferably the application of forceps will be required.

Abnormal Presentations

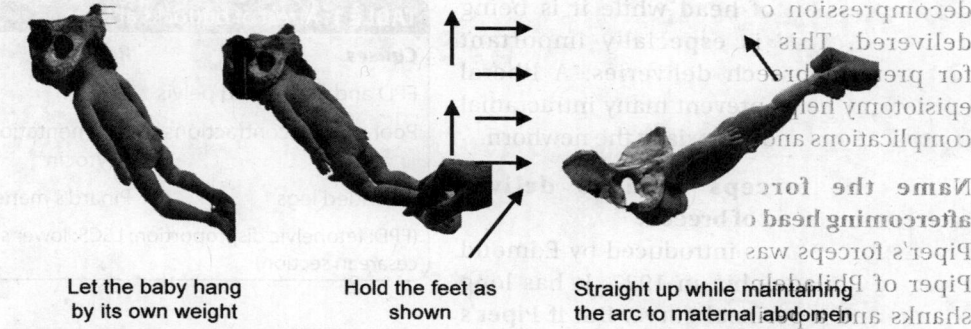

Let the baby hang by its own weight | Hold the feet as shown | Straight up while maintaining the arc to maternal abdomen

Fig. 1: Burns–Marshall technique. *(For color version, see Plate 1)*

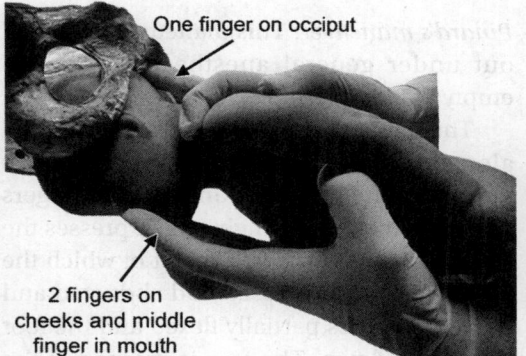

Fig. 2: Original Mauriceau–Smellie–Veit method. *(For color version, see Plate 1)*

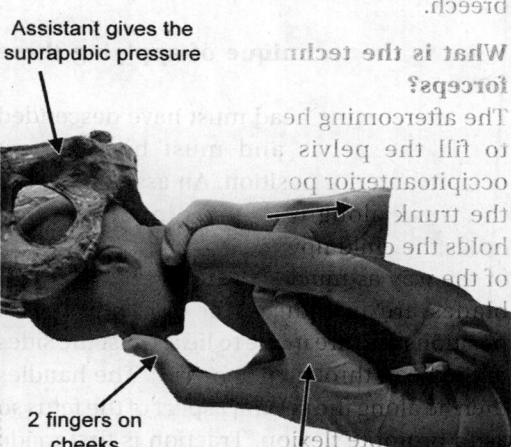

Fig. 3: Modified Mauriceau–Smellie–Veit method. *(For color version, see Plate 1)*

Flexion and shoulder traction (Mauriceau–Smellie-Veit technique)
The baby is placed on the supinated left forearm with the limbs hanging on either side and with the index finger of left hand placed in the mouth to maintain flexion (original method) **(Fig. 2)**. In modified method, the middle and the index fingers of the left hand are placed on the malar bones on either side **(Fig. 3)**. This maintains the flexion of the head. The ring and the little fingers of the pronated right hand are placed on the child's right shoulder, the index finger is placed on the left shoulder, and the middle finger is placed on the suboccipital region. Traction is now given in downward and backward direction till the nape of the neck is visible under the pubic arch. The assistant gives suprapubic pressure to maintain flexion of head. The fetus is carried in upward and forward direction toward the mother's abdomen releasing the face and brow. Lastly, the trunk is depressed to release the occiput and vertex. This technique can also be used in case of delayed engagement of fetal head.

Why do we give episiotomy in breech deliveries?
The role of episiotomy in breech vaginal delivery is to avoid rapid compression and

decompression of head while it is being delivered. This is especially important for preterm breech deliveries. A liberal episiotomy helps prevent many intracranial complications and hypoxia in the newborn.

Name the forceps used to deliver aftercoming head of breech.
Piper's forceps was introduced by Edmond Piper of Philadelphia in 1927. It has long shanks and a perineal curve. But if Piper's forceps is not available, a long-curved forceps can be used to deliver aftercoming head of breech.

What is the technique of applying these forceps?
The aftercoming head must have descended to fill the pelvis and must be in direct occipitoanterior position. An assistant wraps the trunk along with arms in a towel and holds the child upward, so that it may be out of the way as much as possible. The forceps blades are introduced at 4 and 8 o'clock positions and are made to lie against the sides of the head through a short arc. The handles then lie along the ventral aspect of the fetus so as to promote flexion. Traction is first made downward and backward till the chin appears and then the forceps and fetus are carried upward toward the mother's abdomen. Very little or no traction is needed for delivery with Piper's forceps. These forceps are used to maintain flexion of head.

Advantages:
- Controlled delivery of head.
- Flexion is well maintained.
- Pull is directly applied over the fetal head contrary to other manual methods, where it is applied via the vertebral column.

Describe the management of arrest of buttocks.
Arrest at brim
One must reassess again to rule out contracted pelvis and FPD. Other reasons for arrest of

TABLE 1: Arrest of buttocks at brim.

Causes	Remedy
FPD and contracted pelvis	LSCS
Poor uterine contractions	Augmentation with oxytocin
Extended legs	Pinard's maneuver

(FPD: fetopelvic disproportion; LSCS: lower segment cesarean section)

buttock at brim are sacrococcygeal teratoma and poor uterine contractions (unrecognized FPD is the most common cause) **(Table 1)**.

Pinard's maneuver: This maneuver is carried out under general anesthesia (GA) with empty bladder.

The palmar aspect of one hand is carried along the ventral aspect of fetus in the uterine cavity. The fore and middle fingers are applied over the thigh, which presses the latter against the trunk, a result of which the popliteal fossa is pressed and abducted and the leg becomes partially flexed and the foot is brought down. The foot is grasped at the ankle by the internal fingers. Next, feel for the cord and maneuver it to take it to the outer side before flexing and bringing down the leg. If not able to do so, go till fundus, until a foot is reached and drawn down, so the leg is flexed on thigh. Once one or both feet have been brought down, extraction of the breech can be accomplished **(Fig. 4 and Table 2)**.

Groin traction: It can be given to single or both groins using forefinger (during uterine contractions, when breech is being forced down) in a downward and forward direction, taking care that the force used is moderate and is directed more toward the trunk than toward the femur. Traction is much more effective when made during a contraction and when combined with fundal pressure. If it fails to shift the breech, a leg must be brought down by Pinard's maneuver.

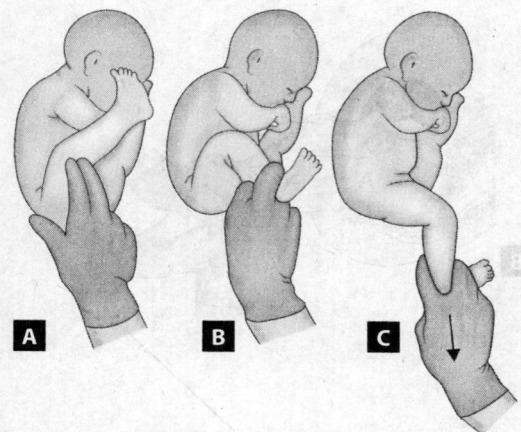

Figs. 4A to C: Pinard's maneuver: (A) Flexion and abduction of popliteal fossa; (B) To catch hold of the ankle; and (C) To pull by movement of abduction.

TABLE 2: Arrest of buttocks at perineum/outlet.

Causes	Remedy
Tight perineum	Pudendal block and liberal episiotomy
Extension of the legs	Groin traction
Poor uterine contractions	Oxytocin augmentation
Outlet contraction/FPD	LSCS

(FPD: fetopelvic disproportion; LSCS: lower segment cesarean section)

What is the management of extended arms during breech delivery?

Causes
- Primary displacement
- Pulling too soon on fetus
- Contracted pelvis
Following are the methods of delivering extended arms:
- Lovset's maneuver
- Classical method

Lovset's maneuver
Principle: It is based on the fact that due to the pelvic inclination, the posterior shoulder enters the pelvic cavity before the anterior shoulder. Thus, if the body of the fetus is turned 180° keeping the back in front, the posterior shoulder will appear behind the pubis. It is attempted when the inferior angle of scapula is visible.

Method: Using a pelvifemoral grip, the fetal trunk is drawn downward with its back in the lateral position. With the visibility of the inferior angle of anterior scapula, the fetal trunk is gently rotated to bring the posterior scapula into an anterior position. The posterior shoulder should be below the promontory, when rotation begins. The back should be kept anterior during rotation and the body is dipped down near completion of rotation. When the rotated shoulder comes below the pubes, hook a finger over the top of the shoulder, free the arm, and slide it down toward the elbow. When the arm is delivered, the fetal trunk is rotated back and the other scapula will appear below the symphysis that arm in turn is now delivered (**Figs. 5A to C**).

Advantages
- No anesthesia is required.
- No intrauterine manipulation is required.

Classical method: Classical method is done under GA with the patient in the lithotomy position. First, the fetus is grasped and drawn downward until the lower angle of scapula is visible or palpable. The fetal thorax is grasped by two hands with thumbs parallel to the fetal spine. Rotate thorax by the shortest route until one shoulder is posterior (if back is lateral, no need to do so). Holding the fetus by legs, lift it forward and toward the side to which its abdominal aspect is directed. This depresses the posterior shoulder still lower. Then slide two fingers of the hand, which corresponds to the arm of the fetus to be brought down, along the back over the posterior shoulder, along the upper arm until the bend of the elbow is reached. Then press the forearm downward across the face until it comes down

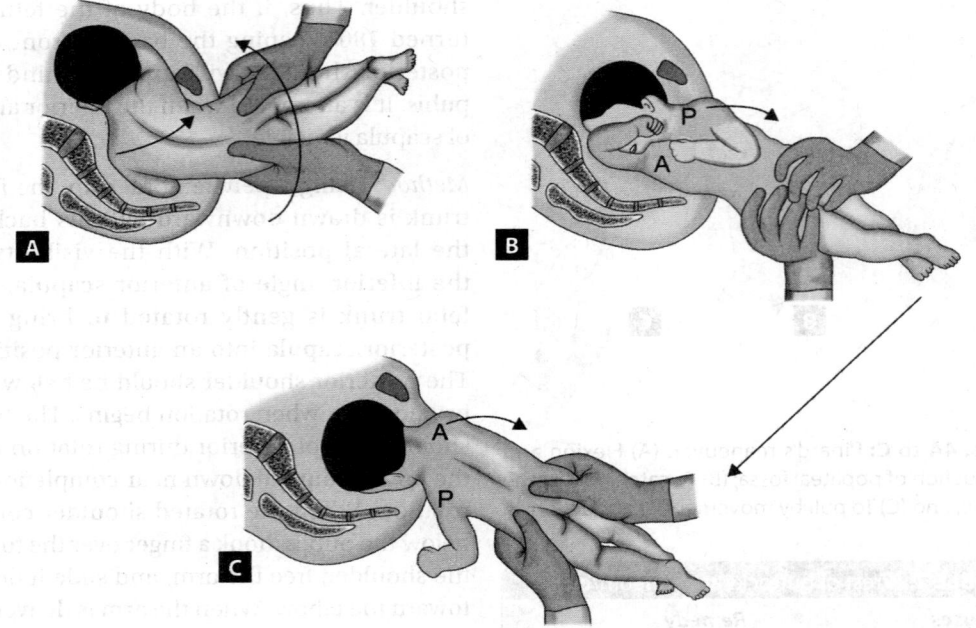

Figs. 5A to C: Lovset's maneuver.

and out between the chest and mother's perineum.

For delivering anterior arm, hold the fetus in downward and slightly lateral direction. Slide two fingers along the back, over the shoulder and along the upper arm until the bend of elbow is reached, and sweep out the arm downward across the face.

The body of the baby is rotated toward the direction where the thumb is pointing. After grasping baby at the pelvic girdle, the trunk is rotated toward the fingertips of the displaced arm until the arm becomes posterior, which is then to be delivered in the usual manner (Fig. 6).

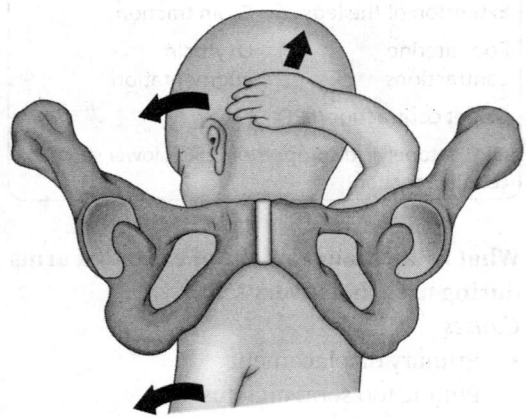

Fig. 6: Direction of movement for releasing arms.

What are the causes for arrest of fetal head in breech delivery?

The causes for arrest of fetal head in breech delivery:

If the above methods fail, symphysiotomy or cesarean section may be required.

What are the causes for arrest of fetal head in vaginal breech delivery?

At the level of pelvic outlet

Rigid perineum: A liberal and generous episiotomy is a good way to overcome this and deliver the aftercoming head of breech. Even better is application of Piper's forceps for delivery of head, as it maintains and aids in keeping the fetal head flexed, keeps traction by the obstetricians off the cervical spine, and offers protection to the fetal head against sudden decompression by allowing a controlled delivery of the head.

Deflexed head: The MSV method will help in causing and maintaining flexion of the fetal head.

At the level of midpelvis
Deflexed or extended head: This can be overcome if premature lifting of the baby is avoided and if proper suprapubic pressure is applied to the fetal head by the assistant. This will maintain the flexion of the fetal head throughout till its delivery. MSV method per vaginally will further aid in keeping the fetal head flexed while delivering it.

Incomplete dilatation of cervix: The two main principles of assisted breech delivery are avoiding rupture of membranes and waiting for full dilatation of cervix. The bag of membranes should be ruptured only when the cervix is fully dilated. The bag of membranes helps in uniform dilatation of the cervix, unlike the irregular breech. For cases with spontaneous ruptured membranes earlier on, the cervix can be manually stretched or Duhrssen's incision made on the cervix—both done under anesthesia—to complete the fetal head delivery. Duhrssen's incision on the cervix are made at 10 and 2 o'clock positions, and if further needed, then at 6 o'clock position, avoiding the descending cervical artery and its injury. In cases of intrauterine fetal death (IUFD), wait for full dilatation.

Occipitoposterior position: This should be diagnosed earlier on and corrected by turning the fetus by keeping the baby's back uppermost always. Using femoropelvic grip, rotate the baby and bring its back to the front anteriorly; it is an important step in assisted vaginal breech delivery. If this may not seem possible, then anesthesia may help. Push the baby's head up and rotate the baby under anesthesia. This is easier said than done and hence prevention is always better.

At the level of pelvic inlet
Disproportion: In modern obstetrics, there is no place for diagnosing cephalopelvic disproportion (CPD) in a breech presentation as late as this. Ideally, it should be diagnosed before the patient goes into labor utilizing all the scoring methods and radiological techniques, if needed, and the patient counseled for a scheduled LSCS if there is the slightest doubt. This is because in breech delivery there is no potential for molding of fetal head to happen, so there is no ground for trial of labor in breech presentation with CPD or macrosomia or contracted pelvis.

Hydrocephalus: Again, this should be diagnosed before labor begins. It can be managed by perforation and draining of cerebrospinal fluid (CSF) to reduce the size of head and accomplishing vaginal delivery. Destructive operations can be attempted by a skilled obstetrician.

Enumerate the incidence and causes of hyperextended head in breech.
The incidence of hyperextended head in term breech presentations is 5%. Causes are:
- Primary posture
- Multiple loops of nuchal cord
- Fetal neck masses
- Torticollis
- Uterine myomas/septae

How is hyperextension of head assessed?
X-ray abdomen showing anterior angle between mandible and cervical spine >105° is suggestive of hyperextension of head. This is also called star-gazing fetus.

What care should be taken in performing rotation at cervical spine?

Remember that the vertebral arteries are susceptible to compromise at this point and excessive rotation (>105°) may result in torsional injury to cervical spine.

What is the role of augmentation of labor in breech presentation?

It is controversial. Augmentation of labor may be considered, if breech is engaged in the pelvis and if pelvimetric dimensions are fulfilled. Oxytocin augmentation with intact membranes is safer, as rupture of membranes increases chances of cord prolapse. Intensive fetal heart rate (FHR) monitoring is required.

Describe Kristeller pressure.

Suprapubic pressure, which helps in maintenance of flexion of aftercoming head of breech, is known as Kristeller pressure. This allows the smallest diameter of the aftercoming head of breech to present for delivery.

What are the high-risk factors in preterm breech fetuses?

- Increased chances of footling/complete breech presentation with increased chances of umbilical cord prolapse
- Increased incidence of premature rupture of membranes (PROM), which may compromise umbilical cord and placental blood flow as well as loss of an effective dilating wedge
- Decreased ability to tolerate stress of labor
- Entrapment of the aftercoming head of breech through partially dilated cervix (lateral incision on the cervix also called Duhrssen's incision) can be given to deliver the head.

How does the outcome of preterm breech delivered vaginally versus preterm breech delivered by cesarean section compare?

Preterm breech delivered vaginally has a:
- 10-fold greater risk of developing neurologic abnormalities
- Four times greater incidence of intracranial bleed
- Low APGAR (appearance, pulse, grimace, activity, and respiration) score (<7 at 5 minutes) due to difficulty in aftercoming head of breech
- Peripheral nerve injury and perinatal mortality are greater in breech vaginal delivery (weight <1,500 g).

A separate consideration may be given to extremely low-birth-weight fetuses (<750 g/ 24–29 weeks) because cesarean section does not seem to improve the survival. In them, multiple factors related to prematurity appear to play a more significant role in determining the neonatal outcome.

What is the role of imaging techniques in breech vaginal delivery?

Antenatal scans are usually available with the patient, but if the patient reports for the first time at term, a quick scan must be done to rule out fetal malformations like hydrocephalous or anencephaly. Attitude of head (flexion or extension) should be noted and estimated fetal weight should also be ascertained at the same time. All these points will guide toward the correct mode of delivery.

There is no role of routine radiological pelvimetry. However, on ultrasound scan, an inlet anteroposterior diameter ≥105 mm, inlet transverse diameter ≥120 mm, and midpelvic interspinous diameter ≥100 mm grossly describe an adequate pelvis. This again will guide toward the choice of mode of delivery.

Describe the procedure of delivering a breech infant by the abdominal route.
Both uterine and abdominal wall incisions should be large enough to permit atraumatic delivery of the breech fetus. The breech extraction must be performed carefully and with optimum speed, not too fast and not too slow. After delivering the legs and/or pelvis, the baby should be held gently by a pelvifemoral grip with a dry warm towel. With gentle traction, the arms are released and the shoulders delivered. The head is delivered by the same movement as in Burns–Marshall technique. A concomitant steady fundal pressure by assistant facilitates flexion of head of baby. Lastly and importantly, the uterus is explored to rule out any uterine anomaly.

What are the factors responsible for poor perinatal outcome in breech presentation?
- Prematurity
- PROM
- Cord prolapse, cord compression, and delay in delivery of aftercoming head of breech during assisted breech delivery lead to perinatal asphyxia
- Traumatic birth injury
- Congenital malformations.

Enumerate possible fetal injuries during breech delivery.
Intracranial injuries
- Tear in tentorium cerebelli
- Intracranial hemorrhage
- Skull fractures

Intra-abdominal injury
- Injury to liver, spleen, kidney, and intestines

Bone injuries
- Fractures of humerus, femur, clavicle, and skull (spoon-shaped depression)
- Avulsion of upper cervical spine and roots
- Occipital bone diastasis

- Epiphyseal separation of scapula, humerus, and femur

Nerve injuries
- Cervical plexus
- Brachial plexus—Erb's paralysis (Duchenne's paralysis) (C5, C6 ± C7)
- Sixth and seventh nerve paralysis

Asphyxia
- Cord prolapse
- Cord compression
- Delay in delivery of head

Others
- Sternocleidomastoid hematoma
- Abrasion over face and body
- Genital organ damage in male fetuses
- Pharyngeal tears and pharyngeal pseudodiverticula as a result of MSV procedure
- Torticollis

Describe Prague maneuver.
Prague maneuver is the technique used to deliver the aftercoming head of breech when occiput is posterior (when the fetus's back fails to rotate anteriorly). The baby is laid with his back on the operator's forearm. The index and middle fingers of the hand hook into the either side of the fetal neck from behind with the other hand grasping the legs above ankles. An assistant uses two fingers over facial bones to maintain an attitude of flexion. By this, the occiput passes forward over the sacral concavity and then over the perineum. The fetal larynx serves as a fulcrum in this type of delivery. The modification of Prague maneuver involves use of two fingers of one hand to grasp shoulder and other hand draws the feet and leg over the maternal abdomen.

Mention incidence of cord prolapse in breech deliveries.
- Frank breech—0.5%
- Complete breech—5%
- Footling breech—15%

What are the ACOG recommendations for breech delivery?

Recommendations of ACOG:
- The decision regarding mode of delivery should consider patient wishes and the experience of healthcare provider.
- Obstetrician-gynecologists and other obstetric care providers should offer ECV as an alternative to planned cesarean section for a woman who has a term singleton breech fetus, desires a planned vaginal delivery of a vertex presenting fetus, and has no complications. ECV should be attempted only in settings in which cesarean section services are readily available.
- Planned vaginal delivery of a term singleton breech fetus may be reasonable under hospital-specific protocol guidelines for eligibility and labor management.
- If a vaginal breech delivery is planned, a detailed informed consent should be documented including risks that perinatal or neonatal mortality or short-term serious neonatal morbidity may be higher than if a cesarean delivery is planned.

■ OCCIPITOPOSTERIOR POSITION

Define occipitoposterior position.

In a vertex presentation, when the occiput is placed posteriorly over the sacroiliac joint or directly over the sacrum, it is known as occipitoposterior position. It is an abnormal position of the vertex rather than abnormal presentation.

What is the incidence of occipitoposterior position?

Occipitoposterior position occurs in approximately 15-20% of all vertex presentations at the onset of labor, but only 5% deliver as occipitoposterior.

What are the causes of occipitoposterior position?
- Shape and inclination of pelvic brim
- Position of trunk
- Shape and size of fetal head

Which is more favorable—left occipitoposterior or right occipitoposterior?

Right occipitoposterior is more favorable because the head engages in right oblique diameter, which has more space than left oblique diameter because of the position of the sigmoid colon on the left side.

What are the clinical diagnostic points for occipitoposterior position?

During pregnancy
- Per abdomen palpation reveals back on either of the flanks or may be difficult to palpate.
- Limbs are felt easily.
- Prominent sinciput may be felt to be directed forward.
- Fetal heart sounds are relatively faint and heard over a wide area.

During labor
- Big forebag of water and early spontaneous rupture of membranes.
- Caput is present.
- Anterior fontanelle is felt more easily because of partial deflexion.
- If flap of ear is felt, it points toward the occiput.
- Premature bearing-down sensation.
- Forceps blades do not lock easily and may slip.
- Peculiar appearance of perineum where anal and vulvar orifices gape unusually and the perineum may tear before the head distends it.

Enumerate the abnormal mechanics in labor leading to failure of anterior rotation of occipitoposterior position.

- When head engages in the pelvis in a primary transverse position or with an occiput in an oblique posterior position and remains unrotated
- When forward rotation of the occiput from an oblique posterior position is arrested in a secondary transverse position
- When a short backward rotation of the occiput from an oblique posterior position into the hollow of the sacrum **(Fig. 7)**.

Enumerate causes leading to failure of anterior rotation of the occiput.

- Partial extension or deficient flexion of head
- Uterine inertia
- Early rupture of membranes
- Android/anthropoid pelvis associated with minor/unsuspected degrees of pelvic contraction
- Big baby
- Anterior placentation

Name the type of maternal pelvis in which occipitoposterior position commonly occurs and why.

Anthropoid or dolichopellic pelvis favors occipitoposterior position. It is a high-assimilation type pelvis (i.e., sacralization of lumbar vertebra) where the anteroposterior diameter at brim is more than the transverse diameter at brim. Here, the delivery may occur by face to pubes mechanism.

Android pelvis has a wedge-shaped brim, which also predisposes to posterior position of the vertex as the bulky occiput cannot find room in the pinched forepart of the pelvis. Here, the position is oblique posterior. It is of poor obstetric value because of lessening of posterior sagittal diameter (i.e., the distance between the midpoint of the widest transverse diameter and sacrum) that affects not only the brim but commonly extends to the plane of least dimensions and pelvic outlet. In this type of pelvis, "deep transverse arrest (DTA)" occurs because impaction of head in pelvis cavity is common, the sacrum is "flat", and there is no room for rotation.

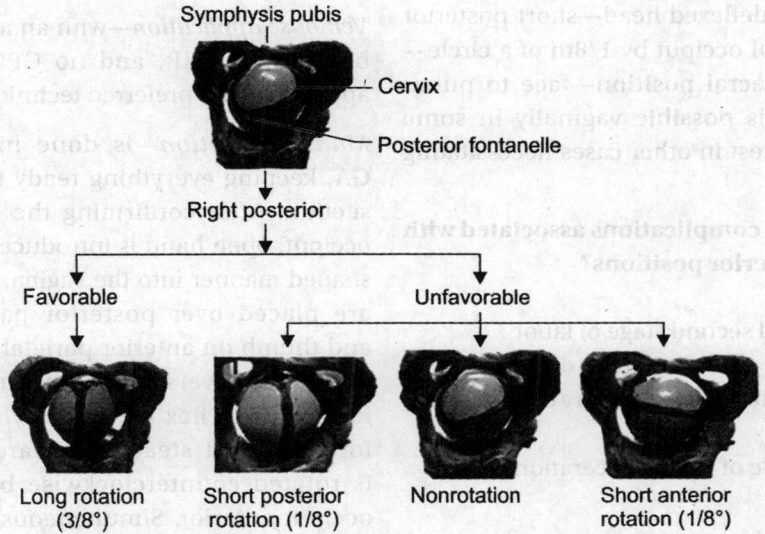

Fig. 7: Diagrammatic representations showing favorable and unfavorable rotation of occipitoposterior position. *(For color version, see Plate 1)*

How does delivery take place in direct occipitoposterior position (face to pubes)?
Anterior fontanelle is part of the head that presents first at vulva. The occipitofrontal diameter engages in the anteroposterior diameter of the outlet. The vertex first passes beneath the pubic symphysis, then the perineum stretches, and the occiput slips over it. Finally, face passes under the symphysis and head delivers by extension. Here, the wide posterior part distends the perineum increasing the risk of severe perineal lacerations.

What are the possible labor outcomes in occipitoposterior positions?
Favorable—long anterior rotation by 3/8th of a circle to occipitoanterior position—in 90% cases. Prolonged labor ensues in these cases.

Unfavorable—nonrotation or malrotation—in 10% cases. Possible scenarios:
- Slightly deflexed head—short anterior rotation of the occiput by 1/8th of a circle—DTA.
- Moderately deflexed head—nonrotation of occiput—oblique posterior arrest.
- Severely deflexed head—short posterior rotation of occiput by 1/8th of a circle—occipitosacral position—face to pubes delivery is possible vaginally in some cases. Arrest in other cases necessitating LSCS.

What are the complications associated with occipitoposterior positions?
Maternal
- Prolonged second stage of labor
- Increased rate of cesarean delivery
- Increased risk of operative vaginal delivery
- Higher rate of vaginal lacerations

Fetal
- Fetal acidosis
- Birth asphyxia—APGAR <7
- Increased birth trauma incidence
- Increased neonatal intensive care unit (NICU) admission

Define DTA (deep transverse arrest).
- *D*—head is *deep* in the pelvis at the level of ischial spines; at 0 station
- *T*—sagittal suture is in *transverse* plane
- *A*—progress is *arrested*, i.e., failure of descent of head beyond the ischial spines with a fully dilated cervix despite good uterine contractions for 1 hour.

How is deep transverse arrest managed?
The management options depending on baby size, FHR, and pelvic assessment are:
- Cesarean section
- Ventouse application
- Manual rotation followed by delivery of baby by forceps application
- Forceps rotation.

Cesarean delivery—should be performed in case of CPD, nonreassuring cardiotocography, fetal distress, maternal distress, and in situations where an experienced obstetrician is not available.

Ventouse application—with an average-sized baby, good FHR, and no CPD, ventouse application is a preferred technique.

Manual rotation—is done in OT under GA, keeping everything ready for cesarean section. After confirming the direction of occiput, open hand is introduced in a cone-shaped manner into the vagina. Four fingers are placed over posterior parietal bone and thumb on anterior parietal bone in left occipitotransverse position. An attempt is first made to flex the head by pushing the forehead end steadily upward and head is rotated counterclockwise bringing the occiput anterior. Simultaneously, the back of fetus is rotated by external hand from flank to midline. Forceps is applied; the right blade should be applied first. In right occipitotransverse, the pronated right hand is introduced in the same manner and rotated clockwise. In modern obstetrics, forceps rotation is not preferred, as it is associated with high neonatal mortality and morbidity and maternal injuries. Specialized skill and training are essential, either Simpson or Tucker-McLane forceps or one of their modifications and specialized Kielland forceps should be available.

Dead fetus—craniotomy through the parietal bone could be done.

■ FACE PRESENTATION

What is the incidence of face presentation?
The incidence of face presentation is 1 in 500 deliveries.

What is the etiology of face presentation?
Box 1 describes the etiology of face presentation.

What are the four positions described in face presentation?
1. Left mentoanterior—most common
2. Right mentoposterior
3. Left mentoposterior
4. Right mentoposterior

What is the denominator in face presentation?
Chin (mentum) is the denominator.

What are the diagnostic points for face presentation?
On abdominal palpation:
- Fetal cephalic prominence is felt on the same side as fetal back.
- The occiput feels prominent, with a groove between head and back.
- Fetal heart is best heard through the fetal chest on the same side as the limbs. In a

> **BOX 1:** Etiology of face presentation.
>
> *Maternal*
> - Disproportion (platypelloid/flat pelvis)
>   Multiparity—pendulous abdomen and flabby abdominal musculature are implicated. Pendulous abdomen permits back of the fetus to sag forward and laterally, often in the same direction in which the occiput points, thus promoting extension of the cervical and thoracic spine
> - Multiple loops of cord around neck
> - Multiple gestation
> - Prematurity
>
> *Fetal*
> - Anencephaly
> - Enlarged fetal thyroid
> - Dolichocephaly
> - Congenital bronchocele/cystic hygroma
> - Meningocele/encephalocele
>
> Intrauterine fetal death—the flaccidity of fetus may attribute to face presentation

mentoposterior position, the fetal heart is difficult to hear because the fetal chest is in contact with the maternal spine.

Face presentation is more commonly diagnosed during vaginal examination.

What is the mechanism of labor in face presentation?
Mentoanterior positions are more common in face presentation. The face engages in the submentobregmatic diameter and descends with increasing extension.

When chin reaches the pelvic floor, there is internal rotation through 1/8th of a circle. The vertex fits in the sacral hollow and the submental region comes to lie under the pubic arch.

After anterior rotation and descent, the chin and mouth appear at vulva and the submentum hinges behind the pubic symphysis. The submentovertical diameter distends the vulva and the head is borne by

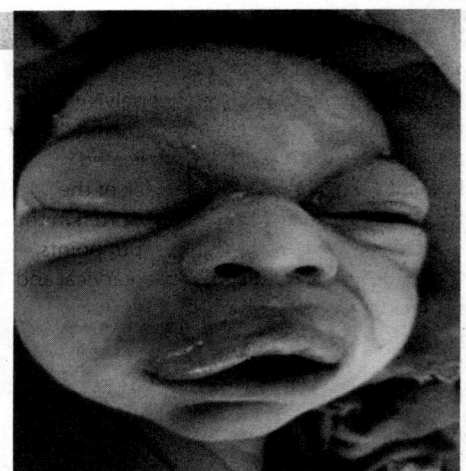

Fig. 8: Edema in face presentation.
(For color version, see Plate 2)

flexion. Nose, eyes, brow, and occiput then appear in succession. Following birth of head, occiput sags backward toward the anus. The chin then rotates externally to the side toward which it was originally directed with and the shoulders are delivered as in vertex presentation.

The rest of the delivery follows the normal mechanism. Labor is usually longer as facial bones do not mold.

Tumefaction: Neonates delivered in the face presentation exhibit significant facial and skull edema, which usually resolves within 24–48 hours **(Fig. 8)**.

How does face presentation differ from other vertex presentations?
Face is made up of cancellous bone, molding does not occur, and it is also a poor dilator of cervix.

What is Beck's Sign?
On pv examination, face presentation may be confused with breech presentation due to facial edema. Here, Beck's sign is helpful—"the anus and ischial tuberosities form a straight line, the mouth and malar bones form a triangle".

What is the incidence of spontaneous rotation in mentoposterior position?
About 30% of mentoposterior presentations rotate to mentoanterior position.

What are the management modalities for mentoposterior position?
Leave for spontaneous conversion to mentoanterior position with a careful watch on progress of labor and fetal heart sounds. Attempts to convert a face manually into a vertex presentation, manual or forceps rotation of a persistently posterior chin to a mentoanterior position, are dangerous and not attempted.

Why mentoposterior cannot deliver vaginally?
The fetal neck is too short to span the length of the maternal sacrum and is already at the point of maximal extension.

The head is in the sacral hollow; the head does not enter the pelvis as the sternobregmatic diameter hits against the pelvic brim and labor is obstructed.

In persistent mentoposterior position, cesarean section is advocated.

What is the incidence of spontaneous vaginal delivery in mentoanterior position?
Labor in mentoanterior position is protracted as facial bones do not undergo molding but spontaneous delivery occurs in 50% of mentoanterior cases or else outlet forceps may be applied.

■ BROW PRESENTATION

What is the incidence of brow presentation?
Brow presentation is the rarest presentation with an incidence of 1:2,000 deliveries **(Fig. 9)**.

What is the etiology of brow presentation?
The etiology of brow presentation is the same as that of face presentation.

Abnormal Presentations

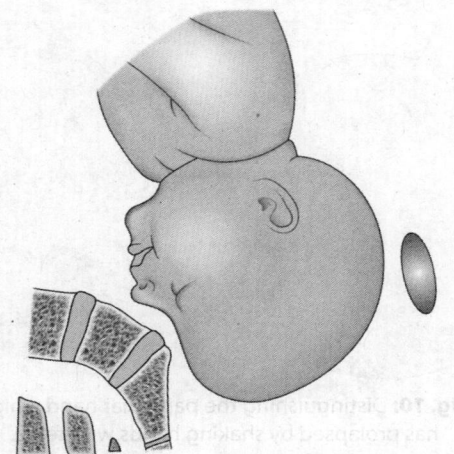

Fig. 9: Brow posterior position.

How often can brow presentation be diagnosed per abdominally?
Clinically, it is not easy to feel for the depression between occiput and back, which is characteristic of face and brow presentations. Because of the rarity of this presentation, labor is often well advanced before the condition is recognized. On pv examination, it may be recognized by the presence of frontal sutures, large anterior fontanelle, orbital ridges, eyes, and root of the nose, which is possible when the cervix is well dilated.

What is the engaging diameter in brow presentation?
When the head lies midway between attitude of complete flexion and complete extension, the brow presents at brim and the longest diameter of head, i.e., mentovertical (13.8 cm), becomes the engaging diameter at brim.

What is the mechanism of labor in brow presentation?
Anterior brow presentations may deliver vaginally, if the head is small, pelvis is of good size, and there are good uterine contractions. Molding then occurs, which causes marked compression of mentovertical diameter causing bulging of frontal bones. Superior maxilla is compressed against the pubes and occiput lies in the sacral hollow. The frontal region first appears at vulva followed by vertex and occiput. Face and chin disengage from the pubes lastly.

If there is persistent brow, cesarean section is the answer.

What are the management options in cases with brow presentation in a dead fetus?
- Craniotomy in experienced hands, otherwise cesarean section.

■ TRANSVERSE LIE

What is the incidence of transverse lie?
The incidence of transverse lie is 1 in 150 births (term and preterm combined).

What is the common presenting part in transverse lie?
The common presenting part in transverse lie is usually shoulder (acromion is the denominator for assigning position in a transverse lie or shoulder presentation) or arm and rarely back or abdomen.

What is the etiology of transverse lie?
Maternal causes
- Multiparity
- Placenta previa
- Polyhydramnios
- Uterine malformations—arcuate uterus and subseptate uterus
- Space-occupying lesion in the lower segment such as fibroid and ovarian cyst
- Marked maternal kyphosis

Fetal causes
- Prematurity
- IUFD
- Multiple gestation
- Fetal malformations

What is the most common position?
Left dorsoanterior (60%) is the most common position.

How can transverse lie be diagnosed?
During pregnancy
Inspection: The uterus is transversely enlarged and therefore even at term, the height of the fundus may only be slightly above the umbilicus. No fetal pole is detected at fundus.

Palpation: Hard round head is felt in one flank and podalic pole in the other. Lower pole feels empty. Back can be easily felt in front of the abdomen in the dorsoanterior position. Irregular nodulations representing small fetal parts are felt in the same location in dorsoposterior position.

Auscultation: Fetal heart sounds are easily heard in lower abdomen in dorsoanterior position and heard high with difficulty in dorsoposterior position.

During labor: Clavicle and ribs are characteristic landmarks. Grid iron feel of ribs in a thin patient in early stages of labor is very distinct. In advanced labor, the shoulder impacts and the characteristic lower pole emptiness on the abdominal palpation disappears. In a considerable number of cases, hand/foot may prolapse. Hand is distinguished from foot by the absence of the projecting heel. Also, fingers are larger than the toes and thumb moves more freely than the large toe. The side of the prolapsed arm, right or left, can be recognized by shaking hands with the fetus **(Fig. 10)**.

What is the mechanism of labor in transverse lie?
There is no mechanism of labor in transverse lie. If the malpresentation is not corrected and the labor continues, fetal shoulder impacts and uterine rupture may occur with concomitant fetal demise. Occasionally, if the fetus is small (usually <800 g) and pelvis

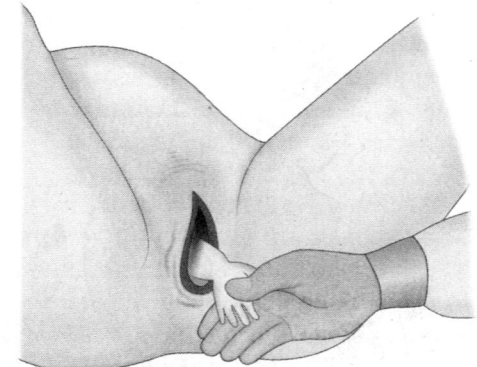
Fig. 10: Distinguishing the particular hand which has prolapsed by shaking hands with fetus.

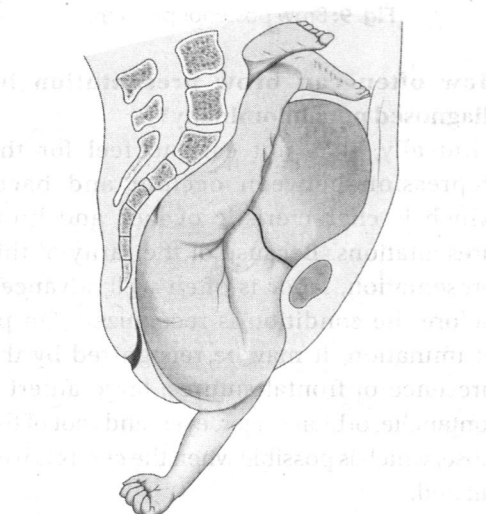
Fig. 11: Spontaneous evolution.

large, spontaneous delivery is possible where the head and thorax pass through the pelvic cavity at the same time and fetus doubles up on itself (birth corpora conduplicata) and gets expelled **(Fig. 11)**.

Explain the management of a case of transverse lie.
When transverse lie is recognized at 36th week of pregnancy
Try ECV with stabilizing induction under cardiotocographic monitoring. A prior ultrasound for placental localization is a must.

When transverse lie is recognized during labor
- Early labor—ECV with stabilizing induction
- Late in labor with fetus live—LSCS
- Preterm transverse lies with salvageable fetus—LSCS
- Late in labor with fetus dead:
  - Internal podalic version under GA
  - Destructive operation (decapitation/evisceration) in experienced hands
  - LSCS in impending rupture or unduly stretched lower segment
- Very preterm transverse lie with fetus not salvageable—can be left for spontaneous vaginal delivery [birth corpora conduplicata (being born doubled up)] after taking all consents duly.

What is neglected shoulder presentation?
After rupture of the membranes in a case of transverse lie, if labor continues unabated the fetal shoulder is forced into the pelvis and the corresponding arm frequently prolapses. The shoulder impacts firmly in the upper part of the pelvis. The uterus then contracts in an attempt to remove the obstacle leading to formation of a pathological retraction ring, which increases higher and becomes more marked. This is referred to as neglected shoulder presentation, which if not timely managed may lead to fetal demise and rupture uterus. In a live fetus, immediate LSCS should be performed. In a dead fetus, decapitation/evisceration may be attempted by skilled and experienced hands after ruling out rupture uterus. In modern obstetrics, LSCS is the only mode of delivery for neglected transverse lie.

COMPOUND PRESENTATION

What is compound presentation?
In compound presentation, an extremity prolapses alongside the presenting part, with both presenting in the pelvis simultaneously (Fig. 12).

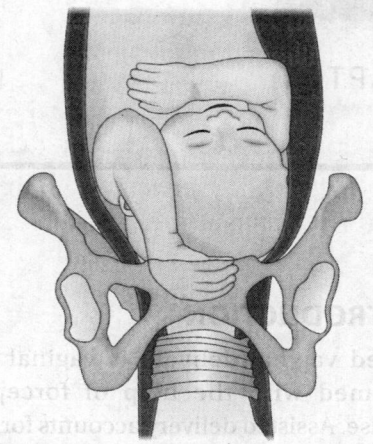

Fig. 12: Compound presentation—the left hand is lying in front of vertex.

What is the incidence of compound presentation?
The incidence of compound presentation is 1 in 1,000.

What are the causes of compound presentation?
Causes of compound presentation are conditions that prevent complete occlusion of pelvic inlet by the fetal head as in premature labor, preterm prelabor ruptured membranes, abnormal presentations, multiple pregnancies, any tumors in the pelvis, and contracted pelvis.

Explain management of compound presentation.
During the second stage, if the hand is presenting alongside the vertex, it could be repositioned back.

In cases of complex compound presentation (i.e., when both arms and legs prolapse) with a live fetus, cesarean section should be considered. In advanced labor with a dead fetus, destructive operation should be considered, if a skilled and experienced obstetrician is available, otherwise perform a cesarean section.

8

CHAPTER

Instrumental Delivery

Sumita Mehta, Sonam Singh

■ INTRODUCTION

Assisted vaginal delivery is vaginal birth performed with the help of forceps or ventouse. Assisted delivery accounts for 3–5% of all deliveries. The main goal of instrumental vaginal delivery is to mimic spontaneous birth without compromising maternal or neonatal morbidity.

The essential conditions for safe assisted vaginal birth include:
- A careful assessment of the clinical situation
- Expertise in the procedure chosen
- Clear communication with the patient.

■ FORCEPS

Identify and describe the instrument (Fig. 1).
- This is the Wrigley outlet forceps.
- It has a marked cephalic area and slight pelvic curve. Its length is 27.5 cm and the widest diameter between blades is 7.5 cm. It consists of two blades, namely left or right, in relation to maternal pelvis when applied. Each blade consists of (1) blade, (2) shank, (3) lock, and (4) handle.

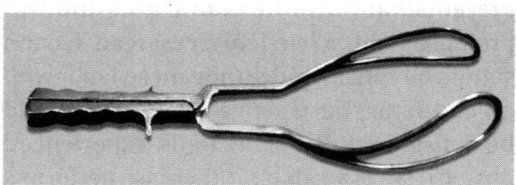

Fig. 1: Wrigley outlet forceps.

How many curves does a forceps have?
Blade has two curves:
1. *Pelvic curve:* This curve is to fit the curve on axis of birth canal. It forms a part of circle whose radius is 17.5 cm. The front of forceps is the concave side of pelvis curve.
2. *Cephalic curve:* This curve lies on the flat surface, which when articulated grasps the fetal head without compression. The radius of curve is 11.5 cm.

How many types of lock are found in obstetric forceps?
There are two main types of locks: Sliding and fixed lock.
1. *Sliding lock:* In this, the blade can move forward and backward independently and can help in delivering the baby by asynclitism, e.g., Kielland's forceps.
2. *Fixed lock:* It can be of two types: English or French type.
   - French lock consists of a threaded bolt screwed into a hole in the left shank and a notch in the right shank, which articulate with this bolt while in English lock the socket is located on the shank at its junction with the handle. The English type is more common and found in Wrigley forceps.

What is the American College of Obstetricians and Gynecologists (2002) classification of forceps application?
Outlet forceps
- Scalp is visible at introitus without separating labia.

- Fetal skull has reached pelvic floor.
- Sagittal suture is in anteroposterior diameter, right occiput anterior (ROA), left occiput anterior (LOA), occiput anterior (OA).
- Fetal head is at or on perineum.
- Rotation does not exceed 45°.

Low forceps
- Leading point of fetal skull is at station more than +2 cm and not on pelvic floor.
- Rotation is 45° or less—LOA or ROA to OA, left occiput posterior (LOP) or right occiput posterior (ROP) to occiput posterior (OP).

Midpelvic forceps: Station above +2 cm but head is engaged.

High forceps: It is not included in this classification.

What are the types of forceps?
- *Long-curved forceps with or without axis traction:* Simpson, Das, Piper's **(Fig. 2B)**, and Barton's forceps
- *Short-curved forceps:* Wrigley outlet forceps and Simpson short forceps **(Figs. 2A and C)**
- *Kielland's forceps:* It is a long, straight forceps with a very slight pelvic curve and a sliding lock. The maximum distance between closed blades is 8.2 cm **(Fig. 2D)**.

Indications of Forceps Application

Maternal indications
- Delay in second stage; nulliparous—4 hours with regional anesthesia and 3 hours without, multiparous—3 hours with regional anesthesia and 2 hours without
- Inadequate bearing-down efforts
- Elective shortening of second stage—severe preeclampsia, eclampsia, pregnancy with heart disease, pregnancy with pulmonary disease, severe anemia, and previous cesarean section.

Fetal indications
- Fetal distress
- Cord prolapse
- Aftercoming head of breech
- Prematurity

What are the prerequisites for forceps application?
According to the American College of Obstetricians and Gynecologists (ACOG), the following prerequisites should be fulfilled before forceps application:
- Maternal consent obtained, risks and benefits thoroughly explained.
- Bladder should be empty.
- Appropriate analgesia.
- Cervix must be fully dilated and fully effaced.
- Presentation must be favorable—vertex, mentoanterior, and aftercoming head of breech.
- Membranes must be ruptured.
- Head should be engaged.
- Fetal weight has been estimated.
- Maternal pelvis adequate for vaginal delivery
- Uterus must be contracting and relaxing.
- A back-up plan if the operative delivery method fails.

What are the types of application of forceps?
Cephalic application: Blades lie along sides of head with long axis of blades corresponding to occipitomental diameter and biparietal diameter (BPD) occupies the widest interval between the blades.

Pelvic application: Forceps are applied symmetrically along the sides of the pelvis irrespective of position of head.

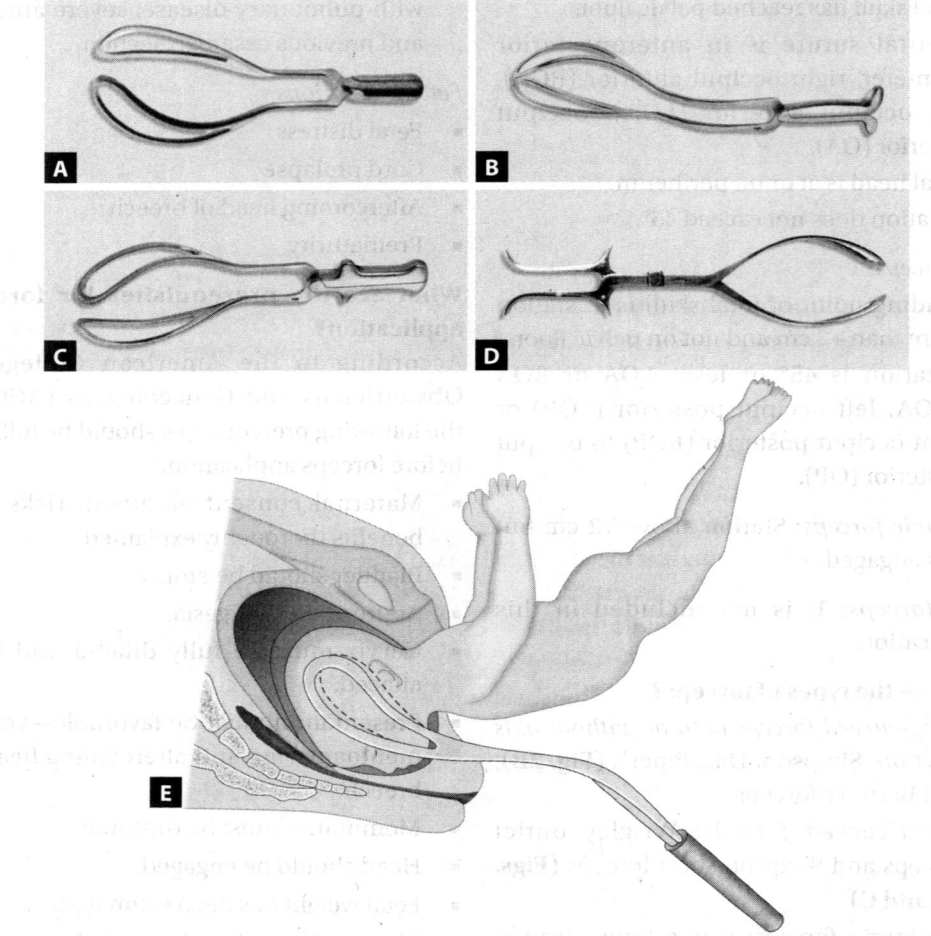

Figs. 2A to E: Types of forceps: (A) Wrigley forceps; (B) Piper's forceps; (C) Simpson–Braun forceps; (D) Kielland's forceps; (E) Delivery of aftercoming head of breech with Piper forceps.

What are axis traction forceps and what are their advantages?

There are three types:
1. Milne-Murray forceps—axis traction mechanism is at the heel of the fenestra.
2. Heigh-Ferguson forceps—axis traction is at the shank.
3. Barnes-Neville forceps—axis traction device is applied at the handle.

Advantages of axis traction
- Force arm of the lever is lengthened, so there is mechanical advantage and less force is required.
- Traction with axis traction coincides with axis of pelvis, so no force is wasted.
- It does not interfere with rotation of the head.
- Axis traction is required when the head is high in pelvis, so it is rarely practiced in modern obstetrics.

What is phantom application of forceps?

Phantom application of forceps is when the forceps are assembled in front of maternal introitus in a position in which they will be after correct cephalic application.

How are forceps applied?
Forceps should be assembled in the correct anatomical position, so that the cephalic curve is facing inward and pelvic curve is facing upward; when so placed, the left blade is in the left hand of surgeon while the right blade is in the right hand of surgeon.

The left blade is applied first because of peculiarity of English lock (slot in left blade faces anteriorly); it is held in pen-holding position and introduced parallel to the opposite ilioinguinal ligament after protecting the vagina with the fingers of right hand.

The blade is pushed up between fetal head and sacral hollow and swept up such that it comes to lie on the left side of pelvis.

The right blade is introduced by holding it in right hand and introducing into vagina under guidance of internal fingers.

The blades are depressed and then locked. There should be no difficulty in locking.

Traction should be given in the axis of the pelvis, for outlet forceps, horizontally and then forward and upward. Traction is given only during uterine contraction and in between traction, the handles can be separated gently. As soon as the head is delivered, blades are removed; right blade first followed by the left.

What is the role of episiotomy in forceps-assisted deliveries?
According to ACOG (2015), Royal College of Obstetricians and Gynaecologists (RCOG) (2011), and Society of Obstetricians and Gynaecologists of Canada (SOGC) (2004) guidelines, routine episiotomies are not recommended in assisted vaginal deliveries; rather a more restrictive approach is advisable. As regards the timing of episiotomy, there are no strict recommendations but various authors advice on giving an episiotomy after applying the forceps, and before giving traction, as the role of an episiotomy is to prevent excessive and extensive perineal trauma.

Discuss epidural analgesia and assisted delivery.
Epidural analgesia is associated with an increased need for assisted vaginal birth though the likelihood of this has decreased with the newer anesthetic techniques [like use of lower concentrations of local analgesic or patient-controlled epidural analgesia (PCEA)].

The risk of assisted vaginal birth is the same whether epidural analgesia is administered in the latent or active phase of labor.

Women using epidural analgesia should be encouraged to adopt lying-down lateral positions rather than upright positions in the second stage of labor to increase the rate of spontaneous birth.

Do not discontinue epidural analgesia during pushing as it has not shown to decrease the incidence of assisted vaginal birth.

Evidence has shown that routine oxytocin augmentation does not decrease assisted vaginal birth in women on epidural analgesia.

There is insufficient evidence to recommend any specific regional anesthesia technique in terms of reducing the incidence of assisted vaginal birth. Evidence has shown that there is no difference between the rates of assisted vaginal birth for combined spinal-epidural, standard epidural technique, or PCEA.

What are the methods of Kielland's forceps application?
There are three methods: (1) Classical, (2) direct, and (3) wandering methods.

What is Scanzoni maneuver or double application technique?
Forceps rotation and delivery with a Kielland's forceps done by wandering method is also called Scanzoni or double application.

In the first application, the blades are applied as in a cephalic application, i.e., correctly in the fetal head irrespective of the pelvis; the occiput is then rotated anteriorly, which makes the blade inverted, so that the pelvic curve faces downward.

What are the contraindications for forceps application?

Absolute maternal contraindications
- Incompletely dilated cervix
- Moderate or severe degree contracted pelvis
- Cephalopelvic disproportion
- Unknown fetal position
- Pelvic tumors causing obstruction

Relative maternal contraindications
- Malpresentation (except planned breech extraction)
- Connective tissue disorders

Absolute fetal contraindications
- Presence of bleeding disorder (hemophilia, thrombocytopenia)
- Bone demineralization (osteogenesis imperfecta)

Relative fetal contraindications
- Prematurity
- Macrosomia

How do you apply forceps in direct occipitoposterior position?

After forceps application, traction is given in the horizontal direction until the root of the nose is under the symphysis. Then forward pull is given to deliver the vertex and occiput by flexion and finally backward pull to deliver the face by extension.

How do you apply forceps in face presentation?

Presentation must be mentoanterior with chin completely rotated to the front. Forceps is applied as in vertex anterior position. First, downward and backward pull is given; this will extend the face fully till the chin comes well below the symphysis pubis. Then handles are lifted upward and delivery is completed by flexion.

Why is Piper's forceps suited for delivery of aftercoming head of breech?

The following features make Piper's forceps ideal for delivery of aftercoming head of breech:
- Long shank with backward curve, so the handles are well below the level of the blades. The dropped handles allow direct application to the baby's head without the necessity of elevating the body above the horizontal.
- Blades have no pelvic curve and so allow direct application to a high head.
- Backward bend of the forceps also gives axis traction.

How is forceps applied in aftercoming head of breech?

Piper's forceps with long shanks and having perineal curve (S shape) is specially designed for this. Forceps is applied from the ventral aspect of the fetus. At first, the baby is allowed to hang unsupported, so that its head is brought down until occiput lies up against the back of symphysis pubis. The assistant holds the trunk upward. The left blade is applied directly to the right side of the baby's face. This blade is always applied first to avoid having to cross the shanks in order to lock the forceps. The opposite blade is then applied and the forceps locked. After checking for accuracy of application, the head is delivered by downward traction. Once the chin appears at the introitus, the forceps handles are elevated forward and upward delivering the head by flexion. Since the blades have no pelvic curve, a deep episiotomy should be performed to prevent damage to the vagina and perineum.

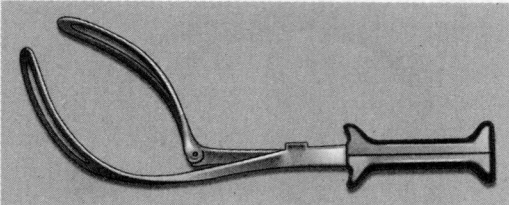

Fig. 3: Barton's forceps.

Describe Barton's forceps (Fig. 3).
The forceps has two fenestrated blades with a sliding lock. The posterior blade has a deep cephalic curve and the anterior blade is hinged, which is flexible over an arc of 90°. The blades are attached to the shank at about a 50° angle.

What is the role of forceps during cesarean section?
Single blade can be used as a vectis or both the blades can also be used.

The lower blade is applied first followed by anterior blade and then the head is delivered by controlled traction.

Trial forceps is an attempt at forceps delivery when anticipating difficulty and ready to abandon the procedure in favor of cesarean section. It is done in the operating room equipped for cesarean delivery.

What is failed forceps?
Failed forceps refers to an unsuccessful attempt to deliver with forceps even after three pulls.

Causes
- Undiagnosed occipitoposterior
- Cervix not fully dilated
- Constriction ring
- Cephalopelvic disproportion
- Hydrocephalus
- Soft-tissue obstruction—lower segment fibroid and ovarian tumor.

What factors are associated with higher rates of failure of assisted delivery?
Higher rates of failure of forceps or ventouse are associated with:
- Maternal body mass index (BMI) >30 kg/m^2
- Short maternal stature
- Large fetus or estimated fetal weight >4 kg
- Head circumference above 95th percentile
- Occipitoposterior position

When should attempted forceps delivery be discontinued?
The forceps delivery should be discontinued if:
- The forceps cannot be applied easily
- The handles do not approximate easily
- If there is no progressive descent even with moderate traction
- If birth is not imminent following three pulls of a correctly applied instrument.

It is important to be aware of the increased risk of fetal head impaction at cesarean section following a failed forceps delivery attempt.

What are the complications of forceps delivery?
Maternal complications
- Vaginal and cervical tears—13% for outlet and 22% with low forceps
- Extension of episiotomy
- Injury to rectum or bladder
- Postpartum hemorrhage
- Sepsis
- Urinary retention and sphincter dysfunction

Fetal complications
- Birth asphyxia
- Intracranial hemorrhage
- Depressed fracture of skull
- Tears of tentorium cerebelli
- Cephalhematoma
- Nerve injuries—facial nerve palsy (0.9% for outlet, 1.7% for low, 9.4% for midpelvic forceps).

Should prophylactic antibiotics be given after forceps delivery?
The RCOG recommends a single dose of intravenous amoxicillin and clavulanic acid following assisted vaginal delivery as it been shown to decrease maternal infection as compared to placebo.

■ VENTOUSE

Identify the instrument (Fig. 4).
The instrument is a metallic ventouse cup.

What are the types of ventouse cups available (Fig. 5)?
There are two types of cups available:
1. *Metal cup (Malmstrom):* A stainless steel and rigid cup
2. *Soft cup—Silastic cup (Kobayashi):* Disposable polyethylene or combined polyethylene and disposable plastic cups (Mityvac).
   They come in four sizes—30, 40, 50, and 60 mm **(Fig. 5)**.

What is Bird's modification of the vacuum cup?
In this modification, the vacuum tube is placed eccentrically on the suction cup and a separate traction chain with handle is used. The vacuum tube is placed eccentrically in Bird's anterior cup (used for occipitoanterior position) and shifted to the side wall of the cup in Bird's posterior cup (used for occipitotransverse and occipitoposterior positions) **(Fig. 6)**.

How is a vacuum delivery more physiologic than forceps delivery?
- Traction is applied only to the instrument in vacuum delivery.
- Patient assists in delivery. Generally, as only pudendal block is given during vacuum delivery, the patient is able to push when traction is applied during contraction.

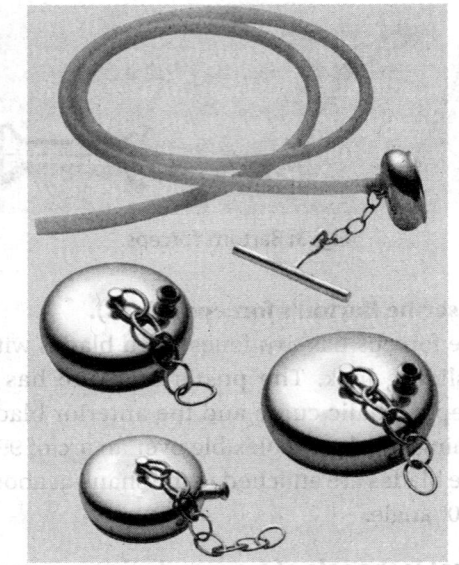
Fig. 4: Metallic ventouse cup.

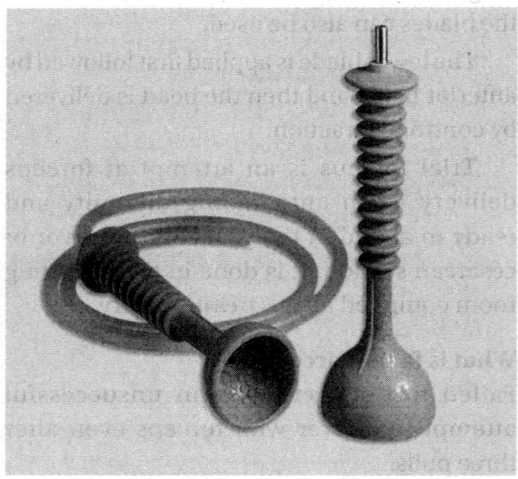
Fig. 5: Ventouse with silastic cups.

What are the advantages of silastic cup?
- Silastic cup can shape to the fetal head.
- It has no sharp edge.
- It causes less scalp trauma.
- Vacuum can be built up and released between contractions with the same effect.

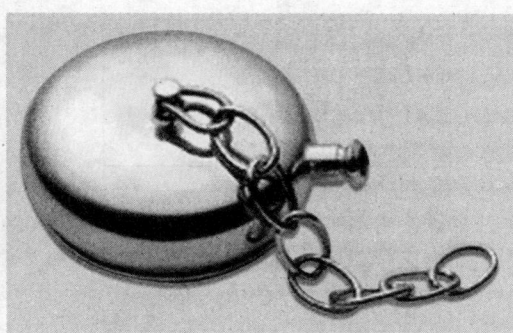

Fig. 6: Bird's modification.

What are the indications for ventouse application?
The indications for ventouse application are the same as those for forceps.

What is chignon?
An artificial caput succedaneum formed after ventouse application is known as chignon.

How much pressure is created by effective vacuum and in how much time?
Pressure is gradually raised at the rate of 0.1 kg/cm^2 per minute until effective vacuum of 0.8 kg/cm^2 is achieved in 5–8 minutes.

What are the advantages of ventouse over forceps?
- It can be applied in unrotated or malrotated occipitosterior position.
- It does not occupy space.
- It can be applied even when head is at high level in comparison to forceps.
- Lesser traction is required.
- Less skill is required.

What are the contraindications for ventouse application?
- Presentation other than vertex (face, brow, and breech)
- Preterm fetus—the risk of subgaleal hemorrhage and scalp trauma is higher with ventouse delivery than forceps at preterm gestational ages. Vacuum birth should be avoided below 32 weeks' gestation and used with caution in fetuses between 32 and 36 weeks' gestation
- High station
- Cephalopelvic disproportion
- Fetal coagulopathy
- Recent fetal scalp blood sampling.

What are the prerequisites for ventouse application?
- There should be no bony resistance below the head.
- Cervix should be fully dilated (RCOG 2011).
- Head should be engaged less than 1/5th palpable per abdomen.

How should ventouse be applied?
- Largest possible cup should be used according to dilatation.
- Episiotomy is optional.
- Proper placement of the cup—center of cup on "flexion point", which is 3 cm in front of posterior fontanelle in midline close to occiput **(Fig. 7)**.
- Ensure that no cervical or vaginal tissue is trapped.
- A vacuum of 0.2 kg/cm^2 is created and increased at the rate of 0.1–0.8 kg/cm^2 till a good chignon is formed.
- Traction must be at right angles to cup and should be applied with uterine contraction.
- Traction is made by one hand and the other hand presses the cup over the fetal head; not more than three pulls are applied.
- Release vacuum after delivery of head; inspect cervix and vagina after delivery.

How many attempts should be made?
If there is no descent after three successive uterine contractions, no further trial should be given [Food and Drug Administration (FDA) approved].

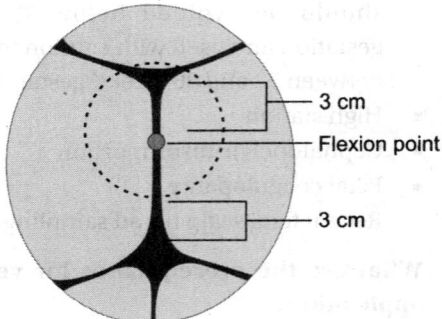 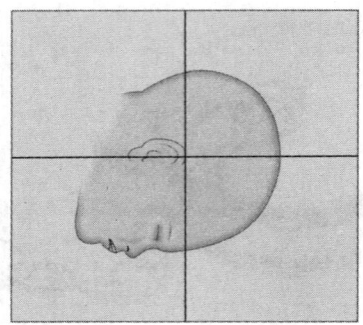

Fig. 7: Pivot point.

Rapid versus slow method of vacuum application—which is better?
- *Slow method:* 0.2 kg/cm² per 2 minutes; vacuum is created in four steps up to 0.8 kg/cm² taking 8 minutes
- *Rapid method:* 0.8 kg/cm²; vacuum is created in single step in <2 minutes.

No significant difference in detachment rate, fetal, and maternal morbidity was found with either method (RCOG 2011).

However, the World Health Organization Reproductive Health Library (WHO RHL) 2013/RCOG 2020 recommend a rapid method, as it reduces duration of procedure to <6 minutes, while there is no evidence of difference in maternal/neonatal outcome.

What are the complications of ventouse application?
Fetal complications
- Scalp injury: 0.8–33%
- Cephalhematoma: 1–26%
- Intracranial hemorrhage
- Subaponeurotic hemorrhage
- Retinal hemorrhage

Maternal complications: Genital tract injuries—cervical tears and vaginal wall lacerations.

What is the mean failure rate of ventouse?
The mean failure rate of ventouse is 9% with rigid cups and about 16% with soft cups.

When should vacuum-assisted birth be discontinued?
If there is no descent of fetal head to the maternal perineum after a maximum of three pulls, the procedure should be discontinued.

Also, if there have been two "pop-offs" of the instrument, the procedure should be discontinued.

How would you compare vacuum extraction with forceps delivery?
Cochrane metanalysis of randomized trials comparing ventouse and forceps delivery concluded that vacuum extraction was:
- More likely to fail at achieving vaginal birth
- Associated with more cephalhematoma
- Increased association with retinal hemorrhage
- Less likely to be associated with significant maternal perineal and vaginal trauma
- Associated with less pain at delivery and at 24 hours
- No more likely to be associated with birth by cesarean section
- Not associated with significantly different neonatal morbidity with respect to low 5 minute Apgar scores or need for phototherapy

How do you compare the maternal outcomes for vacuum and forceps-assisted vaginal birth?

- Episiotomy with vacuum, episiotomy is given in 50–60% women while in forceps it is performed in >90% patients
- Significant vulvovaginal tears—10% with vacuum and 20% with forceps delivery
- OASI (obstetric anal sphincter injuries)—1 to 4% with vacuum and 8–12% with forceps
- Postpartum hemorrhage—10 to 40% with both vacuum and forceps

Discuss the perinatal outcomes with assisted vaginal birth.

- Cephalhematoma—seen in 1–12%; predominantly in vacuum births
- Subgaleal hemorrhage—3 to 6 in 1,000 vacuum deliveries
- Intracranial hemorrhage—5 to 15 in 10,000 vacuum and forceps
- Facial or scalp lacerations—10%
- Retinal hemorrhage—17 to 38%; more common with vacuum
- Jaundice—5 to 15%
- Cervical spine injury—seen mainly with Kielland's rotational forceps
- Facial nerve palsy—rare but mainly seen with forceps.

What conditions are associated with higher failure rates of operative vaginal delivery?

Factors associated with unsuccessful assisted vaginal delivery are:
- Increased birth weight
- Increased duration of second stage of labor
- Attempted rotation of fetal head
- Elderly gravidas
- Increased BMI of mother
- Epidural analgesia.

What is Odon device?

The Odon device is a novel, single-use, new device for assisted vaginal birth that employs an air cuff around the fetal head for traction. The lack of negative pressure on the fetal head which is seen in vacuum delivery is eliminated with Odon device, and thus it lowers the incidence of intracranial hemorrhage. Also, as the pressure applied is less than during a forceps application, it is associated with a lower incidence of adverse events.

■ SUGGESTED READING

1. Dalvi SA. Difficult deliveries in cesarean section. J Obstet Gynaecol India. 2018;68(5): 344-348.
2. Hobson S, Cassell K, Windrim R, Cargill Y. Assisted vaginal birth. SOGC Clinical Practice Guideline 2019;41(6):870-82.
3. Lemos A, Amorim MM, Dornelas de Andrade A, de Souza AI, Cabral Filho JE, Correia JB. Pushing/bearing down methods for the second stage of labour. Cochrane Database Syst Rev. 2017;3(3):CD009124.
4. Murphy DJ, Strachan BK, Bahl R, on behalf of Royal College of Obstetricians Gynecologists. Assisted vaginal Birth. BJOG 2020;127:e70-e112.
5. Operative Vaginal Birth: ACOG Practice Bulletin, Number 219. Obstet Gynecol. 2020;135(4):e149-e159.
6. Suwannachat B, Lumbiganon P, Laopaiboon M. Rapid versus stepwise negative pressure application for vacuum extraction assisted vaginal delivery. Cochrane Database Syst Rev. 2012; CD006636.

9. Obstetric Procedures

Abha Sharma, Sruthi Bhaskaran

■ INTRODUCTION

Obstetrics procedures are maneuvers or surgical interventions done on pregnant women for conditions associated with pregnancy, labor, or puerperium.

■ EXTERNAL CEPHALIC VERSION

What is external cephalic version?
External cephalic version (ECV) is a procedure by which fetal presentation is altered by physical manipulation through maternal abdomen and to bring the favorable cephalic pole as the presenting part to reduce cesarean rates.

What are the recommendations for external cephalic version in modern obstetrics?
External cephalic version is offered to all low-risk women with breech or transverse lie at term. There is no role of ECV before term. According to the Cochrane 2015 review, there is no effect of ECV before term on the rate of breech presentation at delivery, cesarean section, Apgar scores, or perinatal mortality.

In view of lack of evidence of effectiveness and reports of unacceptably high complication rates from ECV before term, there is at present no place for ECV before term in modern obstetrics.

There is sound reason to use ECV at term with caution. The *American College of Obstetricians and Gynecologists (ACOG) (2020) recommends that efforts be made to reduce breech presentation by ECV whenever possible.*

What is the success rate of external cephalic version?
The success rate of external cephalic version is 35–85% (average of about 50%).

What is the best time for version?
- The best time for version is 36–37 weeks, but any point thereafter till early labor.
- *Early version:* Chances of reversion are more.
- *Late version:* Procedure is difficult because of increasing size of the fetus and diminishing liquor; however, use of uterine relaxants (tocolytics) has made version at later weeks easier and, if complications develop, labor can be augmented by artificial rupture of membrane (ARM) or delivered by lower-segment cesarean section (LSCS).

What are the contraindications of external cephalic version?
Any contraindication to vaginal delivery is a contraindication to ECV. Other relative contraindications include:
- Antepartum hemorrhage (previa or abruption)
- Multiple pregnancy
- Ruptured membranes
- Congenital malformation of uterus
- Contracted pelvis
- *Obstetric complications:* Severe pre-eclampsia, obesity, elderly primigravida, and bad obstetric history
- Estimation of fetal weight (EFW) 4 kg or more

- Engaged presenting part
- *Fetal causes:* Congenital malformation, dead fetus, hyperextension of head, fetal compromise, and oligohydramnios.

In which cases is successful version possible?
- Multiparity
- Complete breech
- *Nonlongitudinal lie:* A fetus in oblique or transverse position
- Nonengaged breech
- Sacroanterior position and lateral fetal spine positions
- Adequate liquor [amniotic fluid index (AFI) >10 cm]
- Nonobese patient

What are the causes for failure of version?
- Nulliparity
- Breech with extended legs/engaged
- Scanty liquor
- Big-size baby
- Fetal weight <2,500 g
- *Mechanical:* Obesity, increased tone of the abdominal muscles, and irritable uterus
- Low station of fetal head
- Short cord
- Malformations of the uterus
- Sacroposterior position
- Anterior/cornual placenta

What are the risks of version?
Complications after ECV is <1% and include the following:
- Premature onset of labor
- Premature rupture of membranes
- Umbilical cord prolapse
- Placental separation and bleeding (0.1%)
- Entanglement of cord around the fetal part or formation of a true knot leading to impairment of fetal circulation
- Increased incidence of fetomaternal hemorrhage
- *Fetal heart rate changes:* Usually stabilizes once procedure is discontinued
- Stillbirth
- Amniotic fluid embolism
- Need for emergency cesarean section (0.5%)

Can external cephalic version be attempted in a scarred uterus?
There is limited information regarding ECV in women with previous cesarean section. Majority studies done are on previous one cesarean, and ECV has been found to be safe.

What are the prerequisites for version?
- Rule out contraindications for ECV
- Pelvic assessment
- Reactive cardiotocography (CTG)
- Prior sonography [amount of amniotic fluid, placental localization, and bisphenol S (BPS)]
- Informed consent
- *Tocolytic drugs (250 µg terbutaline subcutaneous preferred):* Contraindicated in significant heart disease, hypertension; side effects–tachycardia, flushing, tremors, and palpitations
- *Spinal/epidural anesthesia (ECV 1.5 times more successful):* May be considered for a repeat attempt
- Availability of fully equipped OT for LSCS, if required.
- Fasting, administration of anesthetic premedication or insertion of intravenous access (unless for tocolysis)—not recommended.

What are the postversion requisites?
- *Recheck CTG:* Fetal heart monitoring to be done for at least 30 minutes or more if indicated. A transient (<3 minutes) fetal bradycardia after ECV is common; continuous fetal monitoring in left lateral position is done, if does not improve after 6 minutes, prepare for cesarean section.

- Anti-D administration (if Rh-negative) 500 IU within 72 hours (ideally after Kleihauer–Betke test for amount of fetomaternal hemorrhage).

What is the management of failed version?
Pregnancy is continued with usual check-up and unexpectedly one may find that spontaneous version has occurred.

Reassess: Age of the mother, especially primigravida, associated complicating factors, size of the baby, and pelvic capacity; accordingly decide mode of delivery.

Elective LSCS:
- Baby >3.5 kg
- Hyperextension of the head
- Footling presentation
- Pelvic contraction
- Associated complicating factors

Vaginal breech delivery
- *Fetal weight:* 1.5–3.5 kg
- Adequate pelvis
- Flexed head
- No other complication
- Frank breech

What are the most consistent factors associated with successful version?
- Increasing parity
- Nonengaged and complete breech with spine in lateral position
- Good amount of amniotic fluid
- Gestational age (earlier attempts increase the chance of success, but chance of reversion is more).

What are the techniques for external cephalic version and how are they performed?
- A forward roll or a backward flip
- For ease of hand movements and maneuvering, ultrasound coupling gel or powder is applied to abdomen.
- The breech is disengaged from pelvis by slowly inserting fingertips of both hands deeply behind pubic symphysis and scooping breech out. ECV may be done by two obstetricians simultaneously.
- The ACOG describes beginning with a forward roll and then attempting a backward roll, if the forward roll fails.
- *Forward roll:* Operator stands on the opposite side of fetal back. For the fetus in the left sacrolateral position, the operator stands on the right side. The breech is held with right palm and pushed toward patients left flank and head with left palm and pushed toward right flank. More pressure is applied to the head than the breech, to maintain flexion of the baby.
- *Backward flip:* Operator stands on the same side as fetal back. For left sacrolateral position, operator stands on left side of patient. The breech is held with the left palm and pushed toward the patient's right flank and upward, taking care to apply most pressure to the breech so that a flexed posture is maintained. Slight back-and-forth movement between the two hands may help promote fetal movement; however, generally, pressure on the fetus should be slow and steady rather than repeated pushing.
- The fetal heart rate is auscultated every 2 minutes.

When should version be stopped?
- Excessive discomfort
- Persistently, abnormal fetal heart rate
- Multiple failed attempts (maximum 4 attempts, with overall 10 minutes' duration)

What are the alternatives to external cephalic version?
- *Expectant:* 3% likelihood of spontaneous conversion

- *Postural maneuvers:* Pelvic elevation by wedge or knee chest position. Not very successful but can be easily done at home
- *Version during labor:* Not very successful because of tense uterus and large baby
- *Moxibustion:* Burning the herbal preparation moxa to generate heat to stimulate acupuncture point BL67 to promote spontaneous breech version
- *Hypnosis:* With suggestion of soft-tissue relaxation
- *Acoustic stimulation:* To startle breech fetus to shift its spine laterally for successful manual version attempts.

INTERNAL PODALIC VERSION

What is internal podalic version?
Internal podalic version (IPV) is a procedure where the accoucheur hand or fingers are inserted through the dilated cervix and one or both lower limbs of the fetus are brought down into the maternal pelvis to expedite vaginal delivery.

Braxton Hicks version is an IPV performed through a partially but not completely dilated cervix; for a nonviable fetus.

What are the indications of internal podalic version?
In current obstetrics, the role of IPV followed by breech extraction is limited to malpresentation or abnormal lie of the second twin.

Rarely, it is done in the case of nonviable or dead singleton fetus in transverse lie at full dilatation in presence of experienced operator.

What are the contraindications of internal podalic version?
- Signs of obstructed labor
- Danger of rupture uterus
- Maternal shock
- Possibility of excessive intrauterine manipulations.

What are the risks of internal podalic version?
- Rupture uterus
- Postpartum hemorrhage (PPH)
- Infection

What are the prerequisites for internal podalic version?
- Informed consent
- Uterus contracting and relaxing
- Small baby with good liquor or just ruptured membranes
- Rule out contraindications
- Good antibiotics and anesthesia.

What are the postversion requisites?
- Check for genital trauma specially rupture
- Prevention of PPH
- Antibiotics

MANUAL REMOVAL OF PLACENTA

What is manual removal of placenta?
Manual removal of placenta (MRP) is the evacuation of the placenta from the uterus by hand.

What are the indications of manual removal of placenta?
- Retained placenta (postdelivery >30 minutes, if active management or >60 minutes for expectant management)
- Severe hemorrhage postdelivery with placenta in situ.

What are the contraindication for manual removal of placenta?
The contraindication for manual removal of placenta is known cases of placenta increta or percreta.

What are the prerequisites for manual removal of placenta?
- Adequate blood replacement
- Anesthesia
- Consent for laparotomy/hysterectomy, if placenta accreta is encountered
- Antibiotics
- Ultrasound (USG) can be used to rule out placenta accreta before shifting the patient for MRP.

What is the technique of manual removal of placenta?
Under anesthesia, a gloved hand is introduced into the uterus, with the other hand on the fundus to control it. The umbilical cord is followed until the lower edge of the placenta is found. The hand is pushed between the placenta and the body of the uterus, and placenta is eased away with a sawing action. When fully detached, the uterine cavity is explored for damage and for other pieces of placenta. The placenta and membranes are removed with the hand in the uterine cavity. Oxytocics are given to contract the uterus. Placenta is examined to be sure that it is complete.

What are the complications of manual removal of placenta?
- Hemorrhage, if try to separate placenta accreta
- Trauma to uterus or cervix
- Atonic PPH
- Inversion uterus
- Infection

What is the management of failed manual removal of placenta?
- The most common cause is undiagnosed placenta accreta. In multiparous patient and in severe hemorrhage, hysterectomy is preferred.
- In patient, who is stable and not bleeding, conservative options (i.e., placenta left in situ) can be tried. This includes—uterine artery embolization, methotrexate, and internal iliac artery ligation. These patients may require hysterectomy at a later date.

PRENATAL DIAGNOSTIC TECHNIQUES
- *Noninvasive (screening tests):* Noninvasive prenatal testing (cell-free fetal DNA and fetal cells circulating in maternal blood), biochemical markers, and USG. (*See* Chapter 3 for details)
- *Invasive:* (Diagnostic tests)
  - Preimplantation genetic diagnosis (PGD)
    - Chorionic villus biopsy
    - Amniocentesis
    - Cordocentesis
    - Fetal tissue biopsy

What are the indications of prenatal diagnostic techniques?
- *A positive screening test [noninvasive prenatal testing (NIPT), double marker, quadruple test] on the maternal blood:* Earlier, advanced maternal age was the most common indication for prenatal cytogenetic analysis. However, now a high risk for aneuploidy on screening test is the most common indication.
- Previous pregnancy resulting in the birth of a child with Down syndrome or other chromosomal abnormalities
- Existence of a chromosomal abnormality in either parent or carrier of balanced chromosomal rearrangement
- History of Down's syndrome or other chromosomal abnormality in a family member
- Birth of a previous child with multiple major malformations
- Pregnancy in women who have X-linked disorders in male relatives

- *Ultrasound markers suggestive of chromosomal aberrations:* The possibility of chromosomal anomaly in a fetus with any single malformation is 5–10%. If two or more malformations are there, the risk increases to >20%. Malformations more likely to be associated with chromosomal anomalies are cystic hygroma (45,X), duodenal atresia (Down syndrome), holoprosencephaly (trisomy 13), omphalocele, and cardiac malformations.
- *Ultrasonographic abnormalities other than malformations (soft markers):* Like increased nuchal translucency, echogenic cardiac focus, echogenic bowel, short femur, renal pyelectasis, etc.
- History of metabolic disorders in the family where enzyme studies may be useful.
- Hematological disorders which can be diagnosed by gene probe techniques.
- Suspected fetal infection.

What is preimplantation genetic diagnosis?
Preimplantation genetic diagnosis is an established alternative to prenatal diagnosis, and involves testing embryos for specific genetic disorders before implantation and selecting preimplantation embryos from a cohort generated by assisted reproduction technology (ART).

What is the sensitivity of diagnosis?
Various studies have reported 95–96% detection rates for numerical chromosomal abnormalities in one blastomere analysis.

What are the indications for preimplantation genetic diagnosis?
- Familial monogenic disease (e.g., cystic fibrosis)
- One partner carries a chromosome rearrangement (e.g., a two-way reciprocal translocation)
- Recurrent failed implantation among women with unexplained infertility [preimplantation genetic screening (PGS) for aneuploidy].

What are the methods used?
Biopsy can be performed on:
- *Blastocyst:* Day 5–6 postfertilization trophoectodermal cells biopsied
- Single blastomere from cleavage-stage embryos on day 3 postfertilization
- *Polar body biopsy:* Polar bodies from oocytes and zygote are biopsied (In countries where biopsy of an embryo is not permitted this is an option). The biopsied cell is tested to establish the genetic status of the embryo.

What testing is done in preimplantation genetic diagnosis?
There are three types of testing done in PGD:
1. *Preimplantation genetic testing for aneuploidy (PGT-A):* To identify embryos with aneuploidy, including subchromosomal deletions and additions
2. *Preimplantation genetic testing for monogenic (single-gene) disorders (PGT-M):* In known heritable pathogenic variant carried by one or both biological parents
3. *Preimplantation genetic testing for structural rearrangements (PGT-SR):* To establish a pregnancy that is unaffected by a structural chromosomal abnormality (translocation) in a couple with a balanced translocation or deletion/duplication.

CHORIONIC VILLUS BIOPSY

When is chorionic villus biopsy performed?
Chorionic villus biopsy is performed between 10 and 13 weeks

What are the cells obtained?
Trophoblast cells:
- *Direct preparation:* 24–48 hours
- *Cultures:* 10–14 days

What are the associated risks?
- *Fetal loss:* Overall 0.22%
  - *Transcervical:* Approximately 0.27% when forceps is used and 3.12% for those done with cannula by a trained operator
  - *Transabdominal:* By appropriately trained operator <0.5%
- Cramping, spotting, and bleeding (32% after transcervical approach)
- *Chorioamnionitis:* 0.2–0.3%
- Rupture of membranes: <0.5%
- Rh-negative immunization
- Incidence of limb reduction defects after 9 weeks is 6/10,000 and the same as background incidence. The frequency of oromandibular and limb hypogenesis; however, it is increased after CVS when performed before 9 weeks.

What is the reliability of the test?
- *False positive:* 2% (amniocentesis—0.06%)
- *False negative:* 0.1% (amniocentesis—1/400,000)

What are the contraindications to chorionic villus sampling?
- Positive *Neisseria gonorrhoeae* culture
- Active genital herpes
- Active bleeding
- Maternal coagulopathy
- Cervical stenosis
- Severe cervicitis
- Uterine myoma
- Intrauterine device (IUD) inside the pregnant uterus

What are the advantages and disadvantages of transcervical chorionic villus sampling?
Advantages:
- Genetic diagnosis is achieved at early gestational age minimizing the anxiety of the parents and facilitating termination of pregnancy at early gestation
- Comfortable for patient
- Technically simple

Disadvantages:
- Slightly higher risk of fetal loss
- Chromosome composition of the chorionic tissue may be different from the chromosome of fetal cells
- Difficult, if placenta is fundal

What are the advantages and disadvantages of transabdominal chorionic villus sampling?
Risk of fetal loss is same as amniocentesis; and literature suggests that risk may be minimized, if transabdominal CVS is performed only after 12 weeks.

Advantages:
- Minimal risk of infection
- Does not cause vaginal bleeding
- It can be performed in second or third trimester.

Disadvantages:
- Amount of tissue obtained is less than with transcervical CVS
- Patient discomfort is greater
- Difficult to perform, if placenta is posterior
- Technically more difficult.

How is the procedure performed?
The procedure is performed under ultrasound guidance and route depends on operator preference, location of placenta (fundal-transabdominal), and retroflexed uterus (transcervical preferred).

Transabdominal: The patient is placed in the supine position and placenta is localized by transabdominal ultrasonography. Under aseptic precautions and after local anesthesia application, 19–20-gauge needle is inserted under ultrasound guidance. Needle is inserted at an angle that allows it to penetrate along the long axis of the placenta. The needle tip is moved back and forth inside the placenta until an adequate sample has been aspirated by the vacuum created in the syringe containing 3 mL of culture medium. The sampling system is then withdrawn under negative pressure. The tissue is put in a plastic tissue culture dish and the content evaluated at a nearby microscope.

Transcervical: The patient is placed in the lithotomy position. Under transabdominal ultrasound guidance and aseptic precautions, plastic cannula is inserted under ultrasound guidance through the canal and into the placenta. The obturator of the cannula is removed and a 20-mL syringe containing medium is attached to the catheter. Chorionic villi are aspirated as the catheter is moved back and forth inside the placenta. The catheter is withdrawn while keeping the syringe under negative pressure. An alternative transcervical method uses a biopsy forceps for sampling. Rest of the procedure is similar to transabdominal.

- At least 5 mg of villus tissue is generally required for genetic studies and should be transported within 24 hours to the laboratory.
- Sampling failure is reported to occur in 2.5–4.8% of procedures.

What are the laboratory aspects?

- A direct cytogenetic analysis and needs only 4 hours
- Useful for detecting numeric abnormalities and major rearrangements
- B-cell culture.
  If direct analysis and culture reveals mosaicism, then confirm it by fetal blood sampling.

■ AMNIOCENTESIS

What are the indications for amniocentesis?

- *Diagnostic*
  - *Early pregnancy:*
    - Sex-linked disorders
    - Karyotyping
    - Inborn errors of metabolism
    - Neural tube defects
    - Fetal infections
  - *Late pregnancy:*
    - Fetal maturity
    - Degree of hemolysis in Rh-sensitized mother
    - Newly diagnosed fetal structural anomaly
    - Early onset fetal growth restriction
    - Meconium staining of liquor
    - Amniography/fetography
- *Therapeutic*
  - *Early pregnancy:*
    - Induction of abortion
    - Repeated decompression in acute hydramnios
  - *Late pregnancy:*
    - Decompression in chronic hydramnios
    - To give intrauterine transfusion
    - Amnioinfusion

When should amniocentesis be performed?

- *Between* 15 weeks and 20 weeks
- *Early amniocentesis:* 11–12 weeks

What are the disadvantages of early amniocentesis?

Currently, early amniocentesis is not recommended due to following disadvantages:

- It is associated with an increased abortion rate.
- Increased incidence of talipes equinovarus (early vs. midtrimester—1.3 vs. 0.1%, respectively)
- Low yield of cells

What are the cells obtained?
On amniocentesis, fetal fibroblast and fluid are obtained for biochemical study.

What are the hazards of amniocentesis?
- *Maternal hazards:*
  - Infection
  - Hemorrhage
  - Preterm labor
  - Premature rupture of membranes ~1.7%
  - Rh isoimmunization
- *Fetal hazards:*
  - Abortion (<1%)
  - Trauma
  - Fetomaternal hemorrhage
  - Oligohydramnios due to leakage of amniotic fluid causes pulmonary hypoplasia, cord compression, and limb contracture deformity.

What are the prerequisites for amniocentesis?
- Maternal blood group and Rh factor
- *Level-2 USG:*
  - To determine the number of fetus
  - To measure the biparietal diameter (BPD), femur length, and abdominal and head circumference
  - To visualize extremities
  - To locate the placenta

How is amniocentesis done?
- Select an adequate puncture site. Avoid placenta and placental cord insertion site for entry. If there is no area free of placenta, a thin area, away from the center of the organ, and its large vessels should be selected and a 22-gauge needle used to withdraw the amniotic fluid. Before amniocentesis is performed, the area selected for inserting the needle should be examined with color Doppler to be certain that a large placental vessel is not present.
- Part preparation
- Local anesthesia, unnecessary although it relieves some of the patients anxiety
- 20–22-gauge needle is used; done under USG guidance
- Needle insertion is in two successive steps: (1) The first step will carry the tip of needle into the subcutaneous tissue; and (2) the second step will place it inside the amniotic cavity, (as the patient involuntary contracts the muscle of the anterior abdominal wall when they feel needle in contact with the skin and this may cause the needle to deviate from its intended route)
- Stylet is removed and connected to a plastic connecting tube, fluid is aspirated with a sterile syringe and the first few mL is discarded because of possible contamination with maternal cells
- Two 10 mL aliquots of fluid are withdrawn (amount of fluid withdrawn should approximately be equal to gestational age, e.g., 15 weeks: 15 mL). Initial 2 mL of fluid should be discarded to avoid maternal cell contamination or can be sent for evaluation of alpha-fetoprotein levels. If bloody fluid is aspirated, a small amount of heparin should be added to reduce clumping of the amniocytes in clotted blood.
- Postamniocentesis, fetal heart is evaluated by real-time USG.

What genetic tests is the amniocentesis sample sent for?
The choice of genetic test to be performed on the cells obtained via amniocentesis depends in part on the indication for testing.
- *Chromosomal analysis (karyotyping):* 7–14 days
- *FISH (fluorescence in situ hybridization):* Limited karyotyping—24–48 hours

- *Chromosomal microarray can identify microdeletions and microduplications:* 3-5 days with direct testing and 10-14 days with cultured cell

Is there a risk of vertical transmission of HIV and HbsAg after amniocentesis?
- Screening for bloodborne viral infections including viral load should be done prior to amniocentesis.
- The risk of mother-to-child transmission (MTCT) of HIV for women on highly active antiretroviral therapy (HAART) with undetectable viral loads is very low.
- Antiretroviral treatment should be optimized to aim for an undetectable viral load prior to amniocentesis or CVS.
- The risk of MTCT of Hepatitis B is low with viral load <6.99 $\log_{10}$ copies/mL but increases with higher viral loads (HBV DNA >500 copies/mL)

CORDOCENTESIS (PERCUTANEOUS UMBILICAL BLOOD SAMPLING)

What are the indications for cordocentesis?
- Fetal anemia
- Chromosomal analysis
- Inborn error of metabolism
- Coagulopathies
- Hemoglobinopathies
- Hematological—for fetal anemia
- Fetal infections—toxoplasmosis and viral infection
- Fetal blood gas and acid–base status
- Fetal therapy

What are the complications of cordocentesis?
- *Fetal loss:* 2-4% (increased risk seen in-fetal structural defects (including hydrops), fetal growth restriction, gestational age < 24 weeks)
- *Hemorrhage:* 30%
- *Fetal bradycardia:* 5% (transient fetal bradycardia is common and recovers spontaneously). In a few percentage of cases, fetal exsanguination could present as persistent fetal tachycardia without bradycardia
- Amniotic fluid leakage
- Preterm labor
- Amnionitis
- Hematoma

Fetal loss depends upon the indication for fetal blood sampling:
- *Low-risk fetus:* Loss rate around 2%
- *High-risk fetus:* Loss rate as high as 43%

How is the procedure done?
- The procedure is done after 18 weeks.
- 20-22-gauge needle and 13 cm in length is used.
- *Done under ultrasonic guidance:* Puncture umbilical vein 1-2 cm from cord insertion at placenta, as it is a fixed point and will not be affected by fetal movement. If the placenta is anterior, puncture of cord is attempted at the level of placental insertion. If the placenta is posterior, a free loop of the cord or the intra-abdominal portion of the umbilical vein is sampled. Advantages of sampling at the intrahepatic vein include absence of cord complications, reduced risk of fetal blood loss and fetomaternal hemorrhage, and certainty of the fetal origin of the sample. Umbilical artery is to be avoided as puncture of the artery increases the incidence of bradycardia and postprocedural bleeding. Flushing with saline may be used to confirm its correct position and around 3–5 mL blood is taken.
- One sample is sent for rapid karyotype, another for Kleihauer–Betke stain and for the determination of mean corpuscular volume (MCV) of the erythrocytes, which

is always higher in fetal blood than in maternal blood >100 (thereby assures that fetal blood has been sampled)
- *Postprocedure:* Real-time USG for fetal heart motion, check for hemorrhage, and anti-D to be given, if nonimmunized Rh-negative pregnancy.

Why is umbilical vein preferred?
As the umbilical vein is larger with a larger lumen, it is less likely to constrict and to cause fetal bradycardia when punctured.

What is the significance of the test?
Test is highly accurate, but due to advances in cytogenetic and molecular studies, the use of fetal blood for diagnosis has diminished.

Use of fetal blood for diagnosis of trisomy 13, 18, and 21 has largely been replaced by FISH, as amniocytes can provide reliable diagnosis within 1–2 days.

For viral infections, polymerase chain reaction (PCR) is done on amniotic fluid.

Increased use of USG for fetal surveillance (biophysical and Doppler) has reduced the need for fetal blood for acid–base status of fetus.

But it is the method of choice in:
- Diagnosis and therapeutic intervention for erythroblastosis fetalis
- Thrombocytopenia (alloimmune and idiopathic), to assess fetal platelet count
- If mosaicism determined in cytogenetic analysis at CVS, knowledge of fetal karyotype in late second or third trimester.

■ FETAL TISSUE BIOPSY

What are the indications for fetal skin biopsy?
- Epidermolysis bullosa
- Epidermolysis atrophica gravis
- Epidermolysis atrophica inversa
- Oculocutaneous albinism
- Incontinentia pigmenti
- Sjögren-Larsen syndrome
- Ehlers–Danlos syndrome
- Ectodermal dysphasia

What are the indications for fetal liver biopsy?
Fetal liver biopsy is done in case of ornithine carbamoyltransferase deficiency.

What are the indications for fetal muscle biopsy?
Genetic myopathies: Duchene muscular dystrophy. Usually, deletion analysis or linkage analysis or DNA isolated from either amniocytes or chorionic villi provides reliable diagnosis, but in rare cases, these methods fail then muscle biopsy serves as a useful option.

Most commonly performed in fetal gluteal muscle.

In which cases is fetal kidney biopsy done?
- Congenital nephrosis
- Fetal liver and kidney biopsy hold a small place in the diagnostic armamentarium of the prenatal geneticist; however, in rare cases, they may be used to relieve the diagnostic dilemma for high-risk families with a previous affected child.

■ SUGGESTED READING

1. Alfirevic Z, Navaratnam K, Mujezinovic F. Amniocentesis and chorionic villus sampling for prenatal diagnosis. Cochrane Database Syst Rev. 2017;9(9):CD003252.
2. External Cephalic Version: ACOG Practice Bulletin, Number 221. Obstet Gynecol. 2020;135(5):e203-e212.
3. Hofmeyr GJ, Kulier R. External cephalic version for breech presentation at term. Cochrane Database Syst Rev. 2012;10:CD000083. doi: 10.1002/14651858. CD000083.pub2. Update in: Cochrane Database Syst Rev. 2015;4:CD000083. PMID: 23076883.

4. Jindal A, Sharma M, Karena ZV, et al. Amniocentesis. [Updated 2023 Aug 14]. In: StatPearls [Internet]. Treasure Island (FL): StatPearls Publishing; 2024 Jan-. Available from: https://www.ncbi.nlm.nih.gov/books/NBK559247/
5. Peddi NC, Avanthika C, Vuppalapati S, Balasubramanian R, Kaur J, N CD. A Review of Cordocentesis: Percutaneous Umbilical Cord Blood Sampling. Cureus. 2021;13(7):e16423.
6. Practice Bulletin No. 162: Prenatal Diagnostic Testing for Genetic Disorders. Obstetrics & Gynecology 127(5):p e108-e122, May 2016.
7. Taylor-Phillips S, Freeman K, Geppert J, Agbebiyi A, Uthman OA, Madan J, et al. Accuracy of non-invasive prenatal testing using cell-free DNA for detection of Down, Edwards and Patau syndromes: a systematic review and meta-analysis. BMJ Open. 2016;6(1):e010002.

10 CHAPTER

Obstetric Drills

Upasana Verma, Sumita Mehta

■ SHOULDER DYSTOCIA

Shoulder dystocia is an obstetric emergency in which gentle downward traction of the fetal head does not lead to delivery **(Fig. 1)**. It is usually due to impaction of the anterior shoulder against the maternal symphysis pubis after delivery of the fetal head. It can be caused by impaction of posterior shoulder against sacral promontory. Bilateral shoulder impaction occurs rarely. Normally, the mean interval between the delivery of head and rest of the body is 24 seconds; whereas in shoulder dystocia, it is >60 seconds. The complications associated with shoulder dystocia are mentioned in **Box 1**.

Risk factors:
- Obesity
- Multiparity
- History of dystocia in previous pregnancy
- Diabetes
- Prolonged pregnancies
- Macrosomia

Algorithm for management of shoulder dystocia is given in **Flowchart 1**.

■ MANEUVERS

McRoberts Maneuver (Fig. 2)

Maternal thighs are hyperflexed and abducted bringing both knees toward the chest and held in that position by two assistants. This rotates the symphysis pubis upward and further opens the pelvic outlet by increasing anteroposterior (AP) diameter of pelvis.

Flowchart 1: Algorithm for management of shoulder dystocia.

Head delivered, body not delivered
↓
Diagnosis: Shoulder dystocia?
- Turtle neck sign
- Fetal face is flushed
- Failure of external rotation of head

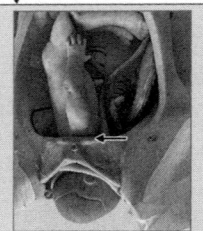

Fig. 1: Shoulder dystocia. *(For color version, see Plate 2)*

↓ Yes
- Avoid further traction over head and neck
- No fundal pressure
↓
- Initiate HELPER drill for shoulder dystocia
- Call for *Help*:
  – Senior obstetrician
  – Two assistants
  – Pediatrician
  – Anesthetist
- *Episiotomy* if not given and *Empty* bladder
  – *First-line maneuver:* McRoberts maneuver—Leg raise and abduct
  Suprapubic *Pressure*
  If fails
- *Second-line maneuver:* Extraction of posterior arm
  Rotational maneuvers: Rubin's II, Wood's corkscrew, reverse Woods corkscrew maneuver
  All fours' position
  If fails
↓
- *Third-line maneuver:* Cleidotomy, symphysiotomy, and Zavanelli maneuver
  Every maneuver is tried for at least 30–60 seconds before going to next
↓
1. Management of maternal complications
2. Neonatal resuscitation and examination for tears

This maneuver should be first used once shoulder dystocia is suspected.

Suprapubic Pressure

If delivery does not occur with the McRoberts maneuver, a firm, steady suprapubic pressure should be applied concurrently in downward or oblique direction just above the symphysis pubis towards the side the baby is facing **(Fig. 3)**. It reduces the fetal bisacromial diameter and rotates the anterior fetal shoulder into the wider oblique pelvic diameter.

BOX 1: Complications of shoulder dystocia.

Maternal:
- PPH
- Obstetric anal sphincter injuries
- Injury to vagina, bladder and urethra
- Uterine rupture
- Lateral femoral cutaneous nerve neuropathy

Fetal:
- Fracture of clavicle and humerus
- Brachial plexus injury*
- Birth asphyxia
- Neonatal death

*Most resolve without permanent disability; however, 10% may result in permanent neurologic injury.

Internal Maneuvers

Delivery of Posterior Arm

Compress all five fingers from the appropriate hand into a "duck-bill" shape, and gently maneuver the hand into the posterior vagina, under the baby. Then, slide the hand along the fetal chest, not the back, up to the fetal hip, or until the posterior hand is identified **(Fig. 4)**. Grasping the wrist of fetus, the posterior arm is swept across the fetus chest followed by delivery of the arm.

If the posterior arm is high up and unable to deliver by above method, the *Menticoglou maneuver* may be applied. It involves placing one finger from each hand under the posterior axilla and applying gentle traction along the curve of the pelvis to deliver the posterior shoulder.

Woods Corkscrew Maneuver

Progressively rotating the posterior shoulder 180° in a corkscrew fashion and causing the impacted anterior shoulder to be released **(Fig. 5)**.

Rubin's 2

Inserting fingers of one hand behind the most accessible fetal shoulder and pushing

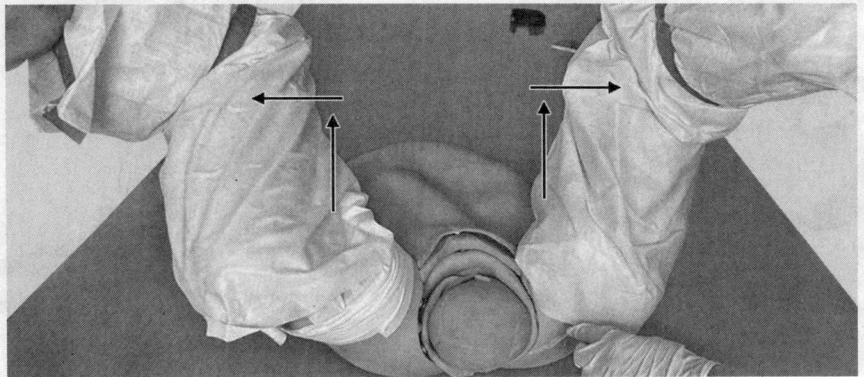

Fig. 2: McRoberts maneuver. *(For color version, see Plate 2)*

toward the fetus chest resulting in collapse of shoulder girdle (**Fig. 6**).

Reverse Woods corkscrew maneuver is same as Rubin's 2.

Gaskins or All Fours Maneuver

It dislodges the anterior shoulder.

Zavanelli Maneuver

Vaginal replacement of head into the pelvis is done, followed by cesarean after giving tocolytics. Performed when there is bilateral shoulder dystocia. Rotate the fetal head to a direct occiput anterior position, flexing the neck so the chin presses against the perineum, and then push the head gently into the vagina.

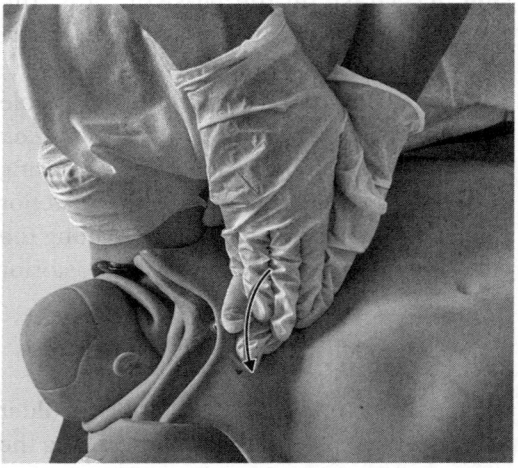

Fig. 3: Suprapubic pressure.
(For color version, see Plate 2)

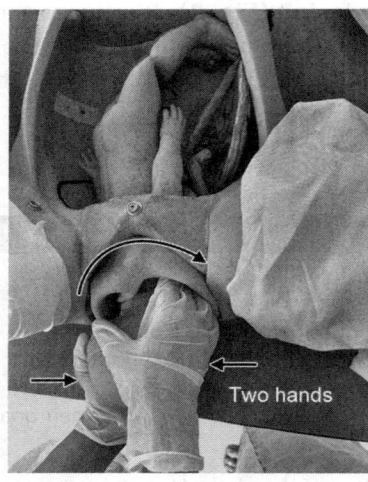

Fig. 5: Woods corkscrew maneuver.
(For color version, see Plate 3)

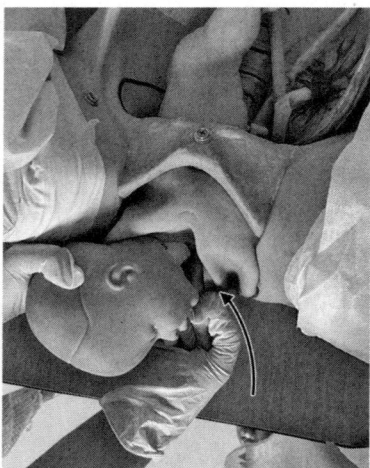

Fig. 4: Posterior arm extraction.
(For color version, see Plate 2)

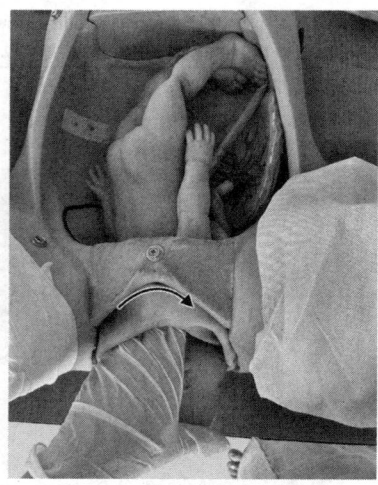

Fig. 6: Rubin's maneuver.
(For color version, see Plate 3)

Cleidotomy

Cleidotomy involves cutting the clavicle with scissors.

Symphysiotomy

The intervening symphyseal cartilage and its ligamentous support are cut to widen symphysis pubis. Urinary tract injury is a complication.

MANAGEMENT OF COMPLICATIONS

Since both traumatic and atonic PPH are expected following drill of shoulder dystocia, PPH management bundle approach should be initiated. Neonate should be examined for injuries by senior neonatologist.

Documentation

Documentation is written series of events and maneuvers applied to be commented upon in the case sheet.

Eclampsia

Eclampsia is commonly defined as a complication of preeclampsia with new onset of grand mal seizure or unexplained coma during pregnancy (≥20 weeks) or postpartum period. It can lead to life-threatening complications such as cerebral hemorrhage, pulmonary edema, abruption placenta, and fetal and maternal death, if not intervened timely.

All patients with convulsions in later half of pregnancy should be treated as eclampsia unless proved otherwise.

Management

- Immediate management
- Subsequent management

Immediate management: Take a quick history and do examination. The first few minutes after convulsions are very crucial; therefore, immediate management plays a very important role to prevent aspiration and cerebral hypoxia, which can lead to serious consequences. The approach to a pregnant woman having convulsions is three pronged and consists of:
1. Stabilize the patient
2. Control convulsions
3. Control blood pressure (BP)

Stabilizing the patient: Call for help (senior obstetrician and assistants) and follow A, B, C of resuscitation. Keep lights dim and minimal noise to prevent further convulsions.

- *Airway:* Place the patient on a railed bed and put her in left lateral position to reduce the risk of aspiration. Put an airway in the mouth and suction out all the secretions.
  Intubate, if necessary in cases of recurrent seizures.
- *Breathing:* Assess the respiratory rate and oxygen saturation with pulse oximeter. Maintain oxygen saturation with oxygen given to the patient at 8–10 L/min. If oxygen saturation falls to <92%, get ABG analysis.
- *Circulation:* Assess the pulse and BP. Secure an intravenous (IV) line with a large-bore cannula (16–18 gauge) and collect blood samples and send for investigations—complete blood count (CBC) with platelet count, serum (S) liver function test (LFT), serum kidney function test (KFT), and serum electrolytes. Start isotonic fluids.
- *Catheterize the patient:* Monitor the urine output and check for urine albumin.

Control convulsions: Injection magnesium sulfate ($MgSO_4$) is the anticonvulsant of choice.

- *Pritchard's regimen:* Loading dose of $MgSO_4$ is given, followed by maintenance dose.
  - *Loading dose:* 4 g of $MgSO_4$ 20% IV over 5–10 minutes and 5 g (50%) deep intramuscular (IM) in both buttocks
  - *Maintenance dose:* 5 g (50%) deep IM in alternate buttocks every 4 hours till 24 hours after the last convulsion or delivery whichever is later.
  - If convulsions recur 2 g (20%) intravenous (IV), $MgSO_4$ is repeated. If refractory to $MgSO_4$ give diazepam (10 mg).
    - During $MgSO_4$ therapy, the following are monitored:
      - *Pulse:* Measured hourly
      - *Blood pressure:* It is measured hourly.
      - *Urine output:* Next dose of $MgSO_4$ is omitted, if output is <30 mL/h for 3 consecutive hours.
      - *Respiratory rate:* Next dose of $MgSO_4$ is omitted, if <12/min.
      - *Patellar reflex:* Stop $MgSO_4$, if unable to elicit reflexes.
      - *Temperature:* It is recorded every 4 hourly.
- Toxicity of $MgSO_4$ leads to suppression of tendon reflexes, respiratory depression, neuromuscular paralysis, and even cardiac arrest.
- Therapeutic dose is 1.5–3.5 mmol/L
- Magnesium sulfate toxicity is dose dependent as shown in **Table 1**.

TABLE 1: Magnesium sulfate toxicity.	
mmol/L	Effects
2.5–5	ECG changes (PR interval prolongation and wide QRS complex)
4–5	Loss of deep-tendon reflexes
>7.5	Respiratory paralysis
>12	Cardiac arrest

- Treatment of toxicity is done with calcium gluconate (10 mL in 10% solution) slow IV over 3–5 minutes.
- *Contraindications* for $MgSO_4$ therapy—renal failure and oliguria, hypocalcemic state, myasthenia gravis, and cardiac conditions such as myocardial damage.
- *Zuspan regimen:* Loading dose is 4 g $MgSO_4$ solution (20%), IV over 5–10 minutes. Maintenance dose is 1–2 g/h by infusion pump for 24 hours.

Control blood pressure: Blood pressure is controlled with injection labetalol 20 mg IV; then repeat measuring BP after 10–15 minutes; if BP is still high, the dose is increased to 40 mg; then 80 mg, and maximum dose is up to 220 mg/day. The aim is to maintain diastolic BP < 100 mm Hg IV.

Hydralazine can also be used to control BP (although it is unavailable in India)—5–10 mg IV/IM initially, then 5–10 mg every 20–30 minutes OR 0.5–10 mg/h IV infusion

Nifedipine is also an alternative drug.

Once stabilization is done, patient is further transferred to tertiary center if multidisciplinary team of senior obstetrician, anesthetist, neurologist, radiologist and blood bank is not available at initial place.

Subsequent management: Meanwhile, the patient is being stabilized, a detailed general, per abdominal, and per vaginal examination is done.

The patient is monitored for:
- Fluid intake and urine output
- Maternal respiratory rate
- Maternal oxygenation
- Continuous fetal monitoring

Termination of pregnancy is done, irrespective of gestational age. Fetal monitoring is done with continuous electronic fetal heart rate (FHR) monitoring. Cesarean section should be done for obstetric indication or if presence of status epilepticus.

ALGORITHM FOR ECLAMPSIA DRILL

- *Protect mother:*
  - Place patient in lateral decubitus position to prevent aspiration
  - Insert padded tongue blade between teeth
  - Elevate bedrails to prevent maternal injury
  - Keep silence, dim lights, and minimal noise to prevent further convulsions
- *Protect airway:*
  - Keep airway clean and patent by frequent oral suctioning
  - Give oxygen by mask at 8–10 L/min
  - Intubation, if necessary (recurrent seizures)
- *Control seizures:*
  - Give MgSO$_4$ (*anticonvulsant of choice*)
    - *Loading dose:* 4 g of 20% solution IV slowly over 5–10 minutes and 5 g of 50% solution IM in each buttock
    - *Maintenance dose:* 5 g IM in alternate buttocks every 4 hourly till 24 hours after delivery or last convulsion.
  - If recurrent seizures refractory to magnesium or intractable seizures—give diazepam (10 mg) or thiopentone (50 mg IV).
- *Control hypertension:*
  - Give injection labetalol or hydralazine
- *Assess:*
  - Mother:
    - Check vitals and oxygen saturation (if less than 92% get ABG)
    - Quick history and examination
    - Laboratory investigations—complete blood count (CBC), liver function test (LFT), kidney function test (KFT), lactate dehydrogenase (LDH), and urine albumin
  - *Fetus:*
    - Fetal heart rate (FHR) monitoring
- *Deliver:* Regardless of gestational age

SUDDEN MATERNAL COLLAPSE

Definition: It is an acute event that involves the cardiorespiratory system or the brain causing reduced or absent conscious levels and potentially death during pregnancy and up to 6 weeks postpartum.

What are the causes for maternal collapse?
Main causes leading to sudden maternal collapse include:
- *4 H:* Hypovolemia, hypoxia, hypothermia, hyponatremia/hypo- or hyperkalemia
- *4T:* Thromboembolism, toxins, tension pneumothorax, tamponade
- Eclampsia
- Intracranial hemorrhage

The common causes of maternal collapse include:
- *Hemorrhage:* Seen in major APH, PPH, uterine rupture and ectopic pregnancy
- Thromboembolism
- *Amniotic fluid embolism:* It presents as collapse during labor or within 30 minutes postpartum and is characterized by acute hypotension, respiratory distress, and hypoxia.
- Cardiac disease
- Sepsis can progress to septic shock and sudden collapse; the most common organisms implicated are streptococcal groups A, B, and D, *Escherichia coli*, and *Pneumococcus*
- Drug toxicity has been seen with local anesthetics either due to inadvertent intravenous injection or systemic absorption of toxic doses administered appropriately.
- Eclampsia
- Intracranial hemorrhage

- *Anaphylaxis:* Mast cell tryptase levels help in confirmation of collapse due to anaphylaxis
- *Electrolyte imbalance:* These include hypoglycemia or hyponatremia and other electrolyte disturbances.

What are the physiological and anatomical changes in pregnancy that affect resuscitation?
- Pregnant women become hypoxic more easily and ventilation is more difficult in them because of changes in lung function, diaphragmatic splinting and increased oxygen consumption during pregnancy.
- Aortocaval compression significantly reduces cardiac output from 20 weeks onwards and decreases the efficacy of chest compressions.
- Pregnant women are more likely to have difficult intubation and higher risk of aspiration.

What is the role of perimortem cesarean section?
If there is no response to CPR within 4 minutes of collapse, or if resuscitation is continued beyond this in a woman who is >20 weeks pregnant, then perimortem cesarean section (PMCS) should be performed to assist maternal resuscitation. It should be done where resuscitation is taking place and the incision, which will facilitate most rapid access, is used; can be midline vertical or suprapubic transverse.

Algorithm for management of sudden maternal collapse is given in **Flowchart 2**.

■ POSTPARTUM HEMORRHAGE

Postpartum hemorrhage (PPH): It is commonly defined as a blood loss of 500 mL or more within 24 hours after normal delivery or more than equal to 1,000 mL following cesarean section. It is the leading cause of maternal mortality in developing countries.

Causes
Four Ts: (1) tone, (2) tissue, (3) trauma, and (4) thrombin; an abnormality in any of these can result in PPH.

Why is drill important?
Postpartum hemorrhage is sudden, unpredictable, and catastrophic, however, death from PPH is avoidable, if immediate and adequate action is taken.

Management of Postpartum Hemorrhage
- Call for help
- Resuscitate
- Monitor and investigate
- Treat the cause of bleeding

Call for Help
Call for senior obstetrician, trained anesthetist, clinical hematologist, and supporting staff.

Resuscitation
- Assess airway, breathing, and circulation.
- Secure two IV lines with wide-bore cannula (14–16 Gauge). Draw blood for blood grouping and cross-matching, complete blood count, LFTs, KFTs, serum electrolytes, and coagulation screen.
- Position the patient flat and keep her warm.
- Administer oxygen at the rate of 10–15 L/min and maintain oxygen saturation.
- Catheterize the patient, empty bladder, and monitor output.
- *Fluid replacement:* Two modes–aggressive approach and hypotensive resuscitative approach—
  - *Aggressive approach:* It restores the circulatory volume, rapidly normalizes the BP and is generally preferred approach in PPH. Crystalloids is the fluid of choice, preferably ringer

Obstetric Drills

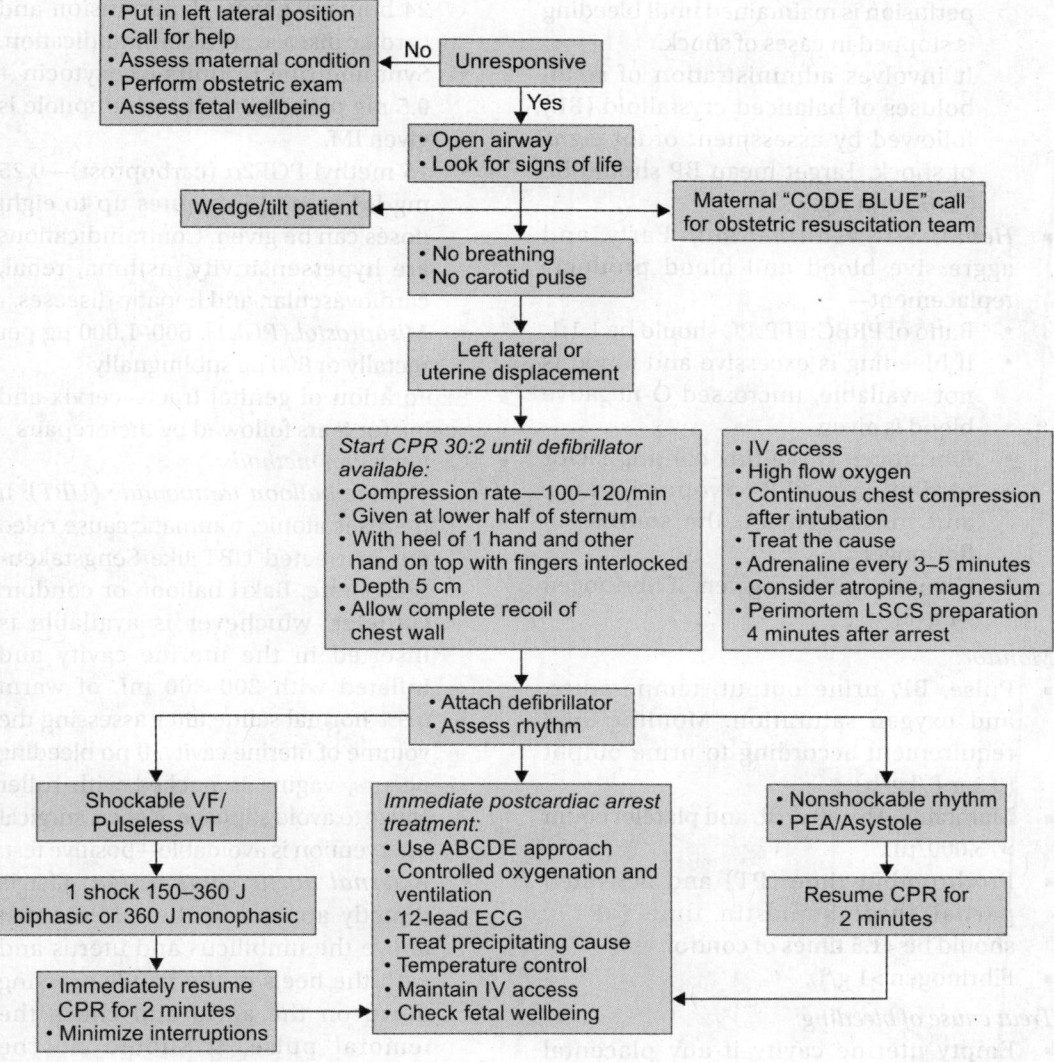

Flowchart 2: Algorithm for management of sudden maternal collapse.

lactate. Rapid infusion of normal saline infusion can lead to hyperchloremic acidosis. 2 L of crystalloids is given until blood is available.
- *Advantages of crystalloids:* Availability, safety, and cost.
- *Disadvantages:* Rapid movement of fluid from the intravascular space to extravascular space may lead to pulmonary, cerebral, and cardiac edema. It may worsen hemorrhage owing to dilutional coagulopathy.
- Colloids stay in the intravascular compartment but are expensive and less available and carry a risk of reaction.
- *Hypotensive resuscitative approach:* This approach is preferred in case of shock. It involves restricting crystalloids in early stage to maintain

lower than normal BP so that organ perfusion is maintained until bleeding is stopped in cases of shock.

It involves administration of small boluses of balanced crystalloid (RL) followed by assessment of for signs of shock. Target mean BP should be 50–60 mm Hg.

- *Hemostatic reanimation:* Early and aggressive blood and blood products replacement—
  - Ratio of PRBC:FFP:PC should be 1:1:1.
  - If bleeding is excessive and blood is not available, uncrossed O-negative blood is given.
  - Fibrinogen is the first clotting factor to diminish. FFP, cryoprecipitates, and fibrinogen are the sources of fibrinogen.
  - Cryoprecipitate is given, if fibrinogen <1 g/L.

Monitor:
- Pulse, BP, urine output, temperature, and oxygen saturation. Monitor fluid requirement according to urine output (0.5 mL/kg/h).
- Maintain—Hb > 8 g/dL and platelet count >75,000/μL.
- Prothrombin time (PT) and activated partial thromboplastin time (aPTT) should be <1.5 times of control.
- Fibrinogen >1 g/L.

Treat cause of bleeding:
- Empty uterine cavity if any placental bits or membranes followed by uterine massage and bimanual compression.
- Give injection tranexamic acid 1 g IV slowly in 10 minutes. Infusion >1 mL/min can cause hypotension.
- *Uterotonics:*
  - *Oxytocin (drug of choice):* 40–60 IU in 500 mL NS at the rate of 60 drops/min in infusion until bleeding stops.
  - *Methergine:* 0.2 mg IV or IM, repeat doses of 0.2 mg can be given IM every 2–4 hours. Maximum of 5 doses in 24 hours is given. Hypertension and cardiac disease are a contraindication.
  - Syntometrine (5 units of oxytocin + 0.5 mg of methergine)—1 ampuole is given IM.
  - 15 methyl PGF2α (carboprost)—0.25 mg IM every 15 minutes up to eight doses can be given. Contraindications are hypersensitivity, asthma, renal, cardiovascular, and hepatic diseases.
  - *Misoprostol (PGE1):* 600–1,000 μg per rectally or 800 μg sublingually
- Exploration of genital tract—cervix and vagina for tears followed by their repairs.
- *Compression methods:*
  - *Uterine balloon tamponade (UBT):* If uterus is atonic, traumatic cause ruled out or treated UBT like Sengstaken-Blakemore, Bakri balloon or condom catheter, whichever is available is inserted in the uterine cavity and inflated with 200–300 mL of warm 0.9% normal saline after assessing the volume of uterine cavity. If no bleeding occurs, vagina is packed with roller gauze to avoid slippage. Hence, surgical intervention is avoidable—positive test.
  - *External aortic compression:* Fist is directly applied in the midline just above the umbilicus and uterus and with the heels of the hands pressing down on the aorta and check the femoral pulse. It should not be palpable, if adequate pressure is applied.
  - *Nonpneumatic anti-shock garment (NASG):* It is a temporary method and provides safe transfer of patient to a higher center for surgical intervention. The garment can apply 30–40 mm Hg of circumferential counter-pressure to the lower body from ankles to diaphragm. The amount of pressure is effective in shunting blood from the

lower extremity and the abdomen to vital organs.
- Lastly, if bleeding continues even after tonicity of uterus, trauma of genital tract, and retained products have been ruled out, coagulopathy is the likely diagnosis. If bleeding occurs, laparotomy is needed.

Surgical management:
- Compression sutures—apposes anterior and posterior wall of uterus.
  - B-Lynch suture
  - Modified B-Lynch suture
  - Vertical suture
  - Square compression suture (Cho's sutures)
- Stepwise uterine devascularization of uterus:
  - Uterine artery ligation
  - Ovarian artery ligation
- Internal iliac artery ligation
- Uterine artery embolization
- Hysterectomy—sooner rather than later.

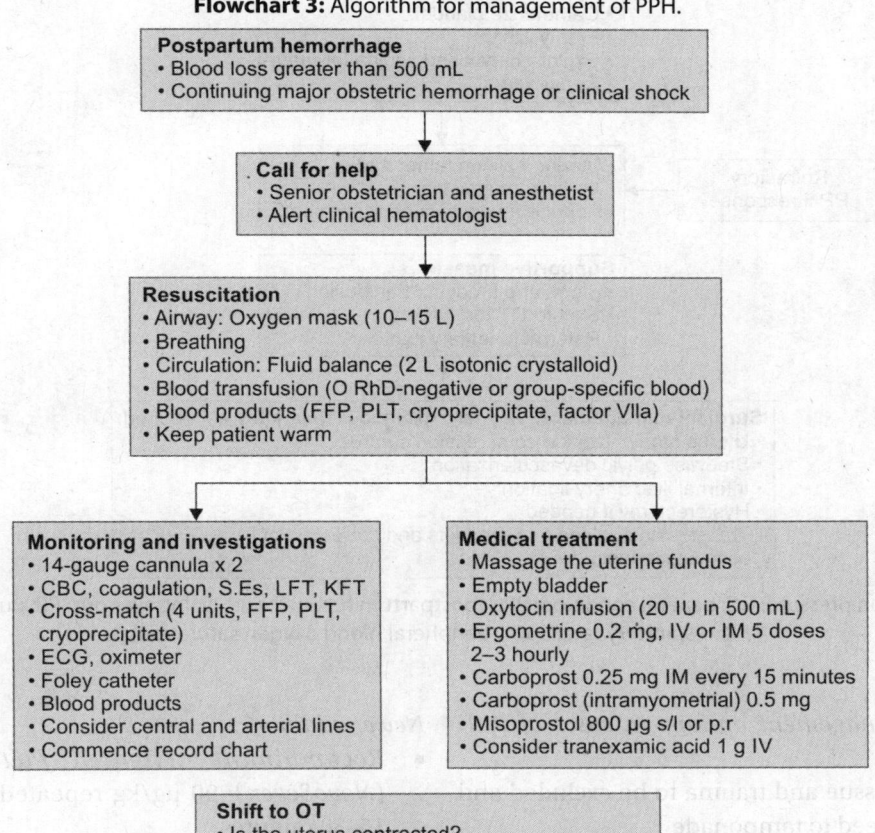

Flowchart 3: Algorithm for management of PPH.

(CBC: complete blood count; ECG: electrocardiogram; FFP: fresh frozen plasma; Hb: hemoglobin; IM: intramuscular; IV: intravenous; KFT: kidney function test; LFT: liver function test; PLT: platelets; PPH: postpartum hemorrhage; RhD: Rhesus D).

Obstetric Drills

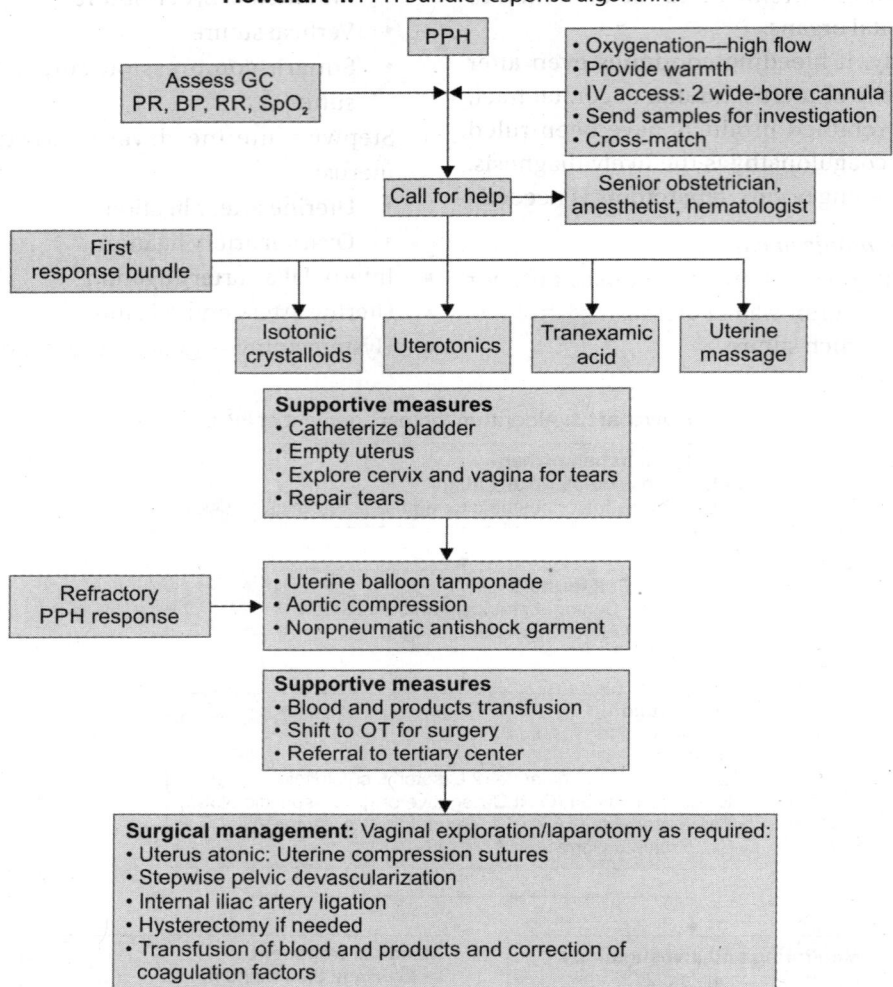

Flowchart 4: PPH Bundle response algorithm.

(BP: blood pressure; GC: general condition; PPH: postpartum hemorrhage; IV: intravenous; PR: pulse rate; RR: respiratory rate; SpO$_2$: peripheral blood oxygen saturation)

The management options in cases of PPH include:
- T—tissue and trauma to be excluded and proceed to tamponade
- A—apply compression sutures
- S—systemic pelvic devascularization
- I—interventional radiology
- S—subtotal hysterectomy

Newer additions:
- *Recombinant activated factor VII (NovoSeven):* 90 µg/kg repeated within 15–30 minutes
- *Carbetocin (oxytocin agonist):* 100 µg IV or IM produces tetanic uterine contractions.
- *Danger signs:* Shock index and rule of 30 are important tools that help in assessment

of amount of blood loss and degree of hemodynamic instability in an emergency.
- *Rule of 30:* It refers to a heart rate increase of >30 bpm, respiratory rate >30/min, fall in systolic BP of 30 mm Hg, urinary output <30 mL/h, hematocrit drop >30%, a 30% fall in hemoglobin (approximately 3 g/dL) and an approximate blood loss of 30% of normal (70 mL/kg in adults; 100 mL/kg during pregnancy).
- *Shock index:* Heart rate/systolic BP
  Normal = 0.5–0.7
  More than 0.9 indicates state of shock and needs immediate resuscitation.
- *The Golden Hour:* It is the time in which resuscitation must begin to achieve maximum survival. As the time elapses between the point of severe shock and start of resuscitation, the percentage of surviving patient decreases.

Algorithm for Postpartum Hemorrhage Management (HEMOSTASIS) **(Flowchart 3)**
- H—*A*sk for help
- A—*A*ssess (vitals and blood loss) and resuscitate
- E—*E*stablish etiology, ecbolics, and ensure blood availability
- M—*M*assage the uterus
- O—*O*xytocin administration
- S—*S*hift to OT

CARE BUNDLES FOR POSTPARTUM HEMORRHAGE (FLOWCHART 4)

In 2017, the World Health Organization developed the care bundles for PPH which include:

First response: It must be implemented at all levels of healthcare including the primary health care. It consists of:
- Uterotonic drugs
- Isotonic crystalloids
- Tranexamic acid
- Uterine massage

Response to refractory PPH bundle:
- Compressive measures
- Intrauterine balloon tamponade
- NASG

(Uterotonics and second dose of tranexamic acid should be administered during the application of this bundle).

SUGGESTED READING

1. Althabe F, Therrien MNS, Pingray V, Hermida J, Gülmezoglu AM, Armbruster D, et al. Postpartum hemorrhage care bundles to improve adherence to guidelines: A WHO technical consultation. Int J Gynaecol Obstet. 2020;148(3):290-9.
2. Giouleka S, Tsakiridis I, Kalogiannidis I, Mamopoulos A, Tentas I, Athanasiadis A, et al. Postpartum Hemorrhage: A Comprehensive Review of Guidelines. Obstet Gynecol Surv. 2022;77(11):665-82.
3. Hill DA, Lense J, Roepcke F. Shoulder dystocia: Managing an obstetric emergency. Am Fam Physician. 2020;102(2):84-90.
4. Madden AM, Meng ML. Cardiopulmonary resuscitation in the pregnant patient. BJA Educ. 2020;20(8):252-8.
5. Practice Bulletin No. 178: Shoulder Dystocia. Obstet Gynecol. 2017;129(5):e123-e133. doi: 10.1097/AOG.0000000000002043. PMID: 28426618.
6. Vogel JP, Nguyen PY, Ramson J, De Silva MS, Pham MD, Sultana S, et al. Effectiveness of care bundles for prevention and treatment of postpartum hemorrhage: a systematic review. Am J Obstet Gynecol; 2024. pp. 7: S0002-9378(24)00042-5.

11 Maternal Resuscitation

Rashmi Salhotra

INTRODUCTION

The latest American Heart Association (AHA) guidelines on resuscitation were released in the year 2020, which also updated the guidelines on maternal resuscitation. This chapter summarizes these recommendations and updates.

Cardiac arrest in pregnancy is a rare event, the incidence being 1:36,000 pregnancies. It is a special situation and uniquely different from adult resuscitation as it involves two lives: The mother and the fetus. An in-depth knowledge of the physiological changes of the pregnancy are vital to the management of maternal cardiac arrest.

What are the causes of maternal cardiac arrest?

The causes of maternal cardiac arrest can be easily memorized by the mnemonic "ABCDEFGH":
- *A:* Anesthetic complications
- *B:* Bleeding
- *C:* Cardiovascular
- *D:* Drugs
- *E:* Embolic
- *F:* Fever
- *G:* General nonobstetric reversible causes
- *H:* Hypertension

The general nonobstetric reversible causes can be memorized as 5Hs and 5Ts. They are as follows:
- *5Hs:* Hypovolemia, hypoxia, hypothermia, hypokalemia, and hyperkalemia
- *5Ts:* Thromboembolism, toxins, tension pneumothorax, tamponade (cardiac), and trauma

Active surveillance for early identification and management of the prearrest conditions can prevent mishaps and improve the outcome of the mother and fetus/neonate. Further, management of the causes of the arrest will aid in the early reversal of cardiopulmonary arrest for improving the outcome of resuscitation. Since cardiac arrest is often sudden in nature, all areas of the hospital catering to pregnant patients (antenatal clinics, antenatal and postnatal wards, labor, and delivery areas) must have a crash cart with all the supplies required for maternal resuscitation.

What are the physiological changes during pregnancy and their implications for maternal resuscitation?

Uterine size: After 20 weeks of gestation, the growing uterus compresses the inferior vena cava and interferes with the venous return to the heart. Therefore, manual left uterine displacement (LUD) or tilt should be given during cardiopulmonary resuscitation (CPR). *Perimortem cesarean delivery (PMCD) should be initiated within 4 minutes and the baby should be delivered within 5 minutes of cardiac arrest.* If the period of gestation (POG) <20 weeks, PMCD is unlikely to significantly aid maternal resuscitation. At POG, between

20 and 23 weeks, the role is doubtful but if the POG is >23 weeks, it is likely to aid both maternal and fetal resuscitation (fetal resuscitation being a secondary benefit).

Respiratory changes: Functional residual capacity is reduced due to uterine enlargement. Oxygen demand is high to meet the requirements of both mother and fetus. Therefore, the demand–supply ratio of oxygen is unfavorable and desaturation occurs rapidly. Thus, *the role of supplementing oxygen during resuscitation cannot be overemphasized.* Oxygen must be supplemented during the resuscitation with a bag-mask device or with the definitive airway device, e.g., endotracheal tube (ETT) or a laryngeal mask airway (LMA). However, time should not be wasted in inserting a definitive airway device if expert help is not available or difficulty is encountered during ETT insertion.

Gastrointestinal changes: The lower esophageal sphincter tone is relaxed and gastrointestinal motility is reduced because of progesterone. The chances of aspiration of acidic contents are high. *Thus, these patients should be considered and treated as full stomach irrespective of the last meal consumption time.* Therefore, cricoid pressure must be applied to prevent aspiration and early securing of airway with the introduction of cuffed ETT should be attempted. Intubation should be attempted by the most experienced person trained in airway management skills.

Airway: All obstetric patients are potential cases for difficult intubation because of presence of upper airway edema. Expert help should be called in early and a difficult airway cart with all the ancillary equipment should always be ready in all areas catering to pregnant population.

■ SURVEILLANCE

Cardiac arrest is a very dramatic situation. In antepartum cases, it becomes all the more unique as it involves two lives. Therefore, identification and continuous surveillance of patients at risk by periodic charting of vital signs such as pulse, systolic and diastolic blood pressure, temperature, respiratory rate, alertness, and urine output should be done. This is known as the Modified Early Obstetric Warning Score (MEOWS). A score of >2 should alarm the physician for a possibility of maternal deterioration and development of cardiac arrest. Multidisciplinary teams should be activated in case the score increases and resuscitation team, anesthesiologists, obstetricians, and pediatricians should be involved for the management of these emergencies.

What are the recommendations for care in maternal collapse?

- Full left lateral decubitus position to relieve aortocaval compression
- 100% oxygen by face mask to treat or prevent hypoxemia
- *Readiness for critical events*: Establishment of a large-bore intravenous (IV) access above the diaphragm
- Active search for the preventable causes of cardiac arrest (ABCDEFGH/5Hs and 5Ts) and appropriate treatment should be instituted.

What is basic life support?

Basic life support (BLS) measures **(Flowchart 1)** should be initiated immediately by the bystander after the recognition of cardiac arrest and should be continued until the expert help arrives or the victim starts responding. Chest compressions followed by provision of breaths should be done. A defibrillator should be used as soon as it is available, wherever indicated, and manual

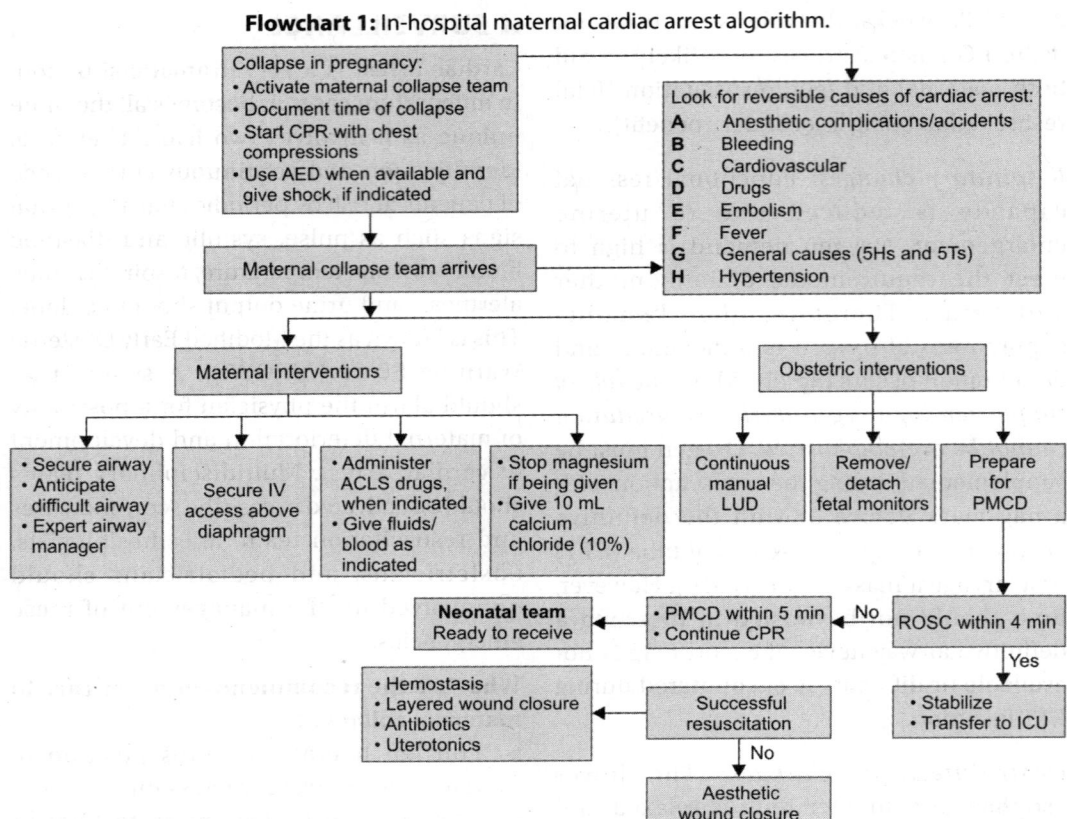

Flowchart 1: In-hospital maternal cardiac arrest algorithm.

(AED: automated external defibrillator; CPR: cardiopulmonary resuscitation; LUD: left uterine displacement; PMCD: perimortem cesarean delivery; ROSC: return of spontaneous circulation)

LUD should be done simultaneously. A minimum of four BLS responders should be present to accomplish all these tasks effectively.

Steps of basic life support: The sequence of resuscitation is C-A-B, where "C" stands for compression, "A" is for airway, and "B" is for breathing. Chest compressions take a priority over establishing an airway and providing breaths.

Scene safety: Ensuring scene safety for the rescuer and the victim is the first step. Universal precautions including the use of personnel protective equipment (PPE) should be taken.

Check responsiveness: Auditory and tactile stimulus should be given to ascertain that the patient is unresponsive.

Check breathing and pulse: The chest should be scanned to look for breathing. Simultaneously, the ipsilateral carotid pulse should also be palpated. All these actions should be performed simultaneously within 5–10 seconds.

Activation of emergency medical services: The emergency medical service (EMS) teams should be activated immediately with a request to bring an automated external defibrillator (AED) or a manual defibrillator.

Chest compressions
- High-quality chest compressions should be initiated immediately. The patient should be lying on a hard surface so that effective chest compressions can be given. A resuscitation board can be used to improve this chest compression efficacy.
- Manual LUD with one hand or two-handed technique (preferred) should be done and must be maintained throughout the resuscitative and the postresuscitative phases to relieve aortocaval compression.
- Chest compressions at the rate of 100–120/min and depth of 5–6 cm at the lower half of the sternum should be initiated. The elbows should be locked. Interruptions should be minimized to <10 seconds, and full chest recoil should be allowed in between compressions. The ratio of compression to ventilation is 30:2. Pressure over the xiphoid process and the ribs must be avoided.

Airway and breathing
- Establishment of airway control and provision of breaths are essential at an early stage as hypoxemia develops more rapidly in the pregnant patient due to increase in maternal metabolism, reduced functional residual capacity, and risk of fetal brain injury.
- Supplemental oxygen must be provided as soon as it is available. Early institution of bag-mask ventilation with 100% oxygen at the rate of 10–15 L/min should be initiated.
- Airway should be secured early during resuscitation because as mentioned earlier, these patients are at an increased risk of aspiration of gastric contents. But intubation should be attempted by an expert only as these patients have an anticipated difficult airway. The standard compression–ventilation ratio of 30:2 should be continued. Hyperventilation should be avoided at all costs.
- Five cycles of 30 compressions and two breaths should be continued over a period of 2 minutes until the multidisciplinary cardiac arrest team takes over or the patient is revived or a defibrillator is available.

Defibrillation
- Prompt defibrillation with 120–200 J when the rhythm is shockable [i.e., ventricular fibrillation (VF) or pulseless ventricular tachycardia (pVT)] maximizes the likelihood of survival. AED may be used, if a manual defibrillator is not available. DC shock has no adverse effect on the fetus.
- Defibrillator pads should be placed in the anterolateral position. The lateral pad/paddle should be placed under the left breast and the other pad should be placed under the right clavicle. Fetal monitors should be removed, if not done earlier.
- Chest compressions should be resumed immediately after shock. Rhythm should be analyzed only after 2 minutes of shock delivery or if the patient begins to respond.

What is advanced cardiac life support?
Maternal cardiac arrest should be treated as a dire emergency and the response should be fast and well coordinated. The cardiac arrest advanced cardiac life support (ACLS) algorithm as recommended by the AHA 2015 guidelines should be followed. The maternal resuscitation team should comprise an adult resuscitation team including critical care physicians and nurses, obstetrician and obstetric nurse, obstetric anesthesiologist, anesthesia assistant, and neonatology team comprising a nurse, a physician, and a neonatal respiratory therapist. Equipment

for management of airway, PMCD (at least a scalpel and clamps), and neonatal resuscitation must be available in all areas where peripartum patients are taken care of.

The ACLS team should continue BLS tasks. A 6.0 to 7.0 sized internal diameter ETT should be inserted by an expert laryngoscopist, if it has not already been done. If intubation fails, a LMA may be inserted. If available, continuous capnography monitoring should be used to confirm the ETT placement, assess the quality of chest compressions, and confirm return of spontaneous circulation (ROSC).

An IV access should be secured above the diaphragm and epinephrine IV/IO (intravenous/intraosseous) should be administered in a dose of 1 mg every 3-5 minutes. The use of atropine is recommended only for treatment of bradycardia.

If the cause of cardiac arrest is refractory (shock-resistant) VF and VT, amiodarone 300 mg infusion should be administered, and 150-mg repeat dose may be administered as needed.

What is the role of fetal assessment during cardiac arrest?
Maternal resuscitation is a priority. As per the AHA 2020 guidelines, evaluation of the fetal heart is not helpful during maternal cardiac arrest, and it may distract the team from necessary resuscitation elements. Also, it is advisable to remove all fetal monitoring before defibrillation.

Discuss perimortem cesarean delivery.
- PMCD should be planned once the obstetric and neonatal teams arrive and ROSC has not been achieved within 4 minutes of the onset of cardiac arrest and in whom the uterus extends to or above the umbilicus.
- PMCD provides a twofold benefit. Firstly, it relieves the aortocaval compression. Secondly, early delivery of fetus may result in a decreased risk of permanent neurological damage from anoxia. In situations where the mother cannot be resuscitated, timely delivery of the fetus becomes all the more essential. The risks of neurological damage to the fetus begin to develop after 4-6 minutes of anoxic cardiac arrest, if there is no ROSC. Therefore, it is recommended that PMCD should begin at 4 minutes so as to deliver the baby at 5 minutes after failed resuscitative efforts.
- The procedure for PMCD should be performed at the site of the maternal resuscitation. No time should be wasted waiting for surgical equipment or abdominal preparation. As soon as the scalpel is available, the procedure should begin. All the resuscitative efforts should be continued, including manual uterine displacement. The use of oxytocin after delivery may precipitate rearrest. Therefore, it should be used with caution.

Can vaginal delivery be tried during maternal cardiac arrest?
Assisted vaginal delivery during a cardiac arrest situation may be tried, if the cervix is fully dilated and the fetal head is at a low station.

What is the role of neonatal resuscitation during maternal cardiac arrest?
In maternal cardiac arrest situations, the neonatologists should be prepared for advanced resuscitation. Neonatal endotracheal intubation may be urgently required. In cases of multiple gestation, each newborn should be resuscitated by a separate resuscitation team.

What should be the immediate postarrest care?

Immediately after ROSC, an integrated postarrest care is a must. A thorough assessment, monitoring, and treatment of complications needs to be done. As per the 2020 guidelines, pregnant women who survive cardiac arrest should receive targeted temperature management, with consideration for the status of fetus that may remain in utero. Antiarrhythmic therapy or implantable cardioverter–defibrillator may be used as required.

SUGGESTED READING

1. Jeejeebhoy FM, Zelop CM, Lipman S, Carvalho B, Joglar J, Mhyre JM, et al. Cardiac arrest in pregnancy: a scientific statement from the American Heart Association. Circulation. 2015;132:1747-73.
2. Link MS, Atkins DL, Passman RS, Passman RS, Halperin HR, Samson RA, et al. Part 6: electrical therapies: automated external defibrillators, defibrillation, cardioversion, and pacing: 2010 American Heart Association guidelines for cardiopulmonary resuscitation and emergency cardiovascular care. Circulation. 2010;122:S706-19.
3. Madden AM, Meng ML. Cardiopulmonary resuscitation in the pregnant patient. BJA Educ. 2020;20(8):252-8.
4. Merchant RM, Topjian AA, Panchal AR, Cheng A, Aziz K, Berg KM, et al. Part 1: executive summary: 2020 American Heart Association Guidelines for Cardiopulmonary Resuscitation and Emergency Cardiovascular Care. Circulation. 2020;142(suppl 2):S337-57.
5. Nirmal D, Goodsell R. Clinical Guidelines for: The use of the Modified Early Obstetric Warning Score (MEOWS) Approved by: Maternity Guidelines Committee 2016 Trust Docs ID: MID33/AO13–817.

Neonatal Resuscitation

Rajeev Kumar Thapar

What is normal transition?

Most newborns (85%) make the transition from intrauterine to extrauterine existence smoothly as they start breathing and neonatal circulation takes over from fetal circulation. The placenta stops facilitating the exchange of gases. Nonfunctional fluid-filled fetal lungs get filled with air beginning the exchange of gases. Blood flow to the lungs increases, thus, further facilitating gaseous exchange with closure of ductus arteriosus.

Failure to initiate breathing or effective respiratory efforts and alveoli not getting filled with air with no gaseous exchange leads to respiratory failure and resultant hypoxia that may be detrimental to the life of the baby **(Fig. 1)**.

Around 10% of babies start breathing in response to drying and stimulation, and about 5% may require positive-pressure ventilation (PPV). 2% of term newborns will be intubated and only 1–3 babies per 1,000 births receive chest compression or medications **(Fig. 2)**.

What is the main aim of neonatal resuscitation?

- Neonatal resuscitation helps to restore a baby from the state of asphyxia. It involves learning the steps necessary to ventilate a newborn who is not breathing and to protect the life of the newborn.
- Perinatal asphyxia is an important preventable cause of neonatal mortality and morbidity and contributes to around 20% of neonatal mortality.

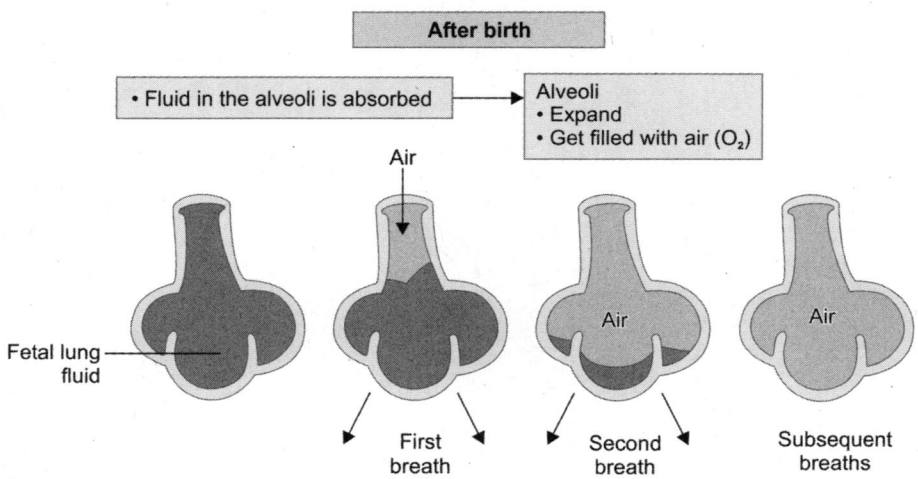

Fig. 1: Air replaces fluid in the alveoli when the baby takes the first breath.

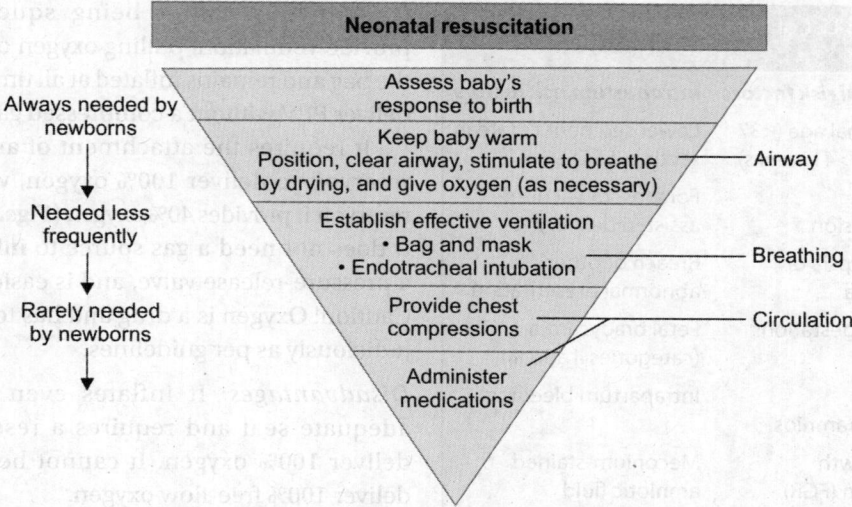

Fig. 2: Inverted triangle of need for resuscitation at birth.

- The Neonatal Resuscitation Program (NRP) is the most effective tool to reduce perinatal asphyxia. The NRP is a standardized, structured program which brings in updated evidence-based practice. The Indian Academy of Pediatrics (IAP) and the National Neonatology Forum (NNF) are aiming at one NRP-trained personnel at all deliveries through the IAP-NNF-NRP-FGM program.
- The common causes of failed resuscitation are the inability to recognize the problem promptly, not reacting quickly and not ventilating the lungs effectively. The correct technique to provide ventilation and assessment of the effectiveness of ventilation are the key points to learn.

Who needs resuscitation?

The need for resuscitation cannot be predicted prior to the birth of a baby. Every birth is to be considered a potential emergency where resuscitation may be required. Therefore, it is the preparedness, and training of healthcare workers involved in the birthing process and a systemic approach to managing afflicted babies at birth that can save many newborn lives. However, with a prior assessment of risk factors, one can anticipate and plan better in terms of personnel and additional equipment.

What are the risk factors that need to be considered?

Table 1 mentions the antenatal and intrapartum risk factors, which need to be considered for anticipation and planning.

What are components of the neonatal resuscitation?

Sequential steps for neonatal resuscitation are shown in **Table 2**.

■ KEY THINGS TO KEEP IN MIND

- *Preparation for birth* is the key to the success of resuscitation. The advantage of preparation is that one can manage resuscitation more smoothly, efficiently, and with great clarity. It will avoid confusion and delay in the initiation of resuscitation of a newborn.
- *Preparation of personnel:* A healthcare professional (HCP) working in the birth

TABLE 1: List of antenatal and intrapartum risk factors.

Antenatal risk factors	Intrapartum risk factors
Gestational age (<37 weeks or >41 weeks)	Lower segment cesarean section (LSCS)
Maternal hypertension	Forceps- or vacuum-assisted delivery
Preeclampsia or eclampsia	Breach or other abnormal presentation
Multiple gestations	Fetal bradycardia (categories II and III)
Poly- or oligohydramnios	Intrapartum bleeding
Fetal growth restriction (FGR)	Meconium-stained amniotic fluid
Significant fetal malformation	Placental abruption
No antenatal care	Maternal general anesthesia or magnesium therapy
Fetal hydrops	Shoulder dystocia

place should be able to initiate bag-and-mask ventilation. In the presence of risk factors, at least two or more HCPs trained in NRP with one person trained in advanced NRP be available at the time of birth.

- *Hand washing:* All the HCPs involved in resuscitation should wash their hands for 40–60 seconds and wear gloves before assembling equipment and supplies.
- *Preparation of equipment and supplies:* All supplies and equipment required for resuscitation must be readily available at every birth. The list of the same is appended in **Table 3**.
- *Infection Prevention:* Universal precautions to be observed **(Flowchart 1)**

What is the most essential equipment to provide positive-pressure ventilation?

It is also known as self-inflating bag **(Fig. 3)**. It is made of silicon material. It fills spontaneously after being squeezed to provide ventilation, pulling oxygen or air into the bag and remains inflated at all times. It can deliver PPV without a compressed gas source.

It requires the attachment of an oxygen reservoir to deliver 100% oxygen, without a reservoir it provides 40% oxygen **(Figs. 4 and 5)**. It does not need a gas source to inflate, has a pressure-release valve, and is easier to use. Caution! Oxygen is a drug and has to be used judiciously as per guidelines.

Disadvantages: It inflates even without adequate seal and requires a reservoir to deliver 100% oxygen. It cannot be used to deliver 100% free-flow oxygen.

What is the process of a successful neonatal resuscitation?

Preparation of delivery and care at birth as appended in the **Table 4**.

What is positive-pressure ventilation?

Positive-pressure ventilation (PPV) is the most important step in neonatal resuscitation. 99% of apneic babies can be revived if PPV is provided correctly at the appropriate time *(within the first golden minute).*

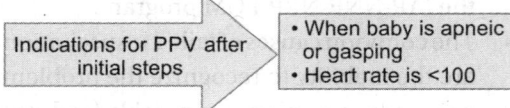

What are the steps to provide effective PPV?
The steps for PPV are discussed in **Table 5**.

When should you intubate the baby?
The indications of endotracheal intubation are given as follows:

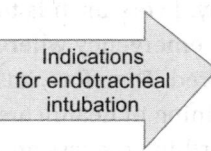

TABLE 2: Sequential steps for neonatal resuscitation.

Preparation for birth	Initial steps	Positive-pressure ventilation (PPV) for 30 seconds	PPV with chest compressions (CC)	Medication along with PPV and CC	Consider other causes
• Predelivery information • Discuss about umbilical cord management	*Breathing well* → Initial steps on mother's abdomen/chest and delay cord clamping (DCC) *Not breathing well* → • Clamp the cord and shift to radiant warmer to provide initial steps *Initial steps*—Warmth, Dry, position, stimulate and suction (if required)	• Indicated after initial steps if baby is apneic, gasping or HR >100 • Effective PPV—chest moves with PPV and HR increases • Breathing well and HR >100, slowly wean PPV • Not breathing and/or HR >60, continue PPV	• HR <60 after 30 seconds of effective PPV • Connect 100% oxygen and intubate if not done already • If HR >60, then stop CC, continue PPV • If HR >100, shift for post-resuscitation care	• Indicated if HR <60, despite 1 minute (60 seconds) of coordinated PPV and CC • Drug: Injection adrenaline 1:10,000 dilution, 0.2 mL/kg intravenously • If HR >60, continue PPV • If HR >100, shift for post-resuscitation care	If no response to adrenaline, consider hypovolemia and pneumothorax

TABLE 3: List of equipment and supplies required for resuscitation.

Preheated radiant warmer	Pulse oximeter
Two clean warm sheets	Laryngoscope with straight blade sizes 0,1
Shoulder roll	Endotracheal tube sizes—2.5, 3.0, 3.5 mm
Plastic bag or wrap for preterm babies (<32 weeks)	Measuring tape for naso tragus length (NTL)
Mucus extractor or 10–12-FG suction catheter	Tape to secure endotracheal tube
Suction machine (80–100 mm Hg)	Scissors
Stethoscope	Injection adrenaline
Air oxygen blender if available	Syringes 1, 2, 5, 20 and 50 mL size
Oxygen source with flow meter able to deliver oxygen at 10 LPM	Normal saline 100-mL bottle
Self-inflating ventilation bag of appropriate size with reservoir and oxygen tube (240 mL for preterm and 500 mL for term babies)	UVC catheter—3.5, 5-FG size with three-way stopcock
Term and preterm masks size 0 and 1	Supplies required for putting UVC
8-FG orogastric feeding tube	

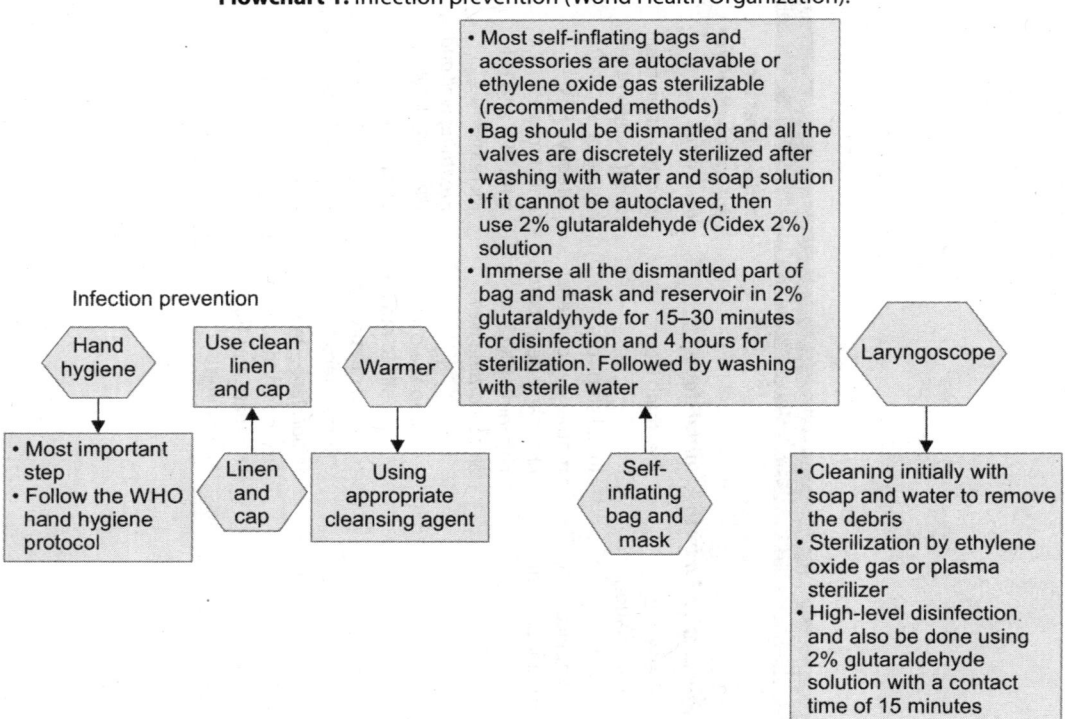

Flowchart 1: Infection prevention (World Health Organization).

Neonatal Resuscitation

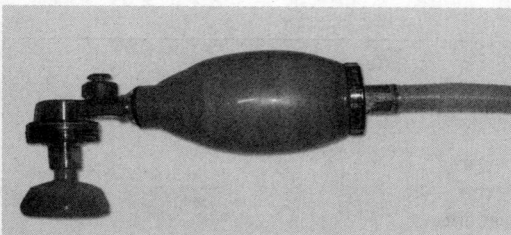

Fig. 3: Self-inflating bag and mask.
(For color version, see Plate 3)

What are the steps of neonatal intubation?
The steps of neonatal intubation are given in **Flowchart 2**.

When to provide chest compressions? (Flowchart 3)
Chest compressions should be provided when HR is <60 per minute post 30 seconds of effective PPV. The aim should be to provide

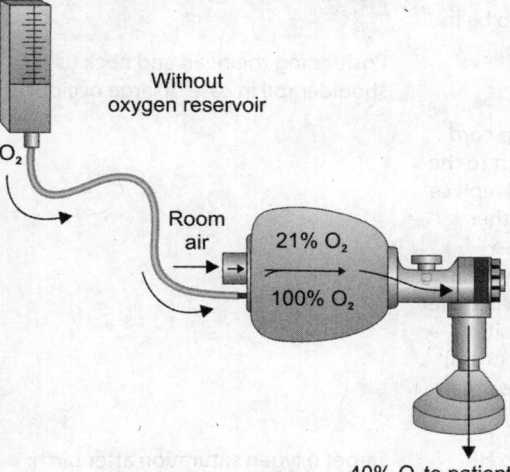

Fig. 4: Ambu bag without reservoir.

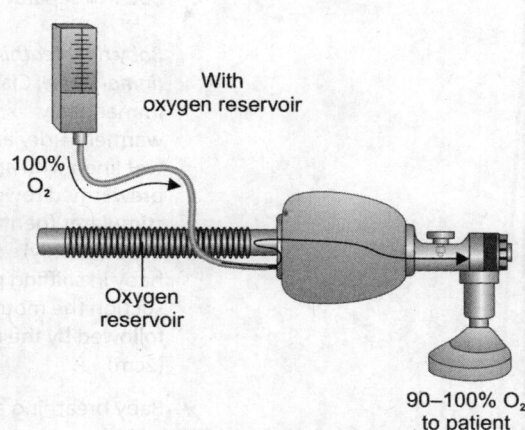

Fig. 5: Ambu bag with reservoir.

TABLE 4: Preparation of delivery and care at birth.			
	Evaluation	*Action*	*Key points*
PREPARE	*Predelivery questions regarding:* • Gestational age • Meconium-stained amniotic fluid (MSAF) • Additional risk factors • Discussion about umbilical cord management with an obstetrician before delivery	Prepare team and team briefing. *Check equipment and supplies:* Functioning of Ambu bag, laryngoscope, and availability of endotracheal (ET) tubes, suction catheter, and pulse oximeter with target saturation table	• Cord clamping should be delayed (DCC) at least 60 seconds if the baby is breathing well • The functioning of the Ambu bag (self-inflating bag) is assessed by squeezing the bag with a palm covering the mask • With an air-tight seal around the mask, the pop-off valve opens and makes a hissing sound • Feel for the air or pressure against the palm. This ensures the opening of the fish-mouth valve • The bag should recoil instantly when pressure is released

Contd...

132 Neonatal Resuscitation

Contd...

	Evaluation	Action	Key points
INITIAL STEPS	Assess for breathing or crying	*Breathing well (routine care):* Deliver to mother's abdomen in skin-to-skin contact (SSC) → dry the baby and remove wet linen and cover the baby with a warm towel → DCC → initiate breastfeeding → Baby and mother to be in SSC (No separation)	Positioning the head and neck using shoulder roll in case of large occiput
		Baby not breathing (initial steps): Clamp cord immediately → shift to the warmer → dry and replace wet linen with another prewarmed towel → stimulates (gently stroking the back only) → place the baby in sniffing position → suction the mouth (5 cm) followed by the nose max (2cm)	
	After initial steps, assess breathing and HR	Baby breathing and HR >100 but appears cyanosed, check for saturation → saturation below target → provide free flow oxygen	Target oxygen saturation after birth: • 1 minute: 60–65% • 2 minutes: 65–70% • 3 minutes: 70–75% • 4 minutes: 75–80% • 5 minutes: 80–85% • 10 minutes: >85% *MSAF does not influence resuscitation. Intubation for tracheal suction in nonvigorous babies born through MSAF is not recommended*
	After initial steps, assess breathing and HR	If the baby has labored breathing—nasal continuous positive airway pressure (CPAP) should be considered	
		Baby not breathing or if breathing but HR <100—provide *positive-pressure ventilation (PPV)*	

TABLE 5: Steps to provide effective PPV.

Initiating PPV	Role of assistant	Ineffective PPV-HR not increasing and chest not moving	After PPV	After care
Self-Inflating Bag	*Effective PPV* • Increasing HR • If HR is not increasing then, chest should move with PPV	Corrective actions • MRSOPA (Mask, Reposition, Suction, Open mouth, Pressure, Artificial airway) • Five rescue breaths with each step to assess chest movement with PPV	Duration • Effective PPV for 30 seconds • Assess for breathing and HR	*Type of care depends on duration of PPV*
• Choose appropriate-size mask **(Fig. 6)** (0 for preterm and 1 for term) • Place the mask covering the chin to bridge of nose, avoiding eyes **(Fig. 7)** • Provide air tight seal **(Fig. 8)** • PPV for 30 seconds with room air in babies >35 weeks of GA and 21–30% O_2 for preterm <35 weeks • Rate of PPV: 40–60/min by reciting "Breath-2-3" synchronizing the squeeze with "Breath" and releasing the bag with "2-3"	Assistant connects pulse oximeter to right hand • After 15 seconds look for effectiveness of PPV by primarily assessing for HR by auscultation and if not increasing, then look for chest movement with PPV	• MR: – Mask readjustment and – Reposition the head and neck • SO: – Suction mouth and nose – Open the mouth • P: Increase the delivered pressure by squeezing the bag harder • A: Alternative airway like intubation • Provide PPV that moves the chest for 30 seconds	• Breathing well • Slowly wean-off PPV and titrate Oxygen for target saturation • HR >100 but not breathing well, continue PPV and add O_2 if saturation below target • If prolonged consider intubation • HR <100, continue PPV, ensure effective ventilation by intubation and add Oxygen if SpO_2 below target ↑	*Effective PPV for 30 seconds only then provide observational care. Observation care* includes monitoring vitals, feeding and activity every 15 minutes for first hour and then 30 minutes in the second hour at mother side only • *Effective PPV >30 seconds, then provide post resuscitation care in the nursery*

Effective PPV given for 30 seconds

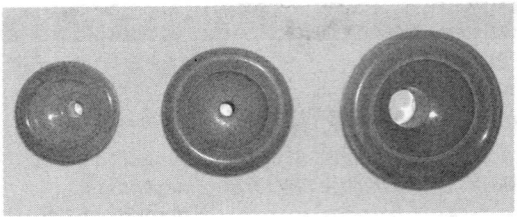

Fig. 6: Various sizes of face cushioned and rounded masks: 00, 0, and 1. *(For color version, see Plate 4)*

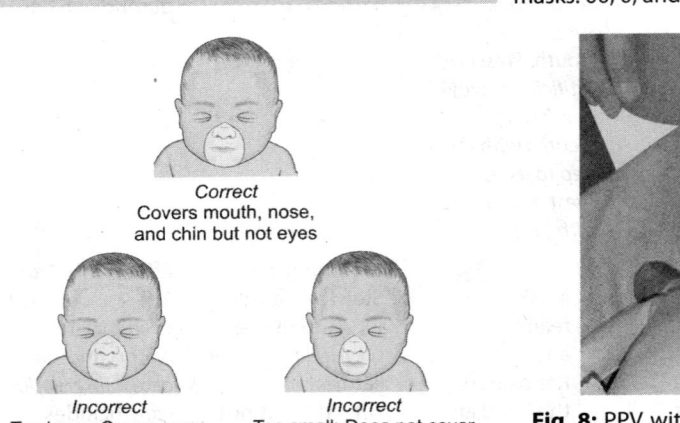

Correct
Covers mouth, nose, and chin but not eyes

Incorrect
Too large: Covers eyes and extends over chin

Incorrect
Too small: Does not cover nose and mouth well

Fig. 7: Correct position of the mask.

Fig. 8: PPV with "C" and "E" clamp to provide tight seal. (PPV: positive-pressure ventilation) *(For color version, see Plate 4)*

Flowchart 2: Steps of neonatal intubation.

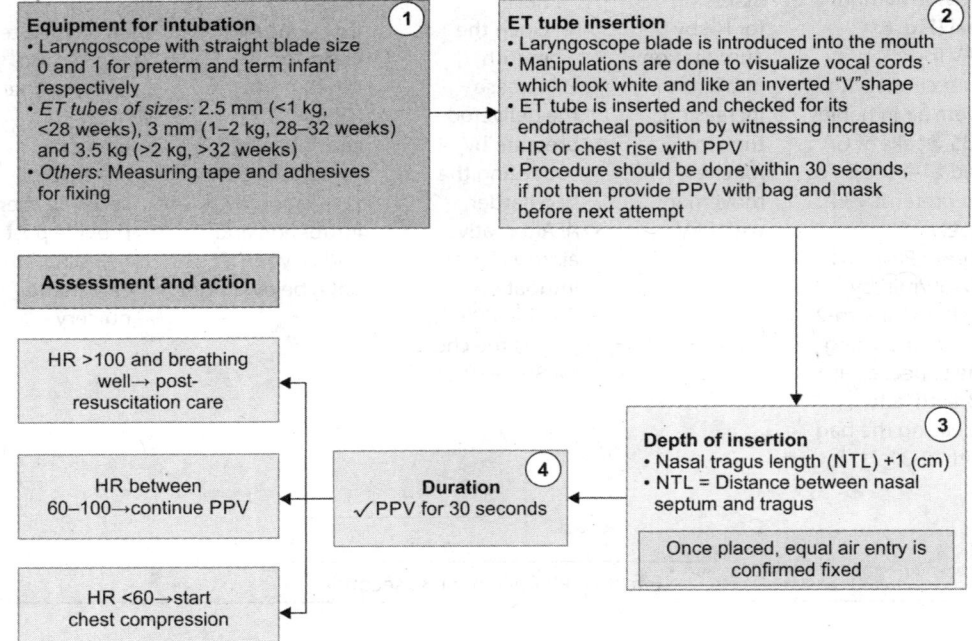

1. Equipment for intubation
- Laryngoscope with straight blade size 0 and 1 for preterm and term infant respectively
- *ET tubes of sizes:* 2.5 mm (<1 kg, <28 weeks), 3 mm (1–2 kg, 28–32 weeks) and 3.5 kg (>2 kg, >32 weeks)
- *Others:* Measuring tape and adhesives for fixing

2. ET tube insertion
- Laryngoscope blade is introduced into the mouth
- Manipulations are done to visualize vocal cords which look white and like an inverted "V" shape
- ET tube is inserted and checked for its endotracheal position by witnessing increasing HR or chest rise with PPV
- Procedure should be done within 30 seconds, if not then provide PPV with bag and mask before next attempt

3. Depth of insertion
- Nasal tragus length (NTL) +1 (cm)
- NTL = Distance between nasal septum and tragus

Once placed, equal air entry is confirmed fixed

Assessment and action

HR >100 and breathing well → post-resuscitation care

HR between 60–100 → continue PPV

HR <60 → start chest compression

4. Duration
✓ PPV for 30 seconds

(ET: endotracheal; HR: heart rate; PPV: positive-pressure ventilation)

Neonatal Resuscitation

Flowchart 3: Heart rate < 60 after 30 seconds of effective PPV.

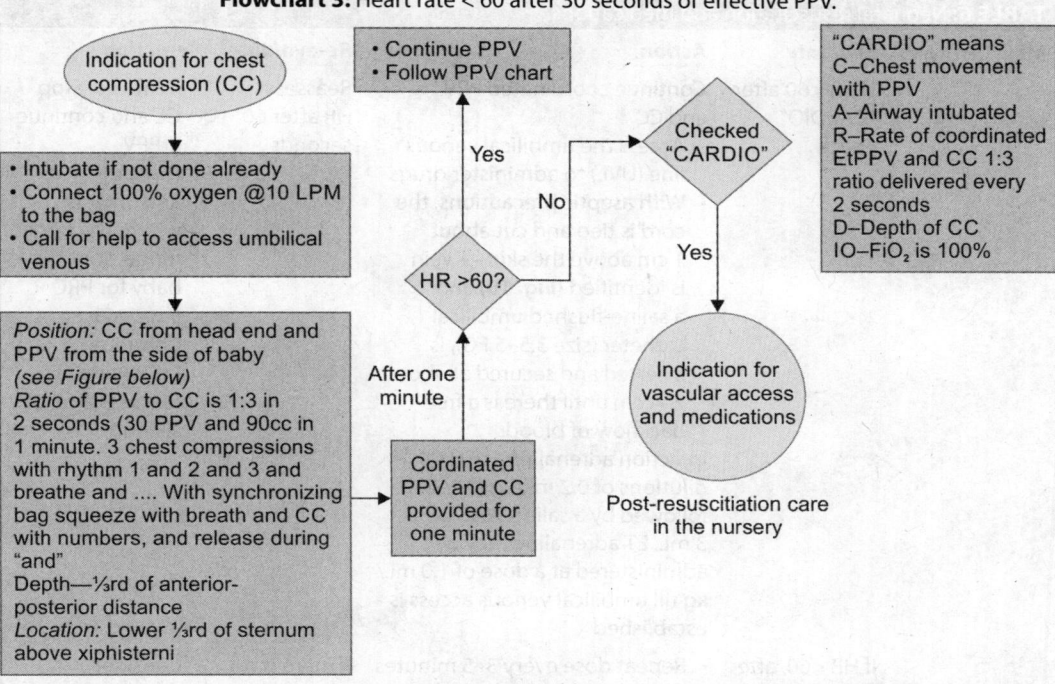

(PPV: positive-pressure ventilation)

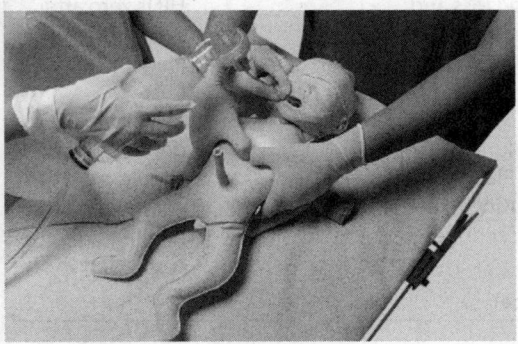

Fig. 9: Chest compression from the head end and PPV from the side of the baby. *(For color version, see Plate 4)*

coordinated chest compressions and PPV (Fig. 9).

What to do next in neonatal resuscitation if HR < 60 after 1 minute of coordinated CC and endotracheal PPV and what is the role of medications in neonatal resuscitation?

Table 6 also mentions the next step to taken in neonatal resuscitation if HR < 60 after 1 minute of coordinated CC and endotracheal PPV.

OVERVIEW OF THE NEONATAL RESUSCITATION PROGRAM

Neonatal Resuscitation Program (NRP) is a standardized evidence-based, structured program. Every person attending delivery should be NRP-trained to improve neonatal care at delivery and to prevent neonatal morbidity and mortality due to birth asphyxia **(Flowchart 4)**.

Reader is suggested to follow the *Performance Checklist from 1 to 7* as appended below for easy recap and skill enhancement. All HCPs working in birthing places should be familiar and thorough with at least bag-and-mask ventilation (equipment and procedure).

TABLE 6: Neonatal resuscitation and medications.

MEDICATIONS	Evaluate	Action	Re-evaluate	Re-action
	If HR <60 after "CARDIO" check	Continue coordinated PPV and CC • Access the umbilical venous line (UVL) to administer drugs • With aseptic precautions, the cord is tied and cut about 1 cm above the skin → vein is identified **(Fig. 10)** and a saline-flushed umbilical catheter (size 3.5–5 FG), is inserted and secured at about 2–4 cm until there is a free backflow of blood. Injection adrenaline 1:10,000 dilutions of 0.2 mL/kg (0.1–0.3) followed by a saline flush of 3 mL. ET adrenaline may be administered at a dose of 1.0 mL/kg till umbilical venous access is established	Reassess HR after 60 seconds	• *If HR >60:* Stop CC and continue EtPPV • Once HR >100 and SpO_2 is within the target range, shift the baby for PRC • *If HR <60:* Continue • EtPPV and CC, reassess after 60 seconds
	If HR <60, after 60 seconds of EtPPV and CC following an intravenous dose of adrenaline	• Repeat dose every 3–5 minutes and assess every 60 seconds for a response • If a history of blood loss and signs of shock are present, then give one bolus of normal saline @10 mL/kg over 5–10 minutes • If the chest transillumination test is positive → Place intercostal drain using a three-way stopcock and syringe	If there is no response to adrenaline	• Consider discontinuing resuscitation, if HR is zero after 20 minutes of life • Post-resuscitation debriefing should be conducted and family should be counseled

(EtPPV: positive-pressure ventilation via endotracheal tube)

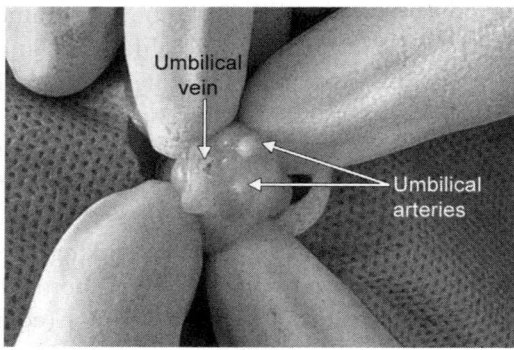

Fig. 10: Umbilical cord showing umbilical two arteries and one vein. *(For color version, see Plate 4)*

Neonatal Resuscitation

Flowchart 4: Neonatal Resuscitation Program Algorithm.

```
                    Perinatal risk assessment
                    Umbilical cord management
                    Team briefing
                    Hand washing
                    Equipment check
                              │
                            Birth
                              ▼
         ┌─────────────────────────────────────┐         ┌──────────────────────────────────────┐
         │  Is the baby breathing/crying?      │── Yes ──▶│ • Continue skin to skin care          │
         └─────────────────────────────────────┘         │ • Ensure open airway                  │
                              │                          │ • Cover baby and mother together      │
                             No                          │ • Clamp and cut cord after one minute │
                              ▼                          │ • Initiate breastfeeding              │
              Warm, dry, stimulate, position             │ • Continue ongoing evaluation         │
              airway, suction if needed                  └──────────────────────────────────────┘
                              │
                              ▼
         ┌─────────────────────────┐   No    ┌──────────────────────────────┐  No
         │ Apnea or gasping?       │────────▶│ Labored breathing or         │─────┐
         │ HR <100 bpm?            │         │ persistent cyanosis?         │     │
         └─────────────────────────┘         └──────────────────────────────┘     │
                     │                                    │                        │
                    Yes                                  Yes                       │
                     ▼                                    ▼                        │
              PPV                                 Positions airway, suction if    │
              Pulse oximeter                      needed                           │
                     │                             Pulse oximeter                  │
                     ▼                             Oxygen if needed                │
         ┌─────────────────────────┐   No         Consider CPAP                    │
         │ Heart rate <100 bpm?    │──────────────────────┐                        │
         └─────────────────────────┘                      │                        │
                     │                                    │                        │
                    Yes                                   ▼                        ▼
                     ▼                        ┌──────────────────────────────────────┐
         If chest not rising take             │ Observational care                    │
         ventilation corrective steps         │ (babies receiving initial steps/brief │
         Ensure adequate ventilation          │ ventilation)                          │
         Consider intubation                  │ Post-resuscitation care               │
                     │                        │ (prolonged ventilation)               │
                     ▼                        │ Team debriefing                       │
   No    ┌─────────────────────────┐          └──────────────────────────────────────┘
  ◀──────│ Heart rate <60 bpm?     │
         └─────────────────────────┘
                     │
                    Yes
                     ▼
         Endotracheal intubation
         coordinated CC with PPV
         100% oxygen, prepare UVC
                     │
                     ▼
   No    ┌─────────────────────────┐
  ◀──────│ Heart rate <60 bpm?     │◀─┐
         └─────────────────────────┘  │
                     │                │
                    Yes               │
                     ▼                │
         IV adrenaline every 3–5 minutes
         if HR remains below 60 bpm
         • Consider hypovolemia
         • Consider pneumothorax
```

FIRST GOLDEN MINUTE

Target oxygen saturation table	
1 minutes	60–65%
2 minutes	65–70%
3 minutes	70–75%
4 minutes	75–80%
5 minutes	80–85%
10 minutes	85–95%
Initial oxygen concentration for PPV	
≥35 weeks of GA	21% oxygen
<35 weeks of GA	21–30% oxygen

Algorithm for neonatal resuscitation
(CPAP: continuous positive airway pressure; GA: gestational age; HR: heart rate; PPV: positive-pressure ventilation)

PERFORMANCE CHECKLIST 1: PREPARATION FOR BIRTH

NAME _____ INSTRUCTOR _____ DATE _____

You have been called in labor room for delivery of a baby, show how would you prepare for birth.

Assesses perinatal risk factors	☐
Expected gestational age	☐
Is amniotic fluid clear	☐
Additional risk factors	☐
Discusses umbilical cord management	☐
Assembles team according to risk factors	☐
Pre-resuscitation team briefing	☐
Washes hands with soap and water for 40–60 seconds along with team	☐
Checks all equipment and supplies	☐
Checks the function of bag and mask	☐

PERFORMANCE CHECKLIST 2: BIRTH AND ROUTINE CARE

NAME _____ INSTRUCTOR _____ DATE_____

You have been called in the labor room to attend delivery, you have already prepared for birth. The baby may be born anytime, demonstrate how you would evaluate and take care of this baby. You may ask me any question you would like to know about the newborn condition's as you progress.

(Instructor: The baby has been born)
Evaluates the baby ☐

Is the baby breathing or crying
(Instructor: Yes the baby is breathing)

Places baby skin to skin with mother ☐

Dries the baby and removes wet linen ☐

Stimulate the baby if needed ☐

Positions head and neck ☐

Clears secretions, if needed ☐

Clamp and cut the cord after one minute ☐

Covers the baby and mother with warm blanket ☐

Continues ongoing evaluation of breathing, activity, color and temperature. ☐
Advises mother to initiate breastfeeding

PERFORMANCE CHECKLIST 3: BIRTH AND INITIAL STEPS

NAME _____ INSTRUCTOR _____ DATE _____

You have been called in the labor room to attend delivery, you have already prepared for birth. The baby may be born anytime, demonstrate how you would evaluate and take care of this baby. You may ask me any question you would like to know about the newborn's condition as you progress.

(Instructor: The baby has been born)

Evaluates the baby ☐

Is the baby breathing or crying ☐
(Instructor: The baby is not breathing)

Cuts the cord and receives baby at radiant warmer ☐

Dries the baby and removes wet linen ☐

Stimulate the baby by rubbing back ☐

Positions airway ☐

Suctions mouth and nose, if baby still not breathing ☐

Assesses breathing ☐
(Instructor: The baby is breathing)

Assesses heart rate ☐
(Instructor: Heart rate 120 bpm)

Returns the baby to mother and places baby in skin to skin contact, covers the baby and mother with warm blanket. Monitors breathing, tone, activity, color, and temperature. ☐
(Instructor: Baby appears cyanotic at 5 minutes)

Checks breathing	*(Instructor: Baby is breathing)*	☐
Auscultates heart rate	*(Instructor: HR 140 bpm)*	☐
Attaches pulse oximeter correctly		☐

(Instructor: SpO$_2$ 72%)

Administers free flow oxygen using correct technique and concentration ☐

Monitors oxygen saturation and take appropriate action ☐

Plans observational care ☐

Neonatal Resuscitation

PERFORMANCE CHECKLIST 4: BAG AND MASK VENTILATION

NAME _____ INSTRUCTOR _____ DATE _____

The baby has just been born and the baby has been provided with initial steps of resuscitation. Demonstrate what you would do for this baby.

- Is the baby breathing
  (Instructor: Baby not breathing) ☐

- Assesses heart rate
  (Instructor: Heart rate 70 bpm) ☐

- Indicates need for PPV and calls for help ☐

- Begins PPV within 60 seconds of birth ☐

- Selects appropriate size mask ☐

- Applies mask correctly ☐

- Starts PPV with room air in term baby ☐

- Requests assistant to place pulse oximeter sensor on baby's right hand or wrist ☐

- Within 15 seconds of beginning PPV requests to check HR to assess if HR increasing ☐
  (Instructor: Heart rate 60 bpm, not increasing)

- Checks for chest rise
  (Instructor: No chest rise) ☐

- Takes ventilation corrective steps ☐
  (Instructor determines how many MRSOPA steps are needed before PPV can result in chest movement)

- Mask adjustment ☐

- Reposition the head and neck ☐

- Gives 5 breaths and assess chest movement ☐
  (Instructor: No chest movement, HR 60 bpm, pulse oximeter no signal)

- Suction the mouth and nose ☐

- Open the mouth ☐

- Gives 5 breaths and assess chest movement ☐
  (Instructor: No chest movement, HR 60 bpm, pulse oximeter no signal)

PERFORMANCE CHECKLIST 4: BAG AND MASK VENTILATION

NAME _____ INSTRUCTOR _____ DATE _____

Increases pressure by squeezing the bag harder ☐

Gives 5 breaths and assess chest movement ☐
(Instructor: Chest moves with the PPV)

Continues ventilation for 30 seconds ☐

Assesses heart rate after 30 seconds of PPV that rises chest ☐
(Instructor: HR 120 bpm, SpO_2 68%)

Continues ventilation, adjusts oxygen concentration as per pulse oximeter, monitors HR and respiratory effort ☐
(Instructor: The baby has spontaneous respiratory effort)

Gradually discontinuous PPV ☐
(Instructor: Heart rate 140 BPM, SpO_2 72% and baby has continuous respiratory effort)

Discontinues PPV ☐

Assesses need for free flow oxygen to maintain oxygen saturation within target range ☐

Initiates free flow oxygen correctly ☐

Assesses heart rate and oxygen saturation and respiratory status ☐
(Instructor: Heart rate 140 BPM, SpO_2 90%, the baby has good respiratory effort)

Weans and discontinuous free flow oxygen ☐

Plans post-resuscitation care ☐

Neonatal Resuscitation

PERFORMANCE CHECKLIST 5: INTUBATION
NAME _____ INSTRUCTOR _____ DATE _____
Demonstrate how you would prepare for and intubate a newborn baby.
Prepares for intubation, requests correct size tube and laryngoscope blade ☐
Assistant checks laryngoscope light and prepares tape for securing tube ☐
Holds laryngoscope correctly in left hand ☐
Opens baby's mouth with finger and inserts blade to base of the tongue ☐
Lifts blade correctly (no rocking motion) ☐
Identify landmarks, takes corrective action to visualize glottis if needed ☐
Inserts tube from the right side without obstructing the vision ☐
Aligns vocal cord guide with vocal cords ☐
Removes laryngoscope while firmly holding tube against baby's palate ☐
Hold tube against baby's palate ☐
Administers PPV ☐
Observes for symmetrical chest movements. Assistant listens for bilateral chest movement and rising HR *(Instructor: Chest is not moving, HR not increasing)* ☐
If the chest is not moving then removes endotracheal tube and resumes PPV by bag and mask ☐
Repeats intubation attempt, observes chest movement. Assistant checks air entry, HR *(Instructor: Chest movement present, air entry present bilaterally)* ☐
Assistant checks tip to lip insertion depth using NTL (Tip to lip = NTL+ 1) ☐
Assistant secures the tube by tape ☐
Continues PPV for 30 seconds ☐

PERFORMANCE CHECKLIST 6: MEDICATION

NAME _____ INSTRUCTOR _____ DATE_____

Demonstrate how you would prepare for and insert umbilical venous cannula in a newborn baby.

Procedure is done in a sterile manner	☐
Attaches three way stopcock to umbilical venous catheter	☐
Flushes catheter and stopcock with normal saline	☐
Closes stopcock to catheter	☐
Cleans lower segment of umbilical cord with antiseptic solution	☐
Ties umbilical tape loosely at base of cord	☐
Cuts cord about 1–2 cm above base	☐
Inserts catheter into vein, open stopcock and gently aspirate syringe, advances catheter approximately 2–4 cm until backflow of blood is detected	☐
Flushes catheter and closes stopcock toward catheter	☐
Ensures catheter is being held in place; may secure with clear adhesive dressing	☐

Neonatal Resuscitation

PERFORMANCE CHECKLIST 7: INTUBATION, CC, MEDICATION
NAME _____ INSTRUCTOR _____ DATE _____

The baby has just been born and the baby has been provided with initial steps of resuscitation. Demonstrate what you would do for this baby.

Is the baby breathing
(Instructor: Baby not breathing) ☐

Assesses heart rate
(Instructor: Heart rate 70 bpm) ☐

Indicates need for PPV, applies mask correctly and begins PPV within 60 seconds of birth ☐

Starts PPV with room air in term baby ☐

Requests assistant to place pulse oximeter ☐

Within 15 seconds of beginning PPV requests to check HR to assess if HR increasing ☐
(Instructor: Heart rate 60 bpm, not increasing)

Takes ventilation corrective steps ☐
(Instructor determines how many MRSOPA steps are needed before PPV can result in chest movement)

Mask adjustment, reposition the head and neck ☐

Gives 5 breaths and assess chest movement ☐
(Instructor: No chest movement, HR 60 bpm, pulse oximeter no signal)

Suction the mouth and nose, opens the mouth ☐

Gives 5 breaths and assess chest movement ☐
(Instructor: No chest movement, HR 60 bpm, pulse oximeter no signal)

Increases pressure to squeeze the bag ☐

Gives 5 breaths and assess chest movement ☐
(Instructor: No chest movement HR 60 bpm, pulse oximeter no signal)

Intubates with correct size tube ☐

Checks for bilateral breath sound and chest movement with PPV ☐

Checks tip to lip insertion depth using NTL ☐

PERFORMANCE CHECKLIST 7: INTUBATION, CC, MEDICATION

NAME _____ INSTRUCTOR _____ DATE _____

Asks assistant to secure endotracheal tube	☐
Continues ventilation for 30 seconds	☐
Assesses heart rate after 30 seconds of PPV that rises chest *(Instructor: HR 30 bpm, pulse oximeter no signal)*	☐
Call for additional help	☐
Asks assistant to increase oxygen to 100%	☐
Administers chest compressions from head of the bed with coordinated ventilation (3 chest compressions to one ventilation every 2 seconds)	☐
Continues coordinated chest compression and ventilation for 60 seconds	☐
Assesses heart rate after 60 seconds *(Instructor: HR 30 bpm, pulse oximeter no signal)*	☐
Ask assistant to prepare umbilical venous catheterization	☐
Requests estimated baby weight *(Instructor: Estimated baby weight 3 kg)*	☐
Requests adrenaline via endotracheal tube	☐
Orders 0.3 mg adrenaline (3 mL of 1:10000 adrenaline) from assistant	☐
Assistant uses closed loop communication with confirmation of medication and dose	☐
Assistant provides the desired amount of adrenaline	☐
Assistant administers the dose via endotracheal tube and announces that ET dose of 3 mL of adrenaline given	☐
Continues coordinated chest compression and ventilation for 60 seconds	☐
Assesses heart rate after 60 seconds *(Instructor: HR 30 bpm, pulse oximeter no signal)*	☐

Neonatal Resuscitation

PERFORMANCE CHECKLIST 7: INTUBATION, CC, MEDICATION
NAME _____ INSTRUCTOR _____ DATE _____

- Assistant places umbilical venous catheter in place ☐
- Requests adrenaline 0.6 mL to be given by umbilical venous catheter ☐
- Uses closed loop communication ☐
- Assistant delivers 0.6 mL adrenaline by umbilical vein and flushes cannula with 3 mL NS and announces, 0.6 mL of adrenaline given followed by 3 mL flush of normal saline ☐
- Assesses heart rate after 60 seconds
  (Instructor: HR 50 bpm, pulse oximeter no signal, the baby is pale) ☐
- Continues coordinated chest compression and ventilation ☐
- Checks for history of blood loss
  (Instructor: Retroplacental clot present/antepartum hemorrhage) ☐
- Requests 30 mL of NS to be given in 5–10 minutes by UVC ☐
- Assesses heart rate after 60 seconds
  (Instructor: HR 80 bpm, pulse oximeter 67%) ☐
- Discontinues chest compressions ☐
- Continues PPV ☐
- Assesses heart rate, breathing and saturation after 30 seconds
  (Instructor: HR 100 bpm, pulse oximeter 80%, no spontaneous respiration) ☐
- Continues PPV and adjusts oxygen concentration as per saturation target ☐
- Assesses heart rate, breathing and saturation after 30 seconds
  (Instructor: HR 130 bpm, pulse oximeter 92%, some spontaneous respiration present) ☐
- Supports baby with PPV and supplemental oxygen as per target oxygen saturation table ☐
- Prepares to move baby to post-resuscitation care setting ☐
- Updates parents and inform them of next steps ☐
- Team debriefs the resuscitation done ☐

SUGGESTED READING

1. Bharti LK, Prakash A, Jain M; Indian Academy of Pediatrics (IAP). Standard Treatment Guidelines 2022, Neonatal Resuscitation Program. [online] Available from https://iapindia.org/pdf/Ch-104-Neonatal-Resuscitation-Program.pdf. [Last accessed April, 2024].
2. Berkelhamer SK, Kamath-Rayne BD, Niermeyer S. Neonatal resuscitation in low-resource settings. Clin Perinatol. 2016;43(3):573-91.
3. Indian Academy of Pediatrics. Advanced NRP Workshop Manual: A Joint Initiative by IAP and NNF. Mumbai: Indian Academy of Pediatrics; 2021.
4. Weiner GM, Zaichkin J. Textbook of Neonatal Resuscitation, 8th edition. Itasca: American Academy of Pediatrics; 2021.

CHAPTER 13

Instruments

Shalini Rajaram, Sandhya Jain, Om Kumari, Vashudha Gupta

■ OBSTETRICS

Describe Sim's speculum (Fig. 1).
Sim's speculum is the most commonly used speculum in obstetrics and gynecology and is used to retract the vaginal walls, particularly the posterior vaginal wall. Because of its peculiar shape, it is also called duckbill speculum. It is either double-ended or single-ended; if it is double-ended, each end is of different size. Three sizes are available: (1) 26 and 31 mm, (2) 31 and 36 mm, and (3) 36 and 42 mm.

What are the different parts of the instrument and specific functions of each?
The speculum has a handle in the center and the blades at right angles to the handle. The blades are rounded at the end, so as to be atraumatic. A trough runs along the entire length of the instrument, so that blood or secretions collecting in the concave blade drain off along the trough in the handle.

What is the technique of use of this instrument?

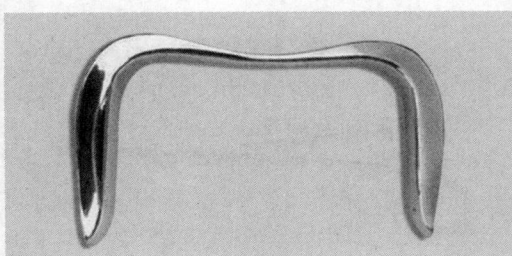

Fig. 1: Sim's speculum.

The blade is lubricated with an antiseptic solution or sterile jelly. The labia minora are held apart by thumb and index finger of the left hand and the blade is inserted in-between, its transverse axis in the long axis of the labia. Once in the vagina, it is rotated through 90° such that the blade retracts the posterior wall of the vagina. The posterior vaginal wall is examined as the speculum is withdrawn.

What are the disadvantages of this instrument?
- Sim's speculum is not a self-retaining instrument; therefore, the assistant is needed to hold it in position.
- Since it moves with the movement of the hand, it is not suitable for colposcopy and colpomicroscopy.
- To use this instrument, the patient needs to be at the edge of the table.

Discuss the indications.
To examine the cervix and vagina:
- Discharge per vaginam
- Cervicitis/cervical erosion/polyps
- Cervical carcinoma and vaginal carcinoma
- *Prolapse:* Uterine, cystocele, urethrocele, rectocele, and enterocele
- Urinary stress incontinence
- Vesicovaginal fistula, rectovaginal fistula
- Congenital malformations of the cervix and vagina

Carrying out procedures:
- Pap smear
- Cervical and vaginal biopsy
- Endometrial biopsy (EB)
- Insertion or removal of intrauterine contraceptive device (IUCD)
- Dilatation and curettage
- Polypectomy
- Hysterosalpingography (HSG)
- Hysteroscopy/colposcopy
- Vaginal surgeries—vaginal hysterectomies/nondescent vaginal hysterectomy (NDVH)
- Culdocentesis/colpotomy

Obstetrical indications:
- To examine and repair for cervical tears/vaginal tears
- Packing the uterine cavity

What is Sim's anterior vaginal wall retractor (Fig. 2)?

Sim's anterior vaginal wall retractor is a long instrument with spoon-shaped ends with transverse serrations on either surface. The loops make an angle of 15° with the shaft and are angled in opposite directions. The transverse serrations provide friction against rugous vagina and aid in efficient retraction.

What are the indications of its use?

It is used for retraction of the anterior vagina for exposure of cervix in conjunction with Sim's speculum.

Describe the sponge-holding forceps (Fig. 3).

Sponge-holding forceps is a long instrument with ring-shaped ends with transverse serrations on the inner surface of ends, which prevent it from slipping. A ratchet catch is on the handles to lock the blades in sponge holder.

What are the indications of its use?
- Preparation of vagina, vulva, and abdominal wall with antiseptic solutions before surgery
- To hold cervix during pregnancy for:
  • Insertion of Foley's catheter in extra-amniotic space for second-trimester pregnancy termination using ethacridine lactate
  • Removal of products of conception during incomplete and inevitable abortions and medical termination of pregnancy (MTP)
  • Diagnosis and repair of cervical tear. Here, two to three sponge holders are required. The first one holds the cervix at a fixed point and the other two are rotated to identify the tear.
  • Holding and steadying the cervix of a pregnant uterus during any procedure, as it is less traumatic
  • Holding cut edges of the lower uterine segment during cesarean section in place of green Armytage
  • Inserting a Cu-T for postpartum insertion
  • Packing uterus in postpartum hemorrhage (PPH) before transferring the patient to the tertiary center
  • Removing retained bits of placenta and membranes

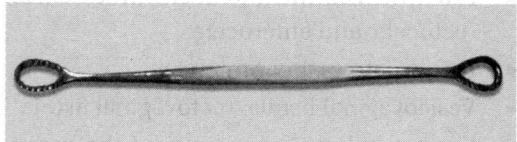

Fig. 2: Anterior vaginal wall retractor.

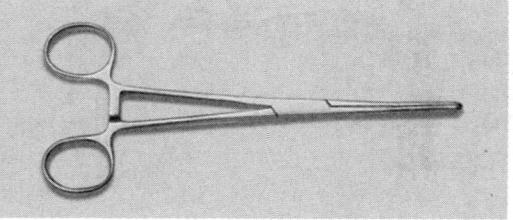

Fig. 3: Sponge holder.

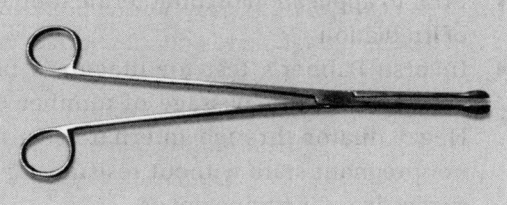

Fig. 4: Ovum forceps.

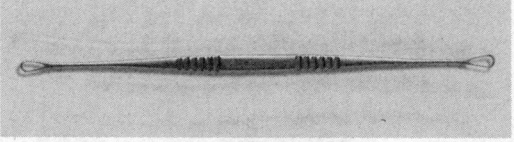

Fig. 5: Uterine curette.

- To hold a sponge to swab blood from a distance during surgery
- For blunt dissection by a folded gauze piece, i.e., separation of bladder from the anterior surface of cervix during abdominal hysterectomy—vaginal hysterectomy
- As a nontraumatic clamp over the ovarian vessels during conservative surgeries, such as myomectomy and metroplasty

Describe Heywood Smith's ovum forceps (Fig. 4).
This instrument has spoon-shaped, blunt, and fenestrated ends, which just come in contact with each other when the forceps is closed. There is no lock on handles, so that the instrument has no crushing action and any structure inadvertently held (like the uterine wall) should not be damaged.

What are the indications of its use?
- First-trimester pregnancy termination—to remove products of conception after cervical dilation
- Removal of bits of placenta and membranes after second-trimester pregnancy termination
- Removal of pedunculated uterine polyps

What can be the complications with its use?
- Uterine perforation
- Injury to intra-abdominal structures, such as small bowel, colon, and secondary to uterine perforation, if the latter has not been diagnosed

- Intrauterine infection
- Incomplete abortion

What is Blake's uterine curette (Fig. 5)?
The instrument has a central shaft and one small oval loop at each end. One end of curette is sharp and the other blunt. The loops are set at an angle, so that it can curette endometrial cavity.

What are the indications for its use?
For curetting the endometrium for biopsy in the following conditions:
- Abnormal uterine bleeding (AUB)
- Diagnosis of endometrial carcinoma
- Diagnosis of endometrial tuberculosis
- Infertility; premenstrual sample for documentation of ovulation
- Fothergill's operation
- Check curettage for incomplete abortion
- Following dilatation and evacuation of products with ovum forceps in first-trimester pregnancy termination
- After evacuation of hydatidiform mole

What can be the complications of its use?
- Uterine perforation
- Incomplete evacuation of product of conception

What are the different types of cervical dilators (Fig. 6)?
There are three commonly used types of cervical dilators, and none has a distinct advantage over the others.
1. *Hegar dilator:* It is smooth, solid, curved rod, curved, and tapering toward the tip. The dilators are serial beginning at 3 mm

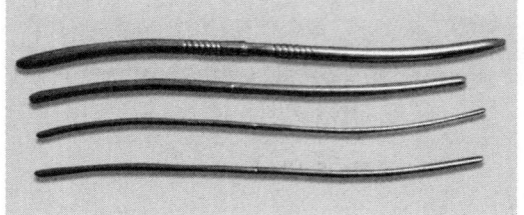

Fig. 6: Hegar cervical dilators.

up to 26 mm, the difference in diameter being 1 mm. Thus, in double-ended instruments, the first dilator will be 3 mm on one end and 4 mm on the other. There is a difference of 3 mm in the diameter near the tip and the maximum dilating portion of the dilator, and so they are numbered from 3/6 to 23/26—numerator signifies diameter at tip and denominator signifies maximum diameter. It may come as either a single- or double-ended instrument.

2. *Hank dilator:* These are similar to Hegar dilators except that they are less curved. The difference in the diameter of successive dilators is 0.5 mm. Thus, it achieves more gradual and hence less traumatic dilatation of cervix.
3. *Pratt dilators:* These are shaped like the Hegar dilator but half graduated; that is, the difference between successive dilators is 0.5 mm and not 1 mm as Hegar dilators. Thus, it achieves less traumatic cervical dilation.

What are the uses of this instrument?
This instrument is used for dilation of cervix prior to:
- Endometrial curettage
- Suction aspiration for first-trimester pregnancy termination
- Evacuation of molar gestation and products of conception
- Hysteroscopic procedures
- Pyometra and hematometra drainage
- Manchester operation
- Prior to application of intrauterine source of irradiation
- Inverse Palmer's test for diagnosis of incompetent os—passage of number 8 Hegar dilator through internal os in a nonpregnant state without resistance is suggestive of incompetent os

Shirodkar's test: When a size 8 dilator, which has been passed through internal os in a nonpregnant woman, is withdrawn, there is a distinct snap, as it passes out of internal os, which is absent in cases of incompetence.

What is the technique of dilating cervix?
The procedure is carried out under paracervical block or general anesthesia. The cervix is exposed and lip held with vulsellum. The uterine cavity is sounded, and the smallest dilator is held like a pen, and its lubricated tip is passed into the cervical canal. Penetration beyond internal os is prevented by the little finger of the surgeon positioned against the patient's perineum. The dilator is held in position for few seconds and then removed so that the next dilator may be passed for serial dilation of cervix.

What are the complications of its use?
- Cervical tears
- Hemorrhage—injury to the descending cervical artery and cervical perforation
- Uterine perforation
- Excessive dilation of cervix may lead to incompetent os
- Introduction of infection

What is green Armytage forceps (Fig. 7)?
Green Armytage forceps is an instrument made of stainless steel and has triangular solid tips with transverse serrations.

What are the indications of its use?
- To hold the cut edges of the lower uterine segment after delivery of fetus

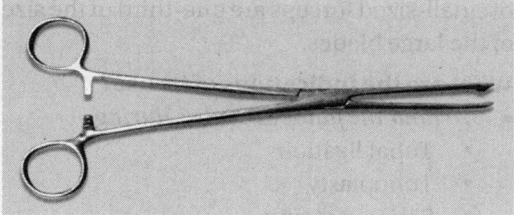

Fig. 7: Green Armytage forceps.

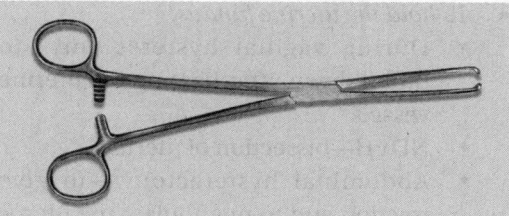

Fig. 9: Allis tissue forceps.

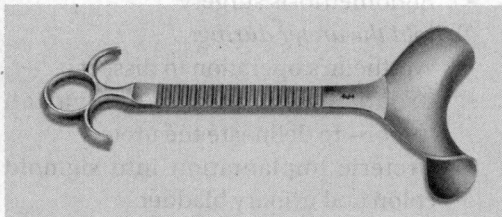

Fig. 8: Doyen's retractor.

- *Advantages:* It holds the edges atraumatically and achieves hemostasis by compressing bleeding edges.

What is Doyen's retractor (Fig. 8)?
This instrument is used for retraction of the abdominal wall suprapubically after opening of the parietal peritoneum. After the uterovesical (UV) fold of peritoneum is opened, it is used to retract the bladder during cesarean section and hysterectomy. It has a sturdy handle with a broad blade with uniform curvature. The broad-retracting surface achieves good retraction. The solid blade achieves reduction in blood loss from cut edges by compression.

What are the indications of its use?
Doyen's retractor is used during procedures, such as:
- Cesarean section
- Laparotomy for ovarian cystectomy, oophorectomy, ruptured ectopic gestation
- Abdominal and peripartum hysterectomies

- Prolapse repairs, e.g., Shirodkar's sling procedure, Khanna's sling operation, Moschcowitz culdoplasty
- Stress urinary incontinence repair surgeries

Describe Allis forceps (Fig. 9).
Allis forceps can be long or short. The longer ones are 17 cm in length and the shorter ones are 12 cm in length. The blades are curved near the tip and are toothed. These have four-in-five teeth or five-in-six teeth. Due to the presence of the teeth, Allis forceps are traumatic and are not used for the skin. The handle of this instrument has a ratchet lock.

What are the indications of its use?
Allis forceps is used:
- *To hold the cut edges of vagina during:*
  - Anterior colporrhaphy and posterior colpoperineorrhaphy—to dissect the vaginal mucosal flaps from the underlying bladder and rectum
  - Abdominal hysterectomy, to hold the vaginal cuff to buttress them
  - Vaginal hysterectomy—to hold the vaginal edges during closure of the cuff of the vagina
  - Excision of the vaginal wall cyst
- *To hold the cervix:*
  - Abdominal hysterectomy—to draw the cervix up after opening the vault of the vagina
  - When vulsellum is not available

- *To hold the uterine fundus:*
  - During vaginal hysterectomy—to pull it down after ligating the uterine vessels
  - NDVH—bissection of uterus
  - Abdominal hysterectomy—to give traction and to manipulate the uterus while clamping the pedicle
- Myomectomy—to give traction on the myoma being enucleated
- Metroplasty—to hold the cut edges of the uterus during suturing
- To hold the rectus sheath during dissecting it from the underlying rectus muscle and also during suturing it
- To hold the angles and the cut edges of the uterine segment during lower segment cesarean section (LSCS)

What is the instrument shown in Figure 10?
The instrument is a Babcock forceps. It is a nontraumatic instrument, which has fenestrated triangular blades and grooved jaws. It is available in three sizes: (1) Large, (2) medium, and (3) small, their lengths being 17, 12, and 10 cm. The blades of large and medium sizes are identical; however, blades of small-sized forceps are one-third of the size of the large blades.

What are the indications of its use?
- *To hold the fallopian tubes during:*
  - Tubal ligation
  - Tuboplasty
  - Salpingectomy
- *To hold the ovaries during:*
  - Ovarian cystectomy
  - Endometriosis surgery
- *To hold the ureter during:*
  - Wertheim's operation to dissect it
  - Broad ligament tumor/ovarian tumor—to delineate the ureter
  - Ureteric implantation into sigmoid colon and urinary bladder
- *To hold the bladder during:*
  - Vesicovaginal repair
  - Bladder repair due to accidental injury
  - Cystostomy
- During internal iliac artery ligation—to dissect the vascular sheath
- *To hold the bowel during:*
  - Rectovaginal repair
  - Third-degree perineal tear—to hold the mucosal edges

Identify and describe the instruments shown in Figures 11A and B.
The instrument shown in **Fig. 11B** is the Braun–Stadler episiotomy scissors.
   The instrument is available in different sizes. The standard size is 16 cm long and is sterilized by dipping into Lysol or glutaraldehyde. The blades are angled on side and tips are round and blunt to reduce the risk of piercing in nearby structures. The shape of the instrument allows easy introduction in the vagina and prevents erratic cutting. Its angle makes it convenient to use, as it prevents butting of the instrument against the patient's buttocks, if the instrument was straight. Busch scissors is another type of episiotomy scissors shown in **Figure 11A**.

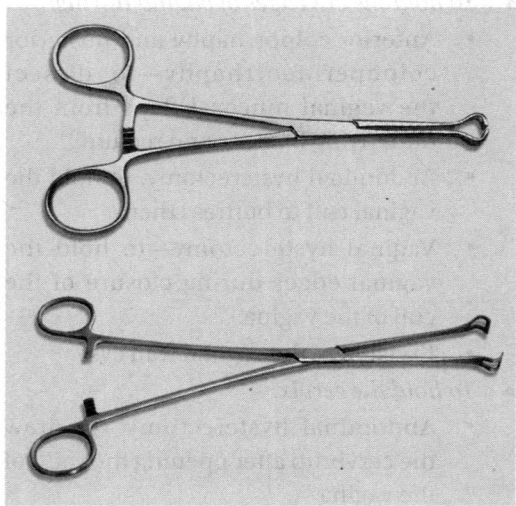

Fig. 10: Babcock forceps.

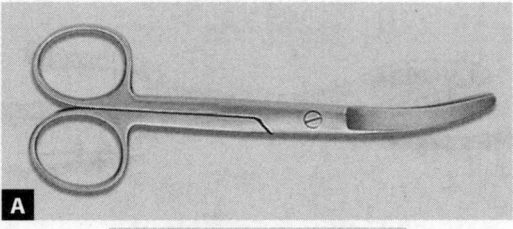

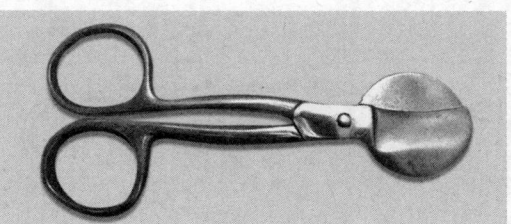

Fig. 12: Umbilical cord scissors.

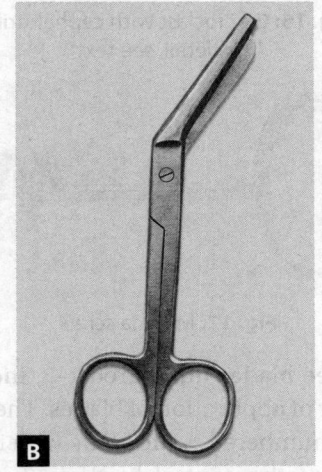

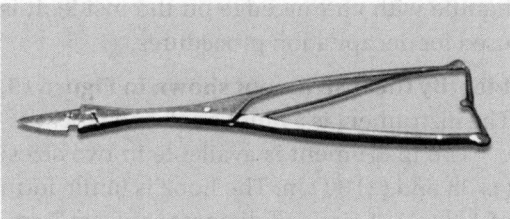

Fig. 13: Simpson's perforator.

Figs. 11A and B: (A) Busch episiotomy scissors; (B) Braun–Stadler episiotomy scissors.

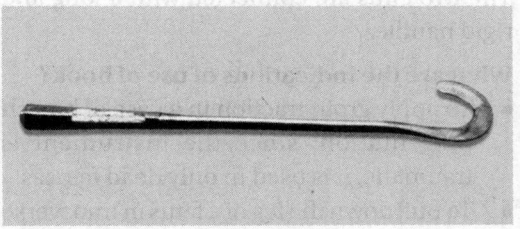

Fig. 14: Decapitation saw.

Identify the instrument shown in Figure 12.
The instrument is the umbilical cord scissors. It is 10.5 cm long with American pattern and is sterilized by immersion in Lysol or glutaraldehyde. Its blades are so curved that on closing, they meet at the tip; this prevents the umbilical cord from slippage during cutting.

INSTRUMENTS FOR DESTRUCTIVE OPERATIONS

What is Simpson's perforator (Fig. 13)?
The instrument is made of stainless steel and is 28.5 cm long. It has blades with triangular tips with outer cutting edges. The blades have two shoulders, distal being proximal to the cutting edge, which prevents the blades from slipping out of fetal head. The proximal shoulder, which lies after a narrow waist, prevents excessive penetration by the blades of the instrument. The blades of the instrument are kept locked by a locking system, which opens by inward pressure and handles are brought together. A flat spring is present between the handles, which is compressed on approximation of handles and on releasing them, goes back to original position.

What are the indications of its use?
- Craniotomy
- Opening fetal thorax or abdomen for evisceration

Identify the instrument shown in Figure 14.
The instrument is the decapitation saw. It has a semicircular blade attached to a long

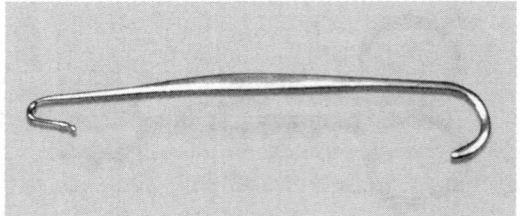

Fig. 15: Hook with crochet.

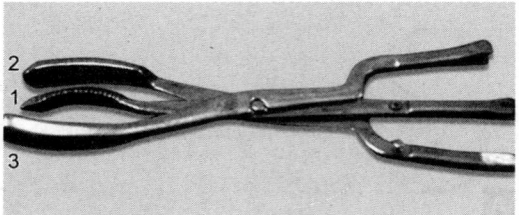

Fig. 16: Cranioclast with cephalotribe (For detail, see text).

handle with cutting edge on the inside. It is used for decapitation procedures.

Identify the instrument shown in Figure 15.
The instrument is a blunt hook and crochet.

The instrument is available in two sizes: (1) 33 and (2) 30 cm. The hook is in the form of 1/3 to 1/2 circle of diameter at least 7 cm. The crochet is small and with a sharp bend. The two ends are connected with a long and rigid handle.

What are the indications of use of hook?
- To apply groin traction in a case of breech presentation; since the instrument is traumatic, it is used in only dead fetuses.
- To pull down the leg of a fetus in transverse lie, provided the fetus is dead, woman is in advanced labor with sufficient cervical dilatation, and there are no signs and symptoms of imminent rupture of uterus.

What are the indications of use of crochet?
- To extract decapitated head by applying traction on fetal lower jaw, orbit, foramen magnum, etc.
- To aid delivery of fetal head after craniotomy by applying traction

What are the uses of embryotomy scissors?
Embryotomy scissors is used for evisceration, cleidotomy, spondylotomy, and decapitation—to cut the soft tissues of fetal neck after dislocation with atlantoaxial joint.

What is the instrument shown in Figure 16?
The instrument is combined cranioclast and cephalotribe. It is a 42-cm, long instrument

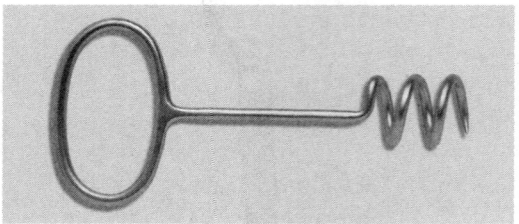

Fig. 17: Myoma screw.

with three blades numbered 1–3, indicating the order of application of blades. The central blade is numbered 1, the blade with its curve parallel to the central blade is 2, and the other is number 3. The central blade is solid; however, 2 and 3 are fenestrated. A long screw is added to the end of the handle of the central blade so that it can be swung into the base of the handle of the other two blades. It is used to crush the vault and base of the dead fetal skull and to extract the fetal head thereafter.

■ GYNECOLOGY

Describe the instrument shown in Figure 17.
The instrument is a myoma screw. It is made of stainless steel. It is shaped-like a threaded screw with a pointed tip while at the other end, there is a shaft ending in a handle. The threads in the screw increase the grip of this instrument.

What are the uses of this instrument?
The instrument holds the myoma during abdominal and vaginal myomectomy. Thus, it can provide traction to the myomas and help in their enucleation.

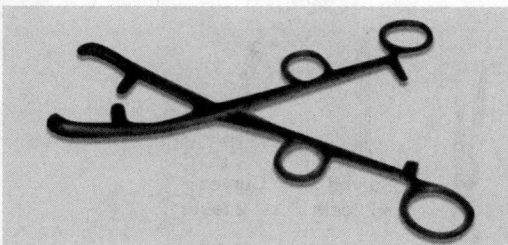

Fig. 18: Bonney clamp.

How do you apply it?
The instrument is applied in an anticlockwise direction with constant screwing motion into the myoma tissue.

Is there any other instrument used for the same purpose?
Myoma hook is used for hooking the myoma during hysterectomies.

Describe the instrument shown in Figure 18.
The instrument is Bonney myomectomy clamp. It has two pairs of finger-grips with a ratchet lock at the proximal end. The blades of this clamp are at an angle of 120° to the handle. The blades are divided into two equal halves by the transverse bars attached to each blade. These blades are covered with rubber caps attached distal to the site of the transverse bars, and this prevents trauma to the tissues.

Why does the clamp have two grips?
The distal grips are used when applying the clamps as the blades can be opened wider with it.

The proximal grips are better suited for tightening and releasing the lock as they give better mechanical advantage.

Discuss the principle of this instrument and its application.
The clamp is applied from the pubic end of the abdominal wound with the angle between the blades and the shanks facing downward. In this manner, the blades go inside the pelvis while the handle remains outside between the patient's thighs. Care is taken to include both the round ligaments when this clamp is applied to the uterus just above the cervix. The round ligament is prevented from slipping by the transverse bars.

By applying the clamp, the blood supply to the uterus and the cervix through the uterine vessels is occluded. The clamp has to be released every 20 minutes for 10 minutes. The reason for its release during an extended myomectomy procedure is that there is accumulation of histamine-like substances due to trauma, and their sudden release into the circulation can lead to postoperative shock. Secondly, the uterus can become anoxic due to the prolonged occlusion of the blood supply.

Can the clamp be applied for cervical leiomyomas?
In case of tumors low in the body of uterus and in cervix, these have to be enucleated first and then the clamp applied.

Is there any other alternative to the clamp?
Yes, red rubber catheter can be used as a tourniquet around the cervix.

Describe the instrument shown in Figures 19A and B.
Hysterectomy clamps are usually 8–9 inches in length and have either curved or straight tips. The curve of the clamps is gentle enough to avoid forcing the bite of tissue laterally. The grasping surface of this instrument has serrations, which can be oblique, longitudinal, or horizontal.

Name the different types of clamps.
Different types of clamps are Heaney clamps, Maingot's clamp, and Kocher's clamp.

How are the clamps applied?
The correct way of applying clamps is with the curve facing the structures to be removed,

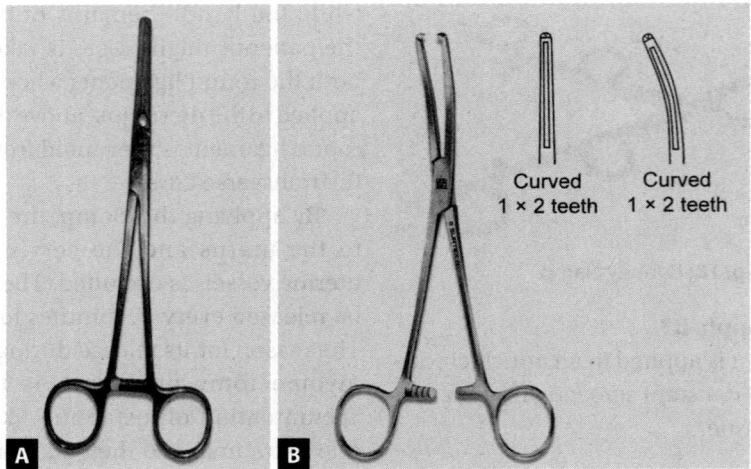

Figs. 19A and B: Hysterectomy clamps. (A) Heaney; (B) Maingot's.

so that the ligature can be passed around the clamped pedicle easily.

Describe the Heaney clamps.
The serration on the blades is oblique and these lack teeth at the tip. Instead, they have a ridge on one blade and a notch on the other blade in which the ridge fits. These ridges and notches can be single or double.

What is the advantage of the oblique serrations?
Since the serrations are oblique, these are at an angle to the structures being clamped and thus the chances of slipping of tissues are minimal. The ridge and the notch add to the security of the pedicle being clamped.

How is Heaney clamp different from Maingot's clamp?
Maingot clamps have a longitudinal ridge in one blade, which fits into the longitudinal groove present on the other blade. The tips of the blades have one on two teeth. These teeth prevent the structures being clamped from slipping and the longitudinal groove and the ridge ensure complete occlusion of the vessels in the pedicle being clamped.

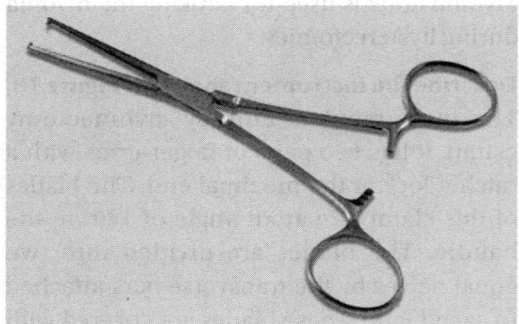

Fig. 20: Kocher's clamp.

What is the instrument shown in Figure 20 and how do you identify it?
The instrument is Kocher's clamp. The blades of this clamp have transverse serrations and are toothed. However, these transverse serrations are less efficient in preventing the slippage of the pedicles than the longitudinal or oblique serrations.

What are the different types of tissue forceps (Fig. 21)?
Tissue forceps come in varying shapes and configurations. Broadly, these can be toothed or nontoothed:
- Smooth nontoothed forceps (Debakey) are commonly used for holding delicate

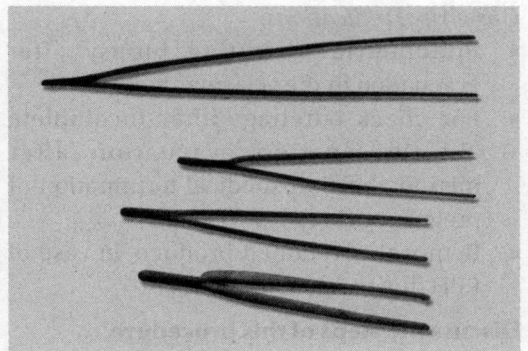

Fig. 21: Tissue forceps.

and friable tissues. They are also used in vascular surgery or for retroperitoneal node dissection.
- The toothed forceps (Adson's) are used to hold the skin while suturing or stapling; that is, they are used for holding firm tissues, such as fascia and rectus sheath. They grip the tissues firmly with minimal pressure.

Artery forceps (Fig. 22A): Artery forceps is used for grasping and compressing an artery to control bleeding. The jaws of the forceps has serrations and handles have a locking mechanism that ensures firm grip on the vessels, aiding in temporary occlusion to manage bleeding effectively.

Lahey's right-angled hemostat (Fig. 22B): It is used for blunt dissection and permits efficient ligature of vessels and organs. The forceps have longitudinal serrations on curved tips and a ratchet lock between the stems.

What are the different types of scissors you know of?
Different types of scissors are Mayo dissecting scissors and Metzenbaum scissors.

Describe the Mayo scissors and discuss its uses (Fig. 23A).
Mayo scissors have rounded tips. They can have either straight or curved blades.

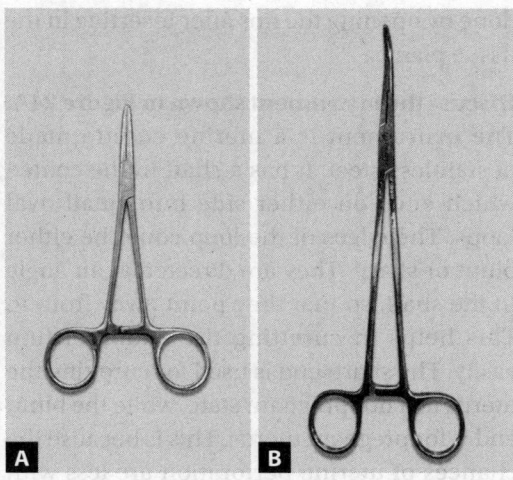

Figs. 22A and B: (A) Artery forceps (hemostat); (B) Lahey's right-angled hemostat.

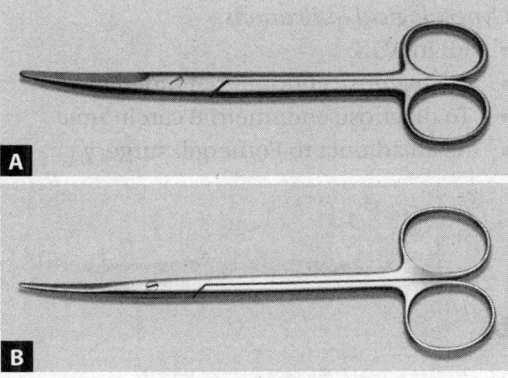

Figs. 23A and B: (A) Mayo's scissors; (B) Metzenbaum scissors.

They are used for dividing the tough tissues, such as rectus fascia, vaginal cuff, and parametrial tissues.

Describe the Metzenbaum scissors and its uses (Fig. 23B).
Metzenbaum scissors have shorter blades proportionate to the shaft. They are used for cutting the delicate tissues, such as the peritoneum. In addition to cutting, they can also be used for retroperitoneal dissection, and in developing planes in areas of adherent or distorted tissues. The blunt dissection is

done by opening the tips after inserting in the tissue planes.

Discuss the instrument shown in Figure 24A.
The instrument is a uterine curette made of stainless steel. It has a shaft in the center, which ends on either side into small oval loops. The edges of the loop could be either blunt or sharp. They are directed at an angle to the shaft, so that they point away from it. This helps in curetting the endometrium easily. The sharp end is used for curetting the uterus in a nonpregnant state, while the blunt end is for pregnant uterus. This is because the chances of uterine perforation are less with the blunt end.

What are the uses of this instrument?
Gynecological indications:
- EB in AUB
- To diagnose endometrial tuberculosis
- To diagnose endometrial carcinoma
- As an adjunct to Fothergill surgery

Obstetrical indications:
- Endometrial curetting biopsy after evacuation in the vesicular mole
- For check curettage after incomplete abortion/suction evacuation after missed abortion/medical termination of pregnancy (MTP)
- Removal of retained products in case of PPH due to retained product

Discuss the steps of this procedure.
This procedure is done under sedation/paracervical block.
- Clean and drape the patient.
- Hold the cervix with a vulsellum and dilate it with Hegar's dilator (generally till 4 mm).
- Introduce the curette and take the curetting from all the walls.
- Send the tissue in formalin (10%) for histopathologic examination (HPE).

What are the different types of endometrial biopsy curette?
Different types of endometrial biopsy curette are Randall's EB curette and Novak's and Pipelle's biopsy curette.

Discuss Randall's endometrial biopsy curette.
Randall's EB curette is a long, thin (external diameter 2 mm) tubular instrument, and it is curved near the tip to facilitate its entry into the uterine cavity. Near its end, it has a notch with a sharp edge in its distal part, so that during the withdrawal of the instrument from the uterine cavity, it presses against the uterine wall and removes a strip of the endometrium. This removed strip enters into the lumen of the instrument and later it can be removed.

What are the advantages and disadvantages of this instrument over the uterine curette?
Advantages: This is a thin instrument. It can be passed into the uterine cavity without

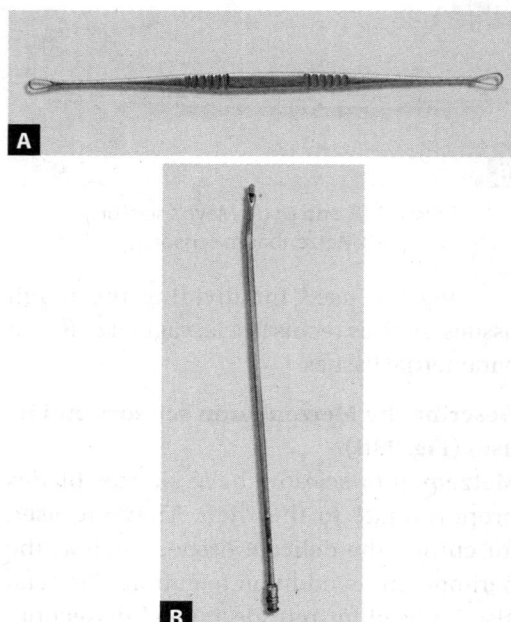

Figs. 24A and B: (A) Uterine curette; (B) Novak's endometrial biopsy curette.

dilating the cervix. Thus, this procedure can be done as an outpatient procedure.

Disadvantages: This instrument removes only a strip of the endometrium. Thus, in cases of focal lesions and suspected carcinoma where we want to sample the entire endometrium, this instrument is not appropriate.

What are the uses of this instrument?
- Diagnosis of the hormonal pattern in infertility and AUB
- For endometrial dating to diagnose anovulation/luteal phase defect/irregular ripening and shedding
- It also acts as a first sound of the uterus.

Discuss Novak's endometrial biopsy curette (Fig. 24B).
This instrument is similar to Randall's EB curette except that instead of a single notch with a cutting edge, it has four notches in succession. This increases the efficiency in curetting the endometrium.

Discuss Pipelle's biopsy curette.
Pipelle's biopsy curette is a long, hollow instrument with a piston at its distal end. After introducing it inside the uterine cavity, the piston is withdrawn. This creates a negative suction pressure, which samples around 98% of the endometrium. It is carried as an office procedure without the need of anesthesia. The tissue is sent in formalin 10%.

Describe the instrument shown in Figures 25A and B.
The instrument is a Leech-Wilkinson cannula. It is a long and tubular instrument with a fixed spiral cone at one end and Luer lock mount at the other end. The spiral cone is so designed that it fits at the external os after the anterior lip is held with vulsellum, and then the cannula is further advanced into the cervical canal by rotating in clockwise motion, so that it fits in the cervix. This forms

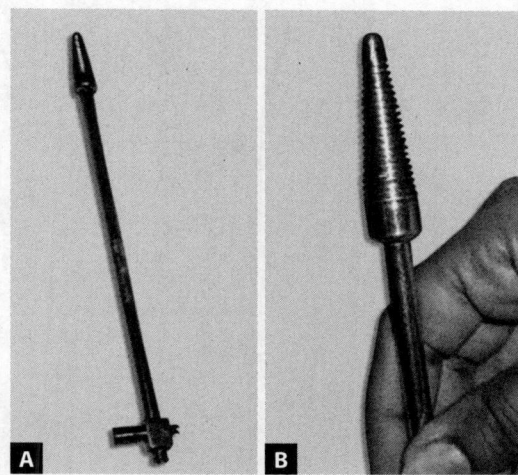

Figs. 25A and B: Leech–Wilkinson cannula.

an airtight fit and prevents any leakage of dye back into the vagina. The dye is introduced from the other end with the help of a syringe.

What are the uses of this cannula?
- HSG to check the tubal patency
- Chromopertubation during laparoscopy
- Rubin's test

What are the complications of the use of this instrument?
- Cervical perforation
- Uterine perforation
- Cervical injury
- Endometritis
- Venous or lymphatic extravasation of dye

Describe the instrument shown in Figure 26.
The instrument is the uterine sound, which is made up of stainless steel and is around 25 cm in length with an olive tip and the rest 5 cm is made up of handle. The instrument is graduated in inches or centimeters at a distance equivalent to normal uterocervical length, i.e., 2.5 inches from its tip, and it is bent at an angle of 150°. This facilitates its entry into the uterine cavity. The tip is around 2 mm, so that it passes the cervical canal without any dilatation.

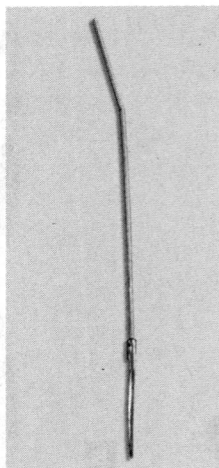

Fig. 26: Uterine sound.

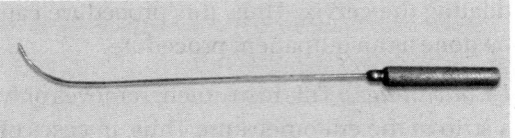

Fig. 27: Bladder sound.

Describe the method of sounding the uterus.

After doing the per vaginal examination, note is made of the position of the uterus. The cervix is held with a vulsellum and the sound is held gently in a pen-holding position and is passed into the canal. At the level of internal os, resistance is felt. Note is made of this length and then it is further passed till it hits the fundus. This gives the uterocervical length. In an anteverted uterus, the instrument is introduced with the angle directed toward the patient while in a retroverted uterus, it faces the floor.

What are the uses of this instrument?
- To measure the uterocervical length
- To measure the supravaginal elongation of the cervix (this is measured by subtracting the length of portio vaginalis from the total cervical length)
- To diagnose and differentiate a polyp from uterine inversion
- To confirm anteversion from retroversion of the uterus determined first by pelvic examination
- To diagnose the missing IUCD
- To diagnose the incompetent os—if the instrument passes the cervix without resistance, diagnosis of incompetent os is made (Shirodkar's test)
- To diagnose cervical stenosis.

Note: This instrument is not to be used in pregnant uterus.

Describe bladder sound (Fig. 27).

This instrument is made of stainless steel and is 25 cm in length with a long, rod-shaped sounding portion and a handle. The sounding portion is curved in its terminal 5 cm.

How does this differ from the uterine sound?
- Bladder sound is not graduated unlike the uterine sound.
- It also does not have any angulations but has a smooth curve.
- It is marked by the absence of olive tip.

What are the uses of this instrument?
- Diagnosis of accidental bladder injury. For this, the sound is passed through the urethra into the bladder and the tip is maneuvered till its tip emerges at the rent in the bladder wall.
- To distinguish the suburethral cyst from the urethral diverticulum. The tip of the sound cannot enter the suburethral cyst.
- During vaginal hysterectomy to know the limits of the bladder on the anterior vaginal wall
- To diagnose suburethral diverticulum
- To sound the bladder for the presence of any foreign body
- For urethral dilatation

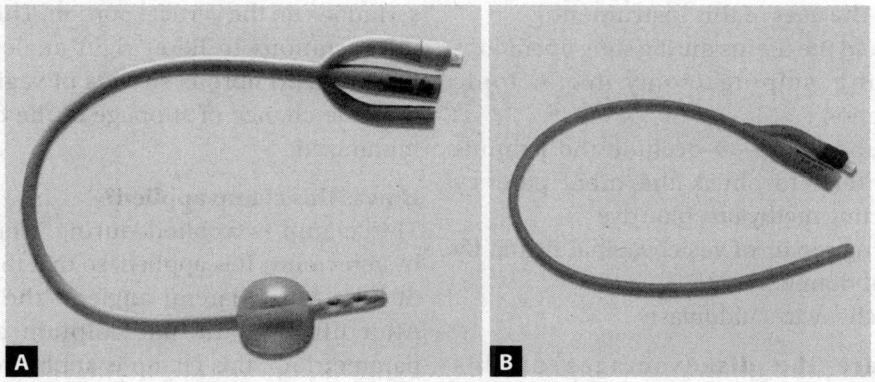

Figs. 28A and B: Foley's catheter image. *(For color version, see Plate 5)*

What is Foley's catheter made up of and how do we sterilize it?
Foley's catheter is made up of latex and is sterilized by gamma rays.

What are the indications of Foley's catheterization (Figs. 28A and B)?
Obstetrics indications:
- During cesarean section—for short-term and long-term during obstructed labor or during bladder injury
- Used in making balloon tamponade in the management of atonic PPH
- To diagnose incompetent os—when no. 12 Foley's catheter can be passed without resistance

Gynecological indications:
- All gynecological surgeries—total abdominal hysterectomy/vaginal hysterectomy/vaginoplasty/colposuspension
- Tourniquet in myomectomy
- HSG
- Saline instillation sonography
- Prolonged bladder drainage—Wertheim's hysterectomy, vesicovaginal repair, Kelly's plication, and bladder injury in any surgery
- Asherman's syndrome—after breaking the adhesions, pediatric Foley's catheter is placed and inflated with 5 mL of saline

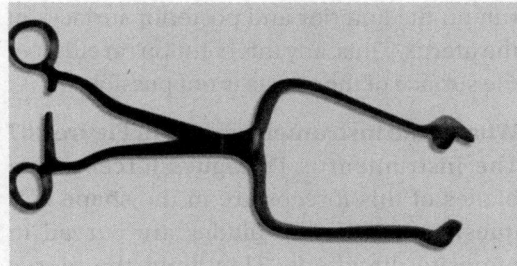

Fig. 29: Shirodkar's forceps.

What are the different types of uterus-holding forceps you know of?
Different types of uterus-holding forceps are Shirodkar's forceps and Dartigues forceps.

Discuss Shirodkar's forceps (Fig. 29).
This instrument has curved blades. The ends of these blades have transverse bars with some degree of mobility. The blades are curved, so that the uterus can be accommodated in-between them. There is a ratchet lock on the handle. This instrument is applied, so that the transverse bar fits on the uterine isthmus anteriorly and posteriorly and the uterus fits in between the curved blades, which similarly fit in the front and behind the uterus. When locked, there is compression of the isthmus and this achieves occlusion of the cervical canal.

Discuss the uses of this instrument.
- To hold the uterus during sling operations
- During salpingectomy for ectopic gestation
- In tuboplasty—to occlude the isthmus and then to check the tubal patency injecting methylene blue dye
- During repair of vesicovaginal fistula by the abdominal route
- Moschcowitz culdoplasty

What are the disadvantages of this instrument?
When this instrument is applied, the blades run on the anterior and posterior surfaces of the uterus. Thus, any intervention on either of the surface of the uterus is not possible.

What is the instrument shown in Figure 30?
The instrument is Dartigues forceps. The blades of this forceps are in the shape of a question mark. The blades are curved in opposite directions. They hold the uterus in the space between the two blades. The disadvantage of this instrument is that it cannot occlude the isthmus. The uses are the same as Shirodkar's forceps, but it cannot be used for tubal patency tests in tuboplasty operations as it cannot occlude the isthmus.

Describe Wertheim vaginal clamp (Fig. 31).
Wertheim vaginal clamp has L-shaped blades. The blades have longitudinal serrations on the horizontal portion of L and transverse serrations on the vertical portion. This makes the serrations to lie at right angles to the muscles and fibrous strands of vagina, and thus the chance of slippage of the clamp is minimized.

How is this clamp applied?
This clamp is applied during Wertheim's hysterectomy. It is applied, so that the angles of L lie at the lateral angle of the vagina. After dividing the paracolpium and the parametrium, this clamp is applied over the vagina on either side and then the vagina is dissected from below the clamp. This prevents the spillage of the malignant cells from the surface of the tumor into the peritoneal cavity during hysterectomy for carcinoma cervix.

Describe Cusco's speculum (Fig. 32).
This instrument has two blades connected by a hinge, so that they can open and close around a transverse axis. The blades, when opened, stretch the anterior and posterior vaginal walls and fix the cervix at the center.

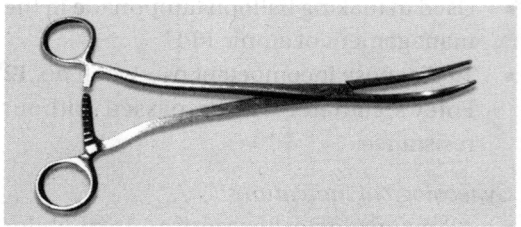

Fig. 31: Wertheim clamp.

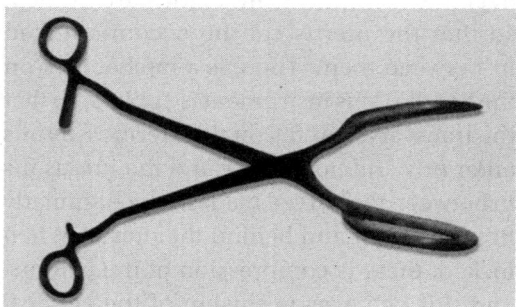

Fig. 30: Dartigues forceps.

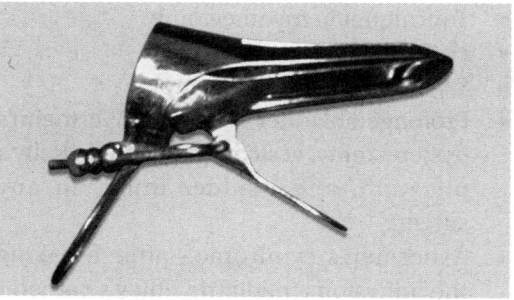

Fig. 32: Cusco's speculum.

What are the indications for the use of this instrument?
- Inspection of the cervix and vagina
- Procedures on the cervix, such as Pap smear and cervical biopsy
- Colposcopy and colpomicroscopy—it is admirable for these procedures, as it fixes the cervix in the center, so that the objective lens may be focused on it.

Discuss its disadvantages.
- Blades cover the anterior and the posterior vaginal walls; therefore, these cannot be used for procedures on these walls.
- The blades occupy space and decrease the maneuverability. Therefore, these cannot be used for procedures such as dilatation and curettage.

Describe the instrument shown in Figure 33.
The instrument is a self-retaining vaginal speculum, which has a weight of lead on its handle. Due to the weight attached on the handle, the blades press on the cut edge of the posterior vaginal wall and achieve hemostasis. The angle between the blades and handle is <90°, so that there is a component of downward force of gravity in the direction toward vagina and this prevents the speculum from slipping out. The length of the blade is such that it can be inserted only after the posterior pouch of peritoneum has been opened.

Discuss the disadvantages of this instrument.
The instrument cannot be used without anesthesia, as it causes severe perineal pain by pressure. Hence, it is not useful for an OPD procedure.

What are the indications for its use?
This instrument is used in various vaginal surgeries:
- Vaginal hysterectomy
- Anterior colporrhaphy
- Vesicovaginal fistula
- Schauta's radical vaginal hysterectomy

■ RETRACTORS

Describe the instrument shown in Figure 34.
The instrument is Langenbeck retractor. It is a hook-type retractor with a teardrop handle and an L-shaped working end. The tip of the retractor has a slight angle for avoiding local injury. It is used to pull back soft tissues and incision or wound edges during laparotomy.

Describe the instrument shown in Figure 35.
The instrument is Deaver's retractor. It has been modified in various lengths and widths to make it useful for both vaginal and

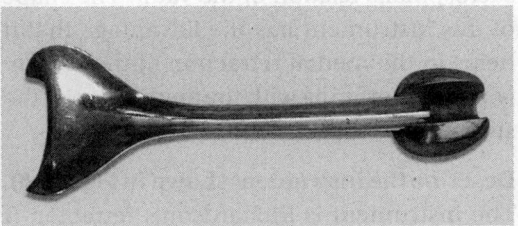

Fig. 33: Auvard speculum.

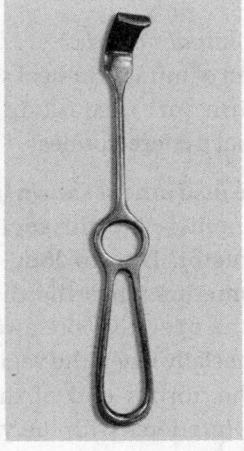

Fig. 34: Langenbeck retractor.

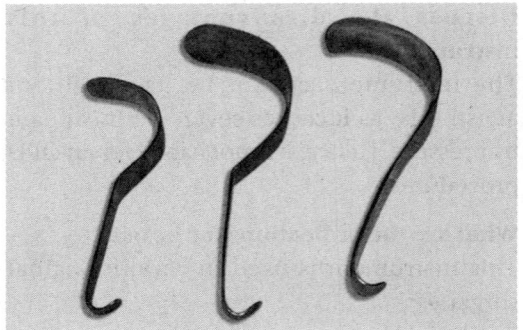

Fig. 35: Deaver's retractor.

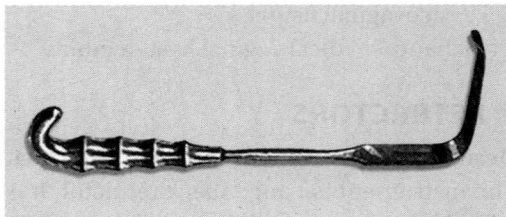

Fig. 36: Heaney retractor.

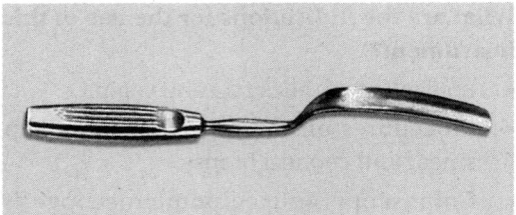

Fig. 37: Breisky–Navratil retractor.

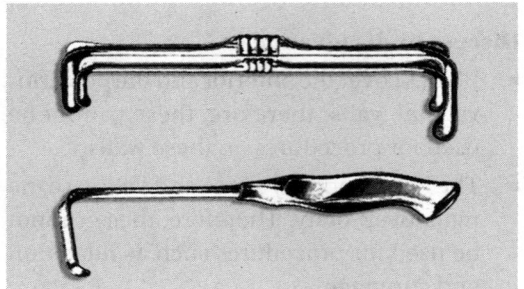

Fig. 38: Richardson's retractor.

abdominal surgeries. Since the blades are thin, it occupies little space and is thus an ideal instrument while operating in depth.

Discuss the indications for the use of this instrument.
During vaginal surgeries: The NDVH/vaginal surgeries to retract the bladder after opening the anterior fold of peritoneum.

During abdominal surgeries:
- Retraction of intraperitoneal structures
- Retraction of the bladder during abdominal hysterectomies

Describe the instrument shown in Figure 36.
The instrument is a right-angled Heaney vaginal retractor. Due to long blade, this retractor sometimes has the disadvantage of pushing the operative site away from the surgeon, especially when the vaginal mucosa is intact. The abrupt end of the retractor occasionally interferes with the visualization of the introitus. In such circumstances, retractors with a rounded curvature are more appropriate.

Describe the instrument shown in Figure 37.
The instrument is a Breisky–Navratil retractor. These retractors are widely used for vaginal exposure. These have the advantage of the curve, which allows the lateral, superior, and inferior tow on the vaginal tissues without the assistant's hand drifting into the operator's field of view.

Discuss the indication for the use of this instrument.
The instrument is used for deep exposure as in sacrospinalis fixation of the vault. The shape of this instrument has the advantage that it helps in the medial retraction of the rectum without interfering with the application of the sutures.

Describe the instrument shown in Figure 38.
The instrument is Richardson's retractor. It can be used for both abdominal and vaginal

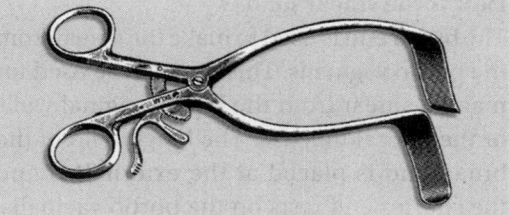

Fig. 39: Rigby retractor.

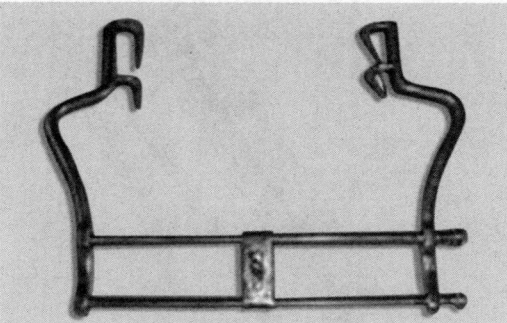

Fig. 40: Balfour retractor.

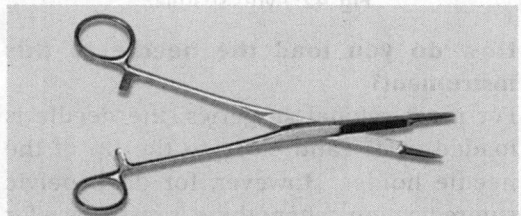

Fig. 41: Needle holder.

operations. The indications for its use are as follows:
- Useful for opening and closing the incisions, when it is desirable to directly visualize the fascial surface
- To lift the abdominal wall for enhancing the exposure to the pelvis

Discuss the instrument shown in Figure 39.
The instrument is a self-retaining Rigby retractor. The two L-shaped blades are connected by a hinge, so that on approximation of the finger-grips the blades open out. The self-retaining retractor has the advantage of obviating the need for an assistant. The disadvantage is that it causes prolonged compression of the retracted tissues, so that their vitality is reduced. Also, the retraction obtained is fixed.

Discuss the instrument shown in Figure 40.
The instrument is Balfour retractor. It has two lateral fenestrated blades, which are connected by a transverse bar. The right blade is fixed and the left blade can slide on the transverse bar and can be fixed at any point by means of a screw. The third blade can also be fixed on the transverse bars such that it retracts at right angles to the two lateral blades.

How do you apply this instrument?
After opening the peritoneum and packing the upper abdominal contents, the retractor is placed with its lateral blades closed together. After placing in the abdominal cavity, the edges of the incision are spread out laterally by opening the blades taking care that bowel and omentum are not included by the blades. Then the third blade is also put and depending on the position, it acts like a suprapubic retractor or an upper abdominal retractor.

Discuss the instrument shown in Figure 41.
The instrument is a needle holder. It can be straight (Wagensteen) or curved (Heaney). At its distal end, it has ring finger-grips and ratchet lock. All needle holders have a broad head with a variety of surfaces to prevent the needle from slipping or rotating. The curved needle holders are especially useful for vaginal surgeries where the angled head allows the placement of curved needles and sutures at almost any conceivable angle with relative ease. These are useful for placing sutures deep within the pelvis.

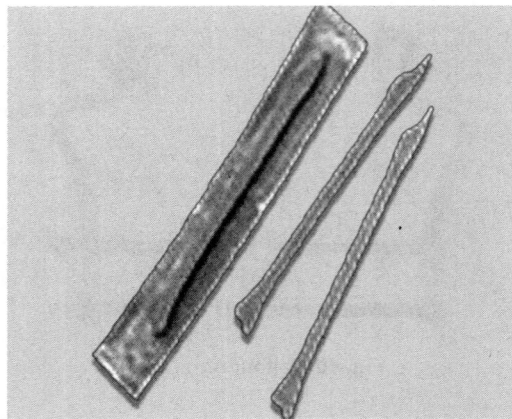

Fig. 42: Ayre's spatula.

How do you load the needle to this instrument?

For most vaginal surgeries, the needle is loaded at 45° and close to the tip of the needle holder. However, for deep pelvic suture ligation, where there is less space for maneuvering, the needle is placed in the jaws of the holder with the curve parallel to the handle. The thenar grip is commonly employed, while the palmer grip is used for the maximal force.

A special type of needle Miya hook is used as a suture ligature for suture insertion in the sacrospinalis fixation.

Discuss Ayre's spatula (Fig. 42).

This instrument can be made up of wood and plastic. This is 15–17 cm long and has two ends. One end is 3 mm broad and 2 cm long. The other broad end has two projections—one of them projecting beyond the other. The wooden spatula is best for cytological smear. Because of its rough surface, it provides enough friction and thus more cells stick onto its surface than the smooth surface of the plastic spatula. This instrument is used for picking exfoliated cells from the cervix, posterior vaginal fornix, upper one-thirds of lateral vaginal walls, or sometimes the buccal mucosa.

How is the smear made?

The broad end is used to make the smear from the portio vaginalis. This can also be used for making smear from the lateral vaginal walls or the buccal mucosa. The longer end of the broad end is placed at the external os and the shorter end rests on the portio vaginalis. Then it is rotated by 360°, so that it picks the exfoliated cells. These cells are used to make cytological smear on the glass slide. Then the long and narrow end is placed into the cervical canal and it is rotated to pick the cells from the cervical canal and another smear is made on the same glass slide.

What are the indications for making the cytological smear?

- Cytological screening for cervical cancer and follow-up in cases of cervical intraepithelial neoplasia (CIN)—exfoliated cells are picked up from ectocervix and endocervix
- Follow-up of carcinoma cervix after Wertheim's, smears are taken from vault
- Hormonal cytology from the upper one-third of the lateral vaginal wall
- Buccal smear for evaluation of Barr bodies

Discuss the instrument shown in Figure 43.

The instrument is Miya hook. Miya hook ligature carrier is an instrument used for sacrospinous ligament suspension of prolapsed uterus and vagina, i.e., hysteropexy. Using it makes the procedure safe and easy. It is also used for transvaginal sacrospinous colpopexy, which consists of sewing vagina to sacrospinous ligament. This procedure is done in posthysterectomy vault prolapse.
- Size—12 inches (30.5 cm)

Discuss the instrument shown in Figure 44.

- The instrument is cervical punch biopsy forceps (Tischler–Kevorkian forceps).
- *Size:* It is a straight instrument with 8 inches shaft and 3 mm × 9.5 mm rectangular bite

Instruments

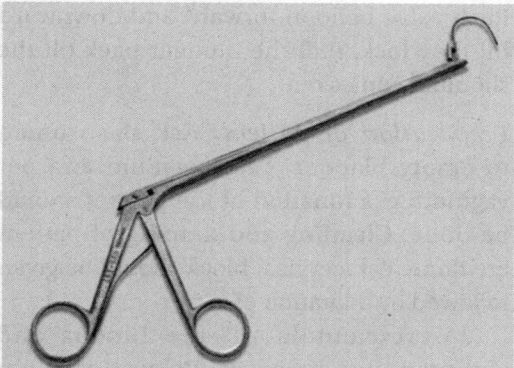

Fig. 43: Miya hook.

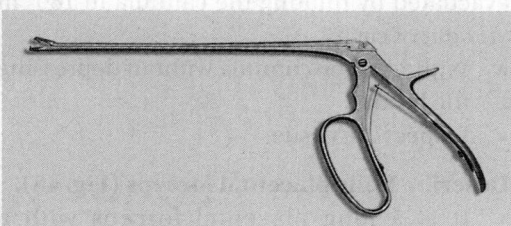

Fig. 44: Cervical punch biopsy forceps.

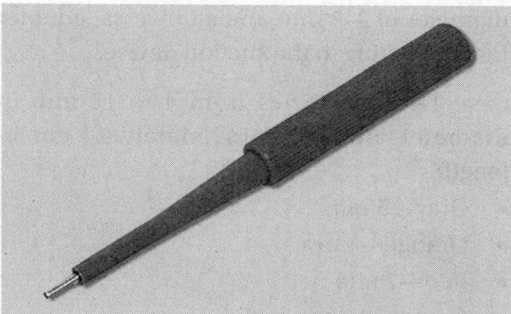

Fig. 45: Keyes punch biopsy forceps.

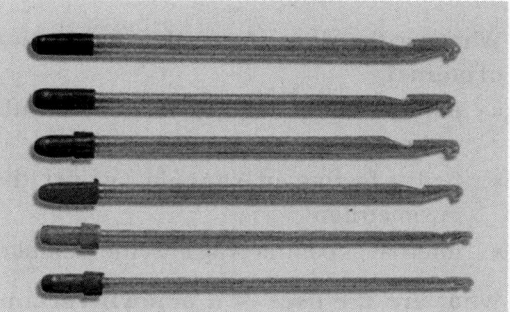

Fig. 46: Karman cannula.

at one end. It has a single lower tooth and a single upper tooth to grasp difficult-to-reach tissue. It has a locking mechanism above the horn on the handle, so that the jaw can lock the tissue sample in place while the instrument is removed from the cervical canal. It has a pistol-style handle with a large ring for multiple fingers. It is made of stainless steel.
- It is useful to obtain cervical tissue, which can be sent for histopathology.

Describe the instrument shown in Figure 45.
- The instrument is Keyes punch biopsy forceps.
- *Uses:* It is useful in obtaining vulval and cervical biopsy.
- *Size:* Its size varies from 3 to 6 mm. It has a sharpened, rounded tip designed to take a vertical core from the epithelium.
- *Procedure:* Firstly, the biopsy site is detected, and skin is cleaned with antiseptic. The skin is stabilized between thumb and index finger. Local anesthesia is given by injecting lignocaine. Keyes punch biopsy forceps is directed inward into the skin in clockwise and anticlockwise directions. This produces a small cylindrical specimen which contains subcutaneous tissue. The tissue is grasped with forceps and elevated above the skin and scissor is used to cut across the base to free tissue from subcutaneous tissue.

Describe Karman cannula (Fig. 46).
Karman cannula is a flexible, disposable, and sterile-packed instrument used for surgical evacuation and endometrial aspiration. It is available in various diameters, which are color coded by size. There is a depth marking in centimeters printed on cannula. There are two opposing apertures on cannula with a

diameter of 4–8 mm and a universal adopter for connecting to the suction device.

Size: The size varies from 4 to 12 mm in diameter and is approximately 24 cm in length.
- Gray—5 mm
- Orange—6 mm
- Red—7 mm
- Green—8 mm
- Blue—10 mm
- Dark blue—12 mm

What are the signs of complete evacuation of uterus?
- Formation of bubbles in the cannula without tissue
- Gritty feeling of cannula against the myometrium
- Internal os contracts against the cannula

What are the uses of a manual vacuum aspirator? How is it used (Fig. 47)?
Manual vacuum aspirator (MVA) is used for suction evacuation till 12 weeks and for endometrial aspiration.

Preparation of aspirator: Position the plunger inside the cylinder. Apply collar stop in place. Push valve balloon forward and downward till they lock. Pull the plunger back till the shoulder comes out.

Preparation of patient: Ask the woman to empty bladder. Per speculum and per vaginum examination of the patient should be done. Cleaning and draping of patient are done. Paracervical block should be given followed by dilatation of cervix.

Insert cannula till the fundus and withdraw just below it. Release vacuum by pressing button. Contents are slowly evacuated by rotating the cannula in 180° in and out of cavity.
- Withdraw the cannula without depressing the button.
- Inspect the tissue.

Describe Kelly placental forceps (Fig. 48).
- It is a long placental forceps with a serrated ring jaw with a slightly curved tip without lock.
- The length of forceps is 31.5–32.5 cm.
- *Procedure:* Sim's speculum is inserted. The anterior lip of cervix is held with sponge-holding forceps. The IUCD is grasped with long-placental forceps in sterile pack with no-touch technique. IUCD should be held

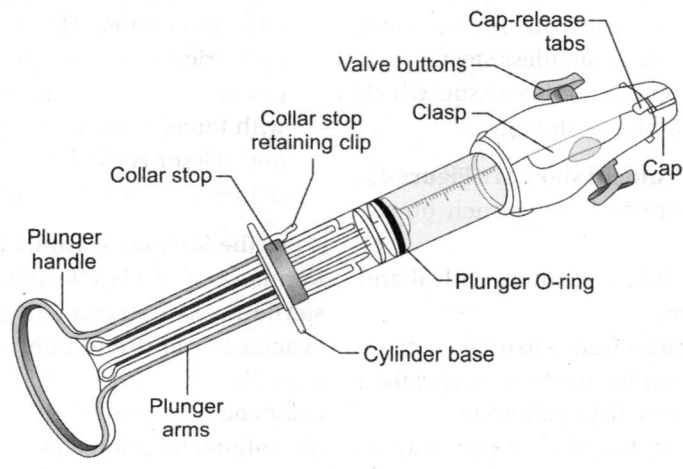

Fig. 47: Manual vacuum aspirator.

Instruments

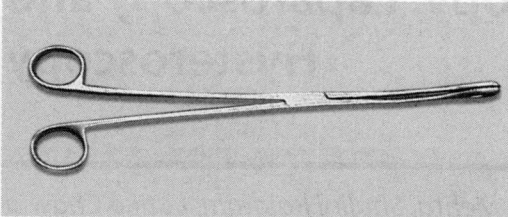

Fig. 48: Kelly placental forceps.

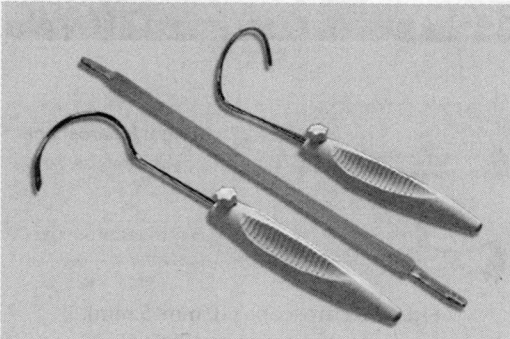

Fig. 49: Synthetic tension-free vaginal tape obturator.

on the edge, once the placental forceps is in the lower uterine cavity, lower the ring forceps that is holding the anterior lip of cervix, and move the left hand to the woman's abdomen and push the uterus superiorly. This is to straighten the angle between vagina and uterus, so that Kelly's forceps can go till fundus. Tilt the forceps slightly anteriorly and release the IUCD and slowly remove the placental forceps taking care not to remove the IUCD.

Describe the instrument shown in Figure 49.
The instrument is a retropubic mid-urethral sling used for the treatment of stress urinary incontinence.

Procedure: The patient is given regional anesthesia and placed in lithotomy position. The bladder is catheterized. The surgeon places the index finger into one vaginal fornix and the thumb lateral to the labia to palpate the ischiopubic ramus, including median margin of obturator foramen at the level of bladder neck and clitoris. A line is marked horizontally at the level of clitoris 1 cm lateral to the groin fold and 2 cm superior to the urethral meatus at an area below the adductor longus muscle. A 2-cm midline incision is made under the mid-urethra with the scalpel. A helical device is placed through the suburethral tunnel until the medial surface of the ischiopubic ramus to exit out through the skin incision and held. The procedure is repeated on the opposite side until the sling is in proper orientation and lying flat underneath urethra. The sling is tensioned and plastic sleeves removed and the skin and vaginal incisions are closed.

CHAPTER 14

Endoscopy: Laparoscopy and Hysteroscopy

Sumita Mehta, Shalini Rajaram, Latika Chawla

LAPAROSCOPY

■ INTRODUCTION

Endoscopic surgery, also known as minimally invasive surgery, involves the use of an endoscope—a thin tube with a light and a camera to visualize and perform surgical procedures inside the human body. It has many advantages as compared to open surgery including minimal trauma, better cosmetic results, shorter hospital stay, and early return to activity. The main endoscopic surgeries in gynecology are laparoscopy and hysteroscopy which can be both diagnostic and operative.

What are the telescopes used in laparoscopic surgery?

There are two basic types of telescopes:
1. With an operative channel
2. Without an operative channel
   - *Size:* 3–12 mm—the larger the caliber and larger the number of fiber bundles, the higher the vision. The most common used in clinical practice are 5 and 10 mm scopes **(Fig. 1)**.
   - *Lens:* It can be straight or angled.
   - Straight is 0°, which provides a panoramic view of the pelvis.
   - Angle is 30°, 45°, or 135°, which assists in evaluating the anterior abdominal wall or working around masses.

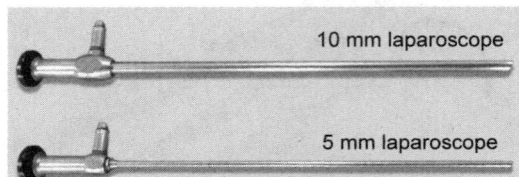

Fig. 1: Laparoscope (10 mm, 5 mm). *(For color version, see Plate 5)*

Trocar and trocar sleeve (cannula): Pneumoperitoneum is created using CO_2 gas and then the trocar sleeve with the trocar is introduced into the abdominal wall. Subsequently, the telescope is introduced into the abdominal cavity through the sleeve after removing the trocar. Trocar sleeve is made up of metal or nonconductive material like fiberglass or Teflon. Trocar is made up of metal and comes in various sizes with a sharp tip. The trocar sleeve has an inlet for the gas with a two-way valve. Disposable plastic trocars are also available. Trocar and cannulas are available in 10, 11, 12, and 5 mm sizes **(Figs. 2A and B)**.

Veress needle (Fig. 3): Veress needle is used for creating pneumoperitoneum. It has two needles. There is an outer needle of 16 gauge, which has a sharp end, and an inner needle inside this, which has a blunt end and a subterminal opening. This opening allows

should not be used at the insertion of Veress needle or the ports as the intestine is anterior and injury is a possibility.

What are the different sites of insertion?
Primary port
- *Infraumbilical:* Abdominal wall is thinnest at the umbilicus and it is cosmetically best.
- *Lee–Huang point:* Midway between xiphisternum and umbilicus in the midline

Secondary port: It is important to identify the inferior and superficial epigastric vessels before insertion of secondary trocars. The inferior epigastric artery, which is a branch of the external iliac artery, lies in close relation to the rectus muscle about 1–2 cm lateral to the obliterated hypogastric artery. The superficial epigastric artery is a branch of femoral vessels and runs toward the umbilicus and can be injured on the rectus muscle **(Fig. 4)**. They can be identified by transillumination in most patients.
- *Palmer's point:* Insertion through this point is preferred in patients with suspected periumbilical adhesions. This point lies on the midclavicular line 3 cm below the costal margin on the left side.
- *Suprapubic laterally (right or left):* 8 cm above symphysis pubis and 8 cm lateral to midline to prevent damage to inferior epigastric vessels
- *Suprapubic midline:* 3 cm above symphysis pubis

It is important to introduce secondary trocars at 90° to the skin. If this angle is not maintained, the trocar may deviate from the preselected site and results in vascular trauma.

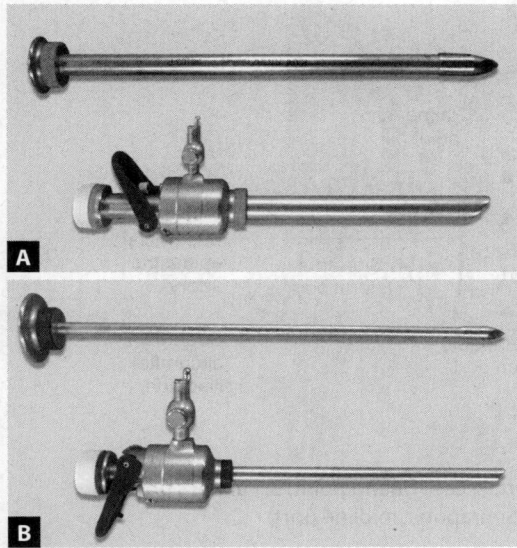

Figs. 2A and B: (A) 10 mm trocar and cannula; (B) 5 mm trocar and cannula. *(For color version, see Plate 5)*

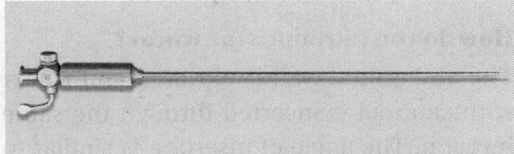

Fig. 3: Veress needle. *(For color version, see Plate 5)*

for the gas to enter into the abdomen to create pneumoperitoneum. There is a spring between the two needles, which allows the withdrawal of the inner needle into the outer needle. The Veress needle will only allow a maximum flow rate of 3 L/min.

How should Veress needle be inserted?
The needle is held gently (pen grip) between index and thumb and inserted through a small subumbilical incision (1.25 cm) at an angle of 45° to the abdominal wall (i.e., toward the hollow of sacrum). In obese patients, the direction of introduction of needle should be 90°. Before insertion, ensure that the needle is patent and bladder is empty and the patient is in supine position. Trendelenburg position

How much pneumoperitoneum should be created?
The abdomen is inflated with about 1–4 L of gas (carbon dioxide). The target intra-abdominal pressure is usually preset to

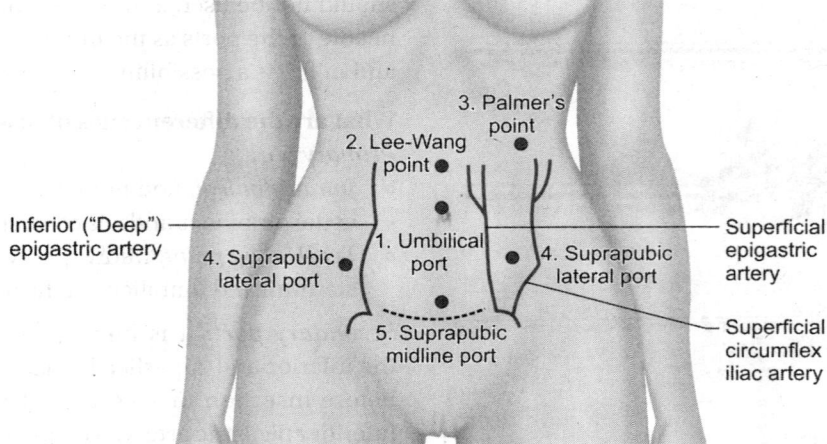

Fig. 4: Sites of various ports (1: Umbilical port; 2: Lee–Huang point; 3: Palmer's point; 4: Suprapubic lateral port; 5: Suprapubic midline port).

12–15 mm Hg. Increased intra-abdominal pressure interferes with diaphragmatic excursion and venous return due to caval obstruction. The necessary volume of gas needed for insufflation is dependent upon the depth of anesthesia, the use of neuromuscular blockade, and the patient's size.

How do you check for the correct placement of the needle?

- *Hanging drop method:* Using a syringe, place a small amount of sterile saline on the open end of Veress needle. Since the intraperitoneal pressure is less than the atmospheric pressure, the saline easily goes into the peritoneal cavity.
- *Syringe barrel test:* Aspiration is done with the help of a syringe to rule out. Blood or bowel contents. The saline is then pushed down and aspiration is again done. If the needle placement is correct, the saline cannot be withdrawn as it goes in the peritoneal cavity.

Intra-abdominal pressure is low (<10 mm Hg) on correct placement and there is free flow of gas

- Obliteration of liver dullness (on percussion)
- Needle moves with respiration.

How do you introduce the trocar?

The abdominal wall is elevated and trocar with cannula is inserted through the same incision. The angle of insertion is similar to that of Veress needle, directed toward the hollow of sacrum.

While introducing the trocar, the index finger acts as a guard and its broad end rests against the thenar eminence and the medial three fingers cradle around the instrument. It is important to hold up the anterior abdominal wall. The direction of insertion depends upon the obesity factor of the patient. In case of an obese patient, it is inserted perpendicular to the abdominal cavity and otherwise at an angle. During introduction, the pressure is applied with the palm of the hand. After introducing into the cavity, the trocar is withdrawn and the sleeve is introduced further to avoid injury to other intraperitoneal structures. Then the trocar is removed and the scope is introduced through the sleeve. During removal of the trocar and the sleeve, it is important that the trocar must be pushed all along the sleeve; otherwise, omentum or bowel may be dragged into the sleeve and will be out along with the trocar sleeve.

What are the indications for laparoscopy?
Diagnostic
- Primary and secondary infertility
- Assessment of pelvis for acute/chronic pain
- Determination of tubal patency (chromo-pertubation test)
- Suspected uterine perforation during hysteroscopy/dilation and curettage (D&C)

Operative
- *Hysterectomy:* This could be total abdominal, radical, or laparoscopic-assisted vaginal hysterectomy.
- Second look surgery after surgical/chemotherapy of malignancy
- Myomectomy
- Tubal sterilization
- Adhesiolysis in cases of prior infection, tubo-ovarian abscess, endometriosis
- Ectopic pregnancy
- Ovarian cystectomy/oophorectomy/aspiration of ovarian cysts after ruling out malignancy. Any spill of malignant cells will lead to dissemination.
- Fulguration of endometriotic implants
- Ovarian drilling for polycystic ovary syndrome (PCOS)
- Removal of foreign bodies from peritoneal cavity [e.g., transmigrated intrauterine device (IUD)]
- Adnexal torsion
- As an adjunct to vaginal hysterectomy as in laparoscopic-assisted vaginal hysterectomy

What are the contraindications for laparoscopy?
Absolute
- *Severe cardiac disease (class IV):* Such patients may not tolerate deep Trendelenburg's position.
- Hemodynamically unstable patient
- Intestinal obstruction with distended bowel
- Massive hemoperitoneum
- Large pelvic tumor
- Ovarian malignancy

Relative
- Multiple previous major surgeries
- Morbid obesity
- Severe chronically ill patients
- Pulmonary disease
- Generalized peritonitis
- Anticoagulation therapy
- Diaphragmatic hernia
- Radical hysterectomy for carcinoma cervix c after the Laparoscopic Approach to Carcinoma of the Cervix (LACC) trial

What are the advantages of laparoscopy versus laparotomy?
- Shorter operative time
- Smaller scar (cosmetic value)
- Faster recovery
- Decreased adhesion formation
- Shorter hospital stay and reduced concomitant cost
- Less postoperative analgesia and reduced need of postoperative analgesia
- Reduced blood loss
- Risk of incisional hernia is less
- Increased patient satisfaction
- Risk of minor complications [fever, wound infection, and urinary tract infection (UTI)] is lower.

What is open laparoscopy (Hasson technique)?

In open laparoscopy, the rectus fascia is incised and the abdomen is entered bluntly using a clamp. It is followed by placing a blunt-tipped trocar and sleeve through this opening. This is done to minimize bowel and vessel injury.

Describe "left upper quadrant insertion" technique.

This technique is done with the patient in supine position and the stomach empty (using a drainage tube). A 5-mm trocar and cannula are introduced in the midclavicular line 3 cm below the costal margin on the left side (Palmer's point). It cannot be used in patients with hepatosplenomegaly or splenomegaly and ascites. It is restricted for use in patients with large pelvic masses and adhesions and patients in the second trimester of pregnancy.

What is the effect of body mass index on laparoscopy?

Low body mass index: In a patient with low body mass index (BMI), the great vessels can be as little as 2.5 cm below the umbilicus. In this group, the abdominal wall should be elevated and the Veress needle should be held on the shaft and not the barrel, thereby increasing the distance from the umbilicus to the aorta and reducing the length of the needle to be inserted. Always direct the needle toward the pelvis, at an angle of 45°.

High body mass index: The average distance from the base of the umbilicus to the aorta in obese patients is approximately 13 cm. In such patients, the Veress needle should be introduced at 90° to the skin.

What are the common complications of laparoscopy?

Primary trocar insertion
- *Bowel injury:* Transverse colon and small bowel
- *Vessel injury:* Inferior epigastric vessels, common iliac arteries or veins, aorta, and inferior vena cava
- Bladder perforation
- Damage to omentum
- Surgical or emphysema
- Vasovagal reflex during gas insertion

Secondary trocar insertion
- Inferior epigastric vessels
- Bowel injury

During the procedure
- *Anesthetic complications:* Ventilatory problems, hypercarbia, and metabolic acidosis (when CO_2 is used for pneumoperitoneum)
- Hypoventilation (pneumoperitoneum and Trendelenburg position lead to basal lung compression and reduced diaphragmatic excursion)
- *Visceral injury:* Recognized, unrecognized, direct, and secondary to diathermy
- *Hemorrhage:* Circulatory compromise
- *Equipment failure:* Cameras, lighting, diathermy, and staples

Postoperative
- Fluid balance
- Thromboembolic
- Unrecognized visceral injury
- Port-site hernia
- Intra-abdominal/wound infection
- Wound dehiscence

What is the management of bowel injuries during laparoscopy?

The risk of bowel injuries during laparoscopy is 0.4/1,000. Small bowel injury presents earlier than large bowel.

Bowel injuries occurring during laparoscopic entry are mainly seen, if there are adhesions. **Table 1** shows the risk of adhesions with various surgeries. These injuries have been classified into two types depending on damage to normally located

TABLE 1: Risk of adhesions.

Previous surgery	Significant periumbilical adhesions
No previous surgery	0.4%
Laparoscopy	0.8%
Pfannenstiel	6.9%
Midline laparotomy	31.5%

bowel (type I injury) or adherent bowel (type II injury).

If there is no tearing of the bowel with Veress needle, then the patient can be managed conservatively with only observation and antibiotics. If the bowel has been penetrated, reparative surgery would be required either laparoscopically or with laparotomy.

What is the management of major vessel injury during laparoscopy?
Major vessel injury occurs in 0.2/1,000 cases, and the right common iliac artery commonly is involved. Generally, the patient in such cases has signs of intraperitoneal bleeding with deterioration in vital signs. The treatment would include doing a laparotomy for vascular repair by a vascular surgeon.

How do you manage abdominal wall vessel injury?
Primary vessels injured are epigastric vessels (inferior and superficial) and superficial circumflex iliac vessels.
- If the vessel ends are visible through the laparoscope and coagulate with diathermy
- Pass a no. 12 Foley's catheter through the port, inflate, remove the port, and use the balloon to create a tamponade, which should be maintained for 4–6 hours.
- A ligating suture can be placed below the injury with the help of Endoclose (Tyco Healthcare).
- If bleeding is brisk, the skin incision around the trocar can be enlarged and both ends of the vessel dissected out and ligated. It is important that both ends of the vessel are ligated because of the anastomosis with the superior epigastric artery.

What is the incidence of incisional hernia in laparoscopy scars?
The incidence of port-site herniation varies up to 0.2%. It occurs through a fascial defect >5 mm, so fascial closure is recommended for an incision >5 mm. Umbilical closure is not required unless a very large incision is made, such as open laparoscopy.

How are laparoscopic instruments sterilized?
Instruments must be dismantled before cleaning. After decontamination, every small piece and space must be cleaned and dried with water and compressed air. For lenses and telescope, alcohol or special soap solution is to be used. Chemical sterilization is done by immersing instruments and telescope in 2% glutaraldehyde (Cidex) solution. Most modern instruments are designed for sterilization in the autoclave at 134°C or can undergo sterilization with EtO (ethylene oxide gas) or with hydrogen peroxide gas plasma.

What do you mean by vessel sealing devices?
Vessel sealing devices are an alternative method to conventional suturing and stapling techniques. This system utilizes a high current and low voltage to collagen and elastin fibers in the vessel wall, thereby causing their denaturation and a permanent seal.
- *Harmonic scalpel* **(Fig. 5):** This device vaporizes as well as coagulates tissues. As high-frequency ultrasonic waves are used, there is minimal sticking of tissue to the transducer tip.

- *LigaSure (Fig. 6):* This is a bipolar vessel sealing system, which works well for both arteries and veins.
- *EnSeal tissue sealing and hemostasis system:* This is also a vessel sealing system, which automatically stops energy delivery when sealing is complete.

Common instruments used in laparoscopy surgery are shown in **Figures 7 to 11**.

What is single-incision laparoscopic surgery?

Single-incision laparoscopic surgery (SILS) is an advanced minimally invasive approach that allows laparoscopic surgery through a single incision in the umbilicus, the pre-existing scar. It is associated with less postoperative pain and better cosmesis, as the number of incisions is less.

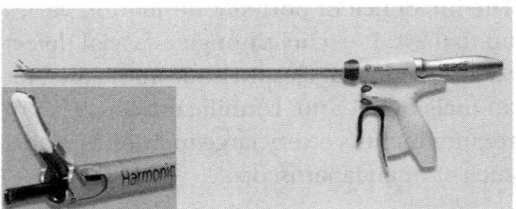

Fig. 5: Harmonic ace. *(For color version, see Plate 5)*

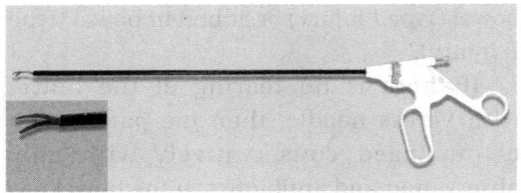

Fig. 9: Laparoscopic scissors. *(For color version, see Plate 6)*

Fig. 6: LigaSure. *(For color version, see Plate 5)*

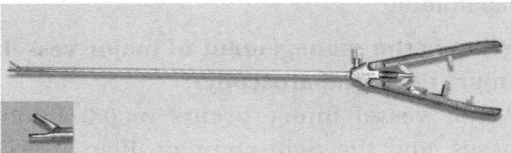

Fig. 10: Laparoscopic needle holder. *(For color version, see Plate 6)*

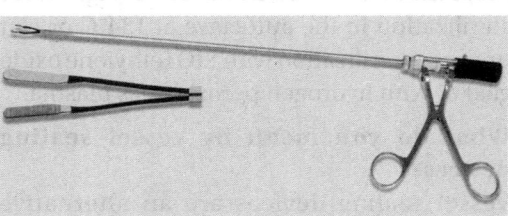

Fig. 7: Bipolar forceps.

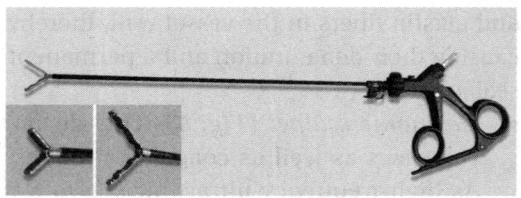

Fig. 8: Laparoscopic tooth and nontooth graspers. *(For color version, see Plate 5)*

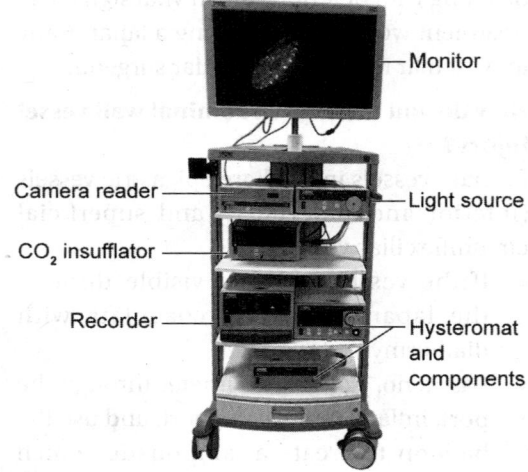

Fig. 11: Overview of a laparoscopy cart, consisting of a monitor, a camera reader, light source, CO_2 insufflator, recorder, and hysteromat. *(For color version, see Plate 6)*

HYSTEROSCOPY

—*"An eye in the uterine cavity is worth much more than a blind curette."*

Identify the instrument shown in Figure 12A.
The instrument shown is a *hysteroscope*.

This is a diagnostic hysteroscope with an outer sheath and the telescope. For diagnostic hysteroscopy, a single sheath for inflow is sufficient and so a smaller outer diameter is required.

Hysteroscope with side channel
There is a side channel on the sheath of a hysteroscope through which instruments (scissors, graspers, cannulation sheaths) can be introduced in operative hysteroscopy **(Fig. 12B)**.

Hysteroscope with working element for operative interventions
The outer diameter of operative hysteroscope using monopolar electrosurgery is up to 10 mm. This includes the telescope with the working element, the inflow sheath, and the outer outflow sheath **(Fig. 12C)**.

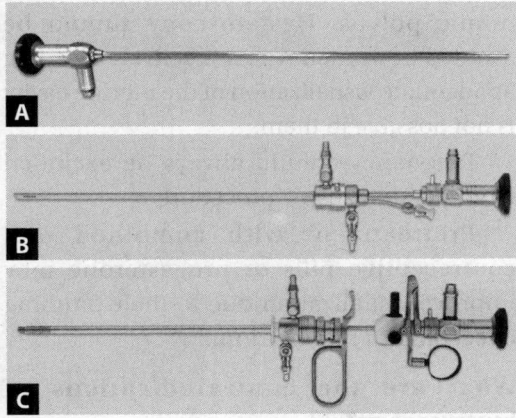

Figs. 12A to C: (A) 5-mm Hysteroscope; (B) Hysteroscope with working side channel; (C) Hysteroscope with working element for operative intervention. *(For color version, see Plate 6)*

Describe the telescopes used for hysteroscopy.
- *Rigid telescopes:* These are commonly used. The telescope may be either straight on (forward view) (0°) or oblique view 30° or 90°.
- *Flexible telescopes:* These have the advantage of easy uterine entry as they have a flexible insertion tube that allows for easier navigation through the curves and contours of the uterine cavity.
- *Microhysteroscope:* High-powered microscope by switching the lens to 150 magnification. Light contact with mucous membrane is needed.
- *Telescope sheath:* A sheath is required to introduce the telescope. Sheath used for diagnostic purposes is smaller (5 mm) than that for operative sheath (7–10 mm). Operative instruments are introduced through the sheath which has an operative channel for French size 7 instrumentation. Operative hysteroscopy needs separate inflow and outflow sheaths. The inflow sheath carries the distension medium to the tip of the telescope, from where it is withdrawn via the outer sheath. This helps to maintain clear view **(Fig. 13)**.

What are the indications for hysteroscopy?
- Abnormal uterine bleeding
- Postmenopausal bleeding
- *Infertility:*
  • Direct visualization of uterine cavity and tubal ostia coupled with targeted EB give specific information
  • Diagnosis and treatment of intrauterine adhesions

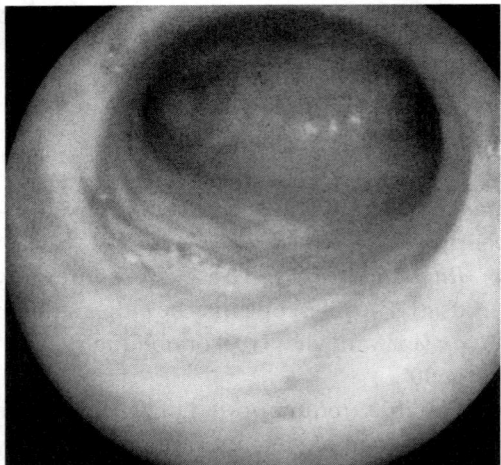

Fig. 13: Panoramic view of uterine cavity with a hysteroscope. Tubal ostium is seen on either side *(For color version, see Plate 6)*

- Fibroids and polyps, which occlude the cervix or tubal ostia, may hamper sperm progression and interfere with implantation.
- Tubal cannulation
- Mullerian anomalies—hysteroscopy may reveal arcuate, subseptate, septate, or bicornuate uterus.
- Assess uterine cavity in cases of repeated abortions
- Unexplained infertility
- Subendometrial PRP/Stem cell injection in women with thin ET or Asherman syndrome
- *Foreign body:* Misplaced intrauterine contraceptive device (IUCD)
- *Chronic pelvic pain:* Concomitant hysteroscopy with laparoscopy can reveal adhesions and septate uterus
- Diagnosis of hemangioma and arteriovenous malformation
- Colpomicrohysteroscopy may be used to visualize the transformation zone in Type III transformation zone
- *Operative hysteroscopy:*
  - Endometrial ablation in cases of heavy menstrual bleeding
  - *Asherman's syndrome:* Synechiolysis
  - Hysteroscopic myomectomy and polypectomy
  - *Metroplasty:* Hysteroscopic resection of septum
  - Removal of foreign body or IUCD in case of missing or coiled-up thread
  - Tubal cannulation and balloon tuboplasty in proximal tubal block
  - *Hysteroscopic sterilization:* STOP (selective tubal occlusion procedure)
    - Essure (interstitial portion of tubes using Nd:YAG laser or electrocoagulation for its insertion)
    - Adiana
  - Laser coagulation of endometrial hemangioma and arteriovenous malformation.

When should hysteroscopy be done?

In premenopausal women with regular cycles, diagnostic hysteroscopy is preferred during the follicular phase; thickened endometrium during the secretory phase of the cycle can mimic polyps. Hysteroscopy should be avoided in women who are actively bleeding as adequate visualization of the uterine cavity is not possible in them.

Pregnancy should always be excluded before hysteroscopic procedure.

Pretreatment with combined oral contraceptive pills or progesterone may improve visualization due to their thinning effect on the endometrium.

What are the contraindications of hysteroscopy?

- Active pelvic infection
- *Cervical cancer:* Hysteroscopy in such patients may cause trauma to lymphatics

and blood vessels leading to systemic dissemination of malignant cells.
- *Pregnancy:* Pregnancy leads to increased softening and vascularity and so is a relative contraindication
- Cervical stenosis
- Recent uterine perforation
- Women with cardiopulmonary disorders are at higher risks of anesthesia as hysteroscopy carries its own risk of gas embolism, fluid overload, and pulmonary edema.

What are the various distending media used?

The anterior and posterior uterine walls are in apposition and the uterine cavity must be distended with gas or fluid to obtain a view.
- *Gas:* Carbon dioxide (CO_2) is delivered via a pressure reduction system or hysteroflator, which is designed to give a flow rate of a maximum of 100 mL/min and maximum pressure of 200 mm Hg pressure control. It is mainly used for diagnostic hysteroscopy because bleeding during operative hysteroscopy obscures visibility.
- *Fluid media:* They allow continuous irrigation during operative procedures and so are preferred during operative hysteroscopy.
  • *Hypotonic fluids:* Solutions such as glycine (1.5%), mannitol, and 3% sorbitol are non-electrolyte distending media and can be used in cases where monopolar energy is being used. As these fluids are hypotonic, so excessive absorption of these fluids can lead to severe complications such as hyponatremic hypervolemia. If unrecognized and left untreated, can lead to bradycardia and hypertension and subsequent pulmonary edema, cardiovascular collapse, and death.
  • *Isotonic fluids:* Solutions such as physiological normal saline of Ringer's lactate are isotonic and so risk of hyponatremia is reduced with their use leads to expansion of the extracellular fluid volume with development of fluid overload, pulmonary edema, and cardiac failure.

While using liquid distension media, volume of fluid instilled and volume of return fluid and the fluid deficit must be calculated. In an ideal setup, a hysteromat (a continuous fluid monitoring device) must be used to monitor fluid input and output. Surgeon must be warned when the fluid deficit exceeds 500 mL as this may cause hyponatremia and hypo-osmolar state. Deficit of >1 L requires measurement of serum electrolytes and diuretic therapy. The American College of Obstetricians and Gynecologists (ACOG) and European Society of Gynaecological Endoscopy (ESGE) recommend use of automated fluid pump and monitoring systems.

What is meant by fluid overload?

While using liquid distension media, volume of fluid instilled, and volume of return fluid and the fluid deficit must be calculated. A decrease is serum sodium levels by 10 mmol/L corresponds to absorption of 1,000 mL fluid and a fluid deficit of >1,000 mL is used as a threshold for defining fluid overload when using hypotonic distension media and it is taken as 2,500 mL or more when isotonic solutions are being used. However, these thresholds apply to otherwise healthy fit women with no other comorbidities. Lower threshold values of 750 mL and 1,500 mL are taken in cases of women who are older or with cardiovascular or renal disease.

The incidence of fluid overload varies according to the type of hysteroscopic surgery, but in general, it should be <5% when using large-diameter resectoscopes.

What are the factors predisposing to fluid overload?
The factors influencing absorption of distension media include the following:
- *Intrauterine pressure:* The absorption of fluid is higher with increased intrauterine pressure.
- *Mean arterial pressure:* If the mean arterial pressure is low, then lower intrauterine pressure is required to cause absorption of fluid into systemic circulation.
- *Depth of myometrial penetration:* With increase in depth of myometrial tissue destruction, absorption of the instilled fluid through open venous sinuses increases.
- *Duration of surgery:* Absorption of fluid increases with increased surgery time.
- *Size of uterine cavity:* Large uterine cavities provide a greater endometrial surface for fluid absorption.

Which is the safest distension media to avoid fluid overload?
Isotonic media are safer than hypotonic media as fluid absorption does not cause hyponatremia. But, nevertheless, fluid deficit must be closely monitored during the procedure, irrespective of the distension media being used.

What is contact hysteroscopy?
In contact hysteroscopy, the uterine cavity is not distended and the endometrium is assessed without any intrauterine pressure. The cellular and vascular patterns are assessed by contact with the hysteroscope and giving high magnification.

What is versapoint?
Versapoint is a bipolar electrosurgical resection system. The electrosurgery generator pulses the electrical energy through the saline irrigation medium from the active electrode tip to the larger return sleeve. This creates a vapor pocket around active electrode and when tissue enters the vapor pocket, the high-density current causes vaporization of the tissue. It is used for vaporizing fibroids and polyps.

What are the various hysteroscopic ablative techniques?
- *First-generation techniques*
  They are done under hysteroscopic guidance:
  - Hysteroscopic laser ablation
  - Transcervical resection of endometrium (TCRE) **(Fig. 14A)**
  - Rollerball endometrial ablation **(Fig. 14B)**
- *Second-generation techniques*
  Hysteroscopy is optional:
  - Thermal balloon ablation
  - Microwave ablation (MEA)
  - Radiofrequency endometrial ablation (REA)
  - Cryoablation
  - Hydrothermal ablation
  - Endometrial laser intrauterine thermotherapy (ELITT)

What is NovaSure?
Endometrial ablation is done using bipolar radiofrequency mounted on an expandable frame. This creates a confluent lesion on the entire endometrial surface. Time required for global endometrial ablation is 90 seconds. Radiofrequency coagulates endometrium up to myometrium. Women with uterine cavity <4 cm, pelvic inflammatory disease (PID), and cesarean delivery are contraindicated.

What is a two-stage procedure for hysteroscopic myomectomy?
Fibroids <2 cm can be resected in one sitting. For larger fibroids or those which

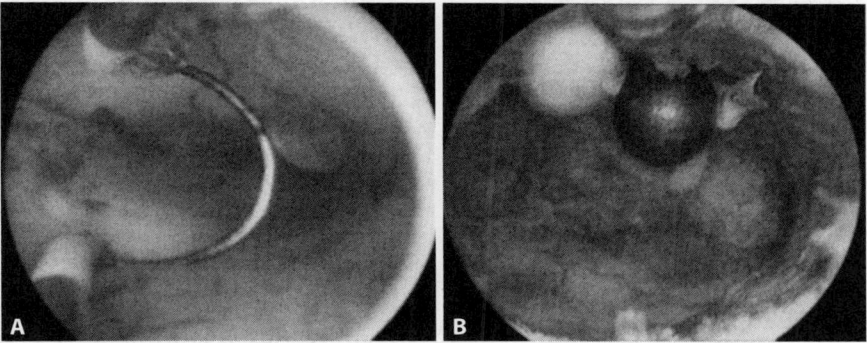

Figs. 14A and B: (A) Endometrial resection with cutting loop; (B) Rollerball endometrial ablation. *(For color version, see Plate 7)*

are more than half intramural, a two-stage procedure is necessary. At stage one, the protruding portion of the fibroid is removed followed by transhysteroscopic myolysis of the intramural portion. Subsequently, gonadotropin-releasing hormone (GnRH) is given for 8 weeks, which shrinks the uterine cavity, thus extruding the intramural portion of the fibroid, which is then easily removed at second stage.

What is the FIGO classification system for uterine leiomyoma? (Fig. 15)
The International Federation of Gynecology and Obstetrics (FIGO) classification of intrauterine myomas:
- *Submucosal group*
  - Type 0: Myoma limited to uterine cavity (pedunculated)
  - Type 1: <50% intramural
  - Type 2: ≥50% intramural
- *Other groups*
  - Type 3: 100% intramural; contacts endometrium
  - Type 4: Intramural
  - Type 5: Subserosal ≥50% intramural
  - Type 6: Subserosal <50% intramural
  - Type 7: Subserosal pedunculated
  - Type 8: Others, e.g., cervical

Myomectomy is suitable for grades 0 and 1.

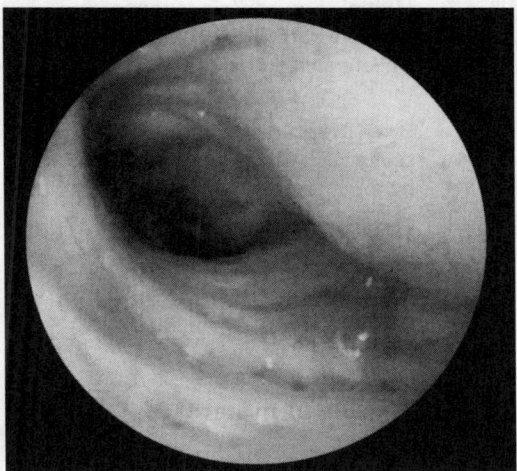

Fig. 15: Submucous fibroid covered by homogeneous endometrium. *(For color version, see Plate 7)*

What is the role of hysteroscopy in Asherman's syndrome (amenorrhea traumatica)?
The classification of intrauterine adhesions as given by the European Society of Hysteroscopy (2010) is as given in **Table 2**.

Hysteroscopic resection of adhesions with postoperative estrogen therapy helps in endometrial regeneration. Role of intrauterine/subendometrial PRP or STEM cell therapy seems promising in the management of Asherman syndrome and thin endometrium in ART setup.

TABLE 2: Classification of intrauterine adhesions.

Grade	Extent of intrauterine adhesions
I	Thin or filmy adhesions easily ruptured by hysteroscope sheath alone. Cornual areas normal
II	Singular filmy adhesions connecting separate parts of the uterine cavity. Visualization of both tubal ostea possible. Cannot be ruptured by hysteroscope sheath
IIa	Occluding adhesions only in the region of the internal cervical os. Upper uterine cavity normal
III	Multiple firm adhesions connecting separate parts of the uterine cavity. Unilateral obliteration of ostial areas of the tubes
IIIa	Extensive scarring of the uterine cavity wall with amenorrhea or hypomenorrhea
IIIb	Combination of III and IIIa
IV	Extensive firm adhesions with agglutination of uterine walls. Both tubal ostial areas occluded

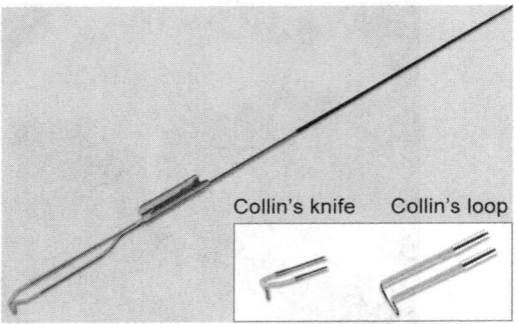

Fig. 16: Collin's knife and loop.
(For color version, see Plate 7)

What is the role of hysteroscopy in tubal cannulation?

Fallopian tube cannulation is a procedure, which is performed hysteroscopically under laparoscopic guidance. It is an excellent alternative for management of patients with cornual obstruction. The uterotubal junctions can be directly visualized with hysteroscopy and this provides easy access for tubal cannulation. Laparoscopy helps in monitoring the procedure and for checking the tubal patency after cannulation. Published studies quote success rates of achieving tubal patency in approximately 70% patients.

Identify the instruments given in Figure 16 that are used in hysteroscopic surgery.

- Collin's knife is used in hysteroscopic septal resection and adhesiolysis **(Fig. 16)**.
- Collin's loop is used for hysteroscopic polypectomy and myomectomy **(Fig. 16)**.

What are the complications of hysteroscopy?

Early complications:
- *Distension media:*
  - *Carbon dioxide gas:* Gas embolism, which can lead to hypotension, tachycardia, and arrhythmia
  - *Glycine:* Fluid overload with hyponatremia. Patient may also develop bradycardia, hypotension, nausea, vomiting, confusion, and agitation. This is due to water moving across the blood–brain barrier leading to cerebral edema. A deficit of 1 L requires caution and surgery is discontinued at 1.5-L fluid deficit.
  - *Dextran 70:* Pulmonary edema, anaphylactic reactions, and coagulopathy consequent to intravasation.
- Hemorrhage
- Uterine perforation—occurs in 1% of women. Extra care should be taken while operating near uterine cornua, as this is the thinnest portion of the uterine wall **(Table 3)**.
- *Infections:* During hysteroscopy, blood and tissue debris become a focus of infection. Also, energy applied to tissue leads to necrosis, which further aggravates infection.

TABLE 3: Complications, incidence, and risk factors of hysteroscopy (ACOG Committee Opinion number 800; 2020)

Potential complication	Incidence	Risk factors
Perforation	0.12–1.61%	• Blind insertion of instruments • Cervical stenosis • Anatomic distortion due to leiomyomas, intrauterine adhesions, congenital anomalies, etc.
Fluid overload	0.20%	• Excessive absorption of distending fluid • Resection of large or deep lesions • High intrauterine pressure
Air and gas embolism	0.03–0.09%	• Excessive intrauterine pressure • Inadequate purging of air from tubing
Hemorrhage	0.03–0.61%	• Uterine perforation • Cervical laceration • Adhesionolysis
Vasovagal reaction	0.21–1.85%	Parasympathetic system activation during manipulation of cervix and instrumentation of cervical canal

- Cervical laceration
- *Air embolism:* It occurs if fluid bubbles are not removed from the tubing prior to start of procedure.

Late complications:
- Infertility
- Abnormal menstrual bleeding hematometra and pyometra
- *Postablation sterilization syndrome:* Endometrial ablation in women with a history of sterilization can lead to postoperative pain. Active endometrium between the scarred uterine cavity and the tubal block leads to hemorrhagic tubal distension during menses. This causes stretching of the intramural and isthmic portion of the tube with resultant pain.

What is the role of antibiotics in hysteroscopic procedures?

Antibiotic prophylaxis is not recommended for routine hysteroscopic procedures. Postprocedural infection rates vary between 0.01% and 1.42% in various studies.

Hysteroscopy is contraindicated during active pelvic infection or in women with prodromal or active herpes infection.

What is office hysteroscopy?

Office hysteroscopy is a minimally invasive procedure which allows direct visualization of uterine pathology using a small-diameter hysteroscope. It has the advantage of allowing visualization without the need for anesthesia and use of an operation theater. With the help of the improved technology, it is now possible to do operative hysteroscopic procedures as well. CO_2 and saline are the most commonly used distension media used for the purpose. Liquid distension is commonly used with an electronically controlled irrigation and suction device so as to obtain <70 mm Hg constant average distension.

What is meant by virtual hysteroscopy?

Virtual hysteroscopy is modified sonohysterography with instillation of special gel inside cavity, which causes adequate distention and ultrasounds are performed in two or three dimensions in real time, creating images almost equal to diagnostic hysteroscopy.

What is vaginoscopic approach to hysteroscopy?

It is a surgical technique which involves the insertion of a hysteroscope to visualize the vagina, cervix, and uterine cavity without the use of a vaginal speculum or holding the cervix with a tenaculum or vulsellum. A small-diameter rigid or flexible hysteroscope is introduced into the vagina and the distension media is used to expand the vaginal canal; the hysteroscope is then directed toward the posterior vaginal fornix and the external cervical os is identified and the hysteroscope is guided into the endocervical and then into the uterine cavity.

The vaginoscopic approach has been shown to reduce procedural pain without any significant difference in the number of failed procedures when compared to traditional hysteroscopy.

Identify the equipment shown in Figure 17.

The equipment shown in the figure is Essure. It is used for hysteroscopic sterilization for which it was approved in 2002. It causes contraception by initiating a chronic inflammatory response and physically occluding the tube. As this takes time, alternative contraceptive methods are to be used for 3 months after the procedure. It is inserted hysteroscopically and when released the outer coil expands and anchors the device in fallopian tube. It has an inner coil made of stainless steel around which is an outer coil

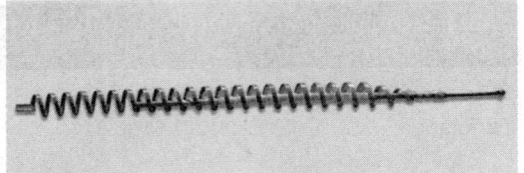

Fig. 17: Essure.

of Nitinol. A hysterosalpingogram (HSG) is required to confirm tubal occlusion 3 months postprocedure.

It was taken off from the market in 2018 after thousands of women experienced severe side effects following Essure insertion. These include heavier or irregular periods, headache, weight fluctuations, fatigue, depression, hair loss and hypersensitivity; many of these reactions are caused by autoimmune reactions to the metal composition of Essure.

■ SUGGESTED READING

1. AAGL practice report: Practice guidelines for the management of hysteroscopic distending media. JMIG 2013;20(2):137-148. https://doi.org/10.1016/j.jmig.2012.12.002.
2. Best practice in outpatient hysteroscopy. Green-top Guideline No. 59; March 2011.
3. Umranikar S, Clark TJ, Saridogan E, Miligkos D, Arambage K, Torbe E, et al. BSGE/ESGE guideline on management of fluid distension media in operative hysteroscopy. Gynecol Surg 13, 289–303 (2016). https://doi.org/10.1007/s10397-016-0983-z.
4. Use of hysteroscopy for the diagnosis and treatment of intrauterine pathology. ACOG Committee opinion No. 800; March 2020.

CHAPTER 15

Robotic Surgery in Gynecology

Latika Chawla, Shalini Rajaram

INTRODUCTION

In the ever-evolving landscape of medical science and technology, robotic surgery has emerged as a ground-breaking advancement, transforming the way surgical procedures are conducted. Robotic surgery is a form of minimally invasive surgery that uses robots to perform surgical procedures. The integration of robotics into the surgical domain represents a paradigm shift, offering unprecedented precision, flexibility, and control to surgeons. This cutting-edge technology not only enhances the capabilities of medical professionals but also holds the promise of improved patient outcomes and a new era in healthcare.

HISTORY OF ROBOTIC SURGERY

The history of robotic surgery dates back to the mid-20th century, with significant developments occurring in the last few decades.
- Idea of using robots in surgery was first conceptualized in the 1950s.
- In 1960, the first robot-assisted surgical procedure was performed using "Arthrobot", a device designed for orthopedic procedures.
- In 1985, PUMA 560, a robotic surgical arm, was used for taking neurosurgical biopsy.
- Automated Endoscopic System for Optimal Positioning (AESOP) introduced in the early 1990s was a robotic arm designed to hold and position an endoscope during surgery, providing surgeons with better visualization. AESOP was modified and later relaunched as the ZEUS.
- da Vinci Surgical System, developed by Intuitive Surgical, was approved by the Food and Drug Administration (FDA) in 2000. It marked a significant breakthrough in robotic surgery. The da Vinci System has remained dominant for over a decade. It is a three- to four-armed system, with a central arm holding a binocular lens that allows for 3D vision. Surgical instruments are articulated at the wrist to provide 7 degrees of freedom.

What are the types of robotic surgical systems?
- *Active systems* essentially work autonomously (while remaining under the control of the operative surgeon) and undertake preprogrammed tasks (e.g., PROBOT, ROBODOC).
- *Semiactive systems* allow for a surgeon-driven element to complement the preprogrammed element of these robot systems.
- *Master–slave systems* are entirely dependent on a surgeon's activity. The surgeon's hand movements are transmitted to laparoscopic surgical instruments, which faithfully reproduce surgeon's hand activity but intracorporeally (e.g., da Vinci, ZEUS).

The da Vinci Xi Surgical System is the latest iteration of the da Vinci robotic surgery platform. It builds upon the success of its predecessors, incorporating advancements in technology to enhance surgical capabilities. This chapter will describe practical aspects of robotic surgery in gynecology using the da Vinci Xi Surgical System.

What are the components of the da Vinci Xi Surgical System?

- *Surgeon console:* The surgeon controls the robotic arms while sitting comfortably at a console located at a distant site in the operating room. The console provides a 3D high-definition view of the surgical site and allows the surgeon to manipulate the camera and instruments with hand and foot controls. The surgeon can also modify the cautery settings sitting at the console **(Figs. 1A and B)**.
- *Patient cart:* This is positioned near the patient during surgery and holds the four robotic arms through which instruments and endoscope are inserted into the patient's body. The cart has a *"Boom"* which is an adjustable rotating support structure that moves the arms into position; a *"Column"* that moves the boom up or down to adjust the height of the system; a *"Helm"* that enables the cart drive functions, boom positioning, and provides a touchpad for system messages and guided menu options; and a *"Base"* that includes a motorized cart drive for positioning and transportation of the cart. The arms are thin and long and offer a greater range of motion. Each arm has a *"Port Clutch"* that controls gross arm movements and raises the boom and an *"Instrument Clutch"* that repositions arm around remote center and advances/retracts the scope and instrument **(Figs. 2A and B)**.
- *Vision cart:* It consists of a 24-inch HD monitor with touchscreen and streamlined controls, an integrated ERBE VIO® dV electrosurgical unit, an endoscope controller where the endoscope is connected, and a video processor with a USB port **(Fig. 3)**.
- *Endo-wrist instruments:* These have a unique design that allows for 7 degrees of motion and 90 degrees of articulation, mirroring the natural movements of

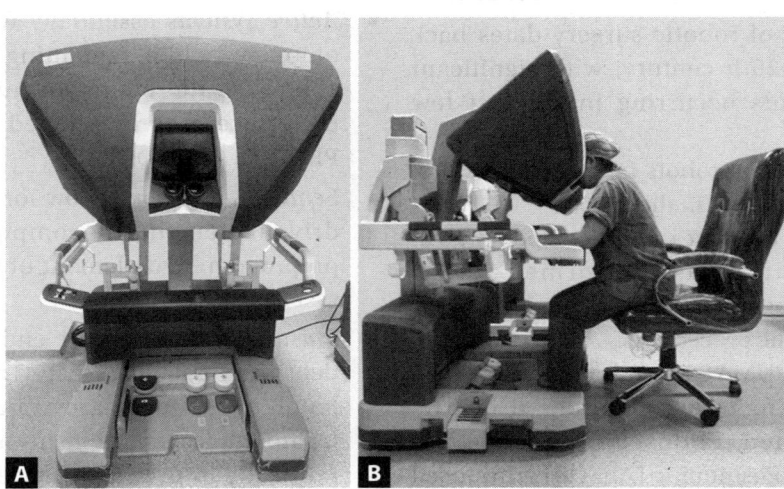

Figs. 1A and B: (A) Surgeon console; (B) Surgeon sitting comfortably at console while operating.
(For color version, see Plate 7)

Robotic Surgery in Gynecology

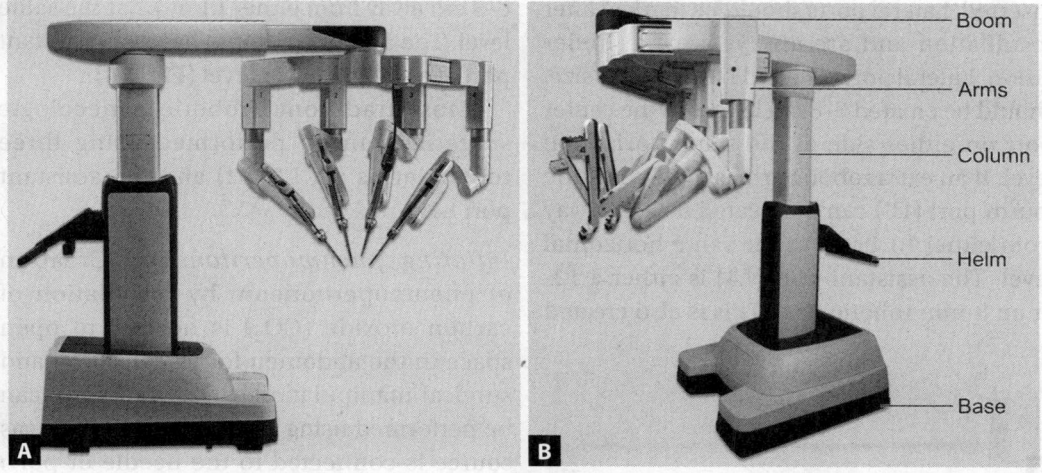

Figs. 2A and B: (A) Patient cart; (B) Components of patient cart. *(For color version, see Plate 8)*

human arm and wrist. Movements are under fingertip control of the surgeon sitting at the console with scaling down of motion and reduction in the tremors. The following endo-wrist instruments are available:

- Bipolar cautery instruments [fenestrated forceps **(Fig. 4A)**, Maryland forceps, curved dissector, long grasper, microforceps, vessel sealer]
- Monopolar cautery instruments [scissors **(Fig. 4B)**, hook, spatula, hot shears]
- Harmonic ace curved shears
- Needle driver **(Fig. 4C)**.

Discuss the steps in robotic surgery.

Anesthesia: Preoperative fitness remains the same as required for laparoscopic surgery. Robotic surgical procedures are done under general anesthesia. Airway pressure should be maintained to ≤25–30 cm of H_2O.

Patient positioning: Steep Trendelenburg position is used for gynecological surgery. Arms are tucked in at the patient's sides. Pressure points should be padded to prevent injuries to peripheral nerves and bony prominences. Cross-body taping may be used to prevent the patient from sliding on the OT table during surgery.

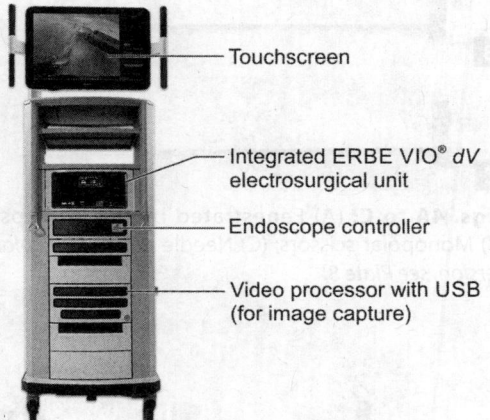

Fig. 3: Components of vision cart. *(For color version, see Plate 8)*

Marking and creation of ports: The center port (C) is marked in the midline, minimum of 15 to maximum of 20 cm from the pubic symphysis. Pneumoperitoneum is created. The center port is created using a 8- or 12-mm robotic trocar and cannula **(Fig. 5A)**, through which an 8- or 12-mm endoscope is inserted. Lateral ports should be marked after insufflation and are always created under vision. Lateral ports (L1 and L2), 8 mm in size, should be created 6–8 cm lateral to the center port on either side at the same horizontal level. If an extra robotic arm is to be used, the fourth port (L3) can be created 6–8 cm away from either L1 or L2 at the same horizontal level. The assistant port (L4) is either a 12- or an 8-mm robotic port. This is also created 6–8 cm away from either L1 or L2 at the same level. The authors prefer to have the assistant port at a slightly lower level **(Fig. 5B)**.

Most traditional robotic gynecologic surgeries can be performed using three robotic arms (C, L1, L2) and the assistant port L4.

Inflating pneumoperitoneum: Creation of pneumoperitoneum by insufflation of carbon dioxide (CO_2) is needed to open space in the abdomen for visualization and surgical manipulation. CO_2 insufflation can be performed using a Veress needle. The gas source is connected to the needle or port; intra-abdominal pressure (IAP) is monitored as gas is insufflate, aiming for a pressure ≤15 mm Hg (ideal around 12–13 mm Hg to minimize physiologic effects).

Docking and targeting: After proper positioning and insertion of ports, the patient cart is brought to the side of the patient. Using a laser line, the cart is aligned to the abdomen and the ports **(Fig. 6A)**. Docking is the process of attaching the robotic arms to the trocar

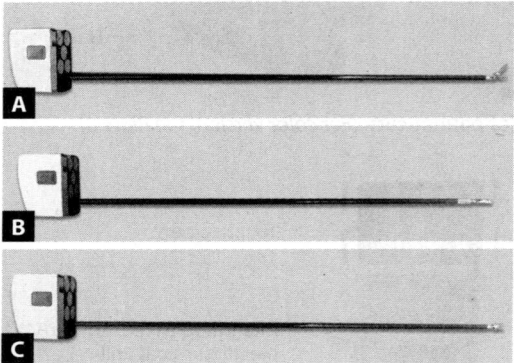

Figs. 4A to C: (A) Fenestrated bipolar forceps; (B) Monopolar scissors; (C) Needle driver. *(For color version, see Plate 8)*

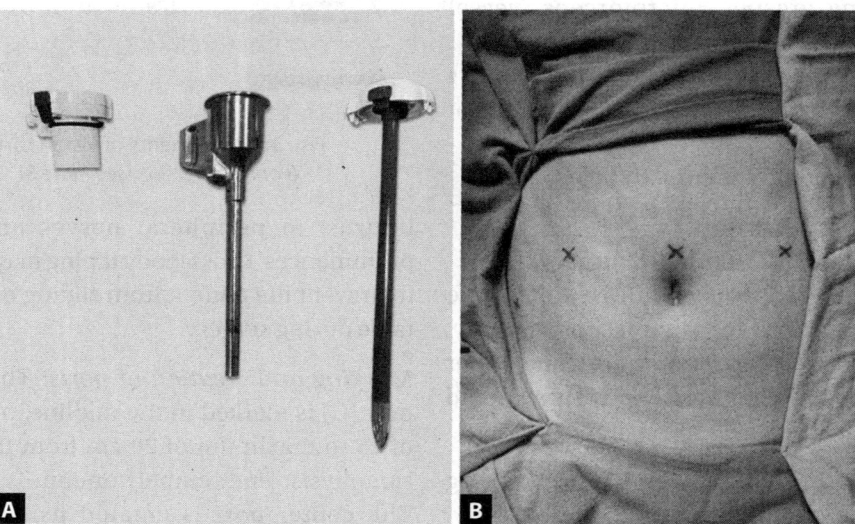

Figs. 5A and B: (A) Robotic trocar and cannula 8 mm; (B) Port placement in robotic gynecological surgery. *(For color version, see Plate 9)*

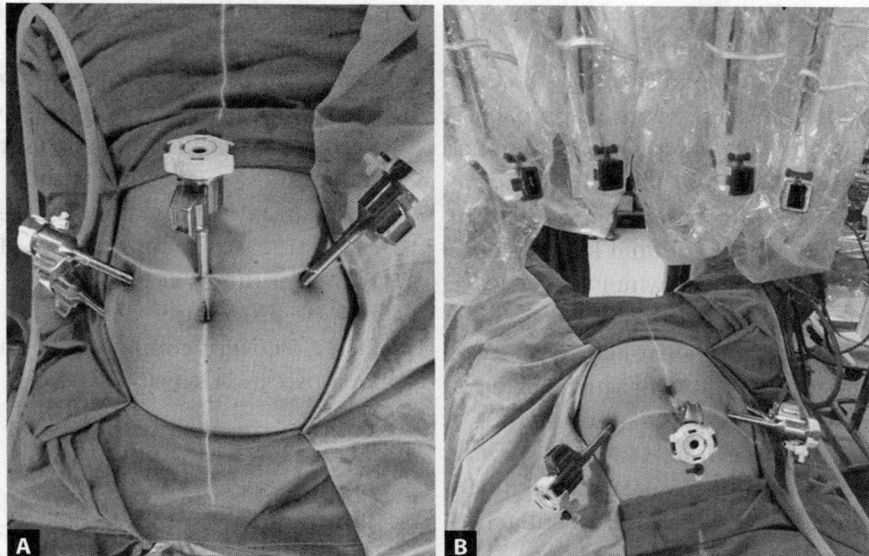

Figs. 6A and B: (A) External targeting using laser line; (B) Robotic arms draped and ready for docking.
(For color version, see Plate 9)

already in place in the patient's abdominal wall **(Fig. 6B)**. The assistant's trocar is not docked. The endoscope is inserted most commonly through the center port (although in Xi, any arm can be used for the camera). An internal targeting system enhances the height of the boom and aligns the robotic arm along the operating field, preventing them from colliding with each other and allows for a smooth procedure. Endo-wrist instruments on either side are then introduced under vision. The cautery leads are connected to the instruments. Once docking is complete, the position of the patient should not be changed to avoid injury to the abdominal wall.

Surgeons can after this begin surgery from the console.

What are the indications for robotics in gynecologic surgery?
- *Procedures that require suturing:* Sacro colpopexy, myomectomy, tubal recanalization
- *Procedures requiring dissection:* Deep infiltrating endometriosis, lymphadenectomy, patients with previous abdominopelvic surgeries where adhesions are expected
- Procedures in obese patients
- *Procedures with large pathology:* Hysterectomy in large size of uterus, myomectomy in large fibroids.

How is tissue retrieval of specimens done after robotic surgery?
Large uterine specimens can be removed by coring or cold knife morcellation through the vagina. Robot allows for minimally invasive hysterectomy in larger uteri; however, removal of the large specimens may take up a lot of time, sometimes more time than the hysterectomy itself. Fibroids after myomectomy can be removed either by colpotomy or may be put in a bag and removed by in-bag cold knife morcellation by extending the center port. The robot will have to be undocked for the same.

What are the advantages of robotic surgery over laparoscopic surgery?

Robotic surgery and laparoscopic surgery are both minimally invasive surgical approaches that offer several advantages over traditional open surgery. While they share some similarities, robotic surgery has distinct advantages over conventional laparoscopic surgery including the following:

- *Enhanced dexterity and precision:* Robotic arms can mimic the wrist-like movements of a surgeon's hands, with a high degree of accuracy and 7 degrees of freedom.
- *Improved visualization:* Robotic surgery provides a three-dimensional, magnified view of the surgical site, offering enhanced depth perception and visualization.
- *Easier learning curve:* Learning curve for robotic surgery is considered to be easy and much smoother as compared to laparoscopic surgery.
- *Reduced surgeon fatigue:* Robotic systems can filter and scale a surgeon's hand movements, reducing the physical strain on the surgeon during long and intricate procedures. This can contribute to less fatigue and allow for longer procedures.
- *Improved ergonomics:* Robotic systems allow surgeons to operate from a console in a comfortable and ergonomically favorable position. This can reduce the physical strain associated with prolonged periods of surgery.
- *Expanded range of motion*: Robotic instruments can rotate 360° providing a wider range of movements than conventional laparoscopic instruments. This can be especially advantageous when working in confined spaces or manipulating organs in challenging anatomical locations and provides ease in suturing (like in myomectomy).
- *Camera:* It is under control of the main surgeon.
- *Shorter hospital stay and quicker recovery:* Minimally invasive surgeries, whether performed with laparoscopic or robotic techniques, generally result in shorter hospital stays and quicker recovery times compared to open surgery. However, some studies suggest that certain robotic procedures may have a slightly faster recovery compared to traditional laparoscopy in specific cases.

Enumerate the disadvantages of robotic surgery over laparoscopic surgery.

- *Cost:* Robotic surgery systems are expensive to acquire and maintain. The initial investment, as well as ongoing costs for maintenance and training, can be significantly higher than those associated with laparoscopic equipment.
- *Training and learning curve:* Robotic surgery requires specialized training for surgeons to operate the robotic system effectively.
- *Size and port placement:* Robotic system itself takes up space in the operating room limiting the available space for the surgical team and instruments.
- *Dependency on technology:* Robotic surgery relies heavily on technology, and technical malfunctions or system failures/ errors can occur. In such cases, there may be a need to quickly switch to an alternative method, such as open surgery or laparoscopy.
- *Lack of tactile feedback:* One of the drawbacks of robotic surgery is the lack of tactile feedback for the surgeon. In laparoscopic surgery, the surgeon can feel resistance and pressure, providing a sense of touch. Robotic systems typically do not provide this tactile feedback, and

surgeons must rely on visual and auditory cues.
- *Procedure time:* Some studies suggest that robotic surgery may take longer than laparoscopic surgery, although in the author's experience, the same surgery may be done quicker with robotic surgery as compared to laparoscopic surgery. Docking is an extra step that may increase the time of surgery as compared to laparoscopy, but with time and experience docking time may be reduced to only a few minutes.

SUGGESTED READING

1. Leal Ghezzi T, Campos Corleta O. 30 years of robotic surgery. World J Surg. 2016;40(10):2550-7.
2. Sood A, Jeong W, Ahlawat R, Campbell L, Aggarwal S, Menon M, et al. Robotic surgical skill acquisition: What one needs to know? J Minim Access Surg.2015;11(1):10-5.

Incisions

Sonia Chawla, Bindiya Gupta

BACKGROUND

Careful selection of incision is one of the essential elements for success of any surgery. The choice of incision is dependent on many factors, which include amount of exposure required, nature of surgery (emergency/elective), indication of surgery, and surgeon's preference. The type of incision also has profound influence on the occurrence of postoperative complications. In this chapter, we will discuss the relevant anatomy, types of incisions, and complications.

The principles of an incision include adequate access, minimal blood loss, preservation of nerve supply, and minimal cutting of muscles, and it should be capable of being extended, if required. Additional considerations in selecting the type of incision include speed of entry, certainty of diagnosis, body habitus, presence of previous scars, potential for problems with hemostasis, and cosmetic outcome.

ANATOMY OF ANTERIOR ABDOMINAL WALL

Before planning any incision, basic knowledge of abdominal wall anatomy and its blood and nerve supply is essential. The anterior abdominal wall is composed of two groups of muscles **(Fig. 1)**:
- Flat (external, internal oblique, and transverse oblique)
- Vertical (rectus abdominis and pyramidalis)

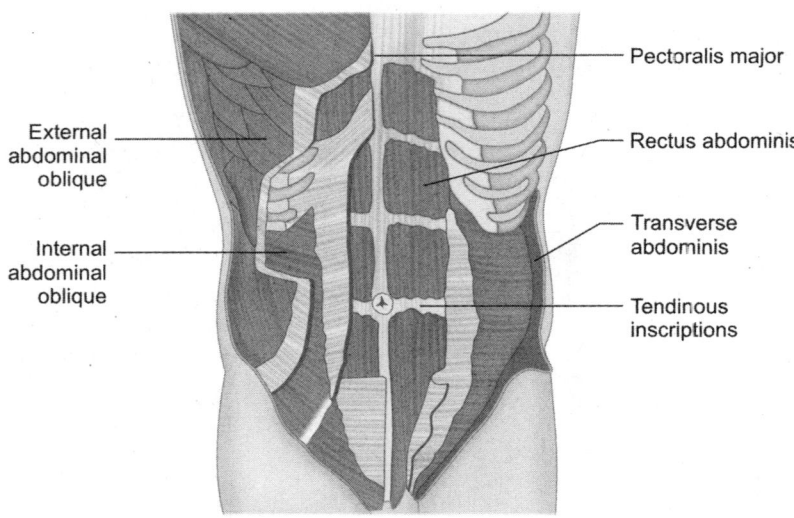

Fig. 1: Anterior abdominal wall muscles.

External Oblique Muscle

External oblique muscle is the most superficial muscle. It originates from lower eight ribs and is attached to the linea alba medially and laterally and downward inserts on iliac crest.

Internal Oblique Muscle

Internal oblique muscle originates from the upper surface of inguinal ligament, iliac crest, and thoracolumbar fascia. The anterior layer fuses with aponeurosis of external oblique while the posterior layer fuses with aponeurosis of transverse abdominis and forms a rectus sheath. Below the arcuate line, the internal oblique aponeurosis does not split and lies anterior to rectus muscle.

Transverse Abdominis

Transverse abdominis originates from the inner surface of 7th to 12th costal cartilage, anterior three-fourth of iliac crest, and lateral one-third of inguinal ligament; moves transversely and medially; and forms aponeurosis to contribute to rectus sheath. Above the arcuate line, transverse abdominis aponeurosis contributes to posterior rectus sheath and below, it passes anteriorly to form anterior rectus sheath.

Vertical Group

Rectus Abdominis

These are paired and long muscles, which run vertically just lateral to linea alba. It originates from pubic crest and runs vertically to insert into fifth, sixth, and seventh costal cartilages and xiphoid process. The rectus sheath covering the muscle is made by the oblique muscles and transverse abdominis aponeurosis.

Nerve Supply

Abdominal skin is innervated in a segmental pattern by the anterior rami of thoracoabdominal nerves (T7–L1).
- T7–T9—innervates the skin above umbilicus
- T10—innervates the skin around umbilicus
- T11 and cutaneous branches of T12, iliohypogastric and ilioinguinal supply the skin inferior to umbilicus

The blood supply to the muscles and skin is summarized in **Table 1**. Knowledge of blood vessels and their distribution is important in planning the incisions in both open and laparoscopic surgeries as damage to these vessels can lead to torrential bleeding and abdominal wall hematomas.

TYPES OF ABDOMINAL INCISION (FIG. 2)

Vertical

Types of vertical abdominal incisions include midline, paramedian, and wide paramedian incisions. The most commonly used is a midline incision, especially in gynecologic oncology surgery. The skin and subcutaneous fat are incised till the rectus sheath using scalpel or electrocautery. The subcutaneous fat is dissected from the rectus until 0.5–1 cm to have better outcomes during incision closure. The rectus muscles are separated vertically in the midline or the space is identified laterally in an avascular plane on one side of the rectus muscle. The peritoneum is opened by blunt dissection or it is grasped between two Allis forceps, pulled up, palpated to rule out any bowel in between the forceps, and opened using scissors and extended.

If the incision needs to be extended above, go around the umbilicus and extend toward

TABLE 1: Blood supply of anterior abdominal wall.

Artery	Source	Supply to	Notes
Circumflex iliac, deep	External iliac artery	Iliacus muscle and the lower abdominal wall	Deep circumflex iliac artery courses along the iliac crest on the inner surface of the abdominal wall
Circumflex iliac, superficial	Femoral artery	Superficial fascia of lower abdomen and thigh	The circumflex iliac after perforating the fascia lata runs parallel to the inguinal ligament and laterally to the iliac crest
Epigastric, superficial	Femoral artery	Superficial fascia and skin of the lower abdominal wall	Turns upward in front of the inguinal ligament and then ascends while spreading out between the two layers of the superficial fascia of the abdominal wall, nearly as far as the umbilicus
Epigastric, superior	Internal thoracic artery	Upper rectus abdominis muscle, upper abdominal wall	Superior epigastric artery is the direct continuation of the internal thoracic artery; it anastomoses with the inferior epigastric artery within the rectus abdominis muscle
Inferior epigastric artery	External iliac artery	–	It originates at the inguinal ligament and ascends upward, perforates the fascia of the musculus transversus abdominis, and climbs upward beyond the arcuate line. Above the umbilicus, it divides into many small branches that anastomose with the superior epigastric artery

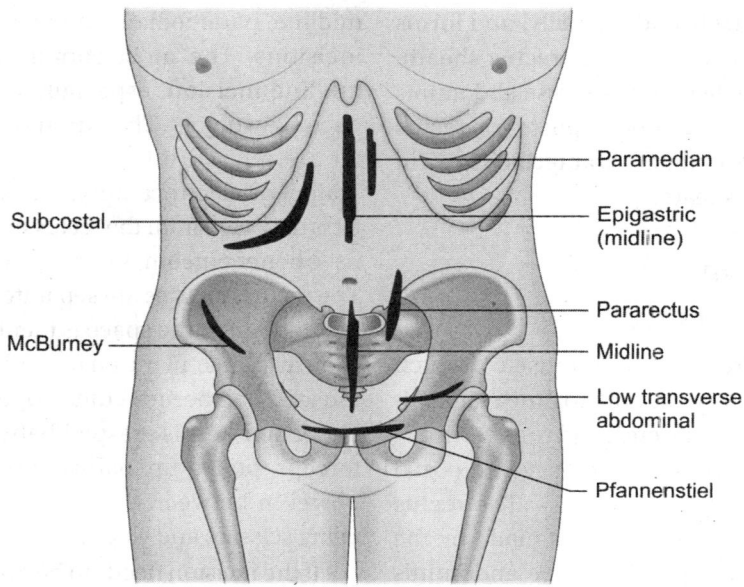

Fig. 2: Laparotomy incisions.

the xiphisternum. Take precaution not to cut through the umbilicus and the incision is taken preferably on the left side to prevent cutting of ligamentum teres.

The advantages of vertical incision include faster entry, minimal blood loss, and easy extensibility vertically upward. The disadvantages include increased incidence of wound dehiscence and incisional hernia formation when compared to a transverse incision. Recent studies suggest that there is a nonsignificant difference in dehiscence rates provided proper surgical closure techniques have been used.

Transverse

Various transverse incisions have been used for cesarean section and gynecologic surgeries, more for benign diseases. Compared to vertical incision, it is less painful, chances of hernia formation are less, and it has better cosmesis. However, the blood loss is more due to more superficial vessels in the skin and fascia, due to which there is an increased risk of abdominal wall hematoma especially due to superficial epigastric artery in high-transverse incision and muscle cutting Maylard and Cherney's incision. Paresthesia due to nerve injuries is more common. Access to the upper abdomen is limited due to limitation of inability to extend.

Pfannenstiel Incision

Pfannenstiel incision is the most frequently used incision, especially for cesarean sections. It is a curved incision about 2 cm above the pubic crest, with lateral apices smiling upward toward anterosuperior iliac spine (ASIS). The incisional length is approximately 10 cm (8–14 cm) depending on the type of surgery. After incising the skin, fat and fascia are incised preferably using cautery. Superficial epigastric vessels may be encountered near the lateral edges of the incision. The rectus sheath is incised transversely and separated from the underlying rectus muscles, which are then split from midline to access the parietal peritoneum. Peritoneum is opened either by sharp or by blunt dissection. Always identify the upper limit of the bladder while opening the peritoneum, especially in cases of previous pelvic surgeries.

During closure, the peritoneum need not be closed as there is no advantage. There is no evidence to support better healing, less infection rate, and wound dehiscence with peritoneal closure. Ensure adequate hemostasis, and closure of fat and superficial fascia is advisable in case depth is >5 cm. Staples or suture are equally effective for skin closure.

Joel–Cohn's Skin Incision

Joel–Cohn's skin incision is a straight transverse incision given 3 cm above the pubic symphysis. Only central subcutaneous fat is incised. Transverse incision in central rectus sheath is widened by craniocaudal stretching. Recti are stretched from midline laterally. Peritoneum is opened by fingers or a small nick and widened craniocaudally.

Maylard Incision

Unlike the Pfannenstiel incision, where the muscles are separated in midline to gain access to peritoneal cavity, Maylard incision is a muscle-cutting incision. It is a curved incision given 3 cm above the pubis symphysis and rectus muscle is cut transversely using cautery to improve the exposure. Ligation of inferior epigastric vessels, which are present on the posterolateral border of each rectus muscle, is done before cutting

TABLE 2: Advantages and disadvantages of various abdominal incisions.

Incision	Advantages	Disadvantages
Midline	Quick, little blood loss, easily extended, minimal nerve damage	Wound dehiscence, hernia formation
Transverse	Less pain, less chance of hernia, better cosmesis	More blood loss, more chance of hematoma formation, more nerve damage, limits exploration of upper abdomen
Paramedian	Better exposure, incisional hernia less	Increased intraoperative bleeding, increased operative time, nerve damage, infection rates are more

the muscle. It should be preferably avoided in patients having clinical evidence of impaired circulation in lower extremities or peripheral arterial disease. In these patients, blood flow from the inferior epigastric artery may be providing the only additional collateral circulation to the lower extremity and its ligation can result in ischemia of the extremity.

Cherney's Incision

After incising the skin and fascia, as in Maylard incision, the tendon of rectus muscle is transected from the pubic bone using electrocautery. Muscles are then retracted in a cephalad direction and the peritoneum is opened. During closure, using nonabsorbable sutures, the rectus muscles are reattached to the distal end of the anterior rectus sheath with interrupted stitches. The muscle cannot be reattached to pubis symphysis due to risk of osteomyelitis. The incision is useful in surgeries for urinary incontinence where a wide exposure to space of Retzius and pelvic sidewalls is required.

Modified Gibson Incision

The incision is marked 3 cm above and parallel to inguinal ligament, up to 3 cm medial to the ASIS to the level of the umbilicus. After entering the peritoneal cavity, round ligament and inferior epigastric vessels are ligated to improve surgical exposure. The incision is used for extraperitoneal lymph node dissection.

Kustner's Incision

Kustner's incision is a slightly curved transverse incision and the fascia is cleaned superiorly and inferiorly until sufficient area is exposed and then a vertical incision is given in the linea alba. Separation of rectus muscles and entrance into peritoneum are done in the same manner as other incisions. This incision has no added advantage and is more time consuming and also its extensibility is limited.

The various incisions of open surgeries are shown in **Figure 2**. The advantages and disadvantages of various abdominal incisions are summarized in **Table 2**. Special precautions need to be taken in obese patients, patients with a history of previous surgery or abdominal Koch's, large cervical fibroids, and ovarian cysts in which the bladder might be pulled high up.

■ SPECIAL CIRCUMSTANCES

Re-entry Incisions

For patients in whom the surgery is planned at the same previous incision site like in repeat cesarean, it is better to make the incision through a previous scar only. If the prior scar is cosmetically not acceptable, then excising the scar and going through it is the preferable approach. The scar can easily by removed by holding and elevating the previous scar with Allis forceps and making an incision around the scar. It is also usually preferred to open the layers a little above the previous incisions so that the peritoneum is opened at a place that is relatively free of adhesions.

Obese Patients

Low transverse incision can be difficult in an extremely obese patient with large panniculus. The incision should not be placed below or within the overlying pad of fat because maceration of skin can increase the risk of infection and thus wound dehiscence.

Incisions in Laparoscopy or Minimal Invasive Surgery

Minimally invasive procedures have largely replaced open surgeries for both benign and malignant conditions due to definitive advantages of reduced operative blood loss, decreased number of hospital days, and patient's improved quality of life.

Relevant Anatomy

It is important to take care of the blood vessels during the placements of the accessory ports as shown in **Figure 3**. The other important intra-abdominal landmarks that need to be identified before trocar insertion are median umbilical ligament that contains the obliterated umbilical artery, obliterated urachus, and upper limit of bladder.

Veress Needle Insertion

- *Subumbilical placement:* A small incision of about 1.0 cm or stab is given at the subumbilical area. The Veress needle is held and inserted at an angle of 45° in nonobese to 90° in morbidly obese women. If an entry is made at an acute angle in very obese women, the needle remains extraperitoneal. The entry pressure can be kept high between 18 and

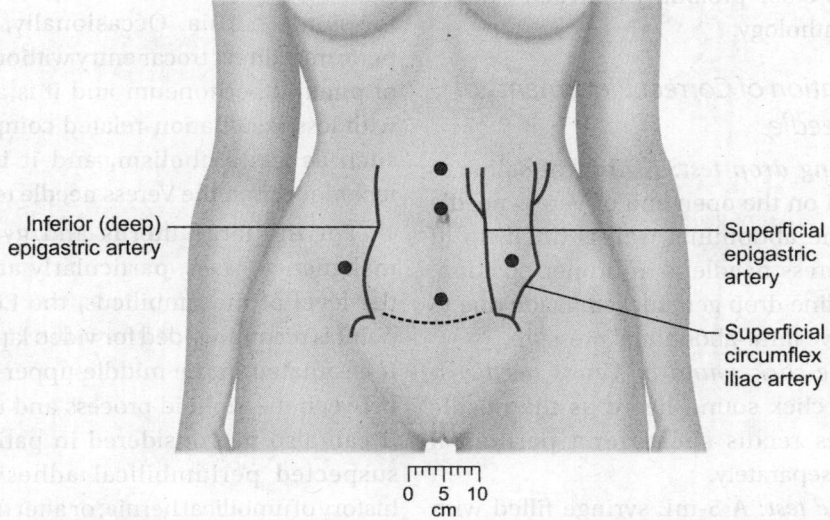

Fig. 3: Port placement with respect to anterior abdominal wall anatomy.

20 mm Hg to reduce the risk of vascular injury. But the pressure should be reduced to 12–15 mm Hg after insertion of primary trocar.
- *Left upper quadrant (Palmer's point):* The point of insertion of Veress needle is in the midclavicular line and 3 cm below the left subcostal border. The technique is especially useful in very obese, very thin, patients with known or suspected periumbilical adhesions and large pelvic masses, and patients in the second trimester of pregnancy and umbilical hernia. Contraindications to Palmer's point include previous gastric or splenic surgery, hepatosplenomegaly, portal hypertension, or gastrosplenic masses.
- *Supraumbilical placement:* This point is generally used if the size of pathology is big, for example, in cases of large bulky uterus or when we are suspecting pelvic adhesions due to previous pelvic surgery, endometriosis, or pelvic inflammatory disease. In cases of large size pathology, placing the primary trocar very near to the pathology can lead to suboptimal vision due to close proximity between camera and pathology.

Confirmation of Correct Placements of Veress Needle

- *Hanging drop test:* A drop of saline is placed on the open end of Veress needle and the abdominal wall is lifted up. If the Veress needle is in proper position, the saline drop gets sucked inside due to negative intra-abdominal pressure.
- *Double-click sound of Veress needle:* It is the click sound heard as the needle pierces rectus sheath and peritoneal cavity separately.
- *Syringe test:* A 5-mL syringe filled with saline is attached to the Veress needle. The plunger is pulled back to aspirate the content, if any, the plunger is taken out to make a water column, the abdomen is lifted to create negative pressure, and the water is sucked inside, if there is proper placement. Also, when aspiration is done, usually nothing is aspirated but in case of an entry in gut or vessel gut, contents or blood can be seen in the syringe.
- Once the Veress needle is attached to an insufflator, the starting pressure should be <10 mm Hg which indicates correct placement.

Primary Trocar Placement (Fig. 3)

After a pneumoperitoneum has been achieved, primary trocar with sleeve (5 mm/10 mm in diameter) is placed at a similar site of the Veress needle. Subumbilical trocar can be inserted using a small curved or a vertical incision. Some surgeons prefer to visualize the trocar entering the abdominal cavity to decrease injury to the intestines or vascular structures using optical trocars and needles. Closure of fascia is recommended for incisions >10 mm, as they have a risk of incisional hernia. Occasionally, surgeons perform a direct trocar entry without creation of pneumoperitoneum and it is associated with less insufflation-related complications, such as gas embolism, and it is a faster technique than the Veress needle technique.

For the large uterus and gynecologic malignancy cases, particularly at or above the level of the umbilicus, the Lee–Huang point is recommended for video laparoscopy. It is situated in the middle upper abdomen between the xiphoid process and umbilicus. It can also be considered in patients with suspected periumbilical adhesions or a history of umbilical hernia, or after three failed attempts of insufflation at the umbilicus.

Open Laparoscopy (Hasson's Technique)

This technique is usually performed at the umbilicus due to close apposition of skin to peritoneum. This involves holding the rectus sheath with Allis forceps and incising the sheath under vision. The peritoneum is then incised to enter peritoneal cavity and a blunt tip trocar with sleeve is then inserted. Some surgeons prefer to take sutures on rectus sheath and peritoneum so that the same can be used for identification of sheath during closure of abdomen. Use of the technique is recommended in cases with previous laparotomy, abdominal tuberculosis, intestinal surgeries, etc., when a blind entry has a higher chance of injury to the gut.

Placement of Side Ports

Lateral

The correct point of insertion is generally approximately two thumbs medial of the ASIS. The distance between two accessory ports should be at least 4–5 cm on the same side.

Ipsilateral port position is favored by many surgeons, especially in gynecologic laparoscopy because the camera person does not physically interfere with the surgeon. Another advantage is that the surgeon does not need to abduct his or her arms that could be difficult, especially for prolonged surgeries.

Midline

A 5–10-mm secondary port is inserted 3 cm above the pubic symphysis. Care should be taken to empty the bladder and in patients with previous cesarean section.

Episiotomy

Episiotomy is a type of surgical incision on perineum and posterior vaginal wall during vaginal delivery.

Types

Mediolateral: The incision is made downward, outward, and extended from midpoint of fourchette to right or left. The direction of incision is diagonal, usually at an angle of 60°.

Structures cut in mediolateral episiotomy:
- Posterior vaginal wall
- Superficial and deep transverse perineal muscles
- Bulbospongiosus and part of levator ani
- Fascia covering these muscles
- Transverse perineal branch of pudendal nerve and vessels
- Subcutaneous tissue and skin
- *Median:* It commences from the center of fourchette and extends posteriorly along midline.
- *Lateral:* It starts around 1 cm away from the center of fourchette and extends laterally. A major drawback is chances of injury to the Bartholin duct.

TABLE 3: Advantages and disadvantages of median and mediolateral episiotomy.

Median	Mediolateral
Advantages: • Muscles are not cut • Blood loss is less • Repair is easy • Postoperative comfort is maximum • Healing is superior • Wound dehiscence is rare	Less chances of involvement of anal sphincter and rectum in case of spontaneous extension
Disadvantages: Extension, if occurs, may involve rectum	• Apposition of tissue is not good • Blood loss is little more • Postoperative discomfort • Relatively increased chances of wound dissection • Dyspareunia more slightly

- *Radical lateral (Schuchardt incision):* This is actually a nonobstetrical incision. It is an extended episiotomy, which is started from midline and extended toward the ischial tuberosity and around the rectum. It is used to facilitate the access to parametrium during radical vaginal hysterectomy.
- *J-shape:* The incision begins in the center of fourchette and dissected downward posteriorly for about 1.5 cm and then directed downward and outward along 5–7 o'clock posterior to avoid anal sphincter.

Advantages and Disadvantages of Median and Mediolateral Episiotomy

Advantages and disadvantages of median and mediolateral episiotomy are given in **Table 3**.

Complications of Episiotomy

Immediate:
- Extension of incision may involve rectum
- Hematoma
- Wound dehiscence
- Infection

Remote:
- Dyspareunia
- Scar endometriosis

■ SUGGESTED READING

1. Barjon K, Mahdy H. Episiotomy. [Updated 2023 Jul 24]. In: StatPearls [Internet]. Treasure Island (FL): StatPearls Publishing; 2024 Jan-. Available from: https://www.ncbi.nlm.nih.gov/books/NBK546675/
2. Carroli G, Mignini L. Episiotomy for vaginal birth. Cochrane Database Syst Rev. 2009 Jan 21;(1):CD000081. doi: 10.1002/14651858.CD000081.pub2. Update in: Cochrane Database Syst Rev. 2017 Feb 08;2:CD000081. PMID: 19160176; PMCID: PMC4175536.
3. Incisions and Closures. In: Yeomans ER, Hoffman BL, Gilstrap III LC, Cunningham F. (Eds). Cunningham and Gilstrap's Operative Obstetrics, 3e. McGraw-Hill Education; 2017.
4. Parshad R, Suhani. Skin Incision for Port Placement in Laparoscopic Surgery-an Often Forgotten Critical Step! Indian J Surg. 2017;79(6):574-575.
5. Pryor A, Bates AT. Abdominal access techniques used in laparoscopic surgery. https://www.uptodate.com>contents>abdominal-access.
6. Sokol ER, Genadry R, Anderson JR. Anatomy and embryology. In: Berek JS, (Ed). Berek & Novak's gynecology. 15th edition. Philadelphia (PA): Lippincott Williams & Wilkins; 2012. pp. 62-111.

CHAPTER 17

Sutures, Needles, and Meshes

Rachna Agarwal, Penzy Goyal

INTRODUCTION

The primary goal of suturing remains the same although the suture materials and techniques have changed over time. The basic principle is supporting and strengthening the wounds till healing takes place to increase its tensile strength. Further, it helps in closing of dead spaces, achieving hemostasis, and approximation of skin edges. This chapter will help in understanding how and why particular sutures are chosen and an appreciation of the basic methods of placing each type of suture.

What are the principles of suture selection?

The principles of suture selection are as follows:

- Suture should be such that it gets absorbed by the time the wound reaches maximum strength.
- Absorbable sutures are used for rapidly healing tissues like intestines and bladder and nonabsorbable sutures for slowly healing tissues like skin, fascia, and tendon.
- Monofilament sutures are preferred in potentially contaminated tissues. The use of multifilament sutures is avoided in such a situation.
- *For cosmetic results:* Inert monofilaments like nylon and polypropylene (PP) are preferred for skin and subcuticular closure with close and prolonged approximation with minimally irritating suture.
- Bladder is preferably sutured with rapidly absorbable suture as nonabsorbable sutures may act as nidus for stone formation.
- The finest size that matches the tissue strength is chosen—this minimizes the tissue trauma when a suture passes through the tissue; it also ensures that a minimum amount of foreign body is left in the body. In case sudden pressure changes are expected, retention sutures should be placed and removed when the patient's condition stabilizes—usually after the skin sutures have been removed.

What is an absorbable suture?

Absorbable suture is defined as "sterile strand capable of being absorbed by living mammalian tissue. It is prepared from collagen derived from healthy mammals or a synthetic polymer, but may be treated to modify its resistance to absorption. It may be impregnated or coated with a suitable antimicrobial agent. It may be colored by a color additive approved by the Federal Food and Drug Administration (FDA)". It generally loses its strength within 60 days.

What is a nonabsorbable suture?

By United State Pharmacopeia (USP) definition, "*nonabsorbable sutures are strands of material that are suitably resistant to the action of living mammalian tissue.* A suture may be composed of a single or multiple filaments of metal or organic fibers rendered into a strand by spinning, twisting, or braiding. Each strand is substantially uniform in diameter throughout its length within USP limitations for each size. The material may be uncolored, naturally colored, or dyed with an FDA-approved dyestuff. It may be coated or uncoated; treated or untreated for capillarity". It maintains its strength even beyond 60 days.

United States pharmacopeia classification:* USP further divides the *nonabsorbable sutures* into various classes:
- *Class I: Silk* (natural) + synthetic fibers of *monofilament*/twisted/braided construction
- *Class II: Cotton or linen* fibers (natural) + *coated natural or synthetic fibers* (coating provides to suture thickness without adding strength)
- *Class III:* Metal wire of monofilament or *multifilament* construction

*http://www.pharmacopeia.cn/v29240/usp29nf24s0_m80200.html

Give examples of absorbable sutures with their sources.
Table 1 shows examples of absorbable sutures with their sources.

What are the examples of nonabsorbable sutures?
Table 2 shows examples of nonabsorbable sutures.

What are the time relations of tensile strength of different sutures?
Time relations of tensile strength of different sutures are given in **Table 3**.

What is the primary suture line?
The suture holding the wound edges in approximation is primary suture line. It may be continuous or interrupted. Continuous suture has more chances of infection; interrupted suture is more secure and better where infection is probability.

Define the following types of sutures.
- *Deep suture:* Under the epidermal skin layer
- *Buried sutures:* Knot protrudes inside, i.e., below the suture line as is used for the rectus sheath
- *Purse-string suture:* Continuous sutures placed around a lumen and tightened like a drawstring to invert the opening, e.g., the stump of appendix.
- *Subcuticular suture:* Continuous or interrupted, placed in the dermis, beneath the epidermal layer, and in parallel to the wound. It is usually applied with monocryl and left to absorb by itself; it can also use vicryl and delayed absorbable suture, which can be removed by pulling through one end.

What is mattress suture?
The mattress suture uses the far–far and near–near systems described in three steps.

Step 1: Far–far suture placement: First, a suture is placed deep in the wound below the dermis, about 4–8 mm from the wound edges. The needle is placed backward in the needle driver and passed across both sides of the wound, and the suture is tied (**Fig. 1**).

Step 2: Near–near suture placement: The suture is placed at a shallow depth (about 1 mm) in the upper dermis. This should be within 1–2 mm of the wound edge (**Fig. 2**).

Step 3: Final suture placement: Suture knotting is to be done on one side of the wound following the near–near passage of the needle. The final knot is on the side where the suture began (**Fig. 3**).

The suture knot should be tied snugly but gently. Excess tension and scarring of the wound could result from eversion of the edges due to excessive pull on the knot. Even tear of the skin and necrosis of the skin

Sutures, Needles, and Meshes

TABLE 1: Absorbable sutures.

Suture	Raw material	Salient points
Surgical gut: Plain chromic Fast absorbing	*Sheep intestine:* Submucosa or *beef intestine:* Serosa	• Ligating superficial blood vessels, suturing of fat • Fast absorbing variety is not to be used inside the body
Polyglactin 910: Uncoated *vicryl* Coated *vicryl* Coated *vicryl plus* Coated vicryl— *RAPIDE*	Copolymer of glycolide and lactide *Coating:* Polyglactin 370 and calcium stearate	• *Vicryl:* Minimum drag, easy to handle, smooth tie down, and unsurpassed knot security • *Vicryl plus:* Prevents bacterial colonization as Triclosan impregnated in the suture • *RAPIDE:* Lower molecular weight, fastest absorbing synthetic suture, and elicits lowest tissue reaction • *Uses:* Skin closure, episiotomy repair, lacerations under casts, etc.
Polyglecaprone 25 (Monocryl)	Copolymer of glycolide and epsilon— caprolactone	• *High-initial strength and rapid absorption:* Monofilament, superior pliability for easy handling and tying. In addition inert in tissues and predictable absorbability • *Uses:* Subcuticular skin closure
Polydioxanone (*PDS II* suture)	Polyester of polyp— dioxanone	• Imbibes mixed features of soft, pliable, and monofilament with absorbability and extended wound support up to 6 weeks • Also has only slight tissue reaction

TABLE 2: Nonabsorbable sutures.

Suture	Raw material	Salient features and uses
Surgical silk	Raw silk spun by silk worms	Represents the standard handling to make into a suture, silk is usually degummed and dyed black. It loses its tensile strength when exposed to moisture, so it should be used dry
	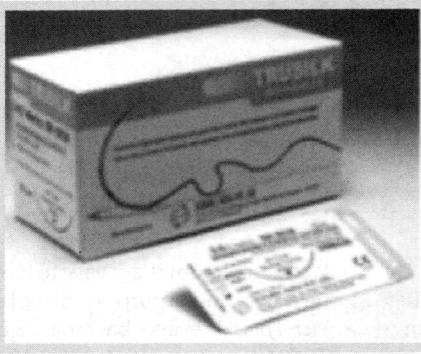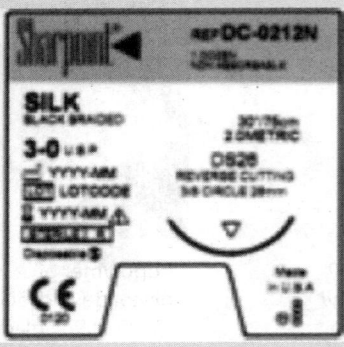	
Stainless steel wire	Specially formulated iron–chromium–nickel–molybdenum alloy	• Absence of toxic elements, flexibility, and fine wire size • *Many discredits:* Difficulty in handling, possible cutting, pulling, tearing of patient's tissues, fragmentation • *Safety issues:* Risk from tearing of gloves and puncture of surgeon's skin
Nylon	Polyamide polymer	• Have a memory, so tend to return to their straight state, so more number of throws are needed • Wet state—it is easier to handle and more pliable • *NUROLON:* Nylon look, feel and handles like silk • Has more tissue strength and elicits less tissue reaction than silk
	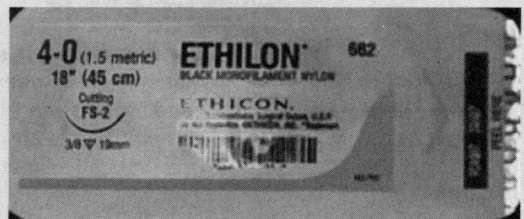	
Polyester fiber Uncoated (*Mersilene*) Coated	Polymer of polyethylene terephthalate	• Precise, consistent suture tension with minimal breakage • Eliminates the need to remove irritating suture fragments, postoperatively
Polypropylene (*Prolene*)	Polymer of propylene	• Relatively biologically inert: Not subject to degradation or weakening by tissue enzymes, minimum tissue reaction • Hold knots better than most other synthetic monofilament materials

Contd...

Contd...

Suture	Raw material	Salient features and uses
		• Proven strength, reliability, and versatility. • *Uses:* Minimal tissue reaction needed, e.g., infected wounds to avoid later sinus formation and suture extrusion
Poly (hexafluoro-propylene-VDF) (*Pronova*)	Polymer blend of vinylidene fluoride and vinylidene fluoride-co-hex-afluoropropylene	*Preferred in infected wounds:* Resists involvement in infection

TABLE 3: Tensile strength of different sutures.

Suture	Tensile strength maintained up to	Strength at 2 weeks	Strength at 3 weeks	5–6 weeks	Absorption time
Plain gut	7–10 days				
Fast absorbing gut (heat treated)	5–7 days				
Chromic gut	10–14 days	Some strength remains			90 days
Monocryl	60–70% at 7 days	30–40%	Almost lost		91–119 days
Vicryl		75%	50%	Lost by 5 weeks	56–70 days
Vicryl RAPIDE	50% at 5 days	Lost			42 days
PDS		70%		50% at 4 weeks, 25% at 6 weeks	6 months
Silk				Loses at 1 year	2 years
Nylon					At the rate of 15–20% per year
Mersilene					

(PDS: polydioxanone)

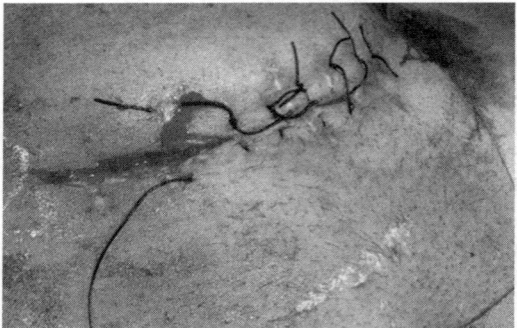

Fig. 1: Far–far suture placement.
(For color version, see Plate 10)

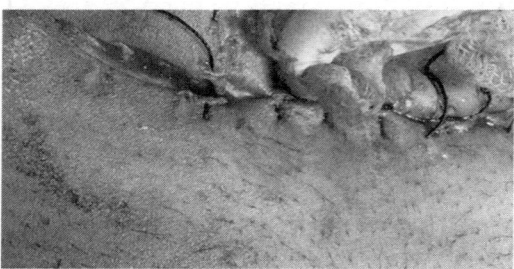

Fig. 2: Near–near suture placement.
(For color version, see Plate 10)

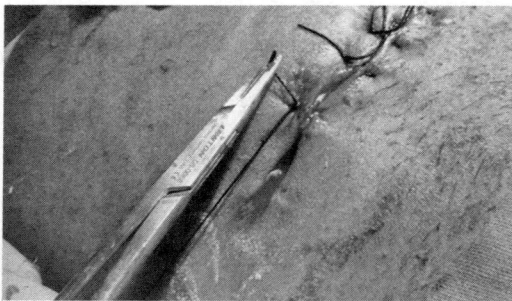

Fig. 3: Final knot is on the side where the suture began. *(For color version, see Plate 10)*

beneath the visible vertical mattress suture may result when the knot is tied too tightly. The natural process of wound inflammation and scar retraction will further pull loops of suture into the skin surface downward.

Scar formation depends on the choice of suture material as large diameter (2-0 or 3-0 absorbable) produces greater skin injury than small-caliber (5-0 or 6-0) suture material.

What is the secondary suture line?

- Suture line is used to reinforce the primary suture where the possibility of wound dehiscence is high (like in obese, debilitated, and patients with large abdominal mass that has been operated upon).
- *Retention sutures or tension sutures:* In an abdominal wound for eliminating the dead space and prevention of fluid accumulation in process of healing by first intention
- As support to wound healing by second intention, especially after burst abdomen
- In cases of healing by third intention for secondary closure following wound disruption

It is to be noted that secondary sutures be placed in opposite fashion from the primary sutures for cases of nonhealing wound, i.e., in an interrupted manner, if primary are continuous and vice versa.

What are the types of secondary sutures?

The major types of secondary sutures are as follows:

Retention sutures: These are inserted around 2 inches lateral from the edge of the wound. This helps to transmit tension lateral to the primary suture line and contributes to the tensile strength of the wound.

Through and through: These sutures are inserted through all layers of the abdominal wall, from inside the peritoneal cavity. They have to be placed before the peritoneum closure by technique of simple interrupted stitch and tied after abdominal closure.

Retention sutures should be removed usually at 3 weeks or between 2 and 6 weeks as these are placed using nonabsorbable materials.

What are the properties of an ideal suture?
The properties of an ideal suture are:
- *Greatest tensile strength* in coherence with size
- *Sterile package* to ensure patient safety along with that of each member of the surgical team
- High *uniform tensile strength*
- High tensile strength retention in vivo, holding the wound securely throughout the critical period, and *rapid resolution thereafter*
- *Uniform diameter throughout*
- Pliable allowing easy handling and *knot security*
- Freedom from impurities for optimum tissue acceptance and least rejection
- Predictable and acceptable performance

What factors decide the choice of suture?
Tissue characteristics: Some tissues repair quickly and regain their strength very fast; hence, suture is used only for a short period of time—the absorbable ones (e.g., catgut for peritoneum)

Some tissues take a long time to regain their strength or may not recover their strength at all; hence, apply nonabsorbable sutures (e.g., silk for implants in bones).

Patient characteristics: In patients with infection, respiratory problems or obesity, delayed absorbable sutures should be applied.

Why cannot we use a single type of long-lasting suture for all tissues?
A suture is required to lose its strength and *dissolve once its function is served* so that the body is saved from the foreign body reaction.

Hence, the suture has to be strong till the tissue is strong and once the tissue is strong, the suture must go.

How does the body react to sutures?
Some amount of foreign body reaction occurs with all sutures. The sutures of biological origin like catgut are lysed by enzymatic degradation. The synthetic sutures like vicryl are broken down by hydrolysis in tissue fluids, hence creating less tissue reaction.

On the other hand, the nonabsorbable sutures like prolene and nylon are encapsulated or walled off by fibroblasts. Thus, they are used in prolapse surgery as mesh or suspension. It is the fibrosis that actually holds together tissues.

How is the suture absorbed?
The initial phase of gradual loss of tensile strength in a linear manner is followed by the second stage of loss of suture mass, i.e., absorption. Thus, loss of tensile strength and absorption of suture material are entirely different. Suture may lose its tensile strength completely and still not be absorbed and vice versa.

What are the indications of nonabsorbable sutures?
- External skin closure—to be removed later
- Prosthesis attachment
- Any elicited history of reaction to absorbable sutures or tendency toward keloid formation/tissue hypertrophy

What determines the choice between monofilament and multifilament sutures?
Monofilament sutures like monocryl resist infection and tie down smoothly. They encounter minimum resistance while passing through tissues. Suture breakage may occur due to weak spot in the strand as a result of crushing or crimping of this suture. Knot security is achieved by more number of throws.

Multifilament suture like vicryl has many filaments twisted or braided in unison.

This contributes to great pliability, tensile strength, and flexibility. Coating helps to negotiate passage through tissues smoothly. Multifilament sutures have microcrevices, which may serve as nidus of infection. But multifilament sutures have excellent handling and knot security.

How is the size of suture determined?
The size is according to the USPs defined criteria. The number 1, 2, 3, and so on denote increasing diameter sutures, whereas 0, 00, 000 denote decreasing diameter of suture thread. The 00 is also denoted as 20, 000 as 3-0, and so on. In usual gynecological practice, no. 1-0 and no. 1 sutures are most commonly used. Number 4-0 and smaller are used for tuboplasty surgery.

How is the tensile strength of sutures measured?
The tensile strength is measured in terms of the pounds of force required to break its strand, especially when it is pulled while tying the knot. The accepted rule is that sutures should be at least as strong as the tissue in which they are applied.

What are antimicrobial-coated sutures?
Triclosan-coated polyglactin 910 antimicrobial sutures are used to decrease the incidence of surgical site infections, especially in clean/contaminated cases. Triclosan is a widely used antibacterial agent and not an antibiotic; hence, the risk of resistance is very low. It acts by nonspecific disruption of the bacterial cell membrane.

■ SURGICAL NEEDLE

What are the parts of a surgical needle?
The needle broadly consists of the point, body, and eye. Other characteristics are the needle radius, needle diameter, and needle length **(Figs. 4A and B)**.

- *Needle diameter* is the diameter of its cross section.
- *Needle radius* is the radius of curvature, i.e., how curved it is.
- *Types of eye* are closed, French eye, or swaged eye.
- *Shape* may vary from being straight, half curved, 1/4 circle, 3/8 circle, or 1/2 circle as shown in **Figure 4B**.

How does the type of needle affect its use (Table 4)? What are the suture less options for wound closure?
They are the topical skin adhesives like DERMABOND and high-viscosity DERMABOND **(Figs. 5A and B)**.

Which kind of wounds can be sealed with topical adhesives?
Low-tension wounds are ideally suited for its application. Wounds on face, torso, and limbs are preferred site of use and used in

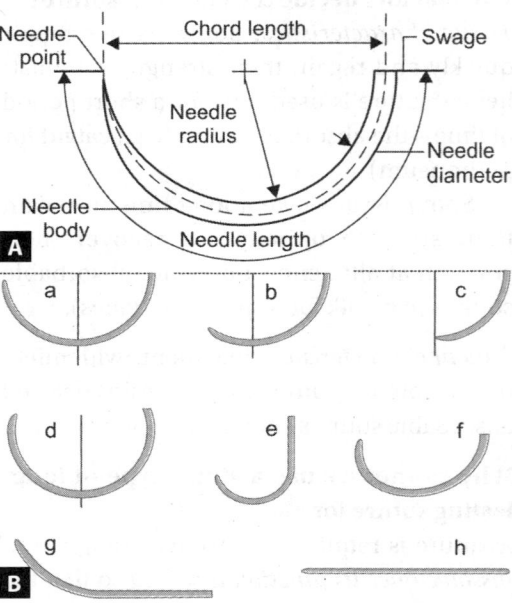

Figs. 4A and B: Parts of surgical needle.
Shapes: a = 1/2 circle, b = 3/8th circle, c = 1/4th circle, d = 5/8th circle, e = j-shaped, f = compound curved, g = half curved, h = straight.

TABLE 4: Types of needles.

Types of needles	Characteristics	Use
Conventional cutting	Sharp point with triangular cross section, square cross section body	Skin, sternum
Reverse cutting	Sharp point at tip with inverted triangle, square cross section body	Fascia, ligament, better for skin as less chances of cut through at the approximated edge
Taper	Pointed with round body	GIT, laparoscopy, urogenital tract, vessels
	40 cm — Tapercut 1/2 Circle — 90 cm	
	40 mm (Heavy) — Tapercut 1/2 Circle — 70 cm / 90 cm	
	40 cm — 1/2 Circle round bodied — 70 cm / 90 cm	
	40 mm (Heavy) — 1/2 Circle round bodied — 70 cm / 90 cm	
Blunt	Blunt tip	Friable tissue, incompetent cervix, liver, spleen

(GIT: gastrointestinal tract)

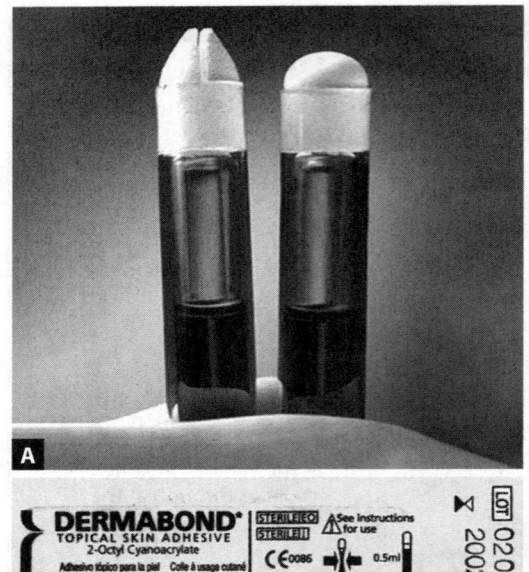

Figs. 5A and B: Topical adhesives.

conjunction with deep-dermal sutures for better results.

What is the ingredient and mechanism of action of these topical adhesives?

Cyanoacrylate tissue adhesives are liquid monomers that undergo an exothermic reaction on exposure to moisture and change to polymers that form a strong tissue bond. The polymer binds the wound edges together to permit normal healing of the underlying tissue. Tissue adhesives should *not* be used for wounds under tension, complex stellate lesions, crush wounds, wounds on the hands and feet or over joints, unless the affected areas are immobilized, because repetitive movements could cause the adhesive bond to break before sufficient wound healing has occurred, wounds on the oral mucosa or other mucosal surfaces (e.g., vagina) or areas of high moisture, such as the axillae and perineum.

Examples of tissue adhesives are:
- 2-octyl cyanoacrylate (e.g., Dermabond, SurgiSeal)
- *N*-butyl-2 cyanoacrylate (e.g., Histoacryl Blue, PeriAcryl)

What are the contraindications to the use of these adhesives?
- Infected wounds or gangrene
- Mucosal surfaces or across mucocutaneous junction
- Surface regularly exposed to body fluids
- Surfaces with dense hair (e.g., scalp)
- In patients with known allergy to cyanoacrylate or formaldehyde

How are the adhesives used?
- The wound must be thoroughly cleaned and debrided.
- The wound edges should be tightly apposed.
- The patient should be positioned so that the wound surface is parallel to the ground.
- Apply two layers of the adhesive, waiting for 30 seconds between the applications
- The adhesive falls off naturally in 5–10 days' time and till that time dry dressing can be applied.
- The patient can take a bath but should keep the wound dry and avoid scratching.

What is fibrin glue?

Fibrin glue creates a fibrin clot for hemostasis, cartilage repair surgeries, or wound healing. It contains separately packaged human fibrinogen and human thrombin.

Mechanism of action

Thrombin fibrinogen into fibrin monomers in 10–60 seconds, which aggregate to form a three-dimensional gel-like structure. It also activates factor XIII from the human body to factor XIIIa, which then cross-links the fibrin monomers to form a stable clot.

Both these processes need calcium to work. As the wound heals, the clot is slowly degraded by the enzyme.

Contraindication

It should be taken care that the glue does not get into blood vessels, as it could lead to clotting in the form of thromboembolism or disseminated intravascular coagulation or to anaphylaxis.

Uses
- For the improvement of hemostasis in liver surgeries, where standard surgical techniques are insufficient
- Repairing dura mater tears
- Repairing bronchial fistulas
- "No sutures" corneal transplantation
- Pterygium excision with amniotic membrane or conjunctival autograft
- In eye trauma for corneal or conjunctival defects
- Skin graft donor site wounds to reduce postoperative pain
- To treat pilonidal sinus disease
- For hemostasis in ovarian cystectomy

What are the recommendations for abdominal wound closure?
- Absorbable suture should be chosen and it should have a caliber that will provide adequate strength to the wound while minimizing foreign body content. Multifilament sutures provide better knot strength, but they are more prone to infection and sinus formation.
- One-half or five-eighths circle, taper point, general closure needles can be used to close most wound incisions.
- Continuous mass closure is the ideal closure method using a suture length to wound length ratio of 4:1 in a simple running technique. The tissue should be reapproximated with low tension to prevent ischemia. A single strand should be tied to another single strand using a square knot or surgeon's knot.
- We suggest not closing the peritoneum, as this appears to confer no benefit.
- To reduce the incidence of incisional hernia following elective midline abdominal closure (first-time closure or repeat closure), we recommend a continuous suture technique using a slowly absorbable monofilament suture. The optimal closure technique in the emergency setting has not been defined. The fascia of nonmidline abdominal incisions can be closed in a similar fashion.

What is a Bogota bag and where is it used?
Laparostomy bag/Bogota bag is a 3 L sterile plastic bag. It is a genitourinary irrigation bag that is sewn to the skin or fascia of the anterior abdominal wall and is also used to close large abdominal wounds. It is a temporary abdominal closure technique and is most commonly used in cases of abdominal compartment syndrome in which decompressive laparotomy is necessary to reduce intra-abdominal pressure to restore blood flow. It is basically used to postpone definite closure until the underlying cause of the elevated intra-abdominal pressure can be resolved. It is a type of tension-free closure that acts as a hermetic barrier that prevents disembowelment and loss of fluids. Also, it allows visual inspection of abdominal contents and hence is particularly useful in cases of ischemic bowel.

What is negative pressure wound therapy?
Negative pressure wound therapy (NPWT), also called vacuum-assisted wound closure, is a wound dressing system that continuously or intermittently applies subatmospheric pressure to the system, which provides a positive pressure to the surface of a wound.

Two systems of NPWT are available commercially:
- Vacuum-assisted closure (VAC) therapy device
- Chariker–Jeter wound sealing kit

Indications
- Nonhealing complex wounds
- Traumatic wounds such as open fractures or open lacerations
- Degloving injuries and burns, which cause partial-thickness skin loss

All these injuries are at a high risk of infection due to contamination from exposure to the surrounding environment. Primary closure of such wounds may entrap the microorganisms in the soft tissue and lead to abscess formation.

Contraindications
- Necrotic tissue or eschar present in the wound bed, such as in full-thickness burns, can exacerbate nonhealing and risk the further spread of necrosis.
- Presence of underlying malignancy due to the hypothetical possibility of tumor propagation and metastasis
- Active osteomyelitis should ideally be treated before the use of NPWT.

Complications
- Pain
- Bleeding
- Infection
- Foam retention
- Unsuccessful therapy delivery due to loss of suction
- Hypersensitivity reaction to the dressing materials
- Intraoperative complications, such as damage to surrounding nerves, blood vessels, and soft tissue

■ MESH

How do you classify meshes? (Table 5)

Meshes are divided into natural and synthetic.

Biological grafts appear to have some advantage of reduced erosion rates, but they have inconsistent tissue strength and source of infection.

A classification of synthetic meshes **(Table 5)** by Amid is based on their physical characteristics.

TABLE 5: Types of meshes.

Natural meshes		
Human	Autologous	Rectus sheath, fascia lata, dermal grafts
	Homograft	Dura mater
Animal	Xenografts	Pelvicol
Synthetic meshes		
Type I (macroporous, i.e., pore size >75 μm)	Prolene, Marlex	Monofilament fibers and have a large pore size: Lower rates of infection and erosion and large pore size admits macrophages and allows rapid angiogenesis
Type II (microporous, i.e., pore size <10 μm in at least one dimension)	Gore-Tex	Using multifilamentous materials and have small pore sizes: can harbor bacteria and promote bacterial growth
Type III (macroporous with either multi- or monofilament)	Teflon, Mersilene, propylene	Properties with mixture of two above
Type IV	Silastic sheets	Relatively solid sheath: not suitable for use in soft tissue

Currently, small diameter, monofilament, macroporous, light weight, and PP type I are the most studied and most preferred meshes. It induces minimal reaction and allows growth of granulation tissues due to its large pores. Type I meshes are made with pore size >90 micrometer, so perimesh inflammatory response soon settles and the mesh is incorporated well by fibrous tissue ingrowth.

There is no evidence-based data about superiority of one over the other, and only case series are available.

Macroporous, monofilament, PP mesh (type I) has been found to have the most favorable biocompatibility profile.

Type 1: Prolene Mesh, see **Figures 6A and B**.

What properties are desired in an ideal mesh?

An ideal mesh should be:
- Biocompatible
- Chemically and physically inert
- Nonallergic
- Noncarcinogenic
- Noninflammatory
- Resistant to infection

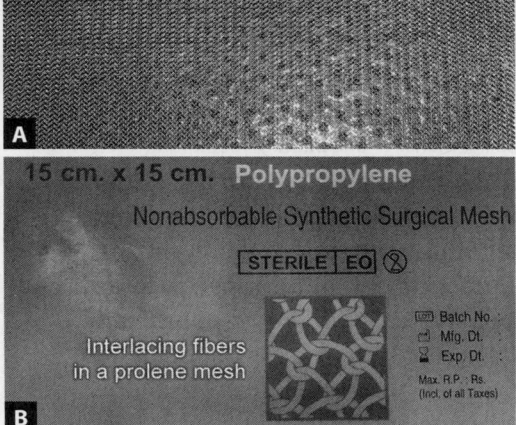

Figs. 6A and B: Prolene mesh with interlacing fibers.

Anisotropy index and security index that allow to easily classify the mechanical performance of commercially available meshes and furnish a novel methodological approach to analyze their performance.

For the abdominal wall meshes, the security index K has been defined to evaluate, if a mesh is able to support the forces that are generated in situ; it is defined as $K = \sigma_m / \sigma_{tissue}$, where σ_m is the maximum stress, which can be sustained by the surgical meshes and σ_{tissue} is the typical stress of the specific tissue. In the case of urogynecological meshes, as precautionary, the same stress used for the abdominal wall could be considered. The bigger the index, the less the probability that the mesh is broken by forces acting normally on natural tissue. Once implanted, the mesh must hold its shape and position and must resist different stresses.

Nylon, Marlex, and Gore-Tex meshes have higher erosion rates, higher stiffness, and also substantial differences in pore size, in manufacturing process, in surface properties, and in mesh topology compared to PP meshes currently marketed. For these reasons, PP mesh is considered the gold standard for urogynecological treatment. Summarizing the type of material that composes the meshes and their biomechanical and topological features plays an important role in the tissue regeneration process and consequently in the implants.

What are Prolift, Perigee, and Apogee?

Surgical repair of pelvic organ prolapse is being augmented using mesh. Perigee and Apogee are single-use needle suspension for mesh or graft-augmented repairs. Perigee uses the transobturator technique for the treatment of anterior prolapse; Apogee uses a posterior vaginal and perianal approach for the treatment of vault and posterior prolapsed.

They are three types of vaginal mesh systems **(Figs. 7A to C)**:
1. *Prolift:* It is a total vaginal mesh reconstructive device. It includes anterior and posterior vaginal meshes. It is anchored to iliococcygeus or sacrospinous ligament apically to the obturator membrane anteriorly and the perineum inferiorly. Mesh erosion is 6.3% and the recurrence rate is 8.3%.
2. *Perigee:* It is a mesh system for anterior wall repair and is anchored to the obturator membrane on both sides.
3. *Apogee:* It is a system for apical and posterior repair, i.e., enterocele and rectocele; it is anchored to the sacrospinous ligament on either side.

A National Institute for Health and Care Excellence (NICE) interventional procedure guidance indicates the use of mesh for apical pelvic-organ prolapse, provided that proper consent, audit, and clinical governance are in place. The surgery should only be performed by surgeons experienced in the management of pelvic-organ prolapse and female urinary incontinence.

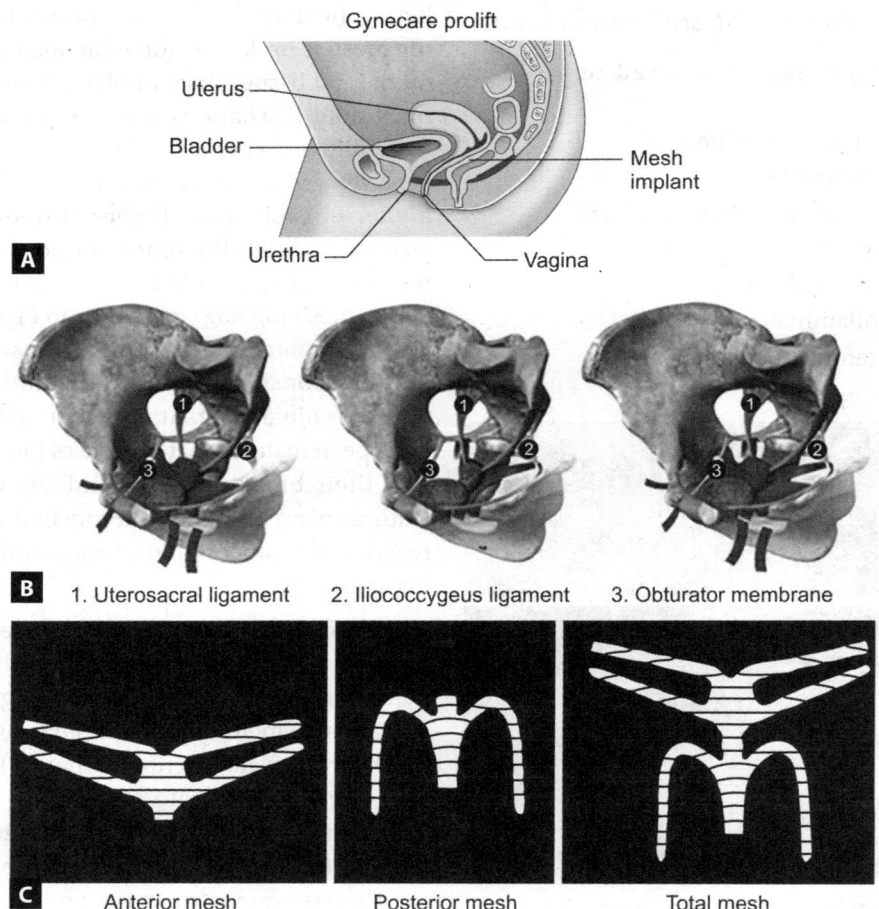

Figs. 7A to C: Vaginal mesh systems.

The newer operations for prolapse (Apogee, Perigee, Prolift, and so on) are transvaginal procedures. They attempt to provide level I and level II (support to the upper and middle aspects of the vagina) support. Evidence in support is based on case series with only relatively short-term follow-up. A recent retrospective multicenter study of these devices (289 women) showed good short-term results in terms of prolapse resolution but with significant morbidity: Buttock pain (52%), vaginal erosion (10%), one case of bladder erosion, and two women with serious infection. Caution must be, therefore, employed before newer operations are introduced into clinical practice. Each new procedure should declare the properties of the grafts and should supply data on erosion and infection rates. Each operation should also supply data on bowel, bladder, and sexual function.

What are the possible complications of meshes?

The complications of meshes are:
- Infection
- Inflammation
- Adhesion formation
- Fistula formation
- Extrusion
- Erosion—is less with natural and Prolene and maximum with Gore–Tex
- Scarring
- Injury to nerves, vessels, bladder, and bowel may occur during placement of Prolift gynemesh.

Some of these consequences could be related also to the surgical procedure, such as the mesh preloading; in other cases, the intraoperative retraction of the mesh could be misinterpreted as shrinkage.

What are the indications of graft in prolapse surgery?

Grafts are indicated in the following situations:
- Recurrent prolapse
- Suboptimal autologous tissue
- To augment the weak or absent endopelvic fascia
- Connective tissue disorders
- Denervated pelvic floor
- Unavoidable stress that increases intra-abdominal pressure—chronic cough and constipation.

SUGGESTED READING

1. Amid PK. Classification of biomaterials and their related complications in abdominal wall hernia surgery. Hernia. 1997;1:15-21.
2. Carmelo DM, Vito S, Giovanni V. Biomechanical, topological and chemical features that influence the implant success of an urogynecological mesh: a review. Bio Med Res Int. 2016;2016:1-6.
3. Gomelsky A, Penson DF, Dmochowski RR. Pelvic organ prolapse (POP) surgery: the evidence for the repairs. BJU Int. 2011;107:1704-19.
4. National Institute of for Health and Clinical Excellence. Sacrocolpopexy using mesh for vaginal vault prolapsed repair. Interventional Procedure Guidance No. 283. London: National Institute for Health and Clinical Excellence; 2009.
5. Saberski ER, Orenstein SB, Novitsky YW. Anisotropic evaluation of synthetic surgical meshes. Hernia. 2011;15:47-52.
6. Slack M, Sandhu JS, Staskin DR, Grant RC. In vivo comparison of suburethral sling materials. Int Urogynecol J Pelvic Floor Dysfunct. 2006;17:106-10.

CHAPTER 18

Disease-specific Investigations in Obstetrics and Gynecology

Sumita Mehta, Rupali Bhatia

INVESTIGATIONS IN GYNECOLOGY

Primary Infertility

- Calculate body mass index (BMI) (normal 18.5–24.9 kg/m^2; both overweight and underweight can affect ovulation)
- *Husband's semen analysis:*
  - Instruct 2–3 days of abstinence before collection
  - The normal values recommended by the World Health Organization (WHO) of semen analysis have been updated in 2021 and are shown in **Table 1**.
- *Rule out tuberculosis (TB):*
  - Mantoux test
  - Hemogram with erythrocyte sedimentation rate (ESR)
  - Chest X-ray [posteroanterior (PA) view]
  - Premenstrual endometrial biopsy (EB)—histopathological examination (HPE) and acid-fast bacilli (AFB) staining/culture, polymerase chain reaction (PCR) for TB, and BACTEC
- *Confirm ovulation by:*
  - Spinnbarkeit test
  - Fern test
  - Mid-luteal phase progesterone. Serum progesterone ≥10 ng/mL on day 21 of menstrual cycle or average of serum progesterone on D-9, D-7, and D-5 > 15 ng/mL in a 28-day cycle confirms ovulation
  - Estimation of luteinizing hormone (LH) surge by LH kit for urine
  - Premenstrual EB—secretory endometrium indicates ovulation
  - Transvaginal ultrasonography for follicular monitoring and ovulation
- *Tubal patency tests done in early follicular phase:*
  - Hysterosalpingogram (HSG)
  - Transvaginal sonography (TVS) with saline sonosalpingography
  - Hysteroscopy with laparoscopy and chromotubation
- *Endocrinal screening test:*
  - Serum follicle-stimulating hormone (FSH), LH on day 2 of menstrual cycle
  - Serum thyroid-stimulating hormone (TSH)
  - Serum prolactin

TABLE 1: The World Health Organization (WHO) reference for semen analysis (2021).

Parameter	Value
Semen volume (mL)	≥1.4
Total sperm number (10^6 per ejaculate)	≥39
Total motility (%)	≥42
Progressive motility (%)	≥30
Nonprogressive motility (%)	≤1
Immotile sperm (%)	≤20
Vitality (%)	≥54
Normal forms (%)	≥4

Polycystic Ovarian Disease (Flowchart 1)

Biochemical Hyperandrogenism

- Total testosterone and free testosterone—if not elevated, then androstenedione (ANSD) and dehydroepiandrosterone sulfate (DHEAS) can be measured; however, they are less specific.

Flowchart 1: Screening and diagnostic assessment of polycystic ovary syndrome (PCOS) (International Evidence-based Guideline 2023).

```
Step 1: Irregular cycles + clinical hyperandrogenism
        Exclude other causes = Diagnosis
                    ↓
Step 2: If no clinical hyperandrogenism
        Test for biochemical hyperandrogenism
        (exclude other causes) = Diagnosis
                    ↓
Step 3: If ONLY irregular cycles OR
        hyperandrogenism
        Adults: Ultrasound for PCOM or AMH
        Adolescents: USG or AMH not required; leads
                     to overdiagnosis
```

(AMH: anti-Müllerian hormone; PCOM: polycystic ovarian morphology; USG: ultrasonography)

- Liquid chromatography with tandem mass spectrometry (LC-MS/MS) assays are very accurate and are recommended for measurement.
- Assessment of biochemical hyperandrogenism is not possible if a woman was on hormonal contraception and the levels should be measured 3 months after stoppage of OCPs.

To exclude other causes (such as congenital adrenal hyperplasia, Cushing syndrome, or androgen-secreting tumors), the following tests are recommended:
- Serum TSH
- Serum prolactin
- *17-OH progesterone:* 20–100 ng/dL prior to ovulation and 100–500 ng/dL during the luteal phase

The polycystic ovary syndrome (PCOS) diagnosis according to the modified Rotterdam is shown in **Table 2**.

- *Free androgen index (FAI) is calculated as:* Total testosterone value × 100 divided by the sex hormone-binding globulin level; values >5 are indicative for PCOS.

TABLE 2: Diagnosis of polycystic ovary syndrome based on the modified 2003 Rotterdam criteria.

Feature	Recommended diagnosis	Considerations
Biochemical hyperandrogenism	• Elevated total or free testosterone, or calculated indices of free testosterone (FAI, bioavailable testosterone; BioT) • DHEAS and ANSD can be considered	High-quality assays should be used for the evaluation
Clinical hyperandrogenism	A modified Ferriman–Gallwey score of ≥4 to ≥8	Threshold level should be considered in the context of patient ethnicity
Oligoanovulation	Oligomenorrhea (cycles >35 days apart or <8 menses a year)	If highly suspicious for PCOS, but does not have oligomenorrhea, consider serum progesterone or LH assessment
PCOM	≥20 follicles per ovary ≥10 cm³ ovarian volume	Based on transvaginal ultrasonography with a transducer frequency of 8 or more MHz

(ANSD: androstenedione; DHEAS: dehydroepiandrosterone sulfate; FAI: free androgen index; PCOS: polycystic ovary syndrome; PCOM: polycystic ovarian morphology)

- *Anti-Müllerian hormone (AMH):* Levels are increased 2–3 fold in women suffering from PCOS compared to normo-ovulatory women. There is still lack of standardization of AMH measurement and diagnostic thresholds and so most recent guidelines do not recommend its measurement as an alternative for detection of polycystic ovarian morphology (PCOM) or as a single test for diagnosis of PCOS.
- *Elevated LH:* FSH ratio is no longer considered to be a diagnostic criterion for PCOS as its value can be inconsistent.
- Insulin resistance is a pathophysiological factor in PCOS, but clinically available insulin assays are of limited value and are not recommended routinely.
- *Cardiovascular disease risk:* Women with PCOS have an increased risk of cardiovascular disease and should be assessed for the same. All women with PCOS regardless of age and BMI should have fasting lipid profile done which includes:
  - Total cholesterol (normal: <200 mg/dL)
  - Triglyceride level
  - Low-density lipoprotein (LDL) (normal: 60–130 mg/dL)
  - High-density lipoprotein (HDL) (normal: 30–70 mg/dL)
- Risk of impaired glucose tolerance and type 2 diabetes is increased in women with PCOS, and this risk is irrespective of their age or BMI. So, glycemic index needs to be measured in all women with PCOS and the 75 g oral glucose tolerance test (OGTT) is the most accurate test to do so.

Hirsutism

- *Serum testosterone—increased (total testosterone:* 20–80 ng/mL, free testosterone: 100–200 pg/mL)
  - Very high levels indicate underlying ovarian neoplasm or adrenal origin.
- *17-alpha-OH progesterone:* Early morning level in follicular phase is done to exclude congenital adrenal hyperplasia (CAH). If 17-alpha-OH progesterone level is >2 ng/mL, then adrenocorticotropic hormone (ACTH) stimulation test is done.
  Adrenocorticotropic hormone stimulation test: 17-alpha-OH levels are measured 60 minutes after intravenous (IV) or intramuscular (IM) administration of 250 µg of ACTH. If level is >10 ng/dL, diagnosis of late-onset adrenal hyperplasia is confirmed.
  Ultrasonography (USG): To rule out ovarian malignancy, polycystic ovarian syndrome (PCOS), and assess adrenal glands.
- *Serum TSH:* If hirsutism associated with irregular cycles
- *Serum prolactin:* If hirsutism associated with irregular cycles
- Investigations for PCOS (if testosterone levels normal or mildly raised)
- *Karyotyping:* It is required in partial androgen insensitivity syndrome.
- 24-hour urine cortisol (if hirsutism associated with symptoms of Cushing's syndrome)

Hyperprolactinemia

- *Serum prolactin levels:* Ideally, a fasting mid-morning sample is recommended (peak level of prolactin is usually between 4 AM and 7 AM).
- Serum thyroid function test
- *Renal function test:* Renal failure is one of the differential diagnoses.
- *Serum FSH and LH:* Women with macroadenoma should be evaluated for hypopituitarism.

- Many patients with acromegaly have prolactin co-secreted with growth hormone and insulin-like growth factor (IGF-1) levels should be measured in them.
- *X-ray skull:* Coned down view of sella turcica.
- Magnetic resonance imaging (MRI) is the imaging study of choice which can detect adenomas as small as 3–5 mm; computed tomography (CT) scan can also be done.
- *Visual field test:* It is usually done in cases of macroadenoma and a tumor that is adjacent to/or compressing optic chiasma.

Genital Tuberculosis

- Hemogram with ESR—lymphocytes increased and increased ESR
- X-ray chest (PA view)
- Mantoux test
- Premenstrual EB/menstrual blood (D1-D3):
  - Biopsy sent in normal saline—for Ziehl–Neelsen (ZN) staining for AFB; for bacilli to be demonstrated by ZN staining—10^5/mL bacilli are required.
  - Culture for AFB sent in formalin—culture is done in LJ medium (Löwenstein–Jensen medium) or agar-based medium. Culture requires as little as 100 organisms/mL to be positive
- *Hysterosalpingography:* It may show radiological features suggestive of genital TB like—
  - Beaded appearance of tubes
  - Stem pipe appearance of tubes
  - Calcification of tubes and ovaries
  - *Golf-club appearance*—only isthmus and proximal ampulla are visualized and the isthmic segment has a rigid, stove-pipe appearance
- Maltese-cross appearance, which shows completely filled tube with rigid and irregular outline
- *Rosette type:* The distal end of the tube is filled with dye giving a rosette-type image
- Leopard skin-like speckled appearance of the ampulla due to the tube being partially filled with dye
- Laparoscopy
- Ultrasonography of pelvic organs for tubo-ovarian masses
- *BACTEC:* This is a radiometric system, which uses fatty acid substrates such as palmitic acid or formic acid labeled with radioactive carbon. As the mycobacteria metabolize these fatty acids, radioactive CO_2 is released, which is measured as a marker of bacterial growth. It has a high sensitivity of 80–90% and shows quicker results (5–10 days).

MGIT (mycobacterial growth indicator tube) is another rapid method for detection of mycobacterial growth that is noninvasive and cheaper than BACTEC.
- *Biochemical markers:* Adenosine deaminase activity; gas chromatography of mycobacterial fatty acids has been utilized for rapid identification of mycobacterial TB
- Enzyme-linked immunosorbent assay (ELISA) for TB
- *PCR for TB:* PCR is a rapid, sensitive, and specific molecular biological method for detecting mycobacterial DNA in both pulmonary and extrapulmonary samples from suspected TB patients. It can detect <10 bacilli per mL of the specimen. Real-time PCR technique is preferred for detection of mycobacterial DNA. It offers added advantage of detecting resistance against various antitubercular drugs.

Ectopic Pregnancy

- Urine for pregnancy test
- Serum beta-human chorionic gonadotropin (hCG) levels for diagnosis, deciding mode of treatment and monitoring; rising or falling trend when the patient is put on conservative/medical management.
- *Ultrasonography:* It is the most important tool for diagnosis. Findings may include gestational sac outside uterus, adnexal mass, tubal ring (echogenic ring like structure outside uterus), free fluid in cul-de-sac or adnexal tenderness with probe palpation.
- *USG Doppler:* "Ring of fire sign" is seen on Doppler, which signifies a hypervascular lesion with peripheral vascularity; can be seen in tubal ectopic pregnancy but also in corpus luteum.
- *Culdocentesis:* Positive in ruptured ectopic pregnancy
- Serum progesterone levels of >25 ng/mL exclude ectopic pregnancy with 97% certainty and values <5 ng/mL indicate a nonviable pregnancy including ectopic or intrauterine.
- Complete hemogram
- Liver function test (LFT) and kidney function test (KFT) for monitoring methotrexate therapy

Müllerian Agenesis

Specific investigations:
- Karyotyping
- Serum FSH
- Serum testosterone
- *Ultrasonography:* Transabdominal/translabial/transrectal two-dimensional or three-dimensional
- *MRI:* Typically can be done without contrast; decision left on discretion of radiologist
- USG KUB (kidneys, ureters, and urinary bladder)
- Look for skeletal abnormalities (scoliosis, vertebral arch disturbances or hypoplasia of wrist); X-ray of concerned part, usually limbs
- Diagnostic laparoscopy

Hormone replacement therapy
- *History:* Personal, medical, gynecological, and family
- *Examination:* Height, weight, BMI, blood pressure (BP), breast, and vaginal examination
- Fasting blood sugar and postprandial blood sugar
- Lipid profile
- Pap smear
- Mammography
- *Transvaginal sonography (TVS):* For endometrial thickness and adnexa
- Workup of relevant symptoms:
  - Urinary incontinence
  - Carbohydrate intolerance
  - Psychoemotional states

Investigations not routinely needed before starting HT:
- *Endometrial sampling:* It is needed only if endometrial thickness is >5 mm.
- *Serum FSH:* It is only done, if diagnosis of menopause is not clear.
- *Bone densitometry:* It is done in women with risk of osteoporosis.

Abnormal Uterine Bleeding

- Urine for pregnancy test to rule out pregnancy
- Complete blood count
- Coagulation panel
- Hemophilia screen (if suggestive personal or family history)
- Thyroid function test

- *Serum prolactin:* To rule out pituitary adenoma
- Investigations to rule out PCOS
- Endometrial tissue sampling (hysteroscopy-guided, if needed); it is considered the first-line test in women >45 years of age. It should be performed in women <45 years and with history of exposure to unopposed estrogen, such as women with PCOS or obesity or women who fail to respond to treatment or continue to have persistent bleeding.
- *Imaging studies:* USG pelvic organs, MRI, and hysteroscopy
- *Saline infusion sonohysterography:* Especially useful in endometrial polyps, submucosal leiomyomas or when images from TVS are inconclusive
- Rule out genital TB (if suggestive personal or family history).

Vesicovaginal Fistula

- *Methylene blue or three-swab test:* Methylene blue solution is instilled in the bladder by Foley's catheter, after three gauze pieces, one above the other, are placed within the vagina. The patient is asked to walk around and void over a period of 20 minutes. The gauze pieces are then examined. The lower swab will be dye stained from voiding or loss of urine from the urethra. If the middle and upper ones are blue, it is vesicovaginal fistula (VVF). If the upper swab is wet but not stained, a ureterovaginal fistula should be suspected. Patients may be given pyridium to detect the presence of a ureterovaginal fistula.
- *Cystoscopy:* To identify VVF, to determine number and location of fistula and the proximity to ureteric orifices
- *Vaginoscopy:* It can be performed using cystoscope and may help in localizing the fistula opening on the vaginal side.
- *Urine:* Culture/sensitivity; a speculum or catheter sample should be sent for culture and sensitivity before surgery. At least three samples should be sterile before surgery.
- Kidney function tests (KFTs)
- Renal USG may show calyceal dilation and ureteric duplication.
- *Intravenous pyelography:* For diagnosis of ureteric fistula, ureteric stricture, and hydronephrotic changes
- Retrograde pyelography
- Examination under anesthesia

Ovarian Malignancy

Routine Investigations
- Hemogram and blood group
- LFT
- KFT
- Fasting and postprandial blood sugars
- *Urine:* Routine/microscopy
- ECG

Specific Investigations
- *Tumor markers:*
  - *Cancer antigen 125 (CA-125):* >35 IU/L in epithelial tumors
  - Carcinoembryonic antigen (CEA) (raised in some epithelial tumors) as well as in bowel primary malignancies. A ratio of >25:1 (CA-125 and CEA) favors an ovarian primary.
  - *Alpha-fetoprotein (AFP):* Increased in embryonal carcinoma and endodermal sinus tumor
  - *hCG:* Increased in choriocarcinoma
  - Placental alkaline phosphatase (PLAP) and lactate dehydrogenase (LDH); increased in dysgerminoma

- *Inhibin B:* Increased in granulosa cell tumor
- *Imaging studies:*
  - USG whole abdomen
  - *Contrast enhanced CT scan abdomen and pelvis:* Gastric or colonic primary with metastases to the ovaries may mimic ovarian cancer and increased CEA points toward GI primary.
  - *X-ray chest (PA view):* It is done to rule out pleural effusion and pelvis.
  - *Mammogram:* These women are usually in the age group in which breast cancer is prevalent.
- Colonoscopy, upper gastrointestinal (GI) endoscopy to rule out metastasis or suspected bowel cancer
- *Endometrial biopsy and endocervical curettage:* If history of postmenopausal bleeding or menstrual irregularities exists
- Ascitic fluid tap for biochemistry and cytology for confirmation of tissue diagnosis

Endometrial Carcinoma

Routine Investigations
As elaborated in ovarian malignancy.

Specific Investigations
- Pap smear
- *Endometrial tissue sampling:* Endometrial biopsy is the most commonly used test using Pipelle aspirate.
- *Dilation and curettage:* If the sample obtained by aspiration is not adequate for histopathological reporting, then D&C is advocated; this may be done under hysteroscopy guidance.

Imaging studies:
- USG whole-abdomen including pelvis
- Saline infusion sonography in some cases
- *Chest X-ray:* To rule out metastasis
- MRI abdomen

Cervical Carcinoma
- Complete clinical examination for staging including P/V/R examination
- Complete blood count
- KFT
- X-ray chest PA view
- *Urine:* Routine/microscopy

Specific Investigations
- Colposcopy; directed cervical biopsy. If the lesion is visible, a punch biopsy is adequate but if it is not satisfactory, then a small loop or cone biopsy may be required.
- *Imaging studies:* The International Federation of Gynecology and Obstetrics (FIGO) 2018 staging permits the use of any imaging modalities (USG, CT, MRI, or PET) to provide additional information on size of the tumor, nodal status, and metastasis.
  - *MRI:* It is the best method of radiologic assessment of primary tumors, which are >10 mm.
  - *USG abdomen:* The diagnostic accuracy of USG is also comparable in expert hands.
  - *Positron emission tomography (PET) scan:* Metastasis >10 mm in lymph nodes is better picked up on PET-CT than CT and MRI with a false-negative rate of 4–15%. It is especially useful in cases of recurrence.
  - *Proctoscopy/barium enema:* Done, if needed, for staging

Vulval Malignancy
- Vulval biopsy from an area where there is transition from normal to malignant

tissue. Poorly differentiated tumors lack laminin production while MIB-1 expression is uniform through the tumor cell population.
- Pap smear
- Colposcopy of cervix, vagina, and vulva
- Cystourethroscopy; if urethra and bladder seem involved
- IVP, if bladder is involved
- Proctosigmoidoscopy
- Barium enema
- Imaging (USG/MRI/CT) for concurrent pelvic pathology and retroperitoneal lymph nodes
- Fine-needle aspiration cytology (FNAC) from lymph nodes
- Routine preoperative investigations

INVESTIGATIONS IN OBSTETRICS

Recommended Routine Laboratory Tests in Antenatal Patients

- Blood group and Rh factor
- Hemoglobin (Hb) (11.0–16.0 g/dL)
- OGTT (75 g glucose load) at first contact and repeat at 24–28 weeks of gestation.
- *Syphilis test (VRDL):* If four-fold change in titer (equivalent change of two dilution, e.g., from 1:16 to 1:4 or from 1:8 to 1:32), it signifies infection
- Hepatitis B surface antigen
- HIV testing
- TSH
- *Urine:* Routine/microscopy.

Premature Rupture of Membranes

- Complete blood count—at least biweekly
  • Leukocytosis (14,000–16,000/µL); sensitivity (29–47%), false-positive rate (5–18%)
- C-reactive protein ≤1.5 mg/dL, slightly elevated in pregnancy; specificity 38–55%
- *Cervical and vaginal secretions:*
  • *Microscopic examination of amniotic fluid:* Ferning or arborization will be seen.
  • pH determination of vaginal fluids (pH of amniotic fluid 7.1–7.3 while pH of normal vaginal secretions is 4.5–6.0). False-positive pH test can be due to presence of semen or blood, alkaline antiseptics, or infections such as bacterial vaginosis.
  • Nitrazine—indicator paper (pH 4.5–7.5)
  • Yellow (4.5)—olive yellow (5.0) × deep olive green (5.5) × blue gray (7.0) × deep blue (7.5)
  • Litmus paper
  • Bromothymol blue
- *Amniotic fluid:*
  • Gram stain
  • Cytokines [interleukin (IL)-6, IL-8]
- *Fetal fibronectin (FFN):* It gets released due to breakdown of cervical extracellular matrix; ≥50 ng/mL is taken as the cut-off. The test has a high specificity but low sensitivity—sensitivity (94%) and specificity (97%). So, a negative test strongly indicates intact membranes but a positive test does not necessarily indicate premature rupture of membranes.
- Measurement of placental alpha-microglobulin-1 in cervicovaginal discharge using various commercially available tests (e.g., Amnisure test).
- *IGF-1 levels:* The sensitivity is 75% and specificity is 97%.
- *High-vaginal swab:* Culture/sensitivity is done weekly, if positive—amniotic fluid culture is positive in 53% cases.
- *Ultrasound:* For evaluation of amniotic fluid index (AFI). If after full evaluation also, the diagnosis is not clear, then indigo

carmine dye is instilled under ultrasound guidance while a tampon or pad is placed in the vagina. If the tampon/pad stains blue, then that is diagnostic of amniotic fluid.
- Biophysical score and S/D ratio—the sensitivity is 25-80% in prediction for clinical chorioamnionitis.

Preterm Labor

- Fetal fibronectin—for prediction and diagnosis. Value of >50 ng/mL is taken as positive. It is done by:
  - ELISA
    - Rapid FFN test:
      - The sensitivity is 94% and specificity is 97%

  Cervical length + FFN or absent fetal breathing movement + FFN—increases the sensitivity to >86% and specificity to >90%.
- USG imaging
  - *Cervical length and dilatation:* Normal cervical length is 35-48 mm. A short cervix is defined as a cervix which is <25 mm at 16-24 weeks POG. If >50% of cervical length replaced by funnel—79% (prediction). The ultrasound can be done vaginally (it is the most accurate), abdominally, or transperineal. *Trust Your Vaginal Ultrasound (TYVU).*
  - *Cervical consistency index (CCI):* Anteroposterior cervical diameter is measured before (AP) and after (AP') application of pressure on the cervix using transvaginal probe and the index is calculated using the formula (AP'/AP) × 100. It is inversely related to gestational age and is lower in pregnancies that deliver preterm.
- Biophysical scoring (BPS)—absence of fetal breathing movement.
- Salivary estriol—by ELISA ≥2.1 ng/mL. Sensitivity (30-40%), specificity (93-98%)
- Increased salivary estriol and progesterone ratio.
- Phosphorylated IGFBP-1 (insulin-like growth factor binding protein-1) is a protein made by the endometrial cells and when delivery is imminent, small amounts of it leak into the cervix. Point-of-care tests are available to measure it.
- Increase corticotropin-releasing hormone (CRH) levels, serum collagenase levels, serum relaxin, and neutrophil collagenase
- *Urine:* Routine/microscopy and culture/sensitivity to rule out asymptomatic bacteriuria
- Vaginal smear for trichomoniasis and bacterial vaginosis
- Tests for sexually transmitted diseases as they can also lead to preterm labor

Pregnancy with Heart Disease

To rule out anemia and thrombocytopenia:
- *Complete hemogram:*
  - Hb (12-16 g/dL)
  - Total leukocyte count (14,000-16,000/µL)
  - Differential leukocyte count
  - Platelet count (150-350 × 10^3/mm^3)
- *Coagulogram:*
  - *Prothrombin time (PT):* 11-16 seconds
  - *Activated partial thromboplastin time (aPTT):* 22-37 seconds
  - *International normalized ratio (INR)—to be maintained:* 2.0-3.0
- Blood urea (10-20 mg/dL)
- *Serum electrolytes:*
  - Serum sodium (136-145 mEq/L)
  - Serum potassium (3.5-5.0 mEq/L)
- *Urine:* Routine/microscopy and culture/sensitivity
- *ECG:* Baseline and to ensure whether cardiac rhythm is normal

- *2-D ECHO:* To rule out valvular thrombus and assess cardiac function
- *Fetal surveillance:*
  - Targeted scan (in patients on anticoagulation therapy)
  - Fetal ECHO, especially in congenital heart disease
- *USG:* For growth monitoring (32 weeks onward)

Cervical Incompetence

Nonpregnant Patients

- Passage of no. 8 Hegar's dilator without resistance
- Passage of no. 16 Foley's catheter without resistance
- Wide or funnel-shaped internal os on HSG

Pregnant Patients

Endovaginal USG: Proposed sonographic indicators of cervical incompetence include:
- Endocervical length <25 mm at <24 weeks
- Cervical canal width >7 mm
- *Internal os dilatation:* First trimester (>15 mm), second trimester (>20 mm)
- Funnel length (>25% of endocervical length)
- Bulging of membranes into cervical canal

Pregnancy with Previous History of Neural Tube Defect

- Ultrasound is the investigation of choice and helps to localize the exact size and site of neural tube defects (NTDs) and vertebrae. Nearly 100% of NTDs are detected by USG. It also helps to identify associated anomalies like cleft palate or cardiovascular abnormalities.
  Early targeted scan is done at 12–13 weeks to look for:
  - *Anencephaly:* Inability to obtain a view of BPD
  - Cephalocele
  - Spina bifida with/without one or more of the following five cranial signs:
    1. Frontal notching (lemon sign)
    2. Small BPD
    3. Ventriculomegaly:
       - Atrial width 7 ± 1 mm constant from 15 weeks onward
       - Atrial width 10–15 mm—mild ventriculomegaly
       - Atrial width more than 15 mm—overt ventriculomegaly
    4. Obliteration of cisterna magna
    5. Elongated cerebellum (banana sign).
- *Maternal serum alpha fetoprotein (AFP):* AFP is formed by the fetal yolk sac, liver, and gastrointestinal tract. Early in gestation, its concentration is higher in amniotic fluid but with increasing gestation, it crosses the placenta and maternal serum AFP levels rise; high level of maternal AFP indicates NTD.
  - *2.0–2.5 MOM:* Upper limit of normal
  - If 2.5–3.5 MOM (indiscriminate zone)—repeat the test
  - More than 3.5 MOM—clearly indicates fetus at risk.
- Amniocentesis—fetal AFP, acetylcholinesterase are measured.
- *Indications:*
  - Maternal serum AFP elevated and USG examination is nondiagnostic
  - Maternal serum AFP elevated
- Fetal karyotyping is indicated, if increased AFP (maternal or amniotic fluid) ± acetylcholinesterase.

Intrauterine Death

- *Blood group:* ABO and Rh factor
- Hemogram with platelet count
- LFT, KFT
- Coagulogram comprising fibrinogen (150–600 mg/dL), PT, and aPTT

- Blood sugar—fasting (<110 mg/dL) and PP (1 hour <140 mg/dL; 2 hours <120 mg/dL)
- Anticardiolipin antibodies [immunoglobulin (IgG) 0-15 GPL; IgM 0-15 MPL], antinuclear antibodies
- Thrombophilia testing
- Serum TSH
- Serology for TORCH [toxoplasmosis, others (syphilis, hepatitis B), rubella, cytomegalovirus, herpes simplex], VDRL (venereal disease research laboratory test)
- Kleihauer-Betke test for quantifying fetomaternal hemorrhage in all patients, irrespective of Rh status.
- *Ultrasound:* Targeted scan for placental malformation, fetal malformation, and growth restriction
- *Amniocentesis:*
  - Fetal infection—cytomegalovirus (CMV), anaerobic, and aerobic infections
  - Karyotype

At delivery:
- Photograph of the child
- Postmortem examination including fetal tissue for karyotyping; sites used for fetal biopsy include skin and fetal cartilage (patella)
- Fetogram (total body radiography)—if dysmorphic stigmata at postmortem examination present
- *Placenta and cord:* For histopathology and culture

Antepartum Hemorrhage

Placenta Previa

- *Blood group:* ABO and Rh factor
- Hemogram with platelet count
- Coagulogram comprising fibrinogen (150-600 mg/dL), PT, and aPTT
- KFT
- *USG:* For placental localization, fetal presentation, and to rule out uterine and fetal malformations:
  - Transabdominal sonography
  - *Transvaginal sonography:* It is especially beneficial for posteriorly situated placenta and decreases scanning time. Sensitivity (87.5%), specificity (98.8%), positive predictive value (PPV) (93.3%), negative predictive value (NPV) (97.6%)

Abruptio Placentae

In addition to above investigations:
- Ultrasound—for confirmation and size of hematoma—sensitivity (24-25%), negative findings in abruption does not rule out the condition.
- Disseminated intravascular coagulation (DIC) profile:
  - *Fibrinogen:* 150-600 mg/dL
  - *PT:* 11-16 seconds
  - *aPTT:* 22-37 seconds
  - *Platelet count:* 150,000-400,000/L
  - *D-dimers:* <0.5 mg/L
  - *Fibrinogen degradation products:* <10 µg/dL
  - Urinary albumin
- Women whose pregnancy is complicated by abruption for which no other clear explanation is evident should be screened for thrombophilias.
  - Factor-V Leiden mutations
  - *Prothrombin* gene mutation
  - Antiphospholipid syndrome
  - Antithrombin-III
  - Hyperhomocysteinemia
  - Protein C and S deficiency

Intrauterine Growth Restriction

To confirm the diagnosis:
- Clinical examination
- *Symphysis:* Fundal height—sensitivity (56-86%), specificity (80-90%)

- *Ultrasound:* Biometry
  - Abdominal circumference (AC) < 10th centile
    - Sensitivity (72.9–94.5%), specificity (50.6–83.8%).
  - *Estimated fetal weight (EFW):* Less than 10th centile
    - Sensitivity (33–89%), specificity (53–90%)
    - Shepard and Aoki formulas are recommended for fetal weight. Hadlock formula may be more appropriate when the fetus is expected to be very small.
  - Head circumference (HC)/AC
  - *Femur length/AC:* Constant after 20 weeks (22 ± 2 weeks); sensitivity (63%), specificity (90%)
  - *Fetal ponderal index:* Gestational age independent 8.325 ± 2.5
    - If <7—significant; NPV (96.4%).
- *AC:* It is the single best measurement, which has the best correlation with fetal weight.

Other parameters:
- *Cerebellar diameter (mm):* 14–24 weeks
- Subcutaneous tissue thickness at the level of fetal mid-calf, mid-thigh, abdominal wall, skinfold thickness, and cheek-to-cheek diameter
- *Placenta:* Volume, weight, and maturity.

To find the cause:
- Complete blood count
- Peripheral smear for malarial parasites
- HPLC
- KFT
- LFT
- *Blood sugar:* Fasting and postprandial
- Antiphospholipid antibody screening, antinuclear antibody, and factor-V Leiden mutation
- TORCH
- HIV testing
- *Urine:* Protein microscopy and culture/sensitivity
- *Ultrasound:* Maternal kidney, ureter, bladder (KUB)
- *Fetal karyotype:* 7% are attributed to aneuploidy

To monitor the growth and further management:
- *Growth monitoring scans:* Fortnightly or more frequent depending upon severity.
- *Doppler:*
  - *Umbilical artery:*
    - Reduced end-diastolic flow
    - Absence of end-diastolic flow
    - Reversal of end-diastolic flow
  - *Middle cerebral artery:* Pulsatility index and peak velocity flow
  - *Inferior vena cava:* Abnormal pulsation/reversal of flow
  - Pulsations in umbilical vein.
- Biophysical profile (NST, liquor, fetal body movements, respiratory movements, and tone).

Gestational Diabetes Mellitus

For screening and diagnosis, the Ministry of Health and Family Welfare, Government of India, recommends (2018):

Universal screening of all pregnant women at first antenatal contact (as early as possible) with 75 g oral glucose tolerance test (OGTT); if negative, repeat OGTT at 24–28 weeks of gestation.

There should be at least 4 weeks' gap between the two tests.

If the pregnant woman presents first time beyond 28 weeks of pregnancy, only one test is to be done at the first point of contact.

OGTT (Methodology):
- Single step test using 75 g glucose ingestion and measuring blood sugar after 2 hours

- The test is done, irrespective of last mealtime.
- 75 g glucose is dissolved in 300 mL of water and the pregnant woman takes it orally. If she vomits within 30 minutes of ingestion, the test is to be repeated the next day. If she vomits after 30 minutes of drinking the glucose load, then the test continues and does not need to be repeated.
- Blood sugar value of ≥140 mg/dL is taken as a cutoff for diagnosis of GDM.

For monitoring:
- Blood sugar fasting and 2 hours postprandial (<120 mg/dL)
- Gain in weight
- Blood pressure levels
- *Glycosylated hemoglobin:* Normal 5–6%; 1% rise—30 mg rise in blood sugar
- KFT
- Lipid profile
- Fundoscopy
- *Urine examination includes:*
  - Routine/microscopy and culture/sensitivity
  - *Urinary ketones:* For caloric deficiency, ketosis in type 1 diabetes mellitus; normal is <20 mg/dL
  - Urinary glucose
  - 24-hour urinary proteins

Fetal surveillance:
- NT/NB scan with dual marker at 11–13^{+6} weeks (CRL between 45 and 84 mm)
- Triple marker at 16–18 weeks
- Level 2 anomaly scan between 18 and 20 weeks period of gestation
- Fetal echocardiogram at 20–24 weeks

Anemia

Diagnosis

- Hemoglobin <11 g% (WHO). It is further classified as:
  - *Mild anemia:* 10.0–10.9 g%
  - *Moderate anemia:* 7–9.9 g%
  - *Severe anemia:* <7 g%

Minimum four Hb estimation tests are required during pregnancy; at 14–16 weeks, 20–24 weeks, 26–30 weeks, and 30–34 weeks of pregnancy.

Types of Anemia

- Complete blood count
- *Peripheral smear:* To look for morphology of RBCs, any abnormal cells or hemoparasites
- *Red blood cell (RBC) indices:*
  - *Mean corpuscular volume (MCV):* 90 ± 8 fL
  - *Mean corpuscular hemoglobin (MCH):* 30 ± 3 pg
  - *Mean corpuscular hemoglobin concentration (MCHC):* 33 ± 2%
- *Serum iron studies:* At least 12-hour fasting; recent blood transfusion gives false elevated readings:
  - *Serum ferritin:* 50–200 µg/L
  - *Total iron binding capacity (TIBC):* 300–360 µg/dL
  - *Serum iron:* 50–150 µg/dL
  - *Saturation:* 30–50%
  - *Protoporphyrin:* 30–50 µg/dL
  - *Transferrin receptors:* Earliest marker to rise and to show the response
- Red cell distribution width
- Reticulocyte count (0.5–2.5%)

To find the cause:
- *Liver function tests:*
  - Total bilirubin (0.3–1.0 mg/dL), direct bilirubin (0.1–0.3 mg/dL)
  - Indirect bilirubin (0.2–0.7 mg/dL)
  - Serum glutamate pyruvate transaminase (SGPT)/ALT (0–35 U/L), serum glutamic oxaloacetic transaminase (SGOT)/AST (0–35 U/L), serum ALP (0–350 U/L)

- Total serum proteins (5.5–8.0 g/dL), serum globulin (2.0–3.5 g/dL)
- Serum albumin (3.5–5.5 mg/dL), albumin:globulin ratio (1.7:1)
- *Coombs test and serum bilirubin:* To diagnose autoimmune hemolytic anemia
- *KFT*
- *HPLC (High-performance liquid chromatography):* To rule out hemoglobinopathies
- *Sickle cell test:* If sickle cell disease is suspected
- *Urine:* Routine/microscopy and culture/sensitivity
- *Stool:* Ova, cyst, and occult blood for 3 consecutive days
- *ECG and ECHO:* Especially if the pregnant woman is breathless and has a cardiac murmur, then cardiac disease needs to be ruled out

In case of refractory anemia:
- Serum folate and red cell folate
- Serum LDH—to rule out hemolysis
- Serum homocysteine
- Blood vitamin B_{12} levels (>90 μg/dL)
- Serum methylmalonic acid
- *Bone marrow aspiration:* This is done in patients of aplastic anemia, refractory anemia and if kala-azar is suspected.

Pregnancy with Hypertension
- Complete blood count
- Platelet count (150–350 × 10^3/mm^3); if platelet count is low, then PT and PTTK are also done.
- KFTs including blood urea, serum creatinine, and serum uric acid
- Liver function test
- Urinary routine and microscopy
- 24-hour urinary proteins (>300 mg/24 hours is significant)
- Fundus examination
- To rule out HELLP (hemolysis, elevated liver enzymes, low platelet count) syndrome:
  - Peripheral smear for hemolysis—burr cell or schistocytes
  - Serum LDH (normal is <600 mg/dL)
  - Platelet count (150–300 × 10^3/mm^3)
  - Liver enzymes.
- Coagulation profile (if deranged platelet count).

Chronic Hypertension
In addition to the above investigations:
- Blood sugar—fasting (<110 mg/dL) and PP (1 hour <140 mg/dL; 2 hours <120 mg/dL)
- Anticardiolipin antibodies (IgG 0–15 GPL; IgM 0–15 MPL)
- Antinuclear antibodies
- ECG
- *Urine:*
  - Culture/sensitivity (to rule out asymptomatic bacteriuria)
  - Routine/microscopy (cast and RBCs)
  - 24-hour urinary protein
  - Analysis of urinary sediments
- Serum creatinine clearance
- Renal sonography/arteriogram

Recurrent Pregnancy Loss

According to the Royal College of Obstetricians and Gynaecologists (RCOG) guidelines, the following investigations should be done:
- *Karyotype of abortus/parental karyotype:* Genetic testing of products of conception is important and can be done by various methods including karyotyping, FISH (fluorescence in situ hybridization), and microarray (most recommended test).
- Antiphospholipid antibodies
- Pelvic ultrasound

Thrombophilia Screening

Inherited thrombophilia:
- Factor V Leiden
- Antithrombin-III

- Protein C and S deficiency
- Activated protein C resistance

However, it is not recommended to undertake routine screening for inherited thrombophilia in cases of RPL.

Acquired thrombophilia (antiphospholipid syndrome)
- *Anticardiolipin antibodies:*
  - *IgG (0–15 GPL):* Better predictor of fetal outcome
  - *IgM (0–15 MPL)*
  - Anti-β_2 glycoprotein I
  - Positive in medium or high titer at more than or equal to two occasions 6 weeks apart
- *Lupus anticoagulant:* Sample must be taken uncuffed and to be centrifuged within 1 hour.
  - dRVVT (dilute Russell Viper venom test)
  - aPTT
  - Kaolin coagulation time
  - A panel of assays should be done; if a single test is to be done, it should be dRVVT.
  - Thrombotic complications are more with lupus anticoagulant positive than patients with positive anticardiolipin antibodies.

Endocrinology:
- Serum TSH and TPO antibodies
- Glycated hemoglobin (HbA1c)
- Serum prolactin

BOX 1: Investigations for luteal phase defect (LPD).

• Serum progesterone level (<10 nmol/L)	Done 3 days before expected period in two consecutive cycles
• Endometrial biopsy	
• Basal body temperature—luteal phase lasting <10 days	

- *Polycystic ovarian disease:* Tests are mentioned earlier in the chapter
- *Luteal phase defect (LPD):* The investigations are shown in **Box 1**.

To rule out uterine malformations (second-trimester losses):

Though uterine malformations do not play an important role in first-trimester pregnancy losses, but still uterine cavity assessment is recommended in them. Imaging studies used to determine anatomical abnormalities include:
- TVS and sonohysterography
- Hysterosalpingography
- Hysteroscopy/laparoscopy
- MRI

To rule out cervical incompetence (second trimester losses):
- Passage of no. 8 Hegar's dilator without resistance
- Passage of no. 16 Foley's catheter without resistance
- Wide or funnel-shaped internal os on HSG

CHAPTER 19

Obstetric Specimens

Pikee Saxena, Archana Mishra, Saloni Chadha

■ HYDATIDIFORM MOLE

Describe the gross specimen shown in Figure 1.
It is a formalin-fixed hysterectomy specimen, which shows tissue resembling grape-like vesicles, which might occur as a result of hydropic degeneration of chorionic villi as seen in case of hydatidiform mole (HM).

What do you understand by gestational trophoblastic disease?
Gestational trophoblastic disease (GTD) comprises benign conditions including complete and partial molar pregnancies, malignant conditions including invasive mole, choriocarcinoma, and placental site trophoblastic tumor (PSTT). If beta-human chorionic gonadotropin (β-hCG) levels continue to be elevated, then the condition is referred to as gestational trophoblastic neoplasia (GTN).

- Pathologic classification of GTD
  - *Benign*
    - Hydatidiform moles
      - Complete
      - Partial
    - Placental site nodule
    - Exaggerated placental site lesion
  - *Malignant*
    - Invasive mole
    - Choriocarcinoma
    - Placental site trophoblastic tumor
    - Epithelioid trophoblastic

What is hydatidiform mole?
Hydatidiform mole is an abnormal conceptus, characterized by trophoblastic proliferation, hydropic degeneration of chorionic villi, and absence of vasculature. It is of two types—(1) complete hydatidiform mole (CHM) and (2) partial mole (PM).

How is hydatidiform mole different from hydropic degeneration of abortus?
Excessive fluid accumulation or liquefaction of placental villous stroma is present in hydropic degeneration of an abortus, but without undue trophoblastic hyperplasia.

What are the distinguishing features of complete mole and partial mole? (Table 1)
- CHM is formed with duplication of a single sperm after fertilization of an empty

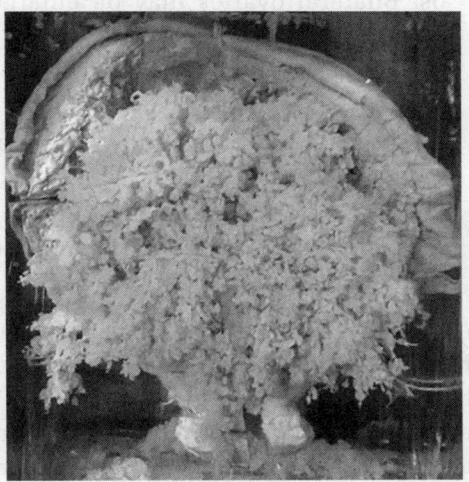

Fig. 1: Hydatidiform mole.
(For color version, see Plate 10)

TABLE 1: Distinguishing features of complete mole and partial mole.

	Complete mole	Partial mole
Fetal or embryonic tissue	Absent	Present
Hydatidiform swelling of chorionic villi	Diffuse	Focal
Trophoblastic hyperplasia	Diffuse	Focal
Scalloping of chorionic villi	Absent	Present
Trophoblastic stromal inclusions	Absent	Present
Karyotype	46XX; 46XY	69XXY; 69XYY

Source: Republished with permission of McGraw Hill LLC, from Berkowitz RS, Goldstein DP. The management of molar pregnancy and gestational trophoblastic tumors. In: Knapp RC, Berkowitz RS, (Eds.). Gynecologic Oncology. New York: Macmillan; 1993. p. 425; permission conveyed through Copyright Clearance Center, Inc.

ovum while PM is formed after dispermic fertilization of an ovum.
- In patients with CHM, the uterus is usually large compared to the gestational age while this is unusual in PM.
- The β-hCG titers are usually higher in patients with CHM and they tend to return to normal slowly as compared to PM.
- Risk of persistent trophoblastic disease (PTD) is 20% after CHM (15% invasive mole and 5% choriocarcinoma). This risk is very low after PM.
- Ploidy status and immunohistochemistry staining for p57 may help in distinguishing PM from complete mole (CM), with former being positive for p57.

What are the symptoms of patients with molar pregnancy?
- Patients present with amenorrhea of varying duration followed by vaginal bleeding "prune juice"–like fluid may leak into the vagina, mostly during the first trimester. Because vaginal bleeding may be considerable and prolonged, half of these patients present with anemia (hemoglobin <10 g/100 mL).
- Persistent positive urine pregnancy test/serum pregnancy test after a pregnancy event.
- Nausea and vomiting are present in one third of patients. They can also have hyperemesis.
- There maybe history of passage of grape-like vesicles per vaginam.

What are the clinical signs in such patients?
- The uterus is large for dates in 50% of cases. It is doughy, external ballottement is absent and fetal parts are not palpable. Fetal heart sound is not heard in cases of CM.
- Molar tissue may be seen coming through os. Bilateral ovaries may be enlarged suggestive of theca lutein cysts.
- Preeclampsia in the first trimester is seen in about 12% patients.
- Clinical features of hyperthyroidism are seen in 5–7% cases.
- Rarely, patients may present with respiratory distress due to trophoblastic pulmonary embolization.

Why are theca lutein cysts formed in molar pregnancy and what is their treatment?
Theca lutein cysts are seen in 20–40% of patients with hydatidiform mole. They form due to the overstimulation of lutein elements by large amounts of β-hCG secreted by proliferating trophoblasts. They are managed

conservatively and majority regress in 2–4 months after molar evacuation.

How do you diagnose molar pregnancy?
Diagnosis involves a good clinical acumen and is by clinical symptomatology and examination. It can be complemented by a quantitative analysis of β-hCG, if it is greater than two multiples of the median (MoM), and ultrasonography (USG), which shows multiple echoes (snow storm pattern) without the normal gestational sac or fetus in cases of complete HM.

In PM, a fetus may coexist with the molar tissue. The ultrasound diagnosis of a partial molar pregnancy includes presence of a live or dead fetus along with soft markers such as cystic spaces in the placenta and a ratio of transverse to anteroposterior (AP) dimension of the gestation sac >1.5. However, final diagnosis can only be made after histopathological diagnosis of the products of conception.

How do you manage a case of molar pregnancy?
All cases of molar pregnancy require suction curettage. Before evacuation, investigations including blood group and Rh typing, complete blood count, baseline serum β-hCG, X-ray chest, abdominal, and pelvic ultrasound are done. Special test such as thyroid function test is done, if there is evidence of hyperthyroidism and blood gas determination, if patient has respiratory distress.

What is the management of a twin pregnancy with a viable fetus and a molar pregnancy?
Twin pregnancy with a viable fetus and a molar pregnancy may be allowed to continue, if the mother desires. But with appropriate counseling that the probability of achieving a live birth is 25% and couple should be informed about increased chances of abortion, hemorrhage, preterm delivery, intrauterine death, fetal growth restriction, pulmonary embolization, preeclampsia, and thyroid storm. She requires monitoring in a multidisciplinary clinic experienced in the management of patients with malignant tumors during pregnancy.

Prenatal invasive testing for fetal karyotype may be done when there is confusion whether the pregnancy is a CHM with a coexisting normal twin or a PM.

What is the role of medical termination in molar pregnancy?
Medical removal of a complete molar pregnancy should be avoided, if possible, irrespective of the agents used. Role of mifepristone for molar pregnancy is not clear.

What is the preferred method of termination in a case of molar pregnancy?
Suction curettage is the method of choice, and it is always better to do under ultrasound guidance if diagnostic facility is there, as this minimizes the chances of perforation and confirms completeness of procedure.

Suction curettage is preferred, except when fetal parts presence and its size affect the process and then medical removal is suggested.

Is it safe to prepare the cervix prior to surgical evacuation?
Preparation of the cervix immediately prior to uterine removal is considered safe as per the recent guidelines. Ripening of the cervix with either physical dilators or prostaglandins can be done if needed.

Can oxytocic infusions be used during surgical evacuation?
Heavy vaginal bleeding may occur during evacuation of a molar pregnancy; therefore,

surgical curettage should be supervised by a senior gynecologist. The use of oxytocic infusion prior to completion of the evacuation is generally not recommended. However, if the woman is experiencing significant hemorrhage before evacuation, surgical evacuation may be done promptly and the need for oxytocin infusion considered against the risk of tumor embolization.

Should anti-D prophylaxis be given for complete mole and partial mole?

In cases of CM, there is no fetal part present, and therefore anti-D prophylaxis is not required. It is, however, required for PMs.

Should products of conception be sent for examination after surgical termination of pregnancy?

If a fetal cardiac activity has been documented on USG, there is no need to routinely send products of conception for histological examination after suction evacuation. However, the histological assessment of material obtained from the medical or surgical management of all miscarriages is recommended to exclude trophoblastic neoplasia if no fetal parts are identified at any stage of the pregnancy.

If after evacuation, patient is symptomatic or ultrasonography shows persistent mass in the uterus, should evacuation be repeated?

Although there is no role of routine second curettage after molar pregnancy, studies have shown that it may be useful in selected patients where β-hCG <5,000 U/L.

What is the follow-up after suction evacuation of molar pregnancy?

- Follow-up after GTD should be tailored as per the patient's condition.
- If β-hCG has reverted to normal within 56 days of the pregnancy, then follow-up will be for 6 months from the date of uterine evacuation. If β-hCG has not reverted to normal within 56 days of the pregnancy event, then follow-up recommended for 6 months after normalization of the β-hCG level.
- All women should get serum β-hCG levels measured 6–8 weeks after the end of any future pregnancy to exclude disease recurrence, whatever the outcome of the pregnancy.

What is the risk of recurrence of hydatidiform mole?

The risk of molar pregnancy after one previous mole is low (1–2%). It increases to 15–25% after two molar pregnancies.

What is the risk of persistent trophoblastic disease after molar pregnancy?

16% after CM and < 0.5% of PM develop PTD.

What is the role of prophylactic chemotherapy in hydatidiform mole?

- Evidence of metastasis to brain, liver, or gastrointestinal (GI) tract or chest X-ray showing more than 2-cm opacities
- Heavy vaginal or intraperitoneal bleeding or evidence of intraperitoneal hemorrhage
- Increasing titer of serum β-hCG after evacuation
- If 4 weeks after evacuation serum β-hCG >20,000 IU/L because of risk of uterine perforation
- High β-hCG 6 months after evacuation, even if still falling

What is high-risk molar pregnancy?

High-risk molar pregnancy is one with any of the following features:
- High β-hCG levels >100,000 IU/L
- Uterus large for dates
- Bilateral theca lutein cysts >6 cm
- Maternal age >40 years

- Associated preeclampsia, coagulopathy, trophoblastic embolization and/or hyperthyroidism

What is safe contraception following a diagnosis of gestational trophoblastic disease?

Barrier methods of contraception till β-hCG levels become normal. Combined oral contraceptives may be initiated once β-hCG levels become normal.

ANENCEPHALY

Describe the specimen shown in **Figure 2**.

This is a formalin-fixed specimen of the fetus showing anencephaly, i.e., absence of cranial vault and cerebral hemispheres.

How does anencephaly develop?

Anencephaly is a part of the neural tube defect (NTD) spectrum. This defect results when the neural tube fails to close during the 3rd–4th week of development. It has a multifactorial cause with interaction of several genes and environment.

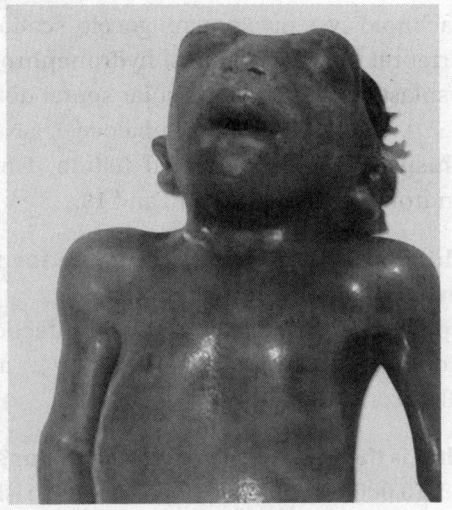

Fig. 2: Anencephaly. *(For color version, see Plate 10)*

How can you make diagnoses of anencephaly?

Screening for NTDs is done during second trimester (16–18 weeks) by estimation of maternal serum alpha fetoprotein (AFP). An elevated AFP is followed by USG in which absence of bony skull vault and of the brain cephalad to the orbits is demonstrated. The diagnosis can be made as early as 11 weeks by transvaginal sonography (TVS) and at ≥14 weeks by transabdominal ultrasound.

What are the associated anomalies in anencephaly?

The incidence of associated anomalies is about 30%. The most frequent is spina bifida (27%), hydronephrosis (16%), cleft lip in 10%, omphalocele in 6%, and cardiac anomalies in 4% of the cases.

Is there any sex predilection in anencephaly?

It has been seen that females are usually affected.

What are the differential diagnoses on ultrasonography?

Severe forms of microcephaly, encephalocele, and exencephaly.

What are the causes of polyhydramnios in these patients?

Hydramnios is present in 35% of anencephaly cases. It is due to diminished fetal swallowing, secretion of cerebrospinal fluid (CSF) directly into amniotic cavity, and excessive fetal micturition.

What is the prognosis of such fetuses?

Anencephaly is uniformly fatal. Most fetuses deliver prematurely. About 30% of them are born live and die within few hours.

What is the management of such patients?

As anencephaly is lethal and its sonographic diagnosis is highly reliable, termination of pregnancy on diagnosis is indicated.

What are the maternal complications?
These are polyhydramnios, preterm labor, abruption, malpresentation (face and brow), postdated pregnancy, and postpartum hemorrhage (PPH).

Why do such patients go postdated?
Uterus-containing anencephaly fetus may be refractory to oxytocin because of low levels of estriol as a result of insufficient production of its precursor cortisol from fetal adrenal.

What is the risk of recurrence in such patients?
Risk of recurrence is 5% after one affected child and 13% after two affected children.

How do you prevent anencephaly?
Preconceptionally folic acid supplementation may decrease recurrence of NTDs. In women with a prior affected pregnancy, supplementation is currently recommended with folic acid 4 mg daily. Women without a history of NTDs should receive 400 μg of folic acid prior to attempting pregnancy and during the first trimester (ACOG 1995).

■ HYDROCEPHALUS

Identify the specimen shown in Figure 3.
This is a specimen of a neonate showing hydrocephalus.

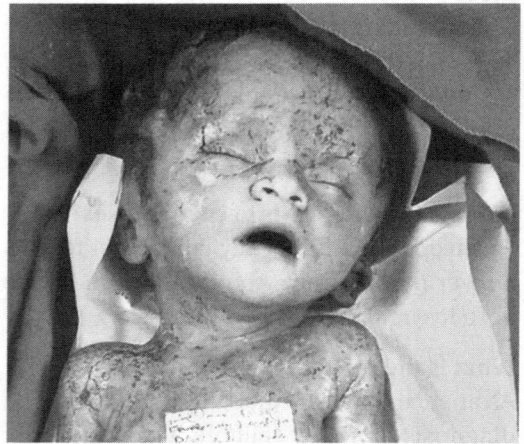

Fig. 3: Hydrocephalus. *(For color version, see Plate 11)*

What is the incidence of hydrocephalus?
The overall incidence varies from 2 to 6 per 1,000 live births.

Is there any sex variation?
There is a greater predilection for males.

Describe ultrasonic features of hydrocephalus antenatally.
- Demonstration of a dilated ventricular system, and ultrasonologically by measuring lateral ventricular to hemisphere width (LVH/HW) ratio in the biparietal and coronal plane. This ratio >0.5 at 24 weeks or more is diagnostic.
- During the second and third trimesters, the transverse atrial diameter is the most accurate measurement, as it remains constant (7.6 mm) at 15–35 weeks and should not be >10 mm.
- Between 10 and 15 mm, it is mild ventriculomegaly and if >15 mm, it is severe.

What are the other associated malformations?
Spina bifida (30%) most commonly occurs in the lumbar area. Others are cephalocele, arachnoid cyst, myelomeningocele, scoliosis, vertebral body anomalies, hydronephrosis, dysplastic kidneys, ventricular septal defect (VSD), Fallot tetralogy, omphalocele, gastroschisis, tracheoesophageal fistula, Down syndrome, and trisomies 13 and 18.

Which infections are attributable for the development of hydrocephalus?
Syphilis, toxoplasmosis, and viral infections such as cytomegalovirus (CMV), and influenza virus.

What is the incidence of hydrocephalus?
3–8/10,000 live births and aneuploidy risk is 3–8%.

What is the risk of recurrence with one affected child?
Risk is 2% but is 25% in X-linked aqueductal stenosis.

What is the usual fetal presentation in hydrocephalus?
It can be cephalic or breech (at least one-third of cases) but cephalopelvic disproportion (CPD) and dystocia may occur.

How do you manage hydrocephalus in labor?
Hydrocephalus fetus with severe associated anomalies should be delivered vaginally by cephalocentesis. With cephalic presentation, transvaginal ventricular tapping should be done at 3–4 cm dilatation. With breech presentation, labor is allowed to progress till delivery of breech and fetal trunk, and then aftercoming head of breech is decompressed by cephalocentesis, transabdominally or transvaginally through a widened suture line. If breech is associated with spina bifida, CSF can be drained by inserting a needle in the spinal canal.

What are the clinical features in hydrocephalus?
Antenatally:
- Head may be felt larger, globular, and softer
- Head may be high-up and nonengaged.

During labor: Pelvic examination may reveal gaping sutures and fontanelle and a crackling sensation felt on pressing the head.

RUPTURE UTERUS

Describe the specimen shown in Figure 4.
It is a specimen of postpartum rupture uterus removed during cesarean hysterectomy. There is a rent in the posterior wall with ragged margins extending from the lower uterine segment on the left side up to the fundus.

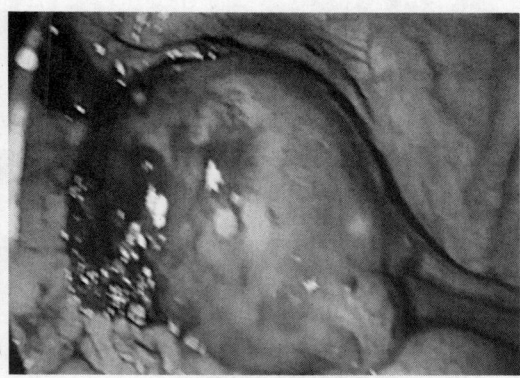

Fig. 4: Rupture uterus.

How is uterine rupture different from dehiscence?
Rupture of the uterus is defined as a rent in the uterine wall, which may be complete or incomplete. Dehiscence is partial separation of the scar with the intact peritoneum and fetal membranes.

What are the causes of rupture uterus during pregnancy?
- *Prior surgical procedures or manipulations:*
  - Almost, all cases occur in previously scarred uterus; usually previous classical cesarean section or hysterotomy. The scar generally gives way in the last 2–3 weeks of pregnancy.
  - Previous curettage in which the uterus may have been inadvertently perforated or myometrium deeply torn
  - Previous perforation of the uterus by an intrauterine device (IUD) may leave a weak area
  - Manual removal of adherent placenta in previous pregnancy, which could lead to damage of myometrium
  - History of myomectomy, especially if the endometrial cavity has been entered during myomectomy or in cases of fundal fibroids.

- *Trauma:* Either direct or indirect. Road traffic accidents increase the risks of uterine rupture and abruption.
- Congenital uterine anomalies
- Rarely, rupture can occur in vesicular mole, and placenta percreta.

What are the causes of rupture uterus during labor?
- Obstructed labor associated with CPD, malpresentation, or hydrocephalus
- Misuse of oxytocic drugs
- High parity
- Cervical scarring after amputation or cone biopsy
- Unrecognized previous injury to the uterine wall
- Manual removal of the placenta
- Trauma due to instrumental delivery
- Breech extraction

How do you clinically recognize uterine rupture?
Symptoms:
- Patient becomes restless and complains of constant pain over lower part of the uterus. Once the uterus ruptures, she may complain of sudden feeling of something giving way followed by loss of uterine contractions.
- *Vaginal bleeding:* It depends on the location of the tear relative to the vessels
- *Hematuria:* A rupture that involves the lower part of the uterus may also include the bladder.

Signs
- Patient may collapse with tachycardia and hypotension.
- If rupture is due to obstruction, vertical stretching of the lower segment and Bandl's ring can be seen.
- Loss of uterine contour
- Superficial palpation of fetal parts

- Fetal distress is the most consistent finding.
- On per vaginam examination, there is loss of station of the presenting part, as it recedes higher after extrusion through the rupture.
- If rupture occurs at end of second stage of labor, the characteristic sign is shortening of the cord.

What is the differential diagnosis of rupture uterus?
- Abruptio placenta
- *Multiple pregnancy:* The uterine outline is often not well demarcated and suspicion of rupture occurs, if patient collapses during labor.
- Impacted shoulder presentation; there may be two swellings with a sulcus in-between.

What is the management of such cases?
Management of rupture uterus:
- Once diagnosis is reached, establish two large-bore intravenous (IV) lines, arrange adequate blood, send baseline investigations (hemogram, coagulation profile, blood urea, serum electrolytes, and random blood sugar); proceed for a laparotomy with blood available [preferably MTP (Massive Transfusion Protocol) kit] for transfusion after taking a written informed consent. And consent for hystrectomy also, if need be.
- Repair of rupture uterus is considered in young women with no living child or low parity in stable conditions and when the wound is clear cut as in lower segment scar rupture.
- Subtotal hysterectomy is preferred in patients of rupture resulting from obstructive spontaneous labor, as patient is in low general condition, is of high parity and anatomy is totally distorted.

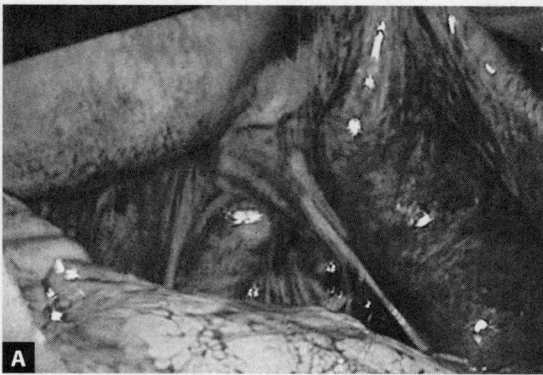 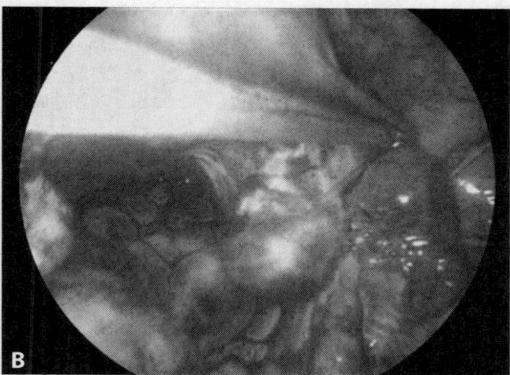

Figs. 5A and B: Ectopic tubal gestation. *(For color version, see Plate 11)*

- Total hysterectomy in a patient of low general condition is more time consuming and may increase the chances of ureteric injury.
- Rupture of anterior lower segment may involve involvement of the urinary bladder. Uterus should be repaired after mobilizing the bladder.
- Lateral lower segment rupture may involve the uterine artery and result in formation of broad ligament hematoma.
- Internal iliac artery ligation may also be required in cases of uncontrolled bleeding.

What are the causes of maternal deaths in cases of rupture uterus?

Uterine rupture is responsible for 5% of maternal deaths, which are due to hemorrhage, shock, disseminated intravascular coagulation (DIC), and sepsis.

What is the incidence of uterine rupture in various scars?

Incidence of scar rupture is:
- *Lower segment cesarean section (LSCS):* 0.4–0.8%
- *Classical:* 4–8%

What is colporrhexis?

Colporrhexis is the rupture of the vault of the vagina. It may be primary where only the vault is involved or secondary when associated with cervical tear. It is said to be complete when the peritoneum is opened up. Treatment is surgical, if accessible repair may be done per vaginam.

ECTOPIC GESTATION SPECIMEN

Identify the specimens shown in Figures 5 and 6.
- These are specimens of fallopian tube with unruptured ectopic pregnancy (Figs. 5A and B).
- This is a specimen of ectopic pregnancy in a ruptured rudimentary horn with a fetus (Fig. 6).

What is the site of ectopic pregnancy in Figures 5A and B?

The site of ectopic pregnancy is in the ampullary part of the fallopian tube, which is widest and longest (4–5 cm).

What is the gestational age at which ampullary pregnancy ruptures?

It is around 8–10 weeks of gestation. Isthmic rupture occurs around 5 weeks and cornual pregnancy may go up to 12–14 weeks.

What is Haas rule?

By this rule, we can make out the period of gestation after measuring the crown-rump length (CRL). The square of the weeks of

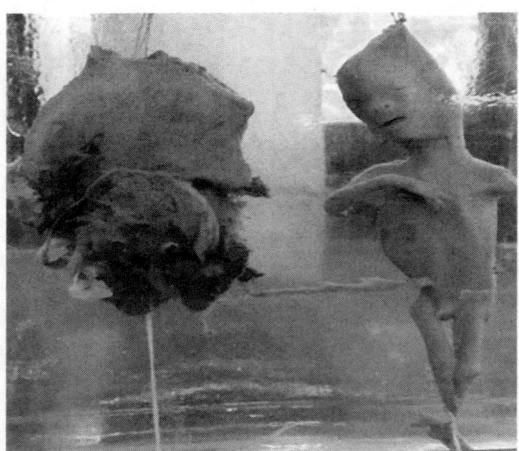

Fig. 6: Ectopic pregnancy in a ruptured rudimentary horn with fetus. *(For color version, see Plate 11)*

gestation is the length of fetus from 2–7 weeks postovulation.

- $2 \times 2 = 4$ mm
- $3 \times 3 = 9$ mm
- $4 \times 4 = 16$ mm
- $5 \times 5 = 25$ mm
- $6 \times 6 = 36$ mm
- $7 \times 7 = 49$ mm

After 2 months, the square of months is the length of fetus in cm till 5 months.

- $2 \times 2 = 4$ cm
- $3 \times 3 = 9$ cm
- $4 \times 4 = 16$ cm
- $5 \times 5 = 25$ cm

After 5 months, the length of the fetus is five times the month of gestation.

- $6 \times 5 = 30$ cm
- $7 \times 5 = 35$ cm
- $8 \times 5 = 40$ cm
- $9 \times 5 = 45$ cm
- $10 \times 5 = 50$ cm.

At term, the length of fetus is 50 cm. This rule is clinically applicable in knowing the gestational age by CRL and vice-versa.

What symptoms can a patient with ectopic present?

If there is a rupture of fallopian tube at ampulla, she would have amenorrhea, history of bleeding per vagina, and pain abdomen with giddiness with/without shock depending on the intraperitoneal hemorrhage.

What are the diagnostic aids?

If ectopic pregnancy is suspected on clinical examination with finding of cervical motion tenderness, presence of an adnexal mass with normal uterine size, fullness in the pouch of Douglas (POD) or with features of shock, transvaginal ultrasound should be done to confirm the diagnosis. Tubal ectopic pregnancies can be visualized as an adnexal mass, which is visualized separate from the ovary with an empty uterine cavity.

Positive culdocentesis gives an idea of intraperitoneal hemorrhage and this aspirated blood does not clot with time.

Serum β-hCG level is useful for planning the management of a suspected ultrasound visualized ectopic pregnancy. In an intrauterine pregnancy, β-hCG level doubles every 48 hours while in ectopic pregnancy, rise will be lower.

Serum progesterone level is not useful in predicting ectopic pregnancy.

How will you diagnose cervical ectopic pregnancy on ultrasonography?

The ultrasound criteria used for identifying cervical ectopic pregnancy include a normal uterus without a sac, a barrel-shaped cervix, a gestational sac visualized below the level of the internal cervical os, and blood flow around the gestational sac using color Doppler.

What are the diagnostic criteria for diagnosing cesarean scar implantation?

The ultrasonic criteria for diagnosing cesarean scar implantation include:

- No gestational sac in the uterine cavity or endocervical canal
- Gestational sac or solid mass of trophoblast located anteriorly at the level of the internal os, embedded at the site of the previous lower uterine segment cesarean section scar.
- Deficient or thinned layer of myometrium between the gestational sac and the bladder.
- Evidence of prominent trophoblastic/placental circulation on Doppler examination.

What are the indications of expectant management?

Expectant management is used for suitably selected and counseled women who can be in close follow-up, have no gestational sac or extrauterine mass, visualized on USG, and have minimal symptoms with low and declining serum β-hCG levels.

What are the indications of medical management?

- Gestational sac <3 cm
- β-hCG <3,000 mIU/mL
- Cardiac activity absent
- Hemodynamically stable patient
- No contraindication to methotrexate

Is there a role of injection of methotrexate in patients with ectopic pregnancy?

There are reports that if bleeding is not active and the rupture is small, after salpingostomy and removing the clots and trophoblastic tissue, one can inject 50 mg of methotrexate.

Injection methotrexate is given as a single intramuscular dose of 50 mg/m^2. Serum β-hCG levels are repeated on days 4 and 7 after injection methotrexate. If the β-hCG level decreases by >15% between days 4 and days 7, β-hCG levels are then measured weekly until <15 IU/L. If the level does not decrease by 15%, a repeat transvaginal ultrasound should be considered to exclude ectopic fetal cardiac activity and the presence of significant hemoperitoneum. Consideration may then be given to repeat a dose of methotrexate.

The National Institute for Health and Clinical Excellence (NICE) recommends that methotrexate should be the first-line management for women who are able to return for follow-up and who have no significant pain, an unruptured ectopic pregnancy with a mass smaller than 35 mm with no visible heartbeat, serum β-hCG between 1,500 and 5,000 IU/L, and no intrauterine pregnancy on USG.

What is the best management of a patient with ectopic pregnancy?

A laparoscopic surgical approach is preferable to an open approach.

In the presence of a healthy contralateral tube, salpingectomy should be performed in preference to salpingostomy.

In women with a history of fertility-reducing factors such as previous ectopic pregnancy, opposite side tubal damage, previous abdominal surgery or pelvic inflammatory disease, salpingostomy should be considered. If a salpingostomy is performed, women should be informed about the risk of persistent trophoblast with the need for serum β-hCG level follow-up. They should also be counseled that there is a small risk that they may need further treatment in the form of systemic methotrexate or salpingectomy.

Injection methotrexate or KCl may be injected directly into the sac under ultrasound/laparoscopic guidance when the diagnosis of live ectopic pregnancy is certain and a viable intrauterine pregnancy has been excluded.

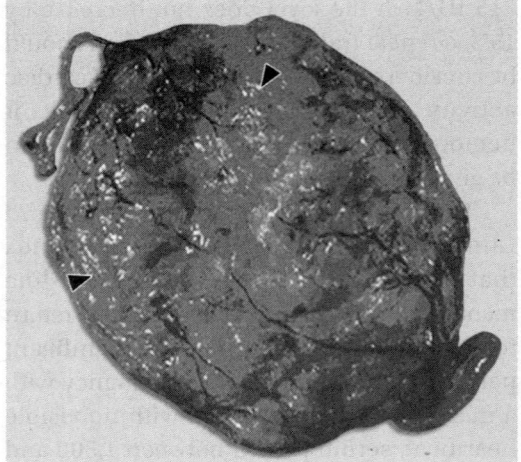

Fig. 7: Placenta of twin delivery.

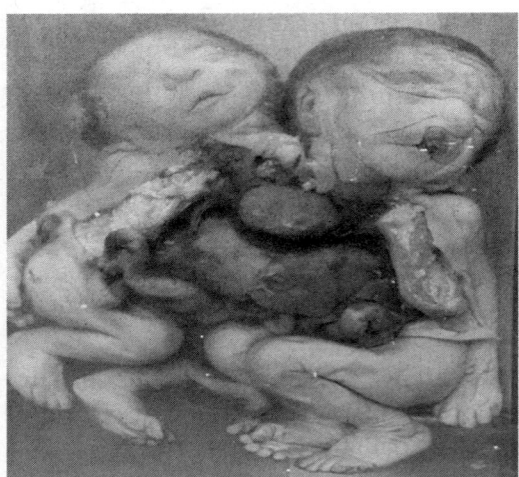

Fig. 9: Conjoint twins. *(For color version, see Plate 12)*

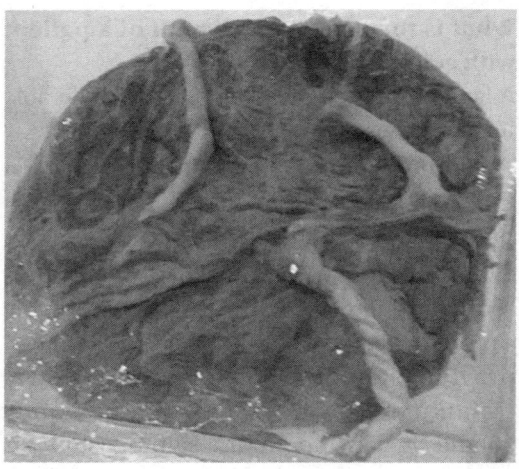

Fig. 8: Placenta of triplet delivery.
(For color version, see Plate 12)

Is oophorectomy advocated with salpingectomy?

No, it is not advocated as the chances of conception decrease with oophorectomy.

What is the rate of recurrence of ectopic pregnancy?

Approximately 13–28% in patients with history of one ectopic; 30% with history of two previous ectopic pregnancies.

■ MULTIPLE PREGNANCY

Identify the specimens shown in Figures 7 to 9.
- It is a specimen showing placenta of a twin **(Fig. 7)** and triplet delivery **(Fig. 8)**.
- It is a specimen of conjoint twins **(Fig. 9)**.

What are the types of twins?
- *Binovular/fraternal/dizygotic twins:* Result from fertilization of two ova, usually of the same or one from each ovary by two sperms.
- *Uniovular twins/identical/monozygotic:* In this, twining occurs at different stages after fertilization:
  - *If division takes place within 72 hours after fertilization:* The embryo will have two separate placenta, chorions, and amnions (diamniotic dichorionic).
  - If twining occurs after the formation of inner cell mass (between 4th day and 8th day), it will result in monochorionic diamniotic twins.
  - *If division occurs after 8th day of fertilization, when the amniotic cavity has already been formed*, it results in monoamniotic monochorionic twins.

How are conjoined twins formed?
If division occurs after the development of embryonic disk, it results in conjoined twins. Four types of fusion occur: (1) Thoracopagus, (2) pyopagus, (3) craniopagus, and (4) ischiopagus.

What is frequency (prevalence) of uniovular twins?
It is constant. It is 1 per 250 births and is independent of race, heredity, age, and parity.

Which factors are responsible for dizygotic twins?
- Race (Negroes)
- Hereditary (especially maternal side)
- Advancing age of the mother
- Increasing parity
- Ovulation inducing drugs
- Nutritional factors (taller and heavier woman)
- Conception within 1 month of stopping oral contraceptive pill (OCP)
- ART

What is superfecundation?
Superfecundation is fertilization of two different ova released in the same cycle by separate acts of coitus within a short period of time.

Superfetation: It is fertilization of two ova released in different menstrual cycles. It is a theoretical possibility up to 12 weeks of pregnancy

What are the complications of twin pregnancy?
Excessive nausea and vomiting, anemia (two-fold), preeclampsia (three-fold), eclampsia (four-fold), polyhydramnios, antepartum hemorrhage (two-fold), malpresentations, preterm labor, discordant growth, and postpartum bleeding (two-fold).

What are the challenges associated with monochorionic pregnancy?
Most complications of monochorionic pregnancies arise on account of vascular placental anastomoses that are almost universal and connect the umbilical circulations of both twins. This results in twin-twin transfusion syndrome, selective growth restriction, twin anemia-polycythemia sequence, twin-reversed arterial perfusion (TRAP), high risk of cord entanglement and although not exclusive to monochorionic twin pregnancy, single intrauterine death is more common.

What is discordant growth and its causes?
A variation of 15–25% in estimated fetal weight of the twins or S/D ratio difference >15% is known as discordant twin. Causes of discordant growth are unequal placental mass, genetic syndromes, and twin–twin transfusion syndrome.

What is vanishing twin syndrome?
After the diagnosis of multiple pregnancy, if there is subsequent disappearance of one or more fetuses resulting in complete reabsorption of a fetus or formation of a mummified fetus papyraceus or development of a subtle abnormality on the placenta such as a cyst, subchorionic fibrin, or amorphous material, it is vanishing twin syndrome.

What is twin reversed arterial perfusion sequence?
Twin reversed arterial perfusion sequence occurs when one twin is acardiac, while the other twin shares its circulation with the acardiac twin. It is a rare and serious complication of monozygotic multiple gestation.

How do you determine chorionicity?
Localization of two separate placenta during the first trimester, a thick (>2 mm) dividing

membrane and fetuses of opposite gender indicates dichorionicity.

What is "twin-peak" sign?

"Twin-peak" sign differentiates between two fused placentas from one large placenta.

On USG, it is visualized as a triangular projection of placental tissue seen to extend beyond the chorionic surface between the layers of the dividing membranes, and it indicates two fused placenta. A T-sign is seen as a right angle relation between membranes and placenta with no extension of placenta between dividing membrane and it indicates two separate sacs and a single placenta.

What is the optimal timing of delivery in a twin and triplet pregnancy?

For uncomplicated dichorionic/diamniotic twin pregnancies, elective delivery may be done at 38 (0/7th) to 38 (6/7th) weeks of gestation, as recommended by the ACOG. Twin pregnancies complicated by fetal growth restriction are delivered earlier than 38 weeks, with the timing dependent on the clinical presentation. In triplet pregnancies, maximum perinatal complications occur at 34 and 35 weeks. Therefore, delivery of triplet pregnancy should be planned at ≥35 weeks. Triplets should be considered post-term at 36 weeks and delivery of triplets should occur by 37 weeks.

What problems are anticipated in a case of intrauterine fetal demise of one twin?

Single fetal demise is common in early pregnancy and has a good outcome for the surviving twin, but if this occurs in late pregnancy, it can have serious consequences for the cotwin including an increased risk of preterm birth, neurologic morbidity, and an increased risk of mortality. This risk is higher in a monochorionic pregnancy because of placental vascular anastomosis.

Death of one fetus may cause ischemic brain damage of the other twin by causing sudden hypotension and disturbing the blood supply to other twin. In diamniotic twins, death of one fetus may cause sudden rupture of the thin membrane between them again leading to sudden hypotension and death of the other twin. Rarely, single fetal death causes release of fibrin and tissue thromboplastins in circulation, causing DIC, which can be fatal both for the mother and the fetus. Another adverse effect of death of one fetus is transchorionic embolization, resulting in death of the other fetus also.

What is twin-to-twin transfusion syndrome?

Twin-to-twin transfusion syndrome (TTTS) occurs due to arteriovenous anastomosis in the shared placenta of monochorionic pregnancy. The donor twin is small and anemic, while the recipient twin is polycythemic, large and at risk for high-output cardiac failure. The mortality rate is 40–90%, with both twins at risk. USG is used to diagnose and score TTTS.

Quintero's TTTS is staged as follows:
- *Stage I:* The bladder in the donor twin is still visible.
- *Stage II:* The bladder in the donor twin is no longer visible, but no critically abnormal findings are observed on Doppler studies.
- *Stage III:* Doppler studies show critically abnormal waveforms.
- *Stage IV:* Hydrops is present.
- *Stage V:* The demise of one or both twins has occurred.

How will you diagnose discordant twins?

On USG, a difference in estimated fetal weight of ≥20% by taking abdominal circumference (AC) and biparietal diameter (BPD) or AC and femur length (FL) to calculate the fetal weight or difference of ≥20 mm in the AC of the two fetuses.

When will you consider cesarean delivery in case of multiple pregnancy?
- Monoamniotic twins
- Noncephalic presentation of first twin
- Conjoint twins
- Interlocking
- Triplets or higher order pregnancy
- Failed version in second twin
- Associated obstetric/medical cause

■ PLACENTAL ABNORMALITY

Identify the specimen shown in Figure 10.
This is a specimen of placenta showing succenturiate lobe.

What is placenta succenturiate?
When one or more small accessory lobes are present in the membranes at a distance from the periphery of the main placenta, with vascular connections between the two, it is known as placenta succenturiate.

What is the clinical importance of this type of placenta?
The accessory lobe may be implanted on the lower segment and may cause antepartum hemorrhage. Sometimes, it may be retained in the uterus after delivery and may cause PPH. In some cases, accompanying vasa previa may cause dangerous fetal bleeding leading to fetal compromise at delivery.

What is an extrachorial placenta?
When the chorionic plate (fetal side) is smaller than the basal plate (located over the maternal side) the placental periphery is uncovered and leads to extrachorial placenta. Such placenta is circumvallate placenta, if the fetal surface of such a placenta appears as a central depression surrounded by a thickened and grayish-white ring.

What is the clinical importance of a circumvallate placenta?
There is increased risk of abortion, abruption, preterm delivery, intrauterine growth restriction (IUGR), and retained placenta or membrane.

What is a membranous placenta/placenta diffusa?
When all fetal membranes are covered as a thin membranous structure occupying the entire periphery of chorion, it may lead to serious hemorrhage due to associated placenta previa or accreta. This is known as membranous placenta/placenta diffusa.

How does a normal placenta develop?
Placenta develops from chorion frondosum, which is the fetal component and decidua basalis is the maternal component.

What is placenta accreta?
Placenta accreta is a condition, when partial or complete placenta, is inseparable from the uterine wall. When there is no plane between the placenta and the myometrium, it is known as placenta accreta, when the chorionic villi invade the myometrium, it is known as placenta increta and when the placenta invades through the myometrium and serosa, and may also invade into adjacent organs, like bladder, it is known as placenta percreta. During delivery, the placenta does

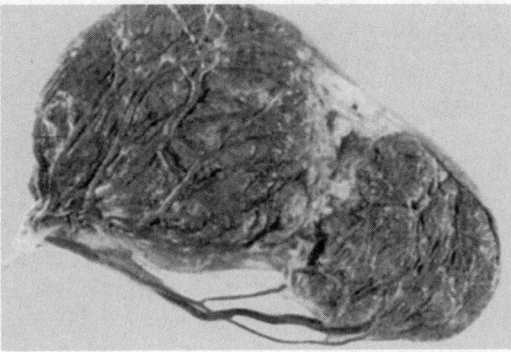

Fig. 10: Succenturiate lobe.

not completely separate from the uterus and is followed by massive hemorrhage and may result in disseminated intravascular coagulopathy; cesarean hysterectomy; injury to the ureters, bladder, bowel, or neurovascular structures; acute transfusion reaction; electrolyte imbalance; renal failure; and even maternal mortality.

How will you diagnose placenta accreta in the antenatal period?
Transabdominal and transvaginal USG is used to diagnose placenta accreta when the placenta is irregularly shaped, placental lacunae (vascular spaces) are seen within the placenta, with thinning of the myometrium overlying the placenta, loss of the retroplacental "clear space," extension of the placenta into the bladder, increased vascularity of the uterine serosa–bladder interface, and turbulent blood flow through the lacunae on Doppler USG. Gray scale USG has a sensitivity of 77–87% and specificity of 96–98% for the diagnosis of placenta accreta. For confirmation of diagnosis, magnetic resonance imaging (MRI) may be done.

CHAPTER 20: Gynecology Specimens

Ruchi Srivastava, Shailza Vardhan, Neerja Goel

■ HYSTERECTOMY

Describe the specimens shown in Figures 1 and 2.

It is a mounted cut specimen of uterus with cervix (total hysterectomy) done for endometrial polyp **(Fig. 1)**.

It is a mounted cut specimen of hysterectomy with bilateral salpingo-oophorectomy (BSO) done for bilateral ovarian tumors **(Fig. 2)**.

What is the type of hysterectomy performed and probable age of patient (Fig. 1)?

The type of hysterectomy is total hysterectomy, and patient is in the reproductive age group since ovaries have been conserved.

What could be the possible indication of total hysterectomy in reproductive age-group women?

Usually, the possible indication of total hysterectomy could be a benign pathology, i.e., polyp, adenomyosis, leiomyoma, endometrial hyperplasia, coagulopathy, ovulatory dysfunction, endometriosis, rupture uterus, and septic abortion.

What are the different routes by which a hysterectomy can be performed?

The different routes are abdominal, vaginal, laparoscopic-assisted vaginal hysterectomy (LAVH), and total laparoscopic hysterectomy.

What are the indications of subtotal/supracervical hysterectomy?

- Obstetric indication—cesarean hysterectomy for atonic postpartum hemorrhage (PPH) and rupture uterus
- Thick adhesion with obliteration of the anterior and posterior cul-de-sac as in endometriosis

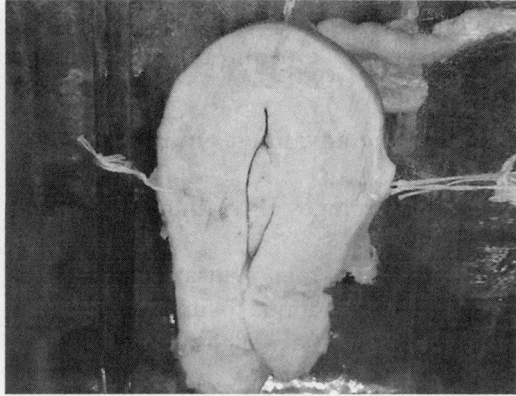

Fig. 1: Total hysterectomy with endometrial polyp.

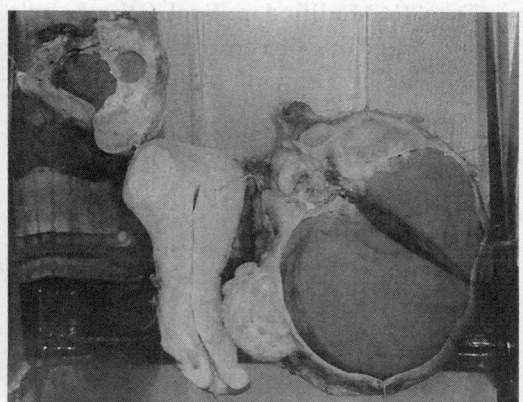

Fig. 2: Hysterectomy with bilateral salpingo-oophorectomy.

- Emergency—when the patient's condition is not good
- Concern for sexual function

What are the advantages of elective subtotal hysterectomy?

There is currently a vogue for subtotal hysterectomy. Its advantages are as follows:
- Prevents vault prolapse
- Prevents abnormal cuff granulations
- Better sexual satisfaction and better orgasmic capability, although no sound scientific data available
- Less vaginal shortening
- But in these, patients need to come for regular follow-up. Cervical smear is important as the chances of carcinoma developing in the cervical stump remain (1%).

What are the different types of hysterectomy?
- Subtotal hysterectomy
- Total hysterectomy
- Hysterectomy with BSO
  - Intrafascial
  - Extrafascial

Piver–Rutledge–Smith classification (1974) is as follows:
- *Type I:* Extrafascial hysterectomy
- *Type II:* Modified radical (Wertheim's hysterectomy)—removal of medial one-half of the cardinal and uterosacral ligament with only selective removal of enlarged pelvic lymph nodes
- The uterine artery is transected at the level of ureter, thus preserving the ureteral branch to the ureter. The anterior vesicouterine ligament is divided, but the posterior vesicouterine ligament is conserved and a smaller margin of vagina is removed.
- *Type III:* Classical radical hysterectomy—involves removal of almost all of uterosacral and cardinal ligaments, upper one-third of vagina and includes pelvic lymph node dissection
- *Type IV:* Extended radical hysterectomy—in this, the periureteral tissue, superior vesical artery, and up to three-fourths of the vagina are removed.
- *Type V:* Partial exenteration—in this, portions of the distal ureter and bladder are resected. Radiotherapy (RT) is preferred over this operation because of its morbidity.

Querleu–Morrow Classification (2017) (**Table 1**)
The Querleu–Morrow classification is based, for the purpose of simplification, on the lateral extent of resection only. Stable anatomic landmarks, such as the crossing of the ureter with the uterine artery and paracervix, and the vascular plane of the internal iliac system are used to define the limits of resection.

What are the indications of total hysterectomy with bilateral salpingo-oophorectomy?
- When the ovary is pathological
- Patient is postmenopausal
- Prophylactic in cases of familial cancer syndrome or where there is strong possibility of carcinoma developing and the patient has finished childbearing
- In surgery for malignancies like cervical cancer in postmenopausal women, carcinoma endometrium, ovarian malignancy, etc.

What are the advantages of retaining the ovaries?

Distinct advantages of retaining the ovaries are:
- Prevention of menopausal symptoms (as the ovaries continue to function normally or occasionally at a slightly reduced level)
- Lesser incidence of osteoporosis and atherosclerosis (as the incidence of osteoporosis is higher in young women

TABLE 1: Querleu-morrow classification of radical hysterectomy.

Dimension Type of radical hysterectomy	Paracervix or lateral parametrium	Ventral parametrium	Dorsal parametrium
A	Halfway between the cervix and ureter (medial to the ureter—ureter identified but not mobilized)	Minimal excision	Minimal excision
B1	At the ureter (at the level of the ureteral bed-ureter mobilized from the cervix and lateral parametrium)	Partial excision of the vesicouterine ligament	Partial resection of the rectouterine–rectovaginal ligament and uterosacral peritoneal fold
B2	Identical to B1 plus paracervical lymphadenectomy without resection of vascular/nerve structures	Partial excision of the vesicouterine ligament	Partial resection of the rectouterine-rectovaginal ligament and uterosacral fold
C1	At the iliac vessels transversally, caudal part is preserved	Excision of the vesicouterine ligament at the bladder. Proximal part of the vesicovaginal ligament (bladder nerves are dissected and spared)	At the rectum (hypogastric nerve is dissected and spared)
C2	At the level of the medial aspect of iliac vessels completely (including the caudal part)	At the bladder (bladder nerves are sacrificed)	At the sacrum (hypogastric nerve is sacrificed)
D	At the pelvic wall, including resection of the internal iliac vessels and/or components of the pelvic sidewall	At the bladder. Not applicable if part of exenteration	At the sacrum. Not applicable if part of exenteration

who undergo bilateral oophorectomy than in older women with natural menopause)

What is opportunistic salpingectomy?
Opportunistic salpingectomy may offer the opportunity to reduce the risk of ovarian cancer in patients who are already undergoing pelvic surgery for benign disease by eliminating the serous tubal intraepithelial carcinoma (STIC lesion) on fallopian tubes where the nidus for ovarian cancer is present.

What are the complications of hysterectomy?
Immediate complications:
- *Intraoperative:* Hemorrhage, injury to adjacent structures like bladder, ureter, bowel, etc., and anesthetic hazards
- *Postoperative period:* Hypovolemic shock, urinary retention, cystitis, vesicovaginal fistula, cystitis, infection in the wound, vault cellulitis, thrombophlebitis, hemorrhage (primary or secondary),

hematoma, wound dehiscence, paralytic ileus, and pulmonary embolism

Delayed complications:
- Vault granulation, vault prolapse, incisional hernia, depression, psychiatric symptoms, and sexual dysfunction

ABNORMAL UTERINE BLEEDING

What is abnormal uterine bleeding? Define the change in terminologies related to abnormal uterine bleeding.

The International Federation of Gynecology and Obstetrics (FIGO) has defined the term abnormal uterine bleeding (AUB) to describe any deviation from normal menstruation or normal menstrual cycle pattern including regularity, frequency, amount, and duration of flow. It includes the following terms for describing various menstrual symptoms:
- *Infrequent menstrual bleeding (earlier termed oligomenorrhea):* One or two episodes of bleeding in a 90-day period. It is recommended that the term oligomenorrhea be abolished.
- *Frequent menstrual bleeding:* More than four bleeding episodes in a 90-day period (this term only includes frequent menstruation and not erratic intermenstrual bleeding)
- *Heavy menstrual bleeding (HMB, earlier defined as menorrhagia):* Excessive menstrual blood loss, which interferes with the woman's physical, emotional, social, and marital quality of life, and which can occur alone or in combination with other symptoms
- *Prolonged menstrual bleeding:* Menstrual periods that are more than 8 days in duration on a regular basis
- *Shortened menstrual bleeding:* Bleeding <2 days in duration. The bleeding is also usually light in volume and is uncommonly associated with serious pathology.
- *Intermenstrual bleeding* (earlier termed metrorrhagia) is defined as irregular episodes of bleeding, between normal menstrual periods.
- *Postmenopausal bleeding* (PMB) is when bleeding occurs more than 1 year after the menopause.

What do you understand by acute or chronic abnormal uterine bleeding?
- *Acute AUB:* Bleeding in a woman of reproductive age, which is of sufficient quantity to require immediate intervention, after pregnancy has been ruled out
- *Chronic AUB:* Uterine bleeding that is abnormal in duration, volume, and/or frequency and has been present for the majority of the last 6 months

Give the Federation of Gynecology and Obstetrics classification of causes of abnormal uterine bleeding (PALM-COEIN) in nonpregnant women?

The acronym PALM-COEIN included polyp, adenomyosis, leiomyoma, malignancy and hyperplasia, coagulopathy, ovulatory dysfunction, endometrial, iatrogenic, and not yet classified.

In general, the components of the *PALM group* are due to *structural entities* that can be measured visually with imaging techniques and/or histopathology, whereas the *COEIN group* is related to *nonstructural or functional entities* that are not defined by imaging or histopathology.

Polyp (AUB-P): These epithelial proliferations comprise a variable vascular, glandular, and fibromuscular and connective tissue component, which may be asymptomatic or may contribute to AUB. These are diagnosed by USG, sonohysterography, and hysteroscopy. Histopathological examination will distinguish benign from malignant.

Adenomyosis (AUB-A): The relationship between adenomyosis and AUB remains unclear, particularly with regard to wide variations in histopathological diagnosis reflecting variations in criteria used and also improved radiological diagnosis. Typically, adenomyosis is associated with increasing age and may co-exist with fibroids. Furthermore, adenomyosis may be both focal and diffuse and it may be harder to establish diagnosis if fibroids are also present.

Leiomyoma (AUB-L): Many leiomyomas are asymptomatic, and frequently their presence is not the cause of AUB. Furthermore, leiomyomas have widely varying rates of growth, even in a single individual.

The primary classification system reflects only the presence or absence of one or more leiomyomas, as determined by sonographic examination, regardless of the location, number, and size. In the secondary system, the clinician is required to distinguish myomas that involve the endometrial cavity (submucosal or SM) from others (O), because SM lesions are those that most likely contribute to the genesis of AUB.

Malignancy and hyperplasia (AUB-M): Although relatively uncommon in reproductive-aged women, atypical hyperplasia and malignancy are important potential causes of or findings associated with AUB. This diagnosis must be considered in any woman in the reproductive years and especially where there may be predisposing factors such as obesity or a history of chronic anovulation.

Coagulopathy (AUB-C): The term "coagulopathy" includes systemic disorders of hemostasis that may be associated with AUB including von Willebrand disease and women on chronic anticoagulation therapy.

Ovulatory dysfunction (AUB-O): It occurs due to endocrine disturbances like polycystic ovary syndrome, hypothyroidism, hyperprolactinemia, mental stress, obesity, anorexia, weight loss, or extreme exercise associated with athletic training. In some instances, the disorder may be caused due to use of gonadal steroids or drugs that impact dopamine metabolism, such as phenothiazines and tricyclic antidepressants. It also occurs due to unexplained ovulatory disorders, which frequently occur at the extremes of reproductive age: Adolescence and menopause transition.

Anovulatory
- Threshold bleeding of puberty menorrhagia
- *Metropathia hemorrhagica:* High-sustained levels of estrogens resulting in episodes of amenorrhea followed by acute heavy bleeding
- Premenopausal dysfunctional uterine bleeding due to atrophic endometrium because of low-estrogen levels.

Ovulatory
- *Irregular ripening:* In this, endometrium receives insufficient support of progesterone from deficient corpus luteal function, and so breakthrough bleeding occurs before the actual menstruation in the form of spotting or brownish discharge. The endometrium reveals incomplete secretory changes. Treatment is to administer progesterone in the premenstrual phase.
- *Irregular shedding (Halban's disease):* It is due to persistent corpus luteum. The menstruation comes on time, but is prolonged and not heavy. Histopathology

picture at the end of menstruation reveals persistence of secretory changes along with proliferative endometrium. Treatment is nonsteroidal anti-inflammatory drugs (NSAIDs) up to 6 months. It is a self-limiting process.

Endometrial dysfunction (AUB-E): It occurs due to imbalance of prostaglandin to prostacyclin ratio, endometrial infection, or inflammation.

What is the management of these patients?
Management depends on the age of the patient, presence of acute heavy bleeding, type of endometrium, and desire for children.

In a young adolescent patient: Investigations are done to rule out bleeding diathesis and thyroid dysfunction, and hormonal treatment is given along with antifibrinolytics and NSAIDs. Combination low-dose oral contraceptive may be advised for 21 days (with 7 days' placebo) for three to six cycles.

Reproductive age group (first rule out pregnancy and infection): A pelvic USG to evaluate the size of the uterus, endometrial thickness, and adnexa, to rule out any endometrial pathology. Treatment with cyclical combined oral contraceptives in patients with no contraindications along with antifibrinolytic and antiprostaglandins is preferred. The course of antibiotics should be given to treat infections.

Peri- or postmenopausal age group: Fractional curettage is undertaken to rule out malignancy. For benign conditions like endometrial hyperplasia and anovulatory bleeding, the patient may be put on progestins.

What is included in polyp category of abnormal uterine bleeding?
Endometrial and endocervical polyps are included in this category. These epithelial proliferations comprise a variable vascular, glandular, and fibromuscular and connective tissue component, which may be asymptomatic or may contribute to AUB. These are diagnosed by USG, sonohysterography, and hysteroscopy. Histopathological examination will distinguish benign from malignant.

How is diagnosis of adenomyosis made?
Besides clinical symptoms of dysmenorrhea, dyspareunia, HMB, pain abdomen, and bloating, criteria of diagnosis are based on histopathologic evaluation of the depth of "endometrial" tissue beneath the endometrial–myometrial interface, as determined via hysterectomy. Diagnosis can be based on sonography and MRI. On USG, adenomyosis is seen as uterine enlargement with cystic anechoic spaces or lakes in the myometrium, localized or global uterine hypertrophy, subendometrial echogenic linear striations or indistinct endometrial/myometrial border.

What are the ACOG recommendations for endometrial biopsy?
The American College of Obstetricians and Gynecologists (ACOG) recommends endometrial biopsy (EB) in all women older than 35 years who have AUB. It is also done in patients aged 18–35 years with risk factors for endometrial cancer, for all women who have been anovulatory for at least 1 year or when necessary to determine ovulatory status.

What are sensitivity and specificity of endometrial aspiration? Name the instrument for aspiration.
Sensitivity 95% and specificity of endometrial aspiration are 98.5%. The instruments used for this procedure are Pipelle, Novak curette, and Karman cannula no. 4.

What is the treatment of endometrial hyperplasia?

Management of endometrial hyperplasia [Royal College of Obstetricians and Gynaecologists (RCOG) 2016]:

Endometrial hyperplasia without atypia:
- Observation alone and 6 monthly follow-up with endometrial biopsies
- Progesterone treatment who fails to respond to observation alone or in symptomatic women with AUB
  - Continuous progesterone—medroxy-progesterone (MPA) 10–20 mg/day for at least 6 months
- Levonorgestrel intrauterine system (LNG-IUS) can be inserted (higher disease-regression rate)

Follow-up is recommended 6 monthly with endometrial biopsies till the two consecutive biopsies are negative.

Indications of hysterectomy in endometrial hyperplasia without atypia:
- Progression to atypia occurs during follow-up of the patient.
- No histologic regression of hyperplasia despite 12 months of treatment
- Relapse of endometrial hyperplasia after completing progesterone treatment
- Persistence of bleeding symptoms
- Woman declines to undergo endometrial surveillance.

Endometrial hyperplasia with atypia:
- *In a woman who wants to retain fertility:* First-line treatment with LNG-IUS is recommended. Oral progesterone is second alternative treatment.
- *Woman with completed family:* Total hysterectomy is first-line management.
- *For postmenopausal woman:* Total abdominal hysterectomy (TAH) + BSO

Follow-up with endometrial biopsies 3 monthly till two consecutive biopsies are negative.

What is the medical management of nonstructural abnormal uterine bleeding?

The medical management can be (1) nonhormonal and (2) hormonal.

Nonhormonal treatment:
- *Antifibrinolytics:* They are the mainstay for ovulatory dysfunctional uterine bleeding (DUB). Decrease blood loss by 50–60%, e.g., tranexamic acid—500 mg, 6–8 hourly, maximum up to 1 g 6 hourly
- *Cyclooxygenase inhibitors:* For example, mefenamic acid and other NSAIDs decrease prostaglandin synthesis.
- Ethamsylate
- Mifepristone (antiprogesterone)

Hormonal treatment:
- Progestin therapy for anovulatory bleeding. Dosage—MPA (10 mg) or norethisterone—for 10 days in luteal phase (D15-D25) or from D5-D26 in case of ovulatory AUB
- Progestin-impregnated intrauterine device (IUD). LNG-IUS (levonorgestrel intrauterine system, Mirena), Progestasert
- Combined oral contraceptive pills (OCPs)
- Depot progesterone preparations
- High-dose estrogen therapy is useful in controlling acute bleeding episodes. Dosage—conjugated estrogens 2.5 mg/day
- *Danazol:* 200–400 mg/day for 3–6 months
- Gonadotropin-releasing hormone (GnRH) analogs for short-term treatment, not >3 months
- Ormeloxifene [selective estrogen receptor modulator (SERM)], antagonizes the effect of estrogen on uterus

What causes bleeding in abnormal uterine bleeding-iatrogenic?

When unscheduled bleeding occurs with cyclic administration of estrogen, progestins, and androgens, the woman may be considered to have breakthrough bleeding and may be categorized as abnormal uterine bleeding-iatrogenic (AUB-I). Combined oral contraceptive preparations may be administered continuously with the goal of achieving amenorrhea.

What may be the causes of bleeding in abnormal uterine bleeding—not yet defined?
Chronic endometritis, arteriovenous malformation, and myometrial hypertrophy are poorly defined as well as some other disorders, which have not been defined as yet.

What are the various methods of endometrial ablation?
First generation
- Endometrial laser resection of endometrium
- Transcervical resection of endometrium
- Rollerball endometrial ablation

Second generation (hysteroscopy is not required)
- Thermal balloon ablation
- Microwave endometrial ablation
- Hydrothermal ablation (circulating hot saline)
- Cryoablation

FIBROID UTERUS

Describe the specimens.
Formalin-preserved specimens of cut section of uterus showing:
- Multiple whorled appearances of fibroids in the myometrium—stages 0, 1, 2, 3, 4, 5 **(Figs. 3A and B)**
- Cervical fibroid—stage 8 **(Fig. 4)** and submucosal fibroid—stage 0 **(Fig. 5)**
- Subserosal fibroid—stage 7 **(Fig. 6)**

Describe the FIGO leiomyoma subclassification system, 2011 (PALM-COEIN).
Refer to **Table 2** for the classification.

What are the main symptoms of fibroids?
The main symptoms are AUB and pain abdomen; pain usually being associated with degeneration, torsion, adenomyosis, or endometriosis. Pelvic pressure, bowel

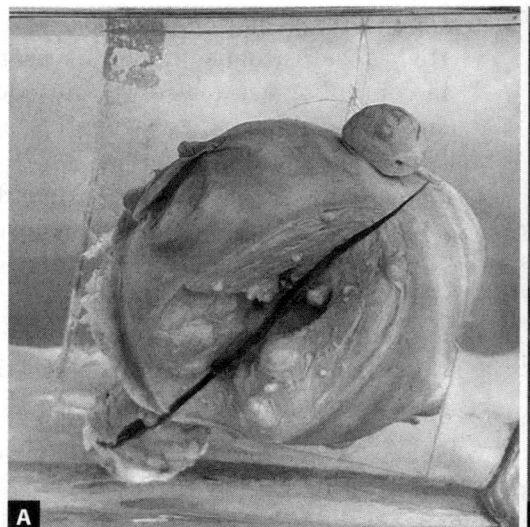
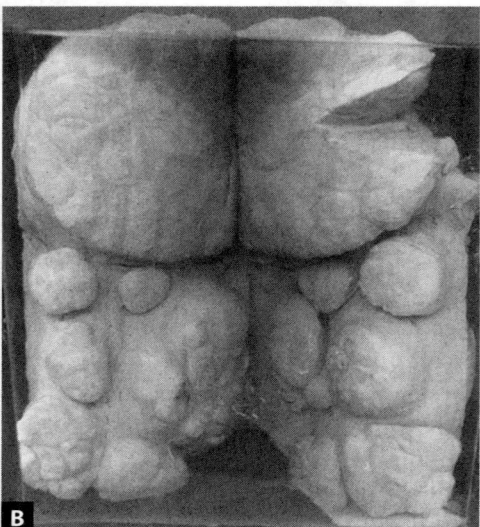

Figs. 3A and B: Multiple leiomyoma. *(For color version, see Plate 12)*

Gynecology Specimens

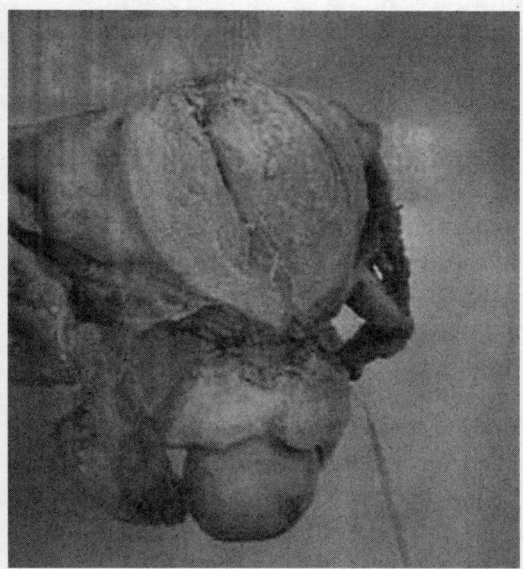

Fig. 4: Cervical fibroid. *(For color version, see Plate 13)*

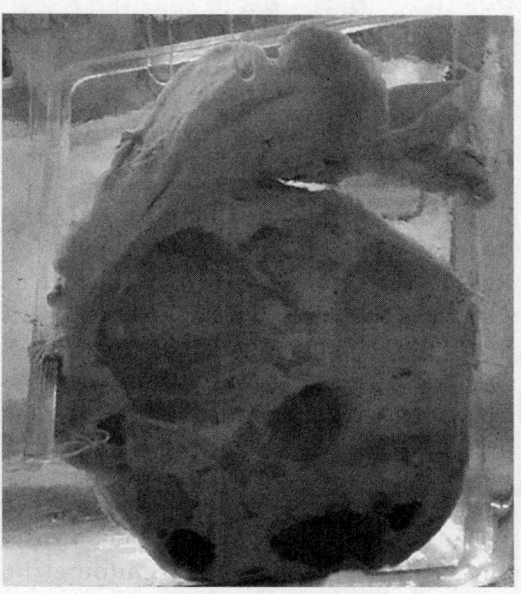

Fig. 6: Subserosal fibroid.

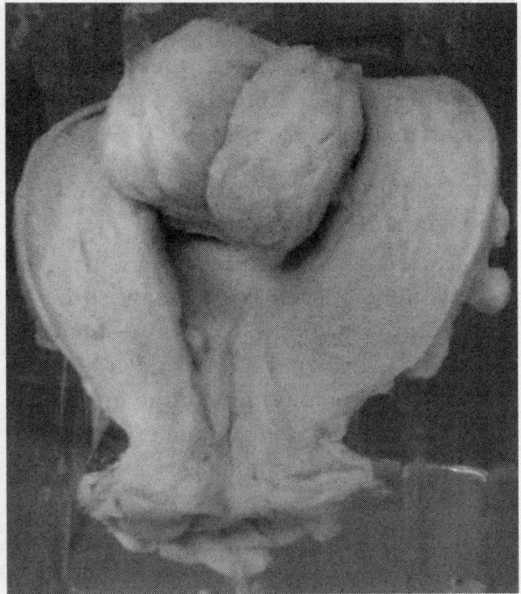

Fig. 5: Submucosal fibroid.
(For color version, see Plate 13)

TABLE 2: International Federation of Gynecology and Obstetrics (FIGO) leiomyoma subclassification system, 2011.

Stage 0	Pedunculated intracavitary
Stage 1	<50% intramural
Stage 2	>50% intramural
Stage 3	Contacts endometrium and 100% intramural
Stage 4	Intramural
Stage 5	Subserosal >50% intramural
Stage 6	Subserosal <50% intramural
Stage 7	Subserosal pedunculated
Stage 8	Others (specify, e.g., cervical and parasitic)

dysfunction, and bladder symptoms such as urinary frequency and urgency may be present with larger fibroids.

What are the causes of abnormal uterine bleeding in patients with fibroid?
Fibroids are associated with anovulation, increased surface area, increased vascularity, estrogen dominance leading to endometrial hyperplasia, and lack of endometrial contractility.

What are the types of degenerations, which occur in fibroids?
Types of degenerations are hyaline, cystic, atrophic, red, fatty, sarcomatous, and calcareous degeneration.

What is the repercussion of red degeneration of fibroid?
Red degeneration of fibroid usually occurs during pregnancy and lactation. There is acute febrile illness but the treatment is symptomatic and conservative.

Name some associated conditions with fibroids
Some associated conditions are pelvic inflammation, endometriosis, adenomyosis, endometrial hyperplasia, endometrial carcinoma, and infertility.

How does fibroid uterus contribute to infertility?
Fibroids may block the cervix or the tubal ostia and prevent ascent of sperms, may increase the uterine contractility, and disturb implantation due to congestion or atrophic changes in the endometrium. They are associated with hyperestrogenic conditions like polycystic ovarian syndrome (PCOS), endometriosis, and adenomyosis and may be anovulatory or have peritoneal factors contributing to infertility.

What are the effects of leiomyoma in pregnancy?
There is an overall increased risk of malpresentation, preterm delivery, placenta previa, abruption, premature rupture of membranes, obstructed labor, cesarean delivery, uterine inertia, PPH, and subinvolution.

How will you diagnose leiomyoma?
Besides symptoms of AUB, the uterus may be enlarged and mobile with irregular contour. Transabdominal and transvaginal USG is able to detect the position, size, and number of fibroids. The fibroid has a whorled appearance on cut section. It is usually well encapsulated and less echogenic than normal myometrium. Associated endometrial hyperplasia, adenomyosis, adnexal masses, hydronephrosis due to pressure effects can also be picked up. For diagnosing submucosal fibroids, sonohysterography has a sensitivity of 98% and specificity of 100%. Hysteroscopy also helps to visualize and remove submucosal fibroids. MRI is also used for accurate fibroid mapping and to define the presence of adenomyosis, adnexal masses, and position of ureters, which helps to plan surgery.

What are some rare complications of fibroid?
Some rare complications of fibroid are polycythemia vera, autoimmune purpura, torsion of subserous fibroid, and sarcomatous changes in 0.2–0.7%.

What are the options of medical management of leiomyoma?
Treatment of women with uterine leiomyomas must be individualized based on symptomatology, size and location of fibroids, age, need, and desire of the patient to preserve fertility or the uterus, the availability of therapy, and the experience of the therapist. Medical management includes the following agents:

- *Antifibrinolytic agents*—reduce HMB but do not reduce size of fibroid.
- *Oral contraceptives*—inhibit ovulation and secretion of estrogen and progesterone.
- *Progestins*—inhibit ovulation and secretion of estrogen and progesterone, decidualize endometrium causing a pseudopregnancy-like state.

- *LNG-IUS*—inhibits ovulation and secretion of estrogen and progesterone and causes endometrial atrophy. It reduces HMB and may reduce the size of fibroid.
- *GnRH analogs with add-back estrogen therapy for not more than 3–6 months*—work by downregulation and desensitization of the GnRH receptors. Another important mechanism is a decrease in the expression of several important effectors of fibroid growth. It controls HMB and also reduces the size of fibroid. Prolonged treatment may cause menopausal symptoms. They are useful in reducing the size and vascularity of fibroid before surgery, but the planes are distorted, which make surgery difficult. Dose—3.75 mg of leuprolide acetate every month.
- *GnRH antagonists*—directly inhibit GnRH without the initial flare-up and cause hypoestrogenism. They control HMB and also reduce fibroid size. Cetrorelix and ganirelix 30–60 mg may be used.
- *Mifepristone*—progesterone receptor modulator with antagonistic properties. It directly reduces the progesterone in the myometrium and leiomyoma. Dose—5 mg daily for 3–6 months.
- *Danazol*—related to 17-α ethinyl testosterone. It is androgenic and reduces estrogen levels by negative feedback action on the hypothalamic–pituitary–ovarian axis. Dose—100–400 mg/day for 4–6 months.
- *Aromatase inhibitors (Letrozole)*—myometrial cells overexpress aromatase P450 and synthesize estradiol to accelerate their own cell growth. Aromatase inhibitors block the aromatase activity and block estrogen production and reduce growth of fibroid. *Dose*—2.5–5 mg/day for 3 months
- *Ulipristal acetate (UPA):* UPA is a selective progesterone receptor modulator (SPRM) that also has antiproliferative effects on leiomyoma cells. It reduces the size of the fibroid and is also useful for fibroids causing pressure symptoms. Of all the hormonal options available for women with fibroids, UPA has the most rapid documented onset of action and control of bleeding, with 80% of women achieving a pictorial blood assessment chart score < 75 within 7 days. *Dose*—5 mg daily for 3–6 months.
- *Cabergoline:* Small studies reported a reduction in fibroid size with cabergoline, a dopamine agonist used to treat hyperprolactinemia. Dose—0.5 mg weekly

What is the surgical management of fibroid?

Women who are symptomatic with HMB or pressure symptoms have repeated pregnancy failure or infertility with submucosal fibroid where other causes have been ruled out, have uterine size ≥14-week pregnant uterus, have cervical/broad ligament fibroids, torsion or uncontrolled bleeding, have completed their family, are more than 40 years of age, are not willing to take medical management, or are not able to tolerate/afford medical management or cannot come back for follow-up should be counseled regarding the alternatives and risks, and the following surgical options may be considered:

- Hysterectomy by any route—abdominal, laparoscopic, or vaginal may be offered as the definitive treatment for symptomatic uterine fibroids and is associated with a high level of satisfaction as there is no risk of recurrence

- Women undergoing myomectomy should be counseled about the risk of bleeding during surgery and about 15% recurrence rate. 10% women undergoing myomectomy will eventually require hysterectomy within 5–10 years. Risk of recurrence is dependent on age, preoperative number of fibroids, uterine size, and associated disease.
- Use of vasopressin, bupivacaine and epinephrine, misoprostol, pericervical tourniquet, or gelatin-thrombin matrix may be used to reduce blood loss during myomectomy.
- Hysteroscopic myomectomy should be considered for the management of symptomatic submucosal fibroids. Submucosal fibroids (types 0, I, and II) up to 4–5 cm in diameter are removed hysteroscopically by experienced surgeons. Type II fibroids may require a two-staged procedure because of the risk of excessive fluid absorption and uterine perforation, and caution should be used particularly with those with <5 mm thickness between the fibroid and the uterine serosa.
- *Laparoscopic myomectomy:* The size or the number of fibroids that can be removed by laparoscopy depend on the surgeon's experience and technique. Operating on multiple fibroids, fibroid size >10 cm, multilayer suturing, identification, and excision of smaller fibroids and removal of fibroids near cervix prolong the duration of surgery, are challenging, and may be removed by laparotomy.
- If morcellation is required to remove the specimen during hysteroscopic/laparoscopic myomectomy, the patient should be informed about possible risks and complications, including the fact that in rare cases, if the fibroid(s) has/have unexpected malignancy, a power morcellation may spread the cancer, potentially worsening their prognosis.
- Magnetic resonance-guided focused ultrasound surgery (MRg-FUS) or high-frequency ultrasound-guided transcutaneous focused ultrasound ablation is another option for treating fibroids. Disadvantages include high-exclusion rate, requirement of an MR machine, prolonged time (minutes to several hours), treatment of one fibroid at a time, and ablation of fibroids centrally, while fibroids seem to grow peripherally. It may cause skin burn, nerve damage, or rarely bowel perforation has been reported.
- Uterine artery embolization may be offered to selected women with symptomatic uterine fibroids who wish to preserve their uterus after counseling about the possible risks of impacted fecundity and pregnancy.

Should myomectomy be done during cesarean delivery?

Elective myomectomy at the time of cesarean delivery is avoided, as it may increase chances of bleeding and is mostly limited only to patients with pedunculated fibroids or to instances in which the lower segment incision for delivering the baby or where the uterus cannot be closed without removal of the fibroid. Centers where cesarean myomectomy is being planned should be adequately staffed, with adequate blood bank services, and the surgery should be attempted only by experienced surgeons.

UTERUS WITH INTRAUTERINE DEVICE

Describe the specimen shown in Figure 7.
The specimen is a formalin-preserved specimen of cut section of a normal size uterus containing an IUD in its cavity.

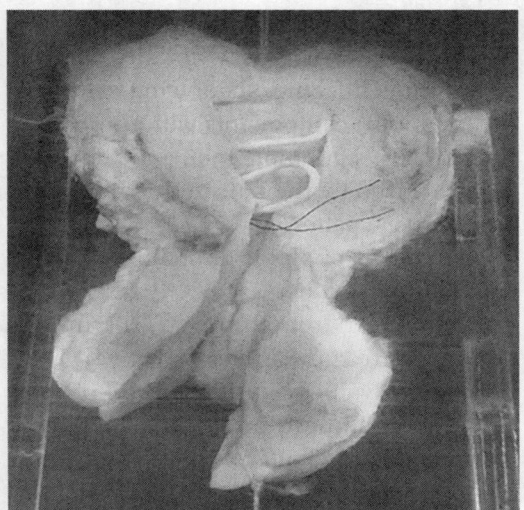

Fig. 7: Uterus with an intrauterine device.

Why did this patient have hysterectomy?
Probably she must have presented with AUB and the preoperative evaluation of IUD may not have been done.

What could be the probable age of this patient?
As the specimen contains only uterus without tubes and ovaries, she must have been <45 years.

What are the ways to manage a case of misplaced intrauterine device when the thread is not seen on per speculum examination?
The possibility of expulsion must be kept in mind. The thread of copper-T (Cu-T) may break or get coiled. In other cases, the IUD may be intra- or extrauterine. Hysteroscopic Cu-T removal is the ideal method for removing IUD. It may also be removed with a hook, an artery forceps, or a curette, if a hysteroscope is not available.

How can you diagnose this condition?
Ultrasonography can be used to locate IUD, which is seen as a bright echogenic shadow. Sometimes, it is difficult to comment on the intramyometrial penetration of one limb in sonography. As all the IUDs are radiopaque, anteroposterior (AP) and lateral views of a plain X-ray abdomen will confirm the presence and probable site, i.e., within or outside the true pelvis. An IUD in the vicinity of ischial spine shows that it is lying in the lower part of uterus.

What is the management of extrauterine intrauterine device?
It is mandatory to remove all intra-abdominal copper-containing devices, as these can cause chemical peritonitis. In this case, laparoscopy may be planned for removal. Laparotomy is needed when it is burrowed in a viscera or not seen on laparoscopy, e.g., has pierced the rectum and is lying on the sacrum or bladder.

What should be done if a woman conceives with intrauterine device in situ?
If a woman wishes to continue with her pregnancy, the physician must remove the IUD. Localization of the IUD is an important first step in this process. When pregnancy occurs with an IUD in place, implantation generally is away from the device and the IUD remains extra-amniotic. USG can localize both the IUD and the gestational sac. If the IUD is left in place, the risk of spontaneous abortion may be as high as 50%. Risks of preterm delivery, septic abortion, and chorioamnionitis are also increased, if IUD is not removed.

DERMOID CYST/MATURE CYSTIC TERATOMA

Describe the specimens shown in Figure 8.
These are formalin-preserved specimens of dermoid cyst of ovary-containing hair.

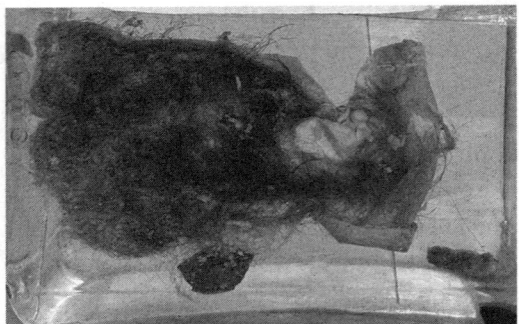

Fig. 8: Dermoid cyst. *(For color version, see Plate 13)*

What are the characteristic features of this cyst?
Dermoid cysts are encapsulated tumors with mature tissue or organ components. They are composed of well-differentiated derivations from at least two of the three germ cell layers, i.e., ectoderm, mesoderm, and endoderm. They contain skin complete with hair follicles and sweat glands, sometimes luxuriant clumps of long hair, pockets of sebum, blood, fat, bone, nails, teeth, eyes, cartilage, and thyroid tissue. Typically, their diameter is smaller than 10 cm and rarely more than 15 cm. Teeth and fragments of bone may be present. It is usually unilateral but can be bilateral in 10–20% of cases.

What is the clinical picture of a patient presenting with dermoid cyst?
The patient may be asymptomatic or may complain of vague pain in abdomen. Acute pain in abdomen may be present in cases of torsion or rupture. It is felt as a cystic mass in the anterior or lateral fornix.

What are the diagnostic aids?
Dermoid cyst can be diagnosed with the presence of teeth or bone on plain X-ray abdomen.

The USG features include diffusely echogenic mass with sebaceous material and hair within the cyst cavity, an echogenic interface at the edge of mass that obscures deep structures (tip of the iceberg sign), mural hyperechoic—Rokitansky nodule, dermoid plug with echogenic, shadowing calcific or dental (tooth) components with presence of fat-fluid levels, multiple thin, and echogenic bands caused by the hair in the cyst cavity: The dot-dash pattern.

On color Doppler examination, internal vascularity is not increased.

Computed tomography (CT) images demonstrate fat (areas with very low Hounsfield values), fat-fluid level, calcification (sometimes dentiform), Rokitansky protuberance, and tufts of hair.

What is struma ovarii tumor?
Struma ovarii tumor is a monodermal, specialized teratoma predominantly composed of mature thyroid tissue comprising >50% of the overall tissue. The patient may present with symptoms of hyperthyroidism.

What is the differential diagnosis of a dermoid cyst?
The differential diagnosis includes endometrioma, tubo-ovarian mass, ovarian abscess, subserous fibroid, and other benign ovarian cysts.

What is the frequency of malignant transformation of this cyst?
A dermoid cyst rarely becomes malignant and the frequency is 1–2%. The counterpart is known as malignant teratoma.

What is the treatment of this cyst?
As a dermoid cyst involves usually the whole ovary, unilateral salpingo-oophorectomy is advocated; however, in the presence of adequate ovarian tissue, ovarian cystectomy can be offered.

What is the role of laparoscopic removal of dermoid cyst?
Laparoscopic removal can be done provided the sebaceous material spill is avoided by

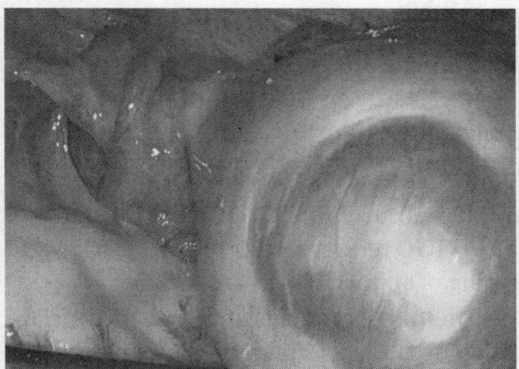

Fig. 9: Twisted dermoid cyst.

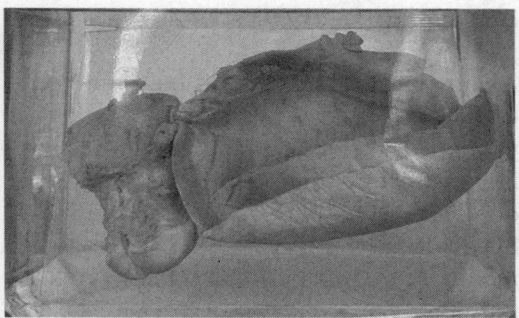

Fig. 10: Serous cystadenoma of ovary.
(For color version, see Plate 14)

proper suction or use of endo-bag, as it can result in peritonitis. If spill occurs, thorough peritoneal wash should be given to avoid peritonitis.

When a patient comes with acute abdomen due to torsion of the cyst, what precautions will you take to apply the clamp over the twisted pedicle?

It is wiser to first untwist the infundibulopelvic ligament and then apply the clamp in order to avoid injury to ureter. However, the previous logic of applying clamp to a twisted pedicle was the risk of embolization of the contents of the cyst **(Fig. 9)**.

■ BENIGN OVARIAN TUMOR

Identify the specimens shown in Figures 10 and 11.

These are specimens of ovarian cysts, probably a serous cystadenoma **(Fig. 10)** and mucinous cystadenoma **(Fig. 11)**.

How did you make this diagnosis?

A serous cystadenoma is usually uniloculated but may be associated with more than one cyst, while a mucinous cystadenoma is usually multiloculated. The fluid is thin in serous tumors, while mucinous tumors have a thick mucoid content.

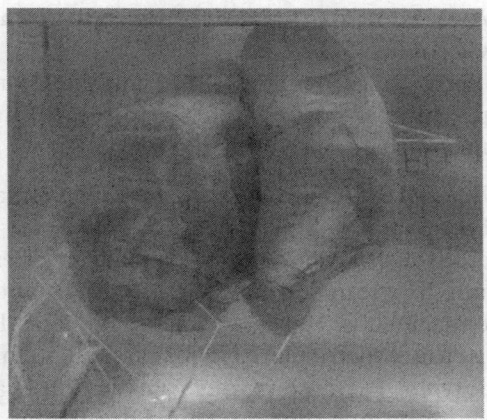

Fig. 11: Mucinous cystadenoma of ovary.
(For color version, see Plate 14)

Do you think this cyst is benign or malignant?

The cyst is probably a benign cyst because the walls and septa are thin and there is no solid component and no papillary excrescences either within or on the surface of the cyst.

What are the features of a benign ovarian mass?

Benign ovarian masses usually occur in the reproductive age group. They are smooth, cystic, unilateral, freely mobile, and not associated with ascites.

What was the surgery done?

The procedure done was an oophorectomy. No part of tube is visualized.

Is a complete staging required in this patient?
A complete staging should be done and if confined to one ovary and the patient is young, a unilateral salpingo-oophorectomy is done. Many a time, complete staging is not done and when malignancy is reported on histopathology, repeat surgery for staging is mandatory. Thus peritoneal fluid cytology, thorough exploration, omental biopsy, and peritoneal biopsies must be done at the primary surgery.

What is the most common epithelial ovarian tumor?
Serous cystadenomas are the most common epithelial ovarian tumors followed by mucinous tumors.

What are the features of serous cystadenoma of the ovary?
Serous ovarian tumors are typically smaller than mucinous tumors, unilocular and homogeneous. They are sometimes bilateral, and this is particularly so for the malignant subtypes. Psammomatous calcification is a feature of serous but not mucinous subtypes.

What are the features of mucinous ovarian cystadenoma?
These tumors are lined by columnar epithelium, typically similar to endocervical or intestinal epithelium. These cells secrete thick, gelatinous mucin which fills the locules. USG shows a typically large cystic adnexal mass, multilocular with numerous thin septations. Loculations may contain low-level internal echogenicity due to increased mucin content. Tumor marker CA-19-9 may be raised even in benign tumors. CA-125 is not raised.

Are there any special features of a mucinous cystadenoma?
Mucinous cystadenomas may reach a very large size and are associated with dermoid cysts and Brenner tumors.

■ MALIGNANT OVARIAN TUMOR

Identify the Specimen shown in Figure 12.
This is a mounted specimen of ovarian malignancy.

What are the various histologic types of epithelial carcinoma?
The FIGO endorses the WHO histologic typing of epithelial ovarian tumors.

The histologic classification of ovarian, fallopian tube, and peritoneal neoplasia is as follows:
- Serous tumors
- Mucinous tumors
- Endometrioid tumors
- Clear cell tumors
- Brenner tumors
- Undifferentiated carcinomas (this group of malignant tumors is of epithelial structure, but they are too poorly differentiated to be placed in any other group)
- Mixed epithelial tumors (these tumors are composed of two or more of the five major cell types of common epithelial tumors. The types are usually specified)

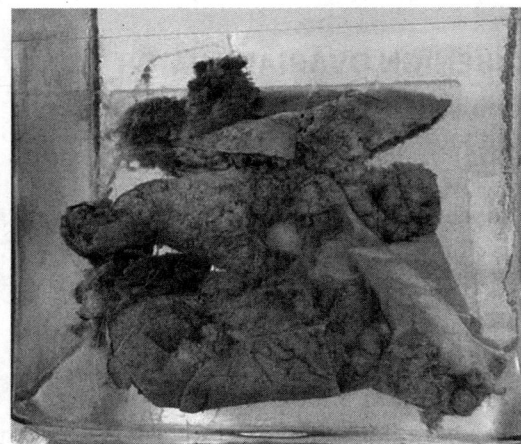

Fig. 12: Papillary serous cystadenocarcinoma of ovary. *(For color version, see Plate 14)*

- Cases with high-grade serous carcinoma in which the ovaries and fallopian tubes appear to be incidentally involved and not the primary origin can be labeled as peritoneal serous carcinoma of undesignated site, at the discretion of the pathologist.

What are the various etiological factors associated with the development of ovarian malignancy?

Ovarian malignancy is associated with early menarche, nulliparity, infertility, use of asbestos and talc, marked premenstrual tension or marked dysmenorrhea, history of pelvic irradiation, history of repeated gonadotropin stimulation, past history of mumps or rubella.

Other high-risk factors are family history of carcinoma ovary, history of breast malignancy, and history of abnormal ovarian function.

Parity, oral contraceptive use, history of breastfeeding, tubal ligation, and hysterectomy have been associated with decreased risk of ovarian cancer.

What is the genetic risk for epithelial ovarian cancer?

Women who have one first-degree relative with ovarian cancer have a 5% risk and women with two first-degree relatives have a 7% risk of developing ovarian cancer. Familial ovarian cancer syndrome comprising three distinct autosomal dominant syndromes, that is, site-specific ovary, breast ovary, and Lynch-II syndrome, is associated with a combination of familial colon cancer (Lynch-I) and a high rate of ovarian, endometrial, breast cancer, and other malignancies of the GI and genitourinary systems. Also, *BRCA-1* and to a smaller extent *BRCA-2* genes have been associated with breast and ovarian cancer.

What is the usual clinical presentation of a patient with ovarian malignancy?

A patient with ovarian cancer may have no symptoms for a long period and when the symptoms develop, they are nonspecific in the form of abdominal discomfort, bloating, and gastrointestinal symptoms. A premenopausal female may develop irregular vaginal bleeding. A pelvic mass compressing bladder or rectum may cause urinary frequency or constipation. Occasionally, lower abdominal pain or distention may develop. In an advanced stage disease, the patient may develop ascites, omental metastasis, or bowel metastases.

On examination, presence of a pelvic mass, which is solid, irregular, and fixed, is highly suggestive of an ovarian malignancy.

What is the role of tumor marker CA-125?

CA-125 has been shown to contribute to the early diagnosis of epithelial ovarian cancer. Elevated levels are found in 82% of patients who have surgically demonstrable epithelial ovarian cancer. Rising or falling levels have correlated with disease progression or regression in more than 90% of the patients. A cutoff of 35 U/mL is chosen for the upper limit of normal. It may rise in other conditions like acute hepatitis, pancreatitis, chronic liver disease, colitis, congestive heart failure, diverticulitis, pneumonia, etc.

What is the risk malignancy index?

Risk malignancy index is calculated after multiplying USG score, menopausal status, and CA-125 level. Malignancy is suspected if score is >250.

What is the workup of malignant epithelial ovarian tumors?

The primary workup for patients with clinical signs or symptoms of ovarian cancer should include an abdominal/pelvic US and/or abdominal/pelvic CT/MRI scan. US is typically used for initial evaluation, as it has been shown to be effective at triaging the majority of adnexal masses into benign or malignant categories. Other imaging modalities may be helpful when the results of US are indeterminate (i.e., either the organ of origin or malignant potential is unclear) and may improve assessment of metastases, staging, and preoperative planning. FDG-PET/CT scan may also be useful for indeterminate lesions. The National Comprehensive Cancer Network (NCCN) panel recommends PET/CT or MRI for indeterminate lesions if they will alter management.

For assessment of abdominopelvic metastases for preoperative staging, estimation of resectability, and surgical planning, abdominal/pelvic CT or MRI is generally more useful than US. All CT/MRI imaging should be performed with contrast unless contraindicated.

Appropriate laboratory studies include complete blood count (CBC) and chemistry profile with liver function test.

Biomarker tests comparing preoperative serum levels to postoperative final diagnosis include serum HE4 and CA-125, either alone or combined using the risk of ovarian malignancy.

What is the role of tumor markers in ovarian malignancy?

Serum CA-125 levels tend to correlate with the clinical course of disease, especially in those with elevated pretreatment levels, so they can be useful for monitoring response to therapy and surveillance for recurrence.

The NCCN guidelines currently do not recommend routine HE4 as part of preoperative workup. In addition to CA-125, the NCCN guidelines mention that other tumor markers may be used as part of preoperative workup, if clinically indicated:

Inhibin, alpha-fetoprotein (AFP), beta-human chorionic gonadotropin (beta-hCG), lactate dehydrogenase (LDH), carcinoembryonic antigen (CEA), and CA19-9.

Alpha fetoprotein (AFP), beta-hCG, and LDH are markers for malignant germ cell tumors that can be helpful in intraoperative diagnosis, preoperative planning, and post-treatment monitoring for recurrence. AFP can be produced by endodermal sinus (yolk sac) tumors, embryonal carcinomas, polyembryomas, and immature teratomas; beta-hCG can be produced by choriocarcinomas, embryonal carcinomas, polyembryomas, and, in low levels, in some dysgerminomas; and LDH can be a marker for dysgerminoma.

Sex cord-stromal tumors of the ovary, particularly granulosa cell tumors, can produce inhibin, and inhibin expression level in tumor tissue and serum have been proposed as diagnostic markers.

Elevated serum CEA is a marker associated with gastrointestinal (GI) primary cancers, but can also occur in patients with ovarian malignancies, particularly mucinous tumors. A ratio of serum CA-125 to CEA > 25 has been proposed for differentiating ovarian cancer from colorectal cancer. CA19-9 is another marker that is elevated more often in mucinous tumors compared with other ovarian cancer types.

What are the treatment guidelines for early stage disease (stages I, II) of ovarian cancer?

Staging laparotomy: A thorough staging laparotomy is an important part of early management. If the preoperative suspicion is malignancy, a laparotomy should be performed. If there is no visible or palpable evidence of metastasis, the following should be performed for adequate staging:

- Careful evaluation of all peritoneal surfaces
- Retrieval of any peritoneal fluid or ascites. If there is none, washings of the peritoneal cavity should be performed.
- Infracolic omentectomy
- Selective lymphadenectomy of the pelvic and para-aortic lymph nodes, at least ipsilateral if the malignancy is unilateral
- Biopsy or resection of any suspicious lesions, masses, or adhesions
- Random peritoneal biopsies of normal surfaces, including from the undersurface of the right hemidiaphragm, bladder reflection, cul-de-sac, right and left paracolic recesses, and both pelvic sidewalls
- TAH and BSO in most cases
- Appendectomy for mucinous tumors if the appendix appears abnormal
- In patients with stage I and favorable histologic grade and desirous of childbearing, unilateral salpingo-oophorectomy may be performed. Complete surgery (TAH with BSO) may be performed after childbearing is complete.

What are the treatment options for advanced-stage disease (stages III and IV)?
Neoadjuvant chemotherapy (NACT) with interval debulking surgery (IDS) should be considered in patients with advanced-stage ovarian cancer who are not good candidates for upfront primary debulking surgery (PDS) due to advanced age, frailty, poor performance status, comorbidities, or who have disease unlikely to be optimally cytoreduced. Patients treated with NACT and IDS should also receive postoperative adjuvant chemotherapy.

Primary cytoreductive surgery is followed by combination chemotherapy. RT (external beam whole abdomen or intraperitoneal instillation of radioactive chromium phosphate) is used after or combined with chemotherapy. Use of RT appears at present to be limited to patients with minimal (<1 cm) residual disease after surgery.

What are the tumor markers specific for germ cell tumors?
Human chorionic gonadotropin, AFP, and LDH are useful in the diagnosis and management of these tumors. AFP is also useful in immature teratomas, endodermal sinus tumor, polyembryoma, and mixed germ cell tumor. hCG is also specific for dysgerminoma **(Fig. 13)**, embryonal carcinoma, and choriocarcinoma. LDH is specific for dysgerminoma.

What is the characteristic feature of sex cord-stromal tumor?
Sex cord-stromal tumors account for 5–10% of all ovarian cancer. Patients present with hormonal symptoms like precocious puberty, amenorrhea, PMB, or virilization. So, patients usually present with stage I disease. Of these tumors, granulosa cell tumors secrete estrogen

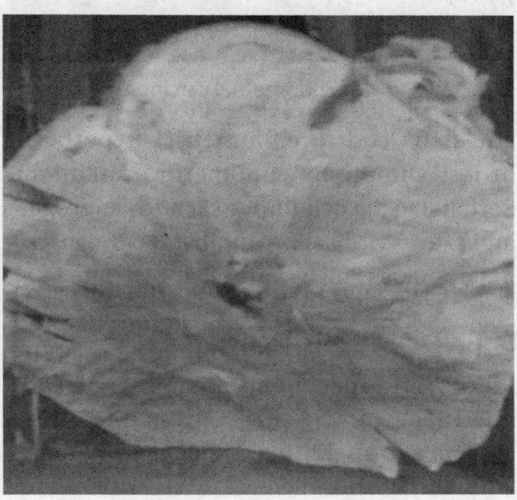

Fig. 13: Dysgerminoma of ovary.

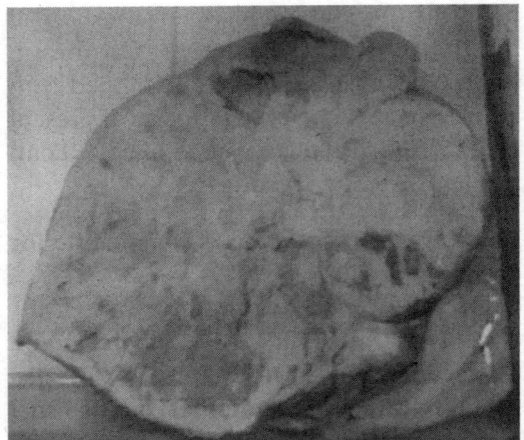

Fig. 14: Granulosa cell tumor of ovary.

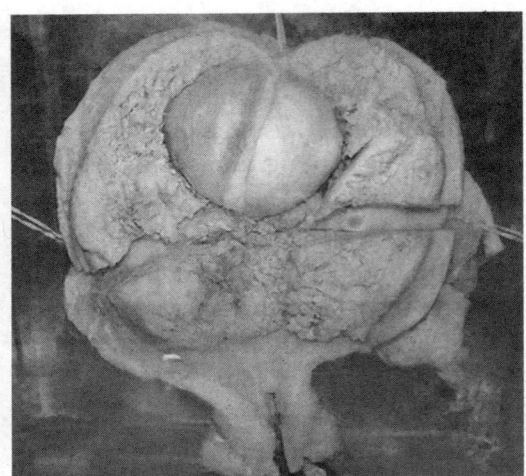

Fig. 16: Endometrial carcinoma with fibroid.

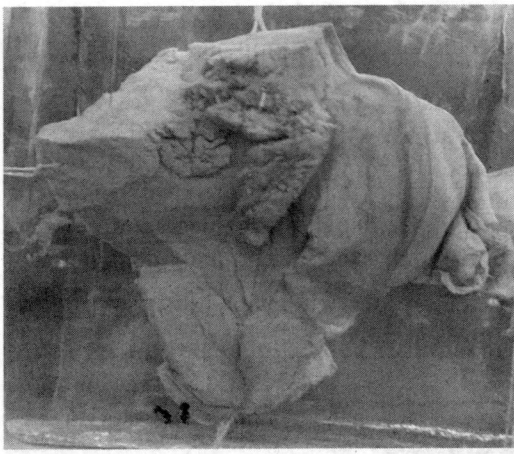

Fig. 15: Endometrial carcinoma.

and may lead to endometrial hyperplasia or less commonly endometrial carcinoma. Sertoli–Leydig cell tumor secretes androgens and causes virilization. Inhibin B is the marker for granulosa cell tumors **(Fig. 14)**.

■ ENDOMETRIAL CANCER

Identify the specimen shown in **Figures 15 and 16**.

It is a formalin-fixed specimen of uterus with cervix and bilateral tubes with ovaries showing endometrial growth.

What was the surgery done?
The surgery done was TAH with BSO.

Is this surgery sufficient for all cases of carcinoma endometrium?
Ideally, the hysterectomy specimen must be subjected to a frozen section analysis. If on frozen section the carcinoma is confined to the endometrium, grade 1 or 2, then the above procedure is sufficient. But any carcinoma, which is above stage 1a G1 or 2 would require a pelvic and paraaortic lymphadenectomy.

What is the staging of carcinoma endometrium (FIGO)?
There is a novel change in the staging of endometrial cancer now and it is based on molecular biology. For details, refer to genital malignancy Chapter 35.

What are the pathogenic types of endometrial cancers?
Refer to genital malignancy Chapter 35.

How is carcinoma endometrium staged?
Carcinoma endometrium, like most other gynecological malignancies, is staged by a surgical pathological system and the final stage is given after the histopathology report

of surgical specimen. However, in patients who are inoperable, the clinical staging system is followed.

What are the risk factors for endometrial cancer?

Endogenous or exogenous estrogen excess is a risk for endometrial cancer. The endogenous risk factors include early menarche, late menopause, nulliparity, PCOS, obesity, estrogen-producing ovarian tumors, etc. The exogenous risk factors would include hormone-replacement therapy and tamoxifen use.

How do you workup a case of carcinoma endometrium?

Histopathologic tumor type and grade in EB is required (IV, A).

Preoperative mandatory workup includes family history; general assessment and inventory of comorbidities; geriatric assessment, if appropriate; clinical examination, including pelvic examination; expert transvaginal or transrectal ultrasound or pelvic MRI.

Depending on clinical and pathologic risk, additional imaging modalities (thoracic, abdominal and pelvic CT scan, MRI, PET scan, or ultrasound) should be considered to assess ovarian, nodal, peritoneal, and other sites of metastatic disease.

Intraoperative frozen section is not encouraged for myometrial invasion assessment because of poor reproducibility and interference with adequate pathologic processing.

What is the treatment of carcinoma endometrium?

Role of minimally invasive surgery in endometrial carcinoma.

Minimally invasive surgery is the preferred surgical approach, including patients with high-risk endometrial carcinoma (I, A).

Any intraperitoneal tumor spillage, including tumor rupture or morcellation (including in a bag), should be avoided (III, B).

If vaginal extraction risks uterine rupture, other measures should be taken (e.g., mini-laparotomy, use of endobag) (III, B).

Tumors with metastases outside the uterus and cervix (excluding lymph node metastases) are relative contraindications for minimally invasive surgery (III, B).

What is the management of early stage endometrial carcinoma?

Standard surgical procedures: Standard surgery is total hysterectomy with BSO without vaginal cuff resection (II, A).

Staging infracolic omentectomy should be performed in clinical stage I serous endometrial carcinoma, carcinosarcoma, and undifferentiated carcinoma. It can be omitted in clear cell and endometrioid carcinoma in stage I disease (IV, B).

Surgical re-staging can be considered in previously incompletely staged patients with high- intermediate-risk/high-risk disease if the outcome might have an implication for adjuvant treatment strategy (IV, B).

Lymph node staging: Lymph node staging should be performed in patients with intermediate-high/high-risk patients.

Sentinel lymph node (SLN) biopsy is an adequate alternative to systematic lymphadenectomy for staging proposes for lymph node staging in stage I/II (III, B).

Sentinel lymph node biopsy can also be considered in low/low-intermediate-risk patients to rule out occult lymph node metastases and to identify disease truly confined to the uterus.

If sentinel lymph node biopsy is performed (II, A):

- Indocyanine green with cervical injection is the preferred detection technique.
- Tracer re-injection is an option if sentinel lymph node is not visualized upfront.
- Side-specific systematic lymphadenectomy should be performed in high-intermediate-risk/high-risk patients if sentinel lymph node is not detected on either pelvic side.
- Pathologic ultrastaging of sentinel lymph nodes is recommended.

How would you screen a woman for endometrial cancer?
All patients at high risk for endometrial cancer should be screened. The best screening modality would be an endometrial aspiration using one of the suction devices like Pipelle. In patients with PMB, hysteroscopy and directed biopsies are preferable.

What is the clinical presentation of patients with endometrial cancers?
Patients present initially with menorrhagia followed by menometrorrhagia or PMB. Pyometra and foul-smelling discharge are rare.

What is the class of hysterectomy done in carcinoma endometrium stage Ia?
Class I hysterectomy, i.e., extrafascial TAH with BSO.

When is postoperative adjuvant radiotherapy indicated?
All patients who are at high risk for locoregional recurrence require RT. These include patients with stage 1B grade 3, stage IC, grades 1 and 2, stage II occult grades 1 and 2, and age over 60 years. Patients with aggressive histologic types such as clear cell and papillary tumors also require RT.

What is the management of advanced-stage endometrial cancer?
In stages III and IV endometrial carcinoma (including carcinosarcoma), surgical tumor debulking including enlarged lymph nodes should be considered when complete macroscopic resection is feasible with an acceptable morbidity and quality of life profile, following full preoperative staging and discussion by a multidisciplinary team. Primary systemic therapy should be used if upfront surgery is not feasible or acceptable.

In cases of a good response to systemic therapy, delayed surgery can be considered. Only enlarged lymph nodes should be resected. Systematic lymphadenectomy is not recommended.

What are the poor prognostic factors?
Apart from stage, histologic grade of tumors, depth of myometrial invasion, status of pelvic and paraaortic lymph nodes, presence of malignant cells in peritoneal washings, histologic type of tumors, cervical invasion, adnexal spread, intraperitoneal disease, estrogen–progesterone receptor status, oncogenes, and DNA-ploidy are all prognostic factors affecting survival.

What is the role of hormone therapy?
Hormone therapy is indicated in patients with a recurrence, and hydroxyprogesterone acetate, medroxyprogesterone acetate, megestrol acetate, and tamoxifen have been used.

■ CARCINOMA CERVIX

Identify the specimen shown in Figure 17.
It is a formalin-fixed radical hysterectomy specimen of uterus with cervix (exophytic growth seen), cuff of vagina, and parametrium, with and without fallopian tubes and ovary (tubes and ovaries may be conserved in a young patient).

What was the surgery done?
Type II or III radical hysterectomy with removal of entire parametrium, upper

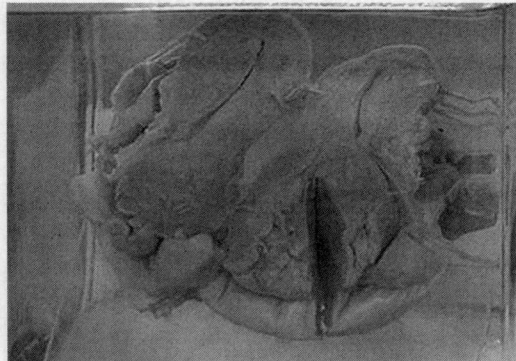

Fig. 17: Cervical carcinoma.
(For color version, see Plate 14)

one-third of vagina, pelvic lymphadenectomy, excision of uterosacrals, and Mackenrodt's ligament. Removal of tubes and ovaries is not part of radical hysterectomy.

What is the incidence of cervical cancer?
Cervical cancer is the most common cancer amongst the Indian women accounting for 23% of all the cancers with an incidence of 19.4–43.5/100,000 women.

Discuss the staging of carcinoma cervix (FIGO).
Refer to genital malignancy Chapter 35.

What are the risk factors for carcinoma cervix?
- Younger age at intercourse
- Multiple sexual partners
- Sexually transmitted disease (STD)
- Human papillomavirus (HPV) infection (16 and 18 being most common)
- Prolonged use of OCP
- Immunosuppression
- Cigarette smoking

What are the investigations allowed by FIGO for staging purposes?
The diagnosis of cervical cancer is established histopathologically from a cervical biopsy [punch, loop electrosurgical excision procedure (LEEP), and cone biopsy]. The next step is to evaluate all pelvic organs to see whether the cancer is confined to the cervix or has extended to vagina, parametrium, bladder, ureters, or rectum. Extension to uterus although disregarded for staging purposes is useful for prognosis. Cervical cancer (apart from vaginal cancer) is the only gynecologic cancer staged clinically. Pelvic examination (per vaginal, per vaginal/rectal or PVR and rectal examination) preferably under general anesthesia (not required in all cases) along with certain diagnostic tests given below will help assign the stage.

For clinical staging, FIGO allows certain diagnostic studies such as intravenous pyelogram (IVP), cystoscopy, proctosigmoidoscopy, barium enema, and colposcopy of vagina and vaginal fornices.

What is the primary management of carcinoma cervix?
The primary treatment of early-stage cervical cancer is either surgery or RT. Surgery is typically reserved for early-stage disease, fertility preservation, and smaller lesions, such as stages IA, IB1, IB2, and selected IIA1.

What are the types of radical hysterectomy?
Types of radical hysterectomy are given in **Table 3**.

What is the role of fertility-sparing treatment of carcinoma cervix?
Microinvasive disease [FIGO stage IA1 with no lymphovascular space invasion (LVSI)] is associated with an extremely low incidence of lymphatic metastasis, and conservative treatment with conization is an option (category 2A) for individuals with no evidence of LVSI. In stage IA1 individuals with evidence of LVSI, a reasonable conservative approach is conization (with negative margins) in addition to SLN mapping algorithm or pelvic lymphadenectomy.

TABLE 3: Types of radical hysterectomy.

	Simple extrafascial hysterectomy	Modified radical hysterectomy	Radical hysterectomy
Diver and Rutledge Classification	Type I	Type II	Type III
Queried and Morrow classification	Type A	Type B	Type C
Indication	Stage IA1	Type IA1 with LVSI, IA2	Stages 1B1 and 1B2, selected cases of stage IIA
Uterus and cervix	Removed	Removed	Removed
Ovaries	Optional removal	Optional removal	Optional removal
Vaginal margin	None	1–2 cm	Upper one-quarter to one-third
Ureters	Not mobilized	Tunnel through broad ligament	Tunnel through broad ligament
Cardinal ligaments	Divided at uterine and cervical border	Divided where ureter transits broad ligaments	Divided at pelvic side wall
Uterosacral ligaments	Divided at cervical border	Partially removed	Divided near sacral origin
Urinary bladder	Mobilized to base of bladder	Mobilized to upper vagina	Mobilized to middle vagina
Rectum	Not mobilized	Mobilized below cervix	Mobilized below cervix
Surgical approach	Laparotomy or laparoscopy or robotic surgery	Laparotomy or laparoscopy or robotic surgery	Laparotomy or laparoscopy or robotic surgery

(LVSI: lymphovascular space invasion)

The panel recommends cold knife conization as the preferred approach to conization. However, LEEP is acceptable as long as adequate margins, proper orientation, and a nonfragmented specimen without an electrosurgical artifact can be obtained. Endocervical curettage should be added as clinically indicated.

Select patients with stages IA2 and IB1, especially for those with tumors of <2 cm in diameter, as they may be eligible for conservative surgery. Radical trachelectomy may offer a reasonable fertility-sparing treatment option for patients with stages IA2 and IB1, and select IB2 cervical cancer with lesions that are ≤2 cm in diameter. In a radical trachelectomy, the cervix, vaginal margins, and supporting ligaments are removed while leaving the main body and fundus of the uterus intact. Laparoscopic pelvic lymphadenectomy accompanies the procedure and can be performed with or without SLN mapping.

Due to their aggressive nature, tumors of small cell neuroendocrine histology are considered inappropriate for radical trachelectomy. Trachelectomy is also inappropriate for treating gastric-type cervical adenocarcinoma and adenoma malignum (minimal deviation adenocarcinoma) due to their diagnostic challenges and potentially aggressive nature.

Vaginal radical trachelectomy (VRT) may be used for carefully selected patients with lesions of 2 cm diameter or less. Abdominal radical trachelectomy (ART) provides a broader resection of the parametria than the vaginal approach and is commonly used in stage IB1 lesions.

What is nonfertility-sparing treatment of carcinoma cervix?

Approaches to hysterectomy include simple/extrafascial hysterectomy (type A), modified radical hysterectomy (type B), and radical hysterectomy (type C). For patients with IA1 disease, cone excision, simple/extrafascial hysterectomy, and modified radical hysterectomy are options. Radical hysterectomy with bilateral pelvic lymph node dissection (with or without SLN mapping) is the preferred treatment approach for patients with FIGO stage IA2, IB1, IB2, and IIA1 cervical cancers. In the United States, definitive chemoradiation is typically preferred over radical surgery for select patients with FIGO IB3 lesions and the vast majority of FIGO stage IIA2 or greater cervical cancers.

The panel agrees that concurrent chemoradiation is generally the primary treatment of choice for stages IB3 to IVA disease based on the results of five randomized clinical trials. Chemoradiation can also be used for patients who are not candidates for hysterectomy.

To preserve intrinsic hormonal function, ovarian transposition may be considered before pelvic RT for select women younger than 45 years of age with squamous cell cancers.

Concurrent chemoradiation, using platinum-containing chemotherapy [cisplatin alone (preferred) or cisplatin/fluorouracil], is the treatment of choice for stages IB3, II, III, and IVA disease based on the results of randomized clinical trials.

What is the role of pelvic exenteration in recurrence?

For recurrent or persistent cervical cancers that are confined to the central pelvis (i.e., no distant metastasis), pelvic exenteration may be a potentially curative surgical option.

What is the role of neoadjuvant chemotherapy before surgery?

In areas where RT facilities are scarce, NACT has been used with the goal of (1) downstaging of the tumor to improve the radical curability and safety of surgery and (2) inhibition of micrometastasis and distant metastasis. There is no unanimity of view as to whether it improves prognosis compared with the standard treatment. The extent of surgery after NACT remains the same, i.e., radical hysterectomy and pelvic lymphadenectomy. However, it must be remembered that NACT may give a false sense of security by masking the pathologic findings and thus affecting the evaluation of indication for adjuvant RT/CCRT. NACT surgery is best reserved for research settings or those areas where RT is unavailable. This is especially true in patients with very large tumors or adenocarcinoma, which have lower response rates.

What are the screening guidelines for Pap's smear?

Screening should be done in women in the age group of 21–65 years of age; repeat every 3 years if Pap's normal. After 30 years of age, HPV DNA testing is added (co-testing) or primary HPV testing can be done; repeat every 5 years, if normal.

What is Sedlis criteria?
The Sedlis criteria defines risk factors for recurrence warranting posthysterectomy radiation for early stage cervical cancer; however, these factors were defined for squamous cell carcinoma at an estimated recurrence risk of ≥30%.

The "Sedlis criteria," which are intermediate risk factors used to guide adjuvant treatment decisions, include:
- Greater than one-third stromal invasion
- Capillary lymphatic space involvement
- Cervical tumor diameters >4 cm

However, potentially important risk factors for recurrence may not be limited to the Sedlis criteria. Additional risk factors for consideration include tumor histology (e.g., adenocarcinoma component) and close or positive surgical margins.

What is the lymph node involvement in various stages?
- *Stage IA1:* 0–0.5%
- *Stage 1A2:* 7–9%
- *Stage IB:* 12–20%
- *Stage II:* 16–35%
- *Stage III:* >35%
- *Stage IV:* >50%

Lymphatic drainage of the cervix
It can be remembered using the acronyms HOPE and SAC:
- *Primary lymph node drainage:*
  - Hypogastric, obturator, parametrial, and external iliac
- *Secondary lymph nodes:*
  - Sacral, aortic (para-aortic), and common iliac

What are the morphologic and histopathologic types of tumor?
Morphologic types:
- Exophytic or cauliflower-like growth
- Endophytic
- Ulcerative

Histopathologic types:
- Squamous cell carcinoma of cervix (70–80%):
  - Large-cell keratinizing
  - Large-cell nonkeratinizing
- Small cell keratinizing
- Adenocarcinoma (20–27%)
- Adenosquamous
- Sarcomas (rare <0.5%)

What is the clinical presentation of cervical cancers?
There are four cardinal symptoms and signs:
Symptoms
1. Foul-smelling discharge
2. Bleeding—postcoital and intermenstrual
3. Pain—advanced stage
4. Cachexia—advanced stage

Signs
1. Contact bleeding
2. Friability
3. Induration
4. Fixity

What are the poor prognostic factors?
Stage of disease is the most important prognostic factor followed by depth of stromal invasion and size of tumor in early stage of disease. These factors are now taken into consideration in FIGO's staging. Other prognostic factors are extension to endometrial cavity, pelvic, and para-aortic lymph node metastases, histologic tumor grade, and lymphovascular space involvement (LVSI).

What are the various sites that the ureter can be injured in radical hysterectomy?
When ureters enter pelvic brim crossing common iliac vessels (retroperitoneal dissection done till common iliac vessels for lymphadenectomy):
- While ligating infundibular pelvic ligaments (ureters lie anteromedial to this ligament)

- At the ureteric tunnel where the uterine artery crosses the ureter
- At the level of uterosacral ligaments
- At the level of vaginal fornix before the ureter enters the bladder

What are the branches of internal iliac artery?

The internal iliac artery is 4 cm long and is a branch of the common iliac artery. It divides into anterior branch and posterior branch. The *anterior branch* is a continuation of the main vessel and divides into five visceral arteries, namely (1) superior vesical (supplies lower ureter and upper bladder and continues as an obliterated umbilical artery), (2) inferior vesical (supplies ureter and bladder base), (3) middle rectal (muscle of lower rectum and anastomoses with superior and inferior rectal arteries), (4) uterine (uterus, ureteric branch, vaginal, and anastomoses with ovarian artery), and (5) vaginal arteries may arise from internal iliac. The parietal branches are obturator, internal pudendal, and inferior gluteal arteries.

The *posterior branch* passes backward and gives an ascending branch; iliolumbar, superior and inferior lateral sacral, and superior gluteal artery.

How does the ureter get its blood supply?

The abdominal part of the ureter is supplied by branches from the renal, aortic, common iliac, and ovarian arteries. The blood supply in this part is from the lateral side. The pelvic part of the ureter is supplied by branches from the uterine, superior and inferior vesical arteries, and is to the medial side of ureter.

■ CARCINOMA VULVA

Describe the specimen shown in Figure 18.

These are specimens of vulva showing clitoris anteriorly, both labia majora laterally and hymenal opening in the center. There is a tumor on the left labia majora.

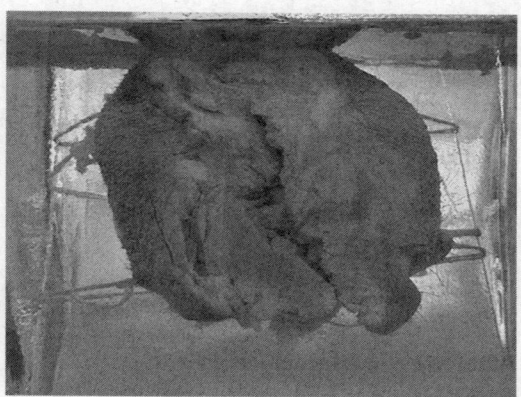

Fig. 18: Vulval carcinoma.
(For color version, see Plate 14)

What is the incidence of vulval cancer?

Vulval cancer represents about 4% of malignancies of the female genital tract. The estimated incidence is about 1–2/100,000 women.

What are the etiologic factors for development of vulval cancer?

- Patients suffering from STD
- Patients with multiple sexual partners
- History of genital warts
- Smoking
- HPV infection
- Patients with lymphogranuloma venereum and granuloma inguinale
- Vulvar dystrophies carry a risk of 0–9% of progression to carcinoma, more commonly squamous cell hyperplasia and lichen sclerosus
- Immunosuppression

How is the disease different in the human papillomavirus-positive group?

These groups of patients are characterized by a younger mean age, more tobacco use, and presence of vulvar intraepithelial neoplasia (VIN) in association with the invasive component. HPV 16 and 33 are the prevalent subtypes.

What are the types of vulval cancer?
The most common is squamous carcinoma (92%), melanoma (2–4%), basal cell (2–3%), Bartholin gland carcinoma (1%), and sarcoma (<1%).

What is microinvasive squamous carcinoma?
Vulval lesions <2 cm with <1 mm stromal invasion are called microinvasive.

What are the clinical features?
Carcinoma vulva is predominantly a disease of postmenopausal women, the mean age being 65 years.
- *Pruritus*—it is the most common symptom
- Vulval bleeding or discharge
- Vulval lump or mass
- Dysuria

What are the investigations that should be done in these patients?
- *Wedge biopsy:* If lesion is <1 cm, excisional biopsy should be done
- Pap's smear
- Colposcopy of the cervix, vagina, and vulva

How does vulval cancer spread?
- Direct extension to include adjacent structures such as vagina, urethra, and anus
- Lymphatic embolization to regional lymph nodes
- Hematogenous spread to distant sites like lung and liver, which is usually late

Describe the lymphatic metastases in these patients.
Initially, spread is to inguinal lymph nodes located between Camper's fascia and fascia lata (8–10 on each side). From these superficial groin nodes, the tumor cells spread to deep femoral nodes, which are located along the femoral vessels (3–4 on each side). Cloquet's node, situated beneath the inguinal ligament, is the most cephalad of the femoral node group. From the inguinal-femoral nodes, cancer spreads to the pelvic nodes, particularly the external iliac group. Lymphatic drainage from the clitoris, centrally located tumors, anterior labia minora, and perineum is bilateral.

What is the incidence of lymph node metastases in vulval cancer?
The actual incidence is 30%. About 20% of patients with positive groin nodes have positive pelvic nodes. The incidence is related to depth of tumor invasion. It is very rare, if tumor invasion is <1 mm, about 7–8, if 1–3 mm, 25% if 3–5 mm, and rises to 35% if invasion is >5 mm.

What is the difference between simple and radical vulvectomy?
In radical vulvectomy, the depth of dissection extends up to the inferior fascia of urogenital diaphragm.

What are the postoperative complications after radical vulvectomy?
Early complications
- Groin wound infection and breakdown
- Seroma—occurs in 10–15% of cases in the femoral triangle. It is managed by periodic sterile aspiration
- Urinary tract infection
- Deep vein thrombosis and pulmonary embolism
- Loss of sensations on anterior thigh due to damage to femoral nerve, which then resolves slowly
- Osteitis pubis

Late complications
- Chronic leg edema in 7% patients
- Recurrent lymphangitis or cellulitis of leg occurs in 10%

- Urinary stress incontinence is seen in 10% cases. It may be associated with genital prolapse
- Introital stenosis, dyspareunia, and psychosexual disturbances
- Femoral hernia
- Pubic osteomyelitis

What are the prognostic factors for vulval cancer?

- Number of positive groin nodes is the single most important variable
- *Stage of the disease:* 5-year survival rates are 95% for stage I, 85% for stage II, 74% for stage III, and 31% for stage IV
- *Poor differentiation on histology:* Tumor ploidy with aneuploid tumor having 23% and diploid tumor 62% 5-year survival
- Tumor size
- Depth of stromal invasion and lymphovascular space involvement

What are the problems associated with the revised International Federation of Gynecology and Obstetrics (FIGO) staging for vulval cancer?

- Patients with negative lymph nodes have a very good prognosis regardless of the size of the primary tumor
- Stage III represents a very heterogeneous group of patients, ranging from those with negative nodes and involvement of the distal urethra or vagina to those with multiple positive groin nodes, who have a very poor prognosis.

What is the treatment of vulval cancer?

- *Stage IA:* <1 mm stromal invasion. In these patients, lymph node metastases are virtually nil. So, radical local excision with 1 cm tumor-free margin is recommended.
- *Stage IB:* >1 mm invasion. Radical local excision with unilateral inguinal femoral (IF) lymphadenectomy. If a lesion involves anterior labia minora or clitoris, bilateral lymph node dissection is done because of the frequent contralateral lymph flow from this region.
  If one microscopically positive groin lymph node—no additional therapy
  If more than two positive lymph nodes—postoperative groin and pelvic radiation
- *Stages II and III:* Radical vulvectomy with bilateral inguinofemoral lymphadenectomy. Pelvic lymphadenectomy is done, if primary lesion includes clitoris or Bartholin gland.
- *Stage IV:* Preoperative radiation with/without concurrent chemotherapy followed by bilateral groin node dissection.

What is the role of radiation therapy in vulval cancer?

- Adjuvant therapy following initial surgery
- Part of primary therapy in locally advanced disease
- For secondary therapy/palliation in recurrent/metastatic disease

Postoperative adjuvant treatment should be initiated as soon as adequate healing is achieved, preferably within 6–8 weeks. Classic indications for treating the primary site include close/positive margin, LVSI, and >5-mm depth of invasion; groin involvement may also be considered a relative indication to include the primary site.

Tumor-directed external beam radiation therapy (EBRT) is directed to the vulva and/or inguinofemoral, external, and internal iliac nodal regions.

What is the role of chemotherapy?

It is mostly used as a neoadjuvant in advanced vulval cancers. Drugs used are bleomycin, cisplatin, and 5-fluorouracil.

How has the treatment of vulval carcinoma changed over the years?
- Individualization of treatment for all patients with invasive disease
- Omission of groin dissection for patients with stage Ia (<1 mm invasion)
- The use of separate groin incisions for groin dissection to improve wound healing, i.e., triple incision technique over en bloc technique
- Omission of contralateral groin dissection with lateral stage IB lesions and negative ipsilateral nodes
- The use of preoperative radiation therapy to obviate the need for exenteration in patients with advanced disease

What is the stage-wise treatment of vulvar cancer?

Stage IA
Microinvasive vulvar cancer

Lesion measuring 2 cm or less in diameter, with a depth of invasion of 1.0 mm or less

Treatment—radical wide local excision and groin node dissection are not necessary (FIGO 2021)

Simple partial vulvectomy, inguinofemoral lymph node (IFLN) evaluation not required (NCCN 2023)

<1% risk of lymphatic metastases

Stage IB
Lateral lesion—radical partial vulvectomy with unilateral IFLND/SLN

Central lesion/(Lateral >4 cm)—radical partial vulvectomy with bilateral IFLND/SLN (NCCN 2023)

Gold standard—radical wide local excision of the tumor (FIGO 2021)

Stage II
FIGO 2021—radical wide local excision with bilateral IFLND/SLN

Small T2 (≤4 cm)—radical partial vulvectomy with bilateral IFLND/SLN

Large T2 (>4 cm)—

Resectable—radical vulvectomy with bilateral IFLND

Unresectable (without removing proximal urethra/bladder/anus)—imaging of LN followed by IFLND.

If positive—EBRT + concurrent chemotherapy to primary tumor/IFLNs/pelvic nodes

If negative—EBRT + concurrent chemotherapy to primary tumor (±selective inguinofemoral LN coverage)

Stage III
Plan EBRT with concurrent chemotherapy followed by pathological response evaluation ± tumor debulking if feasible.

Inguinal femoral lymphadenectomy/imaging may be used to assess nodal metastasis and inform RT treatment planning.

If imaging suggestive of positive positive IFLN, EBRT coverage should include the primary tumor, groin, and pelvic nodes.

If IF lymphadenectomy performed, positive IFLNs on HPE–EBRT coverage should include the primary tumor, groin, and pelvic nodes.

No positive nodes—EBRT with concurrent chemotherapy should be provided with RT coverage of the primary tumor, with or without selective coverage of IFLNs.

In cases where surgery is thought to be inappropriate or exenteration is required for the individual patient, primary chemoradiation is preferred.

Clinically positive nodes, enlarged groin, and pelvic nodes should be removed if possible, and the patient given postoperative groin and pelvic radiation.

Full lymphadenectomy should not be performed because a full groin dissection followed by groin irradiation may result in severe lymphedema.

Surgical excision of the primary tumor with clear surgical margins and without sphincter damage, whenever possible, constitutes the optimum way to treat advanced vulvar cancer, as well as to palliate symptoms such as local pain and offensive discharge (FIGO 2021).

Stage IVA
Ulcerated or fixed groin lymph nodes should be biopsied to confirm the diagnosis and then treated with primary RT, with or without chemosensitization.

If there is an incomplete response to radiation, the nodes may then be resected if appropriate.

An alternative strategy is the use of NACT with cisplatin or carboplatin and paclitaxel, to shrink the nodes prior to RT (FIGO 2021).

Stage IVB
Concurrent chemoradiation

Palliative therapy
Modified radical vulvectomy: Anterior or posterior or lateral hemivulvectomy with clitoral sparing

CHAPTER 21

Imaging: Hysterosalpingogram, X-ray, and CT Scan

Himsweta Srivastava, Richa Aggarwal, Vineeta Rathi

■ HYSTEROSALPINGOGRAM FILMS

Name the investigation shown in Figure 1. What does it show?
This is a hysterosalpingogram (HSG). It shows the uterine cavity and fallopian tubes. Both tubes are patent as free intraperitoneal spill is seen on both sides.

What are the indications for hysterosalpingogram?
- Infertility—primary and secondary
- Recurrent miscarriage
- Congenital abnormalities of the uterus
- Postuterine surgery, e.g., adhesiolysis, myomectomy
- Post-tubal surgery, e.g., assessment of patency after sterilization or reversal of sterilization, reconstructive tubal surgery

What are the absolute contraindications to hysterosalpingogram?
- Pregnancy
- Active pelvic infection
- Bleeding
- Tubal or uterine surgery within last 6 weeks
- Contrast sensitivity

When in the menstrual cycle should hysterosalpingogram be performed?
Hysterosalpingogram should be performed within 10 days of the first day of the menstrual cycle and after bleeding has stopped. The patient should be instructed to abstain from

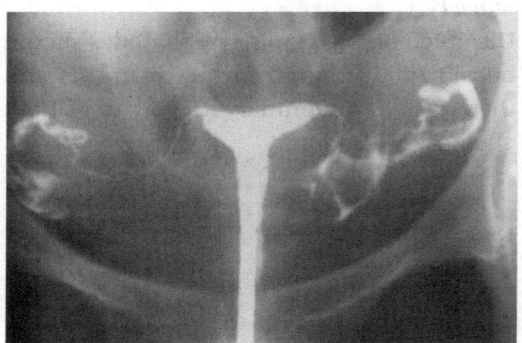

Fig. 1: Normal hysterosalpingogram (HSG).

sexual intercourse from the time menstrual bleeding ends until the day of the study to avoid a potential pregnancy.

What are the complications of hysterosalpingogram?
Pain, bleeding, vasovagal episode, infection, lymphatic or vascular intravasation of dye, irradiation of an early unsuspected pregnancy, allergic reaction, and failure of the procedure are complications of HSG.

Name the parts of the fallopian tube.
Interstitial, isthmic, ampullary, and fimbrial are parts of the fallopian tube.

Which contrast can be used for hysterosalpingogram?
Both oil-based and water-based iodinated contrasts can be used for HSG. Water-soluble dyes have been found to provide better detail of the uterine cavity and mucosal folds of the ampullary portion of the tube and are more

quickly eliminated. Oil-based dyes have been associated with less postprocedure vaginal bleeding, but a higher incidence of lipogranulomas in women as well as a higher rate of allergic reaction. A meta-analysis showed that the most common complication after an HSG with oil-based contrast is intravasation, which was reported in 2.7% of procedures.

Generally, HSG is done using water-soluble contrast, i.e., sodium and meglumine diatrizoate (Urografin 60%, Conray 280, etc.).

How many images are generally taken in a hysterosalpingogram study?

We generally obtain four spot radiographs after the scout radiograph. The first image obtained during early filling of the uterus is used to evaluate for any filling defect or contour abnormality. Small filling defects are best seen at this stage. The second image is obtained with the uterus fully distended. The shape of the uterus is best evaluated at this stage, although small filling defects may be obscured when the uterus is well opacified. The third image is obtained to demonstrate and evaluate the fallopian tubes. The fourth image exhibits free intraperitoneal spillage of contrast material.

What does the investigation in Figure 2 show?

It shows venous intravasation of contrast.

What is the structure marked by the arrow in Figure 2?

The structure is ovarian vein.

When and why does intravasation occur?

- If HSG is undertaken close to either the beginning or the end of the menstrual cycle
- Following recent uterine surgery
- Excessive volume or pressure of contrast medium
- In presence of tubal obstruction

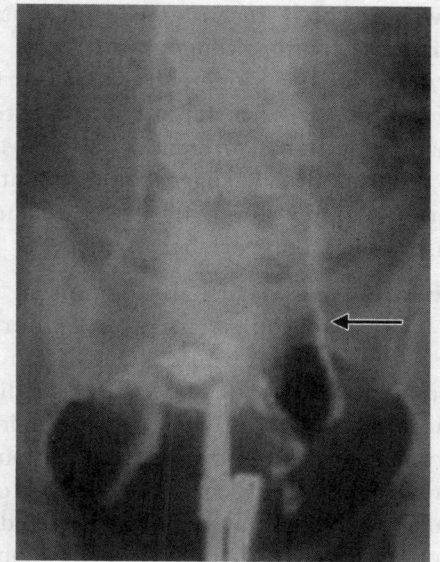

Fig. 2: Venous intravasation.

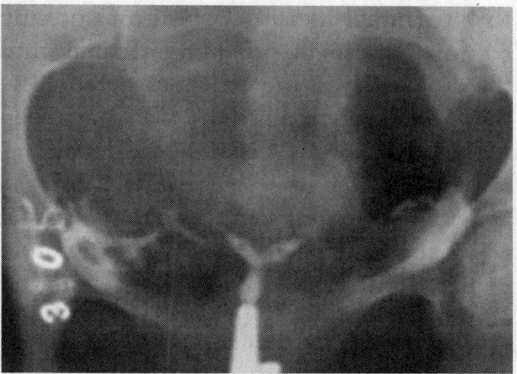

Fig. 3: Bicornuate uterus.

Is the fallopian tube patent?

It is not possible to comment on tubal patency as contrast is flowing into the venous system.

What does the image in Figure 3 show?

It shows a bicornuate uterus.

How does it form or develop?

It forms or develops by the partial fusion of Müllerian ducts.

How can it be differentiated from septate uterus on hysterosalpingogram?
Accuracy of HSG alone is only 55% for the differentiation of a septate uterus from a bicornuate uterus. An angle of <75° between the uterine horns is suggestive of a septate uterus and an angle of >105° is more consistent with a bicornuate uterus.

How would you confirm the diagnosis?
On ultrasonography, in septate uterus, the echogenic endometrial strip is separated at the fundus by the intermediate echogenicity septum (which is isoechoic to myometrium). The external uterine contour is convex, flat, or mildly concave (ideally <1 cm) configuration and may best be appreciated on coronal images of the uterus. Color Doppler may show vascularity in the septum (70% of cases) which, if present, may be associated with a higher rate of obstetric complications. In bicornuate uterus, the external uterine contour is concave or heart-shaped, and the uterine horns are widely divergent. The fundal cleft is typically more than 1 cm deep and the intercornual distance is widened.

On MR images, the septate uterus is generally normal in size and each endometrial cavity appears smaller than the configuration of a normal cavity. The septum may be composed of fibrous tissue (low T2 signal intensity), myometrial tissue (intermediate signal), or both. The bicornuate uterus shows a deep (>1 cm) fundal cleft in the outer uterine contour and an intercornual distance of >4 cm. The uterus demonstrates normal uterine zonal anatomy.

Why is it important to differentiate septate and bicornuate uterus?
The septate uterus is associated with a higher rate of reproductive complications, as the collagenous septum in a septate uterus cannot support a pregnancy as well as the myometrial septum of bicornuate uterus.

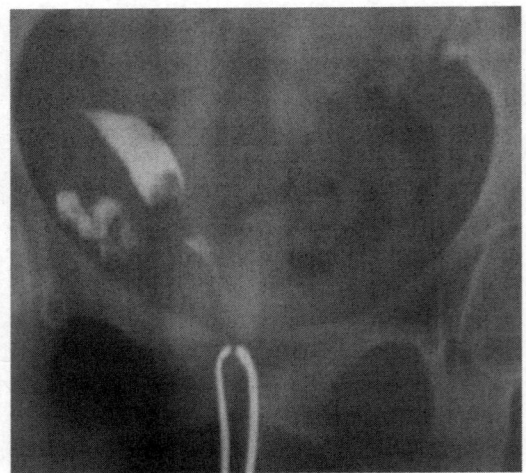

Fig. 4: Unicornuate uterus.

The distinction between a septate uterus and a bicornuate uterus has important management implications. In a septate uterus, the septum can be shaved off during hysteroscopy (metroplasty) to form a single uterine cavity without perforating the uterus. The reproductive outcome has been shown to improve after resection of the septum, with reported decreases in the spontaneous abortion rate from 88 to 6% after hysteroscopic metroplasty. Attempted resection of a bicornuate uterus "septum" leads to a poor outcome.

Figure 4 is a hysterosalpingogram performed with a Foley's catheter in situ. What does it show?
This HSG shows a unicornuate uterus.

What are its developmental associations?
- Failure of development of renal tract on the side of the absent uterine horn
- Presence of a rudimentary horn

How does it form developmentally?
It results from nondevelopment or rudimentary development of one Müllerian duct.

What is the clinical significance of a rudimentary horn?
If a rudimentary horn communicates with the uterine cavity, the patient may benefit from surgical removal of this rudimentary horn.

Figure 5 is a hysterosalpingogram performed with a Foley's catheter in situ. What is the diagnosis?
It shows bilateral hydrosalpinx with loculated peritoneal spill of contrast.

What is the significance of contrast remaining loculated around the tube?
It represents presence of peritubal adhesions.

How can this finding be confirmed?
This finding can be confirmed by laparoscopy with chromotubation or sonohysterosalpingography.

How would you differentiate between hydrosalpinx and loculated peritoneal spill on HSG?
In hydrosalpinx, the tubes appear dilated and tortuous and are folded upon themselves to form a C or S shape. Loculated spillage of contrast in the peritoneal cavity is seen as oval, irregular, or bizarre-shaped collections of contrast near the fimbrial end of the tube. A radiolucent halo may be seen separating the loculated peritubal collection from the dilated tube, known as the "halo sign". This radiolucent halo represents the thickened wall of the tube. On taking delayed HSG films, in loculated spill the contrast may spread out to outline the bowel loops, unlike in a hydrosalpinx.

What does the investigation in Figure 6 show?
This is a HSG showing a well-marginated round filling defect in the uterine cavity.

What is the diagnosis?
There is a filling defect in the uterine cavity; most probably, it can be an air bubble, an endometrial polyp, or a submucosal fibroid.

How can these diagnoses be differentiated?
Care should be taken to flush the catheter thoroughly with contrast material to avoid injecting air bubbles. Air bubbles manifest as well-circumscribed lucencies that collect in the nondependent portion of the uterus. They are often mobile or transient when they are expelled into the fallopian tubes. This fact can help differentiate air bubbles from fixed filling defects. Despite the best efforts, air bubbles are occasionally seen.

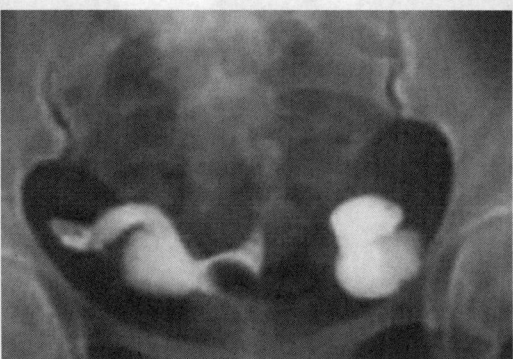

Fig. 5: Bilateral hydrosalpinx with loculated spill.

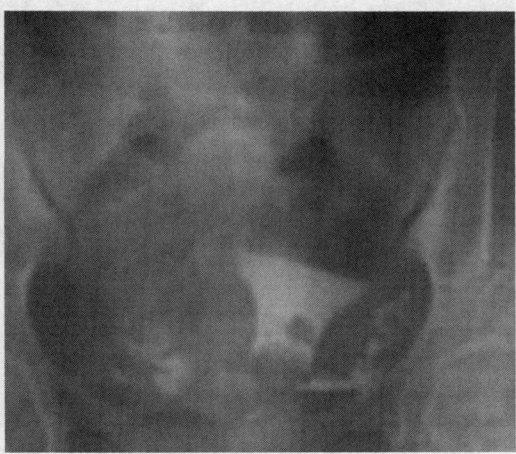

Fig. 6: Filling defect in the uterus.

An endometrial polyp or submucous fibroid is clearly demonstrated on sonohysterosalpingography.

What is the clinical presentation and management of an endometrial polyp?
Endometrial polyp causes intermenstrual bleeding with or without pain. It can be resected after hysteroscopic visualization or conventionally by dilatation and curettage (D&C) and sent for histopathological examination.

What is the film in Figures 7A and B showing?
It is an HSG film showing bilateral cornual block or proximal tubal obstruction (PTO).

What are the common causes of this appearance on hysterosalpingogram?
Proximal tubal obstruction is a common finding on HSG and accounts for approximately 20% of tubal factor cases. Obstruction can be secondary to tubal spasm, thickened mucus plugging of the proximal segment, technical problems, immediate evacuation of contrast from tubes, insufficient injection pressure, and air bubbles.

When does tubal spasm occur?
This condition is associated with a combination of patient anxiety, painful procedure, and rapid contrast injection.

How can tubal spasm be overcome?
Some drugs such as atropine, antispasmodic drugs, and narcotics have been used to suppress tubal muscular spasms. Often, by allowing a small interval of rest before injection of additional contrast slowly into the uterine cavity, talking to the patient gently, and turning the patient toward the nonfilling side or placing her in the prone position, tubal filling is completed. If, even after these maneuvers, the tube remains occluded, it is likely a case of true mechanical cornual obstruction.

What are the causes of tubal occlusion?
The main causes of tubal occlusion include fibrosis secondary to pelvic infection or tubal ligation, salpingitis isthmica nodosa, intramucosal endometriosis, and chronic tubal inflammation. Tuberculosis is an important infectious agent in this part of the tube. The uterine lesion located in the

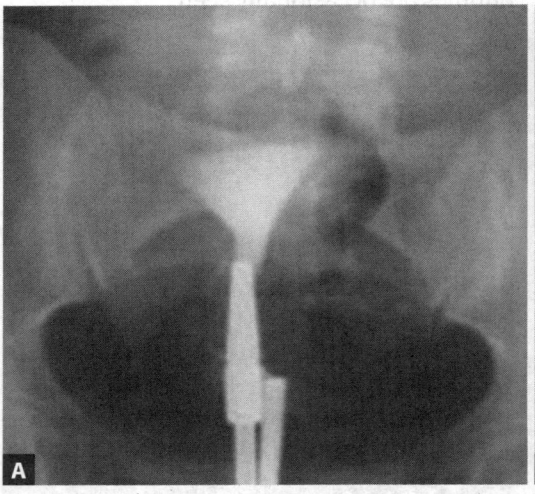 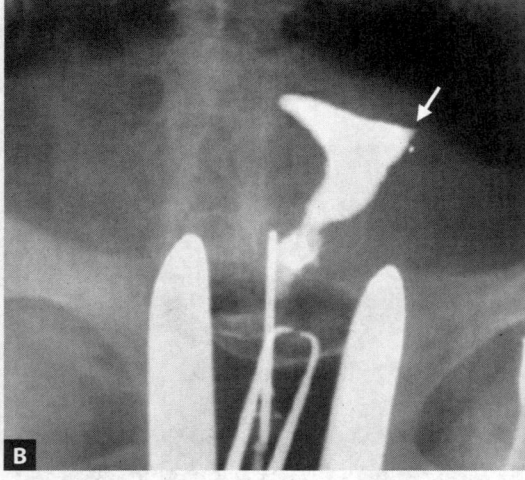

Figs. 7A and B: (A) Bilateral cornual block; (B) Proximal tubal obstruction caused by cornual spasm producing a rounded "breast-like" appearance (arrow).

uterotubal junction such as a uterine polyp, a submucous myoma, endometrial adhesions, or a tumor could rarely obstruct the proximal tube.

How can you differentiate tubal occlusion from tubal spasm on hysterosalpingogram?
Cornual spasm, produced by transient muscular spasm of the interstitial segment, must be differentiated from true organic obstruction of the proximal fallopian tube. On HSG, a rounded "breast-like" shape of the uterine horn suggests cornual spasm. Cornual spasm has been postulated as a more common etiology when the tubal obstruction is unilateral.

How has contrast been introduced in this case?
Contrast has been introduced into the cervix via a Foley's catheter.

What does the hysterosalpingogram in Figure 8 show?
The HSG shows a deformed and distorted uterine cavity.

What is the differential diagnosis?
Asherman syndrome or tubercular endometritis

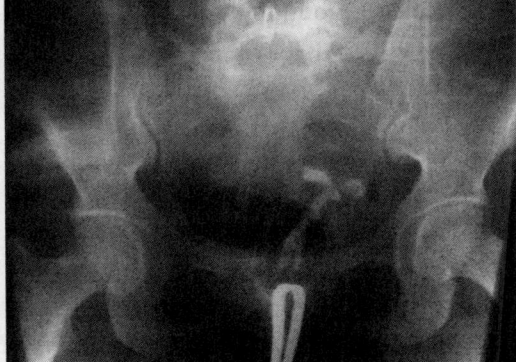

Fig. 8: Distorted uterine cavity.

What is Asherman Syndrome?
Synechiae are intrauterine adhesions that result from scarring, most commonly secondary to the endometrial trauma of curettage. Endometrial infections like tuberculosis and schistosomiasis may also result in synechia formation. Synechiae manifest as irregular filling defects, most commonly as linear filling defects arising from one of the uterine walls. In the worst cases, the uterine cavity appears completely distorted and narrowed, and ostial occlusion may also be evident. Multiple synechiae associated with infertility is known as Asherman syndrome.

Give the clinicohysteroscopic scoring system of Asherman syndrome.

Hysteroscopic findings	
Isthmic fibrosis	2
Filmy adhesions • Few • Excessive (i.e., >50%, of the cavity)	1 2
Dense adhesions • Single band • Multiple bands (i.e., >50% of the cavity)	2 4
Tubal ostium • Both visualized • Only one visualized • Both not visualized	0 2 4
Tubular cavity (sound <6)	10
Menstrual pattern • Normal • Hypomenorrhea • Amenorrhea	0 4 8
Reproductive performance • Good obstetric history • Recurrent pregnancy loss • Infertility	0 2 4
Note: 0–4 = Mild (good prognosis); 5–10 = moderate (fair prognosis); 11–22 = severe (poor prognosis)	

Discuss the management of Asherman syndrome.
The management of Asherman syndrome can be divided into three primary approaches:

(1) Hysteroscopic surgery, (2) re-adhesion prevention, and (3) uterus restoration therapies. The most common treatment for Asherman syndrome is hysteroscopic surgery to cut the adhesions of the uterine wall. A Foley's catheter can be inserted in the uterine cavity for 5–7 days with a bag for removing drainage from the uterus. Another method to prevent adhesions from reoccurring is a uterine balloon stent made from silicon and shaped to fill the uterine cavity. Finally, application of certain chemicals such as hyaluronic acid has been shown to help prevent uterine re-adhesion. Hormone therapy such as estrogen supplements have been proposed to help enhance tissue repair and restore the lining of the uterus. Antibiotic coverage helps to prevent uterine infection and subsequent readhesion formation.

■ X-RAY FILMS

Figure 9 is a plain X-ray of the pelvis showing curvilinear and rounded foci of calcification. What is the diagnosis?
This is a plain X-ray of the pelvis showing curvilinear and rounded foci of calcification on the right side suggestive of calcification in a dermoid cyst.

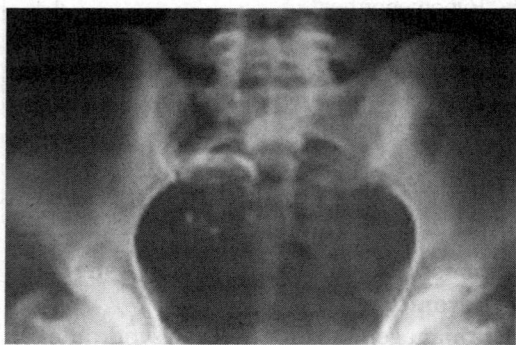

Fig. 9: Calcification in a dermoid cyst.

What are the other imaging features of a dermoid cyst?
Typically, an ovarian dermoid is seen as a cystic adnexal mass with some mural components. Most lesions are unilocular. The signs on USG include the following:

Dermoid plug: It is the most common sonographic feature of a dermoid cyst. It appears as an echogenic mass within the cyst made up of hair, teeth, or fat.

Dermoid mesh: As the name implies, the appearance on ultrasound is of multiple small hyperechoic lines and dots within the cyst forming a "mesh-like" picture. These echogenic foci are small hairs floating in the cystic fluid.

Tip of the iceberg sign: The appearance of a hyperechoic area, the base of which cannot be visualized. This is the result of a mass made up of matted hair and sebum casting an echogenic shadow.

Fat-fluid level, also known as a "hair-fluid level" or "fluid-fluid" level, is believed to be the result of layering of serous fluid and sebum.

Computed tomography (CT) is diagnostic if fat is identified in a solid/cystic lesion.

Can ultrasound estimate the exact size of a dermoid cyst? Why?
No, because fat commonly floats on top of the cyst obscuring deeper structures. Hence, the size of a dermoid cyst may be underestimated with ultrasound.

What is the management of an asymptomatic dermoid cyst?
Previously, it would have been removed, but it is now considered acceptable not to operate on small (<5 cm) incidentally discovered dermoid cysts, provided the ultrasound findings are typical and there is no growth on follow-up scans.

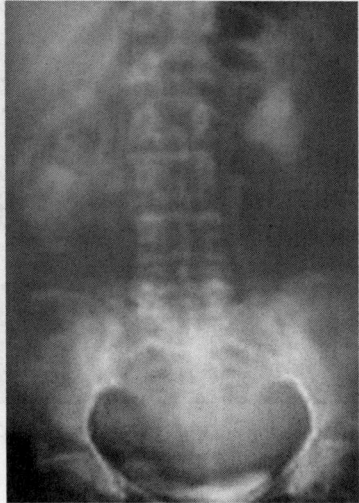

Fig. 10: Ovarian mass with bilateral hydroureteronephrosis.

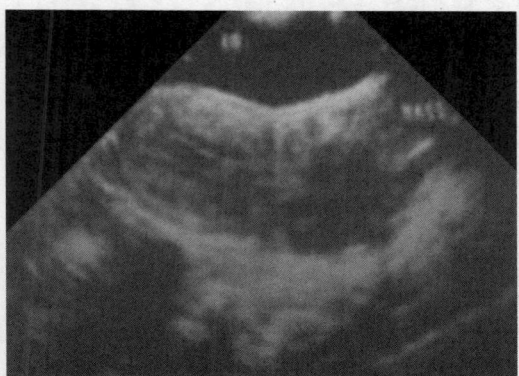

Fig. 11: Fibroid uterus with degeneration.

What is the investigation in Figure 10 and what does it show?
This is an intravenous urography (IVU) showing a soft-tissue density pelvic mass with extrinsic impression on the urinary bladder causing bilateral hydroureteronephrosis.

ULTRASONOGRAPHY

A 35-year-old female presented with polymenorrhagia since 2 years. Per vaginal examination revealed the uterus to be enlarged to 6-week size. What is the sonographic diagnosis shown in Figure 11?
A fibroid is seen in the uterus.

What are the other clinical presentations in a case of fibroid?
Patients may be asymptomatic and present with infertility, recurrent miscarriages, pain, or abdominal distension.

What are the types of fibroids? Discuss the FIGO classification of fibroids based on location of the fibroids.
Fibroids may be submucosal, mural, or subserosal in location.

Submucosal group:
- *Type 0:* Pedunculated intracavitary
- *Type 1:* <50% intramural
- *Type 2:* ≥50% intramural

Other groups:
- *Type 3:* 100% intramural; contacts endometrium
- *Type 4:* Intramural
- *Type 5:* Subserosal ≥50% intramural
- *Type 6:* Subserosal <50% intramural
- *Type 7:* Subserosal pedunculated
- *Type 8:* Others, e.g., cervical, parasitic

Hybrid leiomyoma group:
- Leiomyomas that impact both the endometrium and serosa
- Two numbers listed separately by a hyphen with the first number indicating the endometrial relationship and the second number the serosal relationship

What changes can occur in a fibroid?
A fibroid can undergo fatty change, hemorrhage, cystic degeneration, and calcification and may regress following menopause. It may increase in size during pregnancy.

How will this patient be managed?
If she has completed her family, she may undergo a hysterectomy, otherwise a myomectomy.

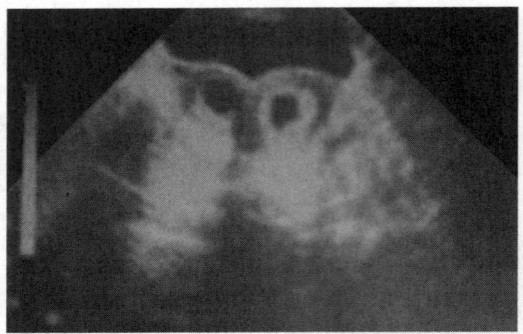

Fig. 12: A transabdominal ultrasound scan in early pregnancy.

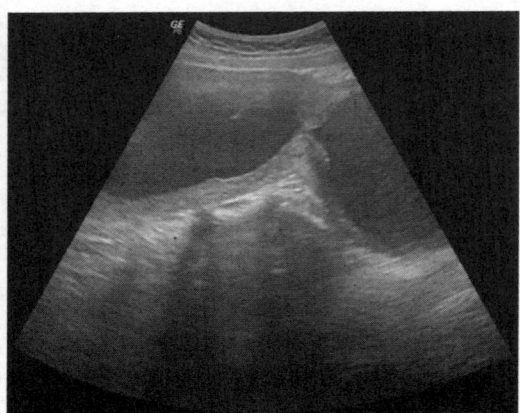

Fig. 13: Sagittal ultrasound scan showing pain in abdomen in a 21-year-old female.

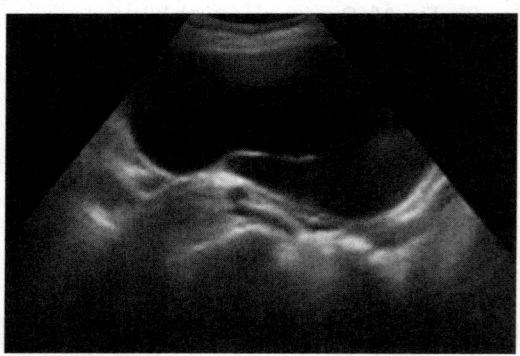

Fig. 14: Serous cystadenoma ovary.

Name the investigation shown in Figure 12.
It is a transabdominal ultrasound scan in early pregnancy.

How can you differentiate this from a transvaginal ultrasound scan?
The full urinary bladder is the anterior-most structure identified in a transabdominal ultrasound.

What does the scan show?
The scan shows an early twin pregnancy in a bicornuate uterus.

What does this sagittal ultrasound scan show in a 21-year-old female with pain abdomen (Fig. 13)?
The uterus and cervix are overdistended with low-level echoes in the lumen. The diagnosis in this unmarried female is hematometrocolpos.

Figure 14 is a sonogram through the right lower abdomen. What is the diagnosis?
There is a cystic mass showing a single thin septa, most probably a serous cystadenoma of the ovary.

What is a simple ovarian cyst?
A simple ovarian cyst is a unilocular, echo-free cyst without solid or papillary projections or septae.

What is the management of a follicular cyst if the patient is asymptomatic?
Cysts up to 3.0 cm in size require no further investigation. Cysts between 3 and 8 cm should be reexamined for decrease in size 3–6 months later. Serum CA-125 may be estimated if necessary. If the size increases, laparoscopy or laparotomy is indicated.

What are the indications of emergency laparoscopy or laparotomy?
Emergency laparotomy is indicated if the patient has symptoms like acute pain due to torsion or hemorrhage within the cyst or signs of intraperitoneal bleeding.

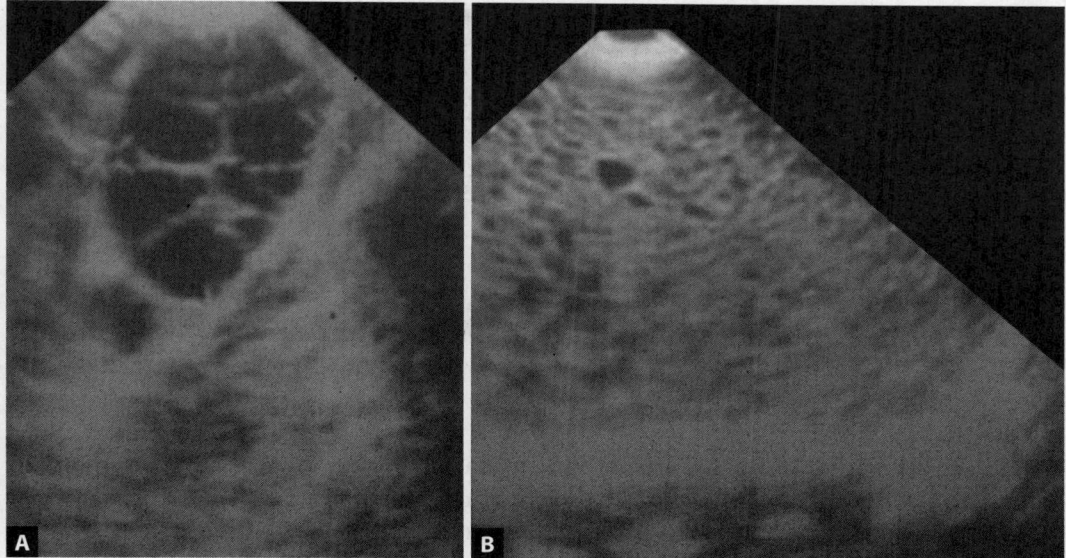

Figs. 15A and B: Hydatidiform mole with theca lutein cyst.

What does the film in Figures 15A and B show?
It shows a hydatidiform mole with theca lutein cyst.

What is the sonographic appearance of hydatidiform mole?
It produces a characteristic snowstorm appearance. There may be absence of fetal parts and heart motion.

How does a patient with hydatidiform mole present clinically?
Bleeding at about 12 weeks, passage of grape-like vesicles per vaginum, hyperemesis gravidarum, preeclampsia–eclampsia before 20 weeks, uterine enlargement out of proportion of duration of pregnancy, and hyperthyroidism.

What is the treatment of choice?
The treatment of choice is vacuum extraction/suction evacuation regardless of uterine size followed by gentle sharp curettage of the cavity to confirm complete removal of trophoblastic tissue. Rh-negative patients should receive Rh-immune globulin at the time of uterine evacuation.

How is a patient with molar pregnancy followed up?
- Weekly human chorionic gonadotropin (hCG) levels, after evacuation until three consecutive normal values are obtained
- Then, monthly hCG levels for a total of 6 months
- Prevent pregnancy for a minimum of 6 months using hormonal contraceptive or barrier method

The sonogram shown in Figure 16 is through the right adnexa in a 42-year-old infertile female complaining of irregular menses, showing a cystic mass with uniform low-level echoes. What is the diagnosis?
The diagnosis is endometriosis.

What is endometriosis?
Endometriosis is the presence of endometrial epithelium and stroma outside the endometrium and myometrium.

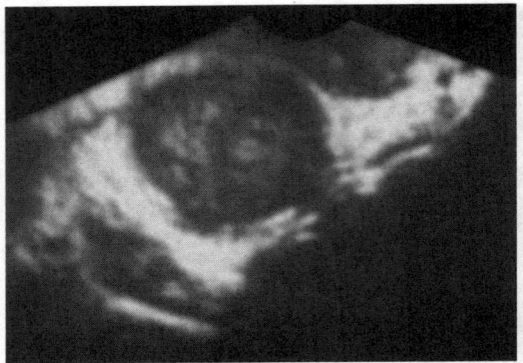

Fig. 16: Endometrioma.

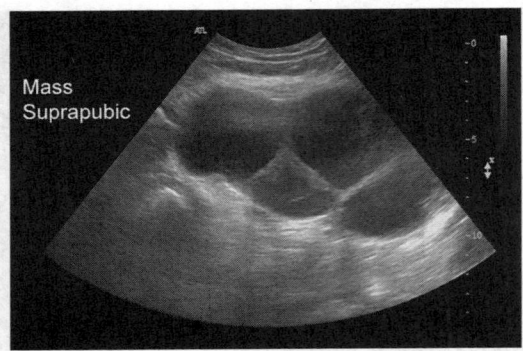

Fig. 17: Malignant ovarian tumor.

What are the common locations of endometriosis?
Ovary, uterine ligaments, fallopian tubes, rectovaginal septum, pouch of Douglas, bladder wall, and umbilicus are common locations of endometriosis.

What are the clinical features of endometriosis?
The patient may be asymptomatic and have dysmenorrhea, dyspareunia, abdominal pain, dysfunctional uterine bleeding, infertility, and/or adnexal mass (endometrioma).

What is the role of laparoscopy in endometriosis?
Laparoscopy is used to look for endometriomas, adhesions, and implants and for staging and follow-up of endometriosis.

The sonogram shown in Figure 17 is of a 55-year-old lady with an adnexal mass. What is the diagnosis?
The diagnosis is a malignant ovarian tumor—mucinous cystadenocarcinoma.

What are the ultrasound features suggesting malignancy in this figure?
Large cystic lesion (>10.0 cm) with thick (1.0 cm), irregular internal septae suggest malignancy.

What are the most common ovarian tumors?
Approximately 85% of malignant ovarian tumors are epithelial in origin and the most common epithelial carcinoma (60–80%) is a serous cystadenocarcinoma.

What is the sonographic appearance of serous tumors?
Serous tumors are predominantly cystic masses. They may show wall thickening, nodularity, septations, and internal solid areas.

Can serous tumors be bilateral?
Between 60% and 70% of serous tumors are bilateral.

What are the risk factors for development of ovarian carcinoma?
- Family history of ovarian, endometrial, breast, and colorectal carcinoma
- Following treatment with ovulation induction agents
- Nulliparous state

Figure 18 is an antenatal sonogram. What does it show?
It shows a fetal head with hydrocephalus.

What is hydrocephalus?
Hydrocephalus is defined as ventriculomegaly and macrocephaly associated with increased

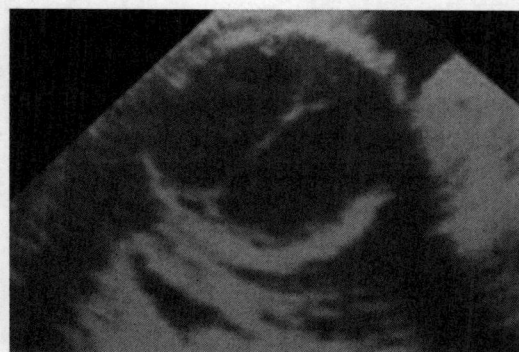

Fig. 18: Fetal hydrocephalus.

intracranial pressure. It results from an abnormal increase in the cerebral ventricular volume compared to brain tissue.

What are its etiological factors?
It may result from abnormal formation of central nervous system (CNS) structures, inherited along a Mendelian pattern or associated with a malformation syndrome. It may result from defects acquired in utero from infection (with subsequent scarring) or inflammation and cerebrospinal fluid (CSF) obstruction from intraventricular hemorrhage or from intracranial tumor. Sometimes, no specific etiology can be found.

What are the associations of fetal hydrocephalus?
A detailed neurosonogram should be performed by a fetal medicine specialist to look for other CNS malformations and extra-CNS anomalies.

How is ventriculomegaly diagnosed on sonography?
A ventricular atrial diameter of >10 mm indicates significant ventriculomegaly.

Name any condition that can be confused with ventriculomegaly.
Choroid plexus cysts. They are typically detected around the second trimester and are seen as sonolucent cysts, particularly around the lateral ventricles. They generally disappear by 26–28 weeks in utero and are of no significance in most cases. However, if one is seen in antenatal imaging it would warrant careful surveillance of the rest of the fetus due to weak associations with karyotypic abnormalities.

What is a lemon sign?
Lemon sign is a classic sonographic sign of Arnold–Chiari malformation besides the banana sign. A lemon-like configuration is seen in the axial section during the second trimester and is caused by scalloping of the cranial contents within a pliable skull and relates to concavity (not just flattening) of the frontal bones.

As the cerebellar hemispheres are displaced into the cisterna magna, they are flattened rostrocaudally and the cisterna magna is obliterated, causing a flattened, centrally curved, banana-like sonographic appearance.

What are the management options in hydrocephalus?
Antenatal:
- Search for other anomalies including karyotype along with MRI (evidence level III).
- Provide cautious counseling regarding prognosis if isolated hydrocephalus is present.
- Interdisciplinary approach is indicated.
- Termination remains an option.
- If pregnancy is continued, serial scans to identify progressive dilation of ventricles, measurement of cortical thickness, and head enlargement.

Labor and delivery:
- Cephalocentesis is destructive and not to be used if optimal survival is the aim (evidence level III).

- Cesarean section is not a priority, but it is done if excessive ventriculomegaly is common.
- Fetuses with isolated disease and moderate-to-severe macrocephaly should be delivered by cesarean section to facilitate the atraumatic delivery of an enlarged fetal head.
- However, cesarean section is not necessary for all cases of hydrocephalus. Vaginal delivery is attempted when the fetus is in vertex presentation and has mild hydrocephalus.

Postnatal:
- Establish cause and type—a postmortem examination is essential. The risk of recurrence is relatively low for sporadic chromosomal abnormalities but is much higher for balanced translocations. Other causes like antenatal infection (i.e., toxoplasmosis), intracranial tumors or cysts, and vascular malformations are unlikely to recur in future pregnancies.
- Provide counseling.
- Provide neurosurgical management.

What do these antenatal images of the fetal abdomen in Figures 19A and B show?
The images show fetal ascites.

What should it be differentiated from?
Fetal ascites should be differentiated from pseudoascites which is seen in the normal fetus and is thought to be due to the hypoechoic abdominal wall musculature or occasionally the hypoechoic fetal omentum can artefactually mimic a small volume of ascites.

What are the causes of fetal ascites?
It is always abnormal, being associated with hydrops fetalis. Other causes include:
- Idiopathic
- Bowel perforation (e.g., meconium peritonitis)

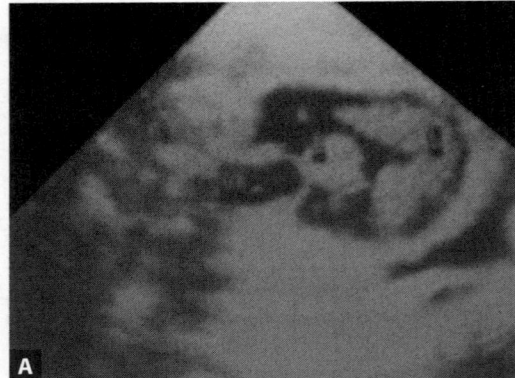
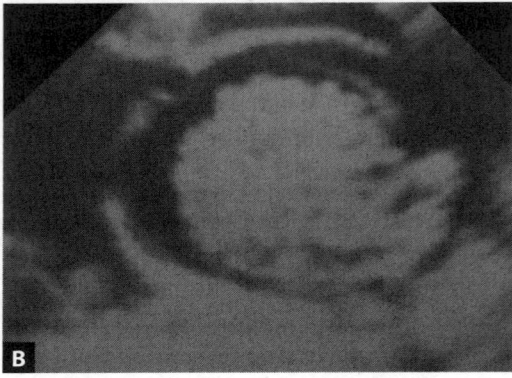

Figs. 19A and B: Fetal ascites.

- Ovarian cyst rupture
- Intrauterine infections
- Hydrometrocolpos
- Fetal urinary ascites
  - Transudation or rupture of the fetal urinary tract
    - e.g., obstruction from posterior urethral valve
  - Persistent urogenital sinus

Figure 20 is an antenatal sonogram of the fetal head. What does it show?
It shows an encephalocele.

What is an encephalocele?
Encephalocele is the least common neural tube defect consisting of herniation of brain and meninges through a bony calvarial defect.

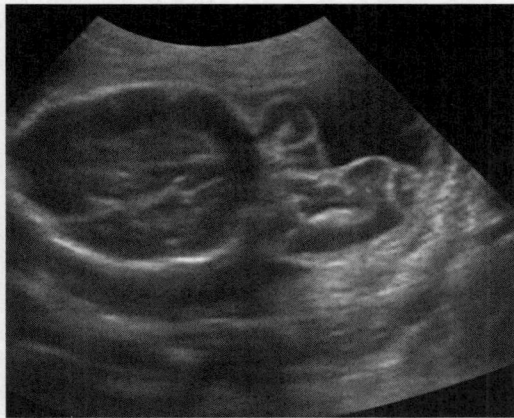

Fig. 20: Encephalocele.

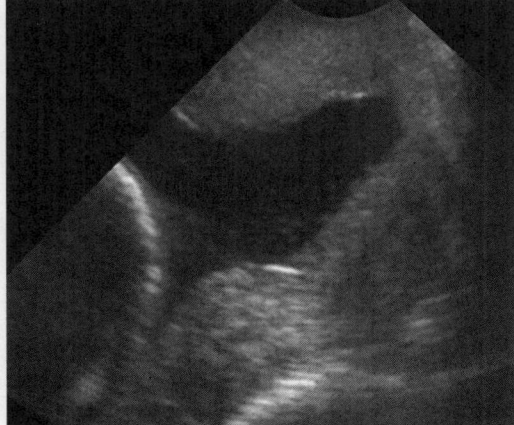

Fig. 21: Cervical incompetence.

What does the antenatal sonographic scan in Figure 21 depict?
It is a transvaginal ultrasound showing endocervical canal dilatation and funneling.

What are the causes of cervical incompetence?
Cervical insufficiency may occur as a result of a functional defect in the cervix, which can be due to an anatomic abnormality (congenital Müllerian anomalies), in utero exposure to diethylstilbestrol (DES), or collagen disorders (Ehlers–Danlos syndrome). Acquired causes of cervical insufficiency include obstetric trauma (e.g., cervical laceration during labor and delivery), D&C, mechanical dilation of the cervix during gynecologic procedures, cervical cauterization or amputation, and conization, which may be performed via cold knife, laser, or loop electrosurgical excision procedure (LEEP).

What is the treatment of cervical incompetence?
Treatment is cerclage procedure. It can be McDonald procedure or Shirodkar procedure if performed vaginally. Cerclage can also be applied transabdominally in cases of severe anatomical defects of the cervix or in cases of prior transvaginal cerclage failure.

What preoperative evaluation should be done before applying cerclage?
- Sonography to confirm a live fetus and to exclude major fetal anomalies
- Cervical samples to rule out gonorrhea and chlamydia. Cervical infections should be treated.
- Restrict sexual intercourse for at least a week before and after surgery

What is cervical index?
Cervical index = 1 + funnel length/cervical length

What is primary, secondary, and tertiary cerclage?
- *Primary cerclage* is prophylactic or elective cerclage applied in patients with high-risk historical factors. It is usually applied between 12 and 16 weeks.
- *Secondary cerclage* is therapeutic or salvage cerclage and is applied in those patients where ultrasonic features are suggestive of cervical effacement (cervical length <26 mm) or dilation.
- *Tertiary cerclage* or emergent or physical examination indicated cerclage is applied

when the cervix is effaced and membranes are exposed in the vagina. (Amniocentesis is strongly recommended prior to such cerclage placement to rule out microbial invasion of the amniotic cavity.)

What does the ultrasonic scan in Figure 22 depict?
This is a transvaginal ultrasound showing polycystic ovarian morphology.

What are the diagnostic criteria of polycystic ovary syndrome?
The most recent criteria were defined by the Androgen Excess Society (AES) 2006, which recommends the following diagnostic criteria for polycystic ovary syndrome (PCOS): (1) Hirsutism and/or hyperandrogenemia, (2) oligo-ovulation and/or polycystic ovaries, and (3) exclusion of other androgen excess or related disorders such as hyperprolactinemia, thyroid disorders, and congenital adrenal hyperplasia.

What are the ultrasonic features for the diagnosis of polycystic ovary?
Polycystic ovaries can be diagnosed when at least one ovary demonstrates the presence of 12 or more follicles in each ovary measuring 2–9 mm in diameter and/or increased ovarian volume (>10 mL), although more recently the importance of ovarian volume over the number of follicles in diagnosing PCOS has been noted.

What are the various metabolic abnormalities associated with polycystic ovary syndrome?
Majority of women with PCOS present clinically with at least one of the following metabolic abnormalities—low high-density lipoprotein cholesterol (HDL-C), elevated body mass index (BMI) and waist circumference, high blood pressure, hypertriglyceridemia, and elevated fasting glucose.

What are the various methods of ovulation induction in polycystic ovary syndrome?
The various methods used are weight loss, clomiphene citrate (CC), CC and metformin, CC and dexamethasone, use of aromatase inhibitors like letrozole and anastrozole, laparoscopic ovarian drilling, and gonadotropins.

Which investigation is shown in Figure 23?
This is a contrast-enhanced CT scan of the pelvis—axial section.

What does it show?
It shows a large, lobulated cystic mass occupying almost the entire pelvis, showing irregular, intensely enhancing solid components within it.

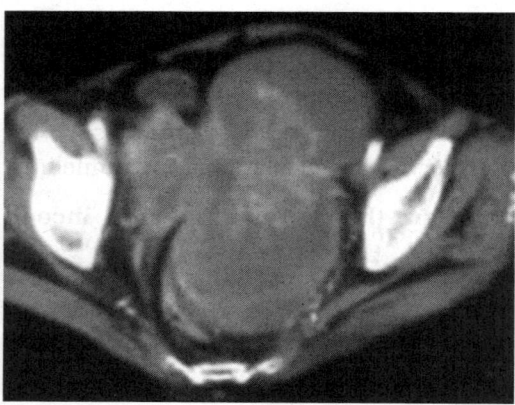

Fig. 23: A contrast-enhanced CT scan of the pelvis—axial section.

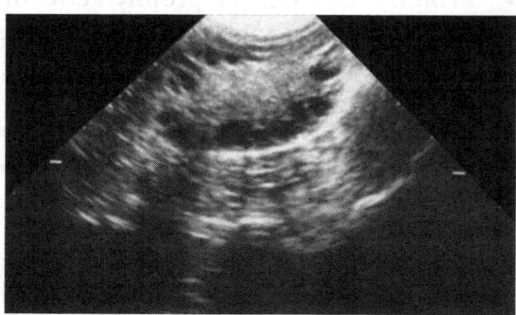

Fig. 22: Polycystic ovary.

What is the diagnosis?
The diagnosis is malignant ovarian tumor.

Name the investigation shown in Figures 24A to D.
This is a contrast-enhanced CT scan of the abdomen and pelvis showing axial sections.

What are the abnormalities shown in Figures 24A to D?
A. The right kidney is normal, but the left kidney shows a dilated pelvicalyceal system (black arrow).
B. The left ureter is dilated (arrowhead).
C. A large lobulated enhancing mass is seen behind the urinary bladder.
D. The heterogeneously enhancing mass involving the cervix is invading the left vesicoureteric junction and also shows loss of fat plane with anterior wall of rectum (arrow).

What is the final diagnosis?
The final diagnosis is carcinoma cervix with rectal and urinary bladder involvement causing left-sided hydroureteronephrosis. (Stage IV).

Which investigation is shown in Figure 25?
It is a contrast-enhanced CT scan showing a sagittal reconstructed image.

What does it show?
The uterus is enlarged and the uterine cavity shows a heterogeneously enhancing mass. The diagnosis is endometrial carcinoma.

What is the investigation shown in Figure 26?
This is a non-contrast CT scan of the pelvis.

Identify the abnormality.
This is a dermoid cyst in the pelvis.

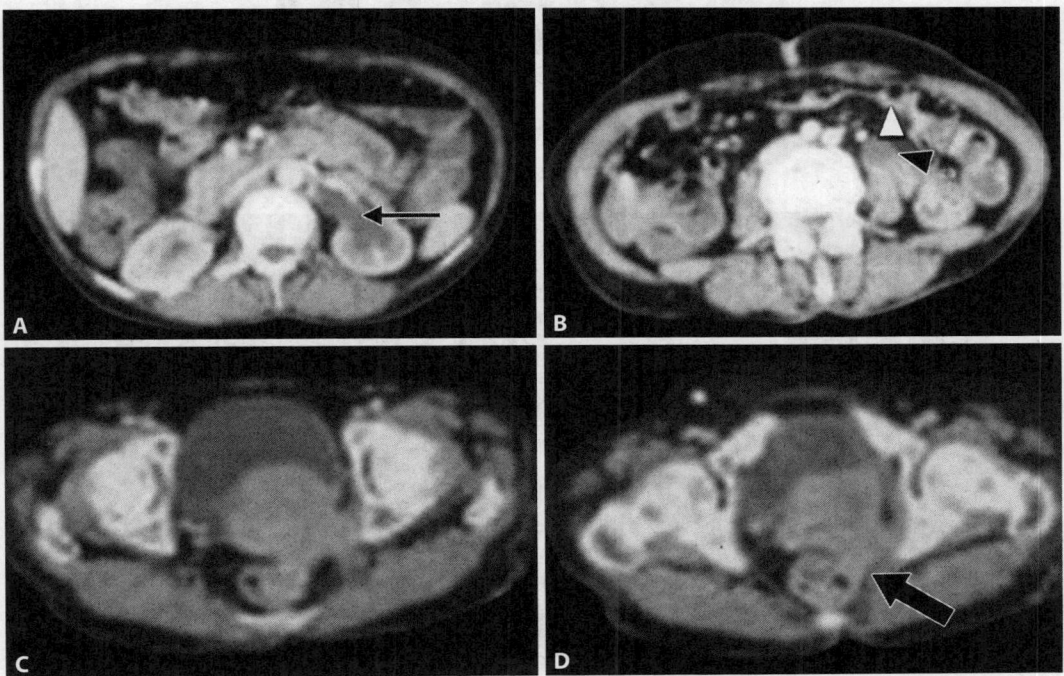

Figs. 24A to D: Contrast-enhanced CT scans of the abdomen and pelvis showing axial sections.

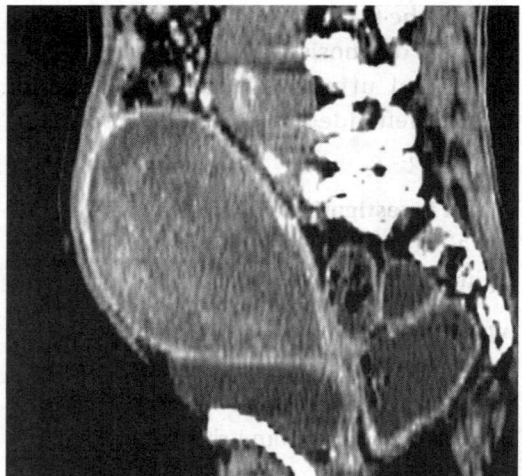

Fig. 25: A contrast-enhanced CT scan showing a sagittal reconstructed image.

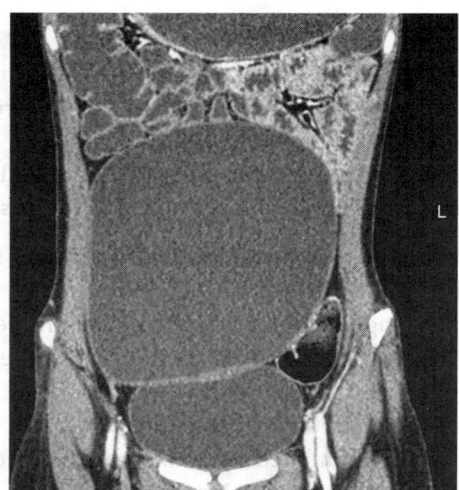

Fig. 27: Coronal reconstructed CT image showing in a teenage female.

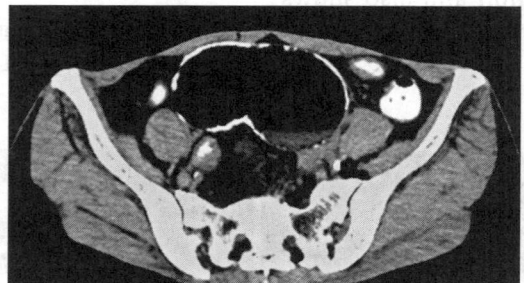

Fig. 26: A noncontrast CT scan of the pelvis.

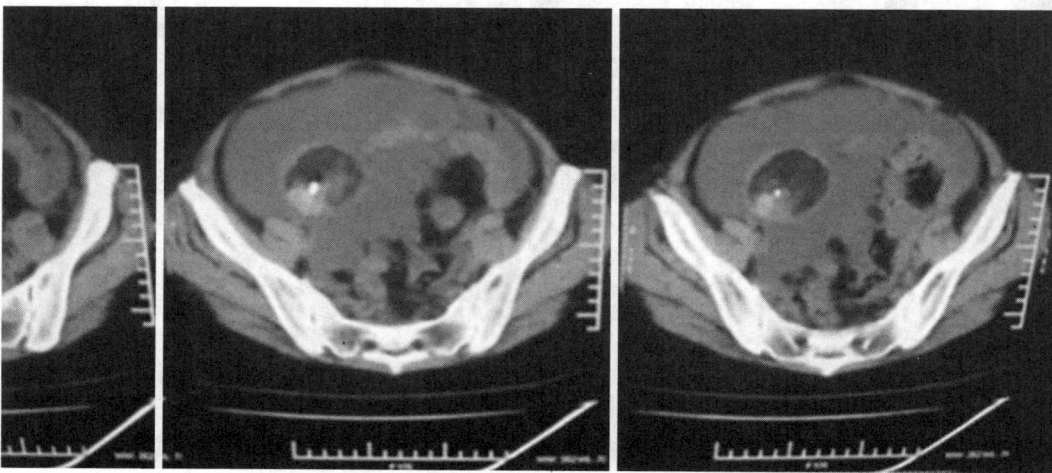

Fig. 28: Contrast-enhanced CT pelvis in a 45-year-old lady with abdominal distention for 2 months.

What are the features favoring this diagnosis?
There is a cystic lesion showing calcification of its wall and a fat-fluid level within.

What does this coronal reconstructed CT image show in a teenage female (Fig. 27)?
This is a large paraovarian cyst displacing the bowel loops into the upper abdomen.

What are the differential diagnoses to be entertained in this case?
Mesenteric cyst, hydatid cyst, and duplication cyst

What is the other cystic structure in the image?
It is the urinary bladder seen above the pubic symphysis.

What are the findings in this contrast-enhanced CT pelvis in a 45-year-old lady with abdominal distention for 2 months (Fig. 28)?
There are ascites and a round lesion showing an enhancing peripheral solid nodule with a central calcific lesion surrounded by fat.

What is the diagnosis?
This is a typical appearance of an ovarian dermoid cyst with malignant transformation.

Ultrasonography in Obstetrics

Vishal Gupta, Ruchi Narayan

■ INTRODUCTION

Since its development, ultrasonography (USG) has rapidly become integrated into the routine clinical care in gynecology and obstetrics. Cost effectiveness, easy availability, good spatial resolution, and real-time nature of the investigation are some of the factors contributing to its immense popularity in addition to it being relatively free of significant adverse effects. The presence of amniotic fluid is an advantage to the radiologist as it provides a good acoustic window through which the fetus can be visualized. However, the interobserver variability of USG demands an experienced radiologist to provide instant interpretation and maximize the information that can be derived from the investigation.

During pregnancy, USG can be done both transabdominally (TAS) and transvaginally (TVS). During TVS, the probe is closer to the region of interest which allows us to use a higher frequency and get a better spatial resolution. However, using a high frequency restricts the use of TVS to the first trimester as the high-frequency sound waves have a limited tissue penetration. On USG, the uterus is localized as a pelvic organ, between the urinary bladder lying anteriorly and the rectum posteriorly. The parts of uterus craniocaudally are fundus, body, and cervix. The fallopian tubes and ovaries are found lateral to the uterus bilaterally and medial to the iliac vessels.

The probes used for TAS are a curvilinear probe (1–6 MHz) and for TVS, a high-frequency probe (7.5–10 MHz) is used.

What are the indications for ultrasonography during pregnancy?

In a uncomplicated pregnancy, a minimum of three ultrasound examinations are recommended, one in each trimester.

- The first-trimester scan (viability scan) provides information regarding viability, number of fetuses, the amniocity and chorionicity and NT (nuchal translucency)/NB (nasal bone). This scan can also be used for dating the pregnancy in cases where the last menstrual period (LMP) is uncertain.

- The second-trimester scan (anomaly scan) is done ideally between 18 and 20 weeks as the fetal parts are well formed by this time and the amount of liquor provides adequate visualization.

- The third-trimester scan (growth scan) is used to ascertain the adequate growth of the fetus. Antenatal Doppler examination can be clubbed with the growth scan and is valuable in cases of intrauterine growth restriction/pregnancy-induced hypertension (IUGR/PIH). More USG/Doppler scans can be added depending upon the specific clinical condition, apart from the three standard scans mentioned above.

Are there any contraindications for doing ultrasound during pregnancy?

There is no absolute contraindication for the USG other than the patient's refusal. The relative contraindications for TVS are term pregnancy and patients with bleeding per vaginum (PV). TVS is considered safe even in the case of placenta previa as angulations of cervix with the probe are sufficient to prevent slipping of the vaginal probe into the cervix and cause placental injury. Also, the vaginal probe lies in the vaginal canal distal to the external os and not into the cervix which also makes the placental injury less likely.

The complication rate associated with ultrasound is relatively low. However, a TVS may cause complications such as anxiety, pain, or vaginal bleeding if done vigorously. The concerns regarding the thermal adverse effects of USG/Doppler are limited to long examinations and have not been systematically characterized or quantified.

Describe the clinical significance of organ formation in a normal fetus.

Fertilization occurs on or about day 14th as the mature ovum and sperm unite to form the zygote in the distal third of the fallopian tube. The cells divide as the zygote travels through the fallopian tube and by the time it enters the uterine cavity (at day 17), it is at a 12–15-celled stage and is known as morula. The blastocyst stage occurs at about day 20 and thereafter implantation occurs by day 23. Subsequent tissue differentiation and organogenesis are rapid. The neurulation process starts at 5th week and gets completed by the end of 6th week. The primitive gut is formed during 6th week and the midgut herniates in the umbilical cord between 8th and 12th week. By the end of 8th week, the heart attains its definite form. The primitive kidneys start ascending by the 8th week and get completed by the 11th week. The external genitalia reaches its mature form by the end of the 14th week.

What is the sonographic appearance of normal intrauterine pregnancy in the first trimester?

Implantation occurs in the fundal region of uterus, between day 20 and day 23, usually ipsilateral to the ovulating ovary. The earliest reliable sign of intrauterine implantation is the visualization of gestational sac (GS) within the thickened decidua (*intradecidual sign*) and can be seen between 4.5 and 5 weeks on TVS. It is visualized on TAS by about 5.5 weeks. These time frames assume a 28-day menstrual cycle (Naegle formula), and necessary adjustments must be made in women with longer/shorter menstrual cycles.

In cases where menstrual history is not accurate or menstrual cycles are irregular, serum beta-human chorionic gonadotropin (hCG) correlation should be done as the serum beta-hCG level becomes positive soon after the implantation, long before the visualization of GS on USG. (Beta-hCG level for GS visualization on TAS is >2,000 mIU/mL and on TVS is >1,000 mIU/mL.)

What is double decidual sign?

The *double decidual sign* refers to the visualization of GS as an echogenic ring formed by decidua capsularis and chorion leave eccentrically placed in the decidua parietalis forming two echogenic rings.

The normal GS contains only two structures, the yolk sac (YS) and the fetal node with the YS first to appear. On TAS, YS should always be visualized when the mean sac diameter (MSD) is 15 mm or more and fetal node must be visualized when MSD is 20 mm or more. YS plays a role in transferring nutrients to the developing embryo during 3rd to 4th week of gestation when placental circulation is developing. Angiogenesis occurs in the walls of YS in 5th week. The vascular channel in the wall of YS joins the fetal circulation via the vitelline duct containing paired vitelline arteries and veins. The YS remains connected to the midgut by the vitelline duct. The number of YS determines the amnionicity of a multifetal pregnancy. The upper limit of YS diameter in the first trimester of gestation is 5.6 mm. The YS is rarely visualized after 12 weeks by which time the primary wave of trophoblastic invasion is complete and the placenta assumes the dominant role in providing fetal nutrition.

What is the double bleb sign?

Double bleb sign represents two blebs, of which one is amnion and the other is YS. It is the earliest demonstration of amnion and can be seen by 5.5 weeks when crown-rump length (CRL) is 2 mm. The amniotic cavity expands and fills the chorionic cavity completely by 14th to 16th week.

On USG, an embryo can be visualized in a GS when MSD is 10 mm and should always be seen when MSD is >20 mm. The cardiac activity should always be visualized if CRL is >5 mm, although it is commonly identified in smaller embryos. A fetal heart rate (FHR) <100 bpm is a poor prognostic sign.

Discuss formation of umbilical cord.

The umbilical cord is formed at around the end of 6th week (CRL = 4 mm) as the amnion expands and envelops the connecting stalk. The cord contains two umbilical arteries, one umbilical vein (the allantois) and the vitelline duct, all of which are embedded in Wharton's jelly.

The umbilical arteries arise from the fetal internal iliac arteries and become the superior vesical arteries and medial umbilical ligament in the newborn.

The umbilical vein carries the oxygenated blood from the placenta to the fetus and it is shunted through the ductus venosus into the right atrium. The umbilical vein forms the ligamentum teres in the newborn, which attaches to the left branch of portal vein. The ductus venosus becomes the ligamentum venosum. The allantois is associated with the urinary bladder development and becomes the urachus and median umbilical ligament.

What is meant by early pregnancy failure?

Fetal development and embryonic growth are highly predictable in the first trimester, and any deviations can be considered abnormal. The term early pregnancy failure is considered in any of the following situations:

- CRL of ≥7 mm and no cardiac activity
- MSD of ≥25 mm and no embryo
- Absence of embryo with heartbeat ≥2 weeks after a scan that showed a GS without a YS
- Absence of embryo (with cardiac activity) ≥11 days after a scan that showed a GS with a YS
- GS with no embryo and an MSD <12 mm on the initial scan that fails to double in size on a scan ≥14 days later
- GS with no embryo and an MSD ≥12 mm on the initial scan with no embryo heart activity on a scan ≥7 days later
- Embryo (irrespective of CRL) without cardiac activity on initial scan and on repeat scan ≥7 days later
- Cessation of a previously documented cardiac activity of embryo (irrespective of CRL)

Other poor prognostic signs in early pregnancy are distorted GS shape, thin trophoblastic reaction (<2 mm), low-lying GS in the endometrial cavity, a FHR <100 bpm, arrhythmias, an abnormally large YS, calcified YS, low beta-hCG, early oligohydramnios, and subchorionic hemorrhage.

ECTOPIC PREGNANCY

The incidence of ectopic pregnancy is increased due to many factors such as increased age and parity, history of infertility, pelvic inflammatory disease (PID), in vitro fertilization (IVF), previous tubal pregnancy, cesarean section, tubal reconstructive surgery, intrauterine contraceptive device (IUCDs), etc. The classical triad of pain, abnormal vaginal bleeding, and palpable adnexal mass is seen in <50% of cases. Other associated features like amenorrhea, adnexal, and cervical motion tenderness also contribute to the diagnosis.

What are the sonographic features of ectopic pregnancy?

The sonographic diagnosis of a chronic ectopic pregnancy rests on the demonstration of three signs in a patient with positive beta-hCG levels:

1. Absence of intrauterine GS
2. Adenexal mass
3. Free fluid in pouch of Douglas (POD)

Care should be taken not to misinterpret a decidual cast as a GS.

The sonographic appearance of live embryo with cardiac activity in the adnexa is an unequivocal sign of ectopic pregnancy.

The negative beta-hCG test essentially excludes the presence of a live pregnancy. If the hCG level is above the threshold level (i.e., 1,000 mIU/mL for TVS and 2,000 mIU/mL for TAS), it is possible to see an intrauterine pregnancy (IUP). If GS is not visualized in the endometrial cavity with an increased hCG level, ectopic pregnancy should be suspected. The doubling time of beta-hCG is approximately 2 days in a normal IUP. Pregnancy with a dead or dying embryo has falling hCG levels. Ectopic pregnancy shows a slow rise in hCG levels.

Evaluation of the Embryo

What is the normal embryonic development mimicking pathology?

Intracranial cystic structures in the first trimester:
- Rhombencephalon (at 6–8 weeks) which forms the 4th ventricle in later life
- Telencephalon and diencephalon (at around 9–11 weeks) which forms lateral ventricles and 3rd ventricles, respectively

Physiological anterior abdominal wall herniation—the midgut herniates in the umbilical cord and returns back (between 8 and 12 weeks) and appears as a small echogenic mass in the cord.

How does anencephaly appear on ultrasound?

Due to failure of the closure of anterior neuropore (which normally occurs at ~42 days), there is absence of bony calvarium. The cerebral lobes appear as two semicircular structures above the orbits, seen floating in the amniotic fluid ("Micky Mouse" sign).

When should fetal renal abnormalities be suspected?

Renal agenesis: Normally, fetal kidneys can be seen at 9 weeks and by 12 weeks, urinary bladder can be seen. Fetal urine production starts at about 11–13 weeks. Nonvisualization of kidneys and bladder suggests agenesis.

What are the first-trimester masses seen on ultrasonography?

Ovarian masses: Corpus luteum cyst (usually <5 cm) is a thick-walled cystic structure with circumferential vascular flow. It secretes progesterone to support pregnancy until the placenta takes over it. It regresses at around 16–18 weeks; however, not all corpus luteum cysts regress. Hemorrhagic corpus luteum cyst can be difficult to differentiate from the pathological lesions on single USG alone.

Torsion, rupture, and dystocia are other complications during pregnancy. Dermoid cyst appears as a mass with fat contents, dermoid plug, tooth formation, focal calcification, or fat-fluid level.

Uterine masses: Uterine fibroid is a common finding during the first trimester. Mostly are painless, but some may rapidly enlarge due to estrogenic effect and undergo infarction and necrosis which causes pain.

What all should be evaluated in first-trimester scan?

If a USG has not been performed in the early first trimester of pregnancy, then it is advised to get scan done at 11 + 0 to 14 + 0 weeks of gestation to confirm viability, number, accurate pregnancy dating, screening for aneuploidies, to identify major structural anomalies, to measure NT and screening of preterm eclampsia. However, major malformation can develop later in pregnancy or may not be detected at this stage.

Fetal biometry in the first trimester is done by measuring CRL (between 45 and 84 mm). The fetus should be in neutral position (i.e., neither flexed nor hyperextended). The measurement of CRL is used for the estimation of gestational age in all cases except in pregnancies with IVF. The image should be magnified enough to cover most of the ultrasound screen **(Fig. 1)**. The CRL should be used as a gestational reference for measurement of NT, uterine artery Doppler pulsatility index (PI), and first-trimester screening.

How is fetal biometry done?

Biparietal diameter (BPD) is measured by two techniques, outer to inner (leading edge) perpendicular to the midline falx. Abdominal circumference (AC) is measured in a transverse section, at the level in which stomach bubble and portal vein are

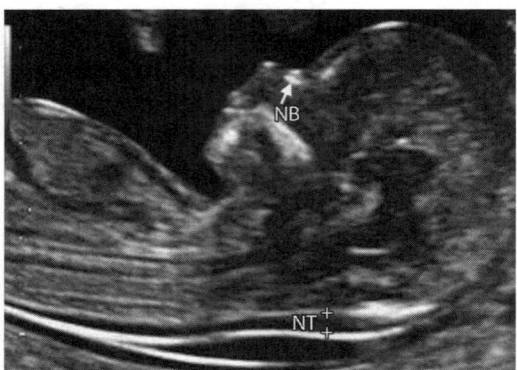

Fig. 1: Nuchal translucency (NT) and nasal bone (NB). *(For color version, see Plate 15)*
Courtesy: The Fetal Medicine Foundation.

visualized, at the outer skin surface. Femoral length (FL) is measured in a plane in which there is continuous linear visualization of shaft of femur till its ossified diaphyseal ends. The triangular spur should not be included for the measurement of FL.

What is the role of midtrimester fetal ultrasound scan?

- It is done between 18 and 24 weeks of gestation. A routine midtrimester fetal ultrasound scan includes evaluation of cardiac activity, fetal number (and chorionicity and amnionicity in cases of multiple pregnancy), gestational age/fetal size, basic fetal anatomy, placental appearance and location, and amniotic fluid volume.
- The cervical length is also measured to predict and prevent cervical causes of fetal loss. If uterine and adnexal masses (fibroids, ovarian cysts) are seen, they should be reported; however, formal assessment of uterine and adnexal anatomy is not part of the routine midtrimester scan.
- For fetal biometry and well-being, head circumference (HC), BPD, AC, and FL are calculated as described above **(Figs. 2A to C)**.

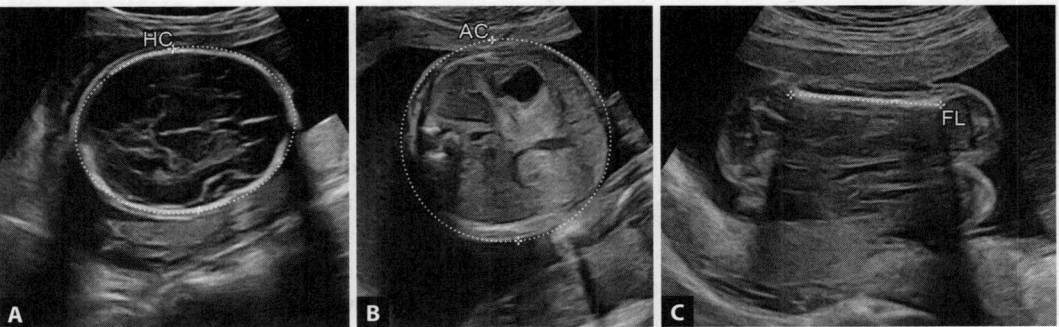

Figs. 2A to C: Standard fetal biometry. Sonographic measurements of (A) head circumference (HC), (B) abdominal circumference (AC), and (C) femur length (FL). *(For color version, see Plate 15)*
Source: ISUOG Practice Guidelines (updated): performance of the routine mid-trimester fetal ultrasound scan.

- A detailed description of the specific anatomic evaluation during an anomaly scan is outside the scope of this chapter. As a rough guide, one should evaluate the fetal head, craniocervical junction, spine, stomach bubble, bilateral kidneys, urinary bladder, and 12 long bones. Fetal echo is recommended at this time for a detailed evaluation of the heart.
- For amniotic fluid volume assessment, amniotic fluid index (AFI) should be used for polyhydraminos whereas deepest vertical pocket (DVP) should be used for oligohydraminos. DPV ≤2 cm is considered as oligohydraminos, DVP between 2 and 8 cm is normal, and DPV >8 cm is considered as polyhydraminos. AFI can be measured 18 weeks onward by measuring all four quadrants. Care should be taken that there should not be any fetal part or umbilical cord included in the pocket while measuring the AFI. For this, color Doppler can be used to rule out any nonvisualized part of umbilical cord lying within the quadrant.
- After 16 weeks, the amnion and chorion are usually fused. Amniotic sheets are benign findings which occur due to uterine synechiae and should be differentiated from amniotic bands which can cause fetal deformities. Biophysical profile is not considered as a routine investigation in midtrimester.
- Whenever possible, TVS measurement of cervix is recommended in midtrimester scan. Cervical length <25 mm before 24 weeks of gestation are prone to preterm birth.
- Umbilical cord assessment is not done as a routine part of midtrimester scan but if marginal (within 2 cm of the placental edge) or velamentous (umbilical vessels' insertion in the amniotic membrane instead of placenta) cord insertion is seen, then it should be mentioned. A velamentous cord insertion may be associated with vasa previa and fetal growth restriction. The pulsed-wave Doppler technique is not recommended as a routine part of the midtrimester scan.
- Chorionicity should be assessed for multifetal pregnancy in the first trimester itself. If no first-trimester scan has been done and it is not possible to visualize two separate placentae and fetal gender is same, then it should be considered as monochorionic pregnancy.

- Placental relation with the internal cervical os should be checked. If the lower placental edge is within 15 mm distance from the internal os on TVS, then follow-up scan is recommended. If placenta accreta is suspected in cases of previous cesarean or lower anterior placenta or placenta previa in midtrimester scan, then detailed evaluation is needed. Lack of the hypoechoic myometrial line below the placenta, large and irregular placental lacunae, interruption of the hyperechoic line between the uterine serosa and the bladder, reduced thickness (<1 mm) of the myometrium underlying the placenta, and placental bulge are the suspicious findings for placenta accreta.
- In the presence of risk factors for vasa previa, a targeted examination using a transvaginal approach is recommended. Vasa previa is defined as unprotected fetal vessels running through the fetal membranes, over or within 2 cm of the internal cervical os. Risk factors for vasa previa include twin pregnancy, conception by assisted reproductive technology, a low-lying or bilobed placenta, succenturiate placental lobes, and velamentous cord insertion. When the transabdominal scan suggests the possibility of placenta previa or shortened/dilated maternal cervix, use of transvaginal sonography with color Doppler imaging is suggested.

What features should be evaluated while doing ultrasound in multiple pregnancy?

In case of multiple pregnancy, specific guidelines are followed which include the following additional elements like determination of amniocity and chorionicity, if feasible (chorionicity better evaluated before 14–15 weeks), visualization of the placental cord insertion, and reporting of distinguishing features (unique markers, position in uterus), as it is critical to label twins correctly.

What is the role of third-trimester ultrasound scan?

- In a pregnant female with no symptoms, third-trimester ultrasound is indicated for the evaluation of different fetal and placental conditions, for example, gestational age, suspected multiple gestations (if no previous reports available), fetal anatomy, fetal anomalies, fetal growth and presentation, placental location, and cervical insufficiency.
- The indications for ultrasound in a symptomatic pregnant female are discrepancy between the uterine size and calculated gestational date, fetal abnormalities/death, placental abnormalities like abruption, placenta previa, hydatidiform mole, premature rupture of membranes, premature labor, vaginal bleeding, amniotic fluid abnormalities, any pelvic mass, uterine abnormalities, abdominal or pelvic pain, etc.
- Transvaginal ultrasound is relatively contraindicated during the third trimester, especially in patients without a prior documented placental location. In those cases, TAS is done to look for placental site and abnormalities. Commonly used dating measurements include BPD, HC, AC, and femur length (FL).
- Fetal movement should be identified and documented. Lack of fetal movement can have different significances and can be affected by the fetal sleep cycle. The fetal heart should be measured using M mode with the caliper placed over the left ventricle.

- The fetal lie (cephalic or breech) and laterality of spine should also be documented. The fetal anatomy should be evaluated for any abnormality. For example, fetal head should be examined for size, symmetry, and normal intracranial structures. Thorax should be looked for both heart and lungs anatomy and abnormalities. The abdominal and limbs should also be looked for as described earlier. The cervical length and effacement, if any, should be evaluated.
- The placenta should be identified; its location (anterior/posterior) and distance from the internal os should be mentioned. If the distance is <3 cm from the internal os, then further evaluation for placenta previa should be done. The placenta should also be evaluated for abnormal masses, hemorrhage, and placenta accreta spectrum with color Doppler studies.
- The umbilical cord should also be evaluated for the vessels and its insertion site.
- The umbilical artery flow should be differentiated from the umbilical venous flow with color and spectral Doppler and should show a "sawtooth" pattern with forward flow throughout the cardiac cycle. If the umbilical artery resistive index is abnormal, further investigation is warranted. The amniotic fluid level should be measured by both AFI and DVP methods if possible. The normal AFI is between 8 and 18.
- Fetal lie and presentation are of higher importance in the third trimester than the first and second trimesters as these parameters determine the course of induction and delivery.
- In the case of multiple gestations, an increased amniotic fluid volume must raise immediate suspicion for a fetal abnormality as most of the cases are related to twin-to-twin transfusion syndrome.

What is the principle of Doppler ultrasound in pregnancy?

Doppler USG is based on the Doppler principle which was first described by Christian Doppler, a Austrian physicist, in the nineteenth century. With the help of this principle, we can determine the direction and speed of blood flow in the vessels, based on the frequency shifts. It helps in evaluation of fetal well-being by insonating the umbilical artery, umbilical vein, middle cerebral vein, ductus venosus, and uterine arteries.

All fetal imaging, including Doppler, should be performed only for valid medical indications and as per ALARA principle, with an appropriate baseline, scale, and sweep speed, angle of insonation, sample volume size and placement, as well as selection of the wall filter to maximize the ease of analysis of the waveform.

Describe fetal circulation.

The umbilical vein carries the oxygenated blood from the placenta through the umbilicus, along the free edge of the falciform ligament to the left portal vein. Some of this blood goes to the liver, but majority of the blood is directed to the right atrium by the ductus venosus. This oxygenated blood crosses the foramen ovale from the right atrium to the left atrium and then to the aorta to preferentially perfuse the coronary arteries and cranial structures with the most oxygenated blood.

The maternal side of the fetoplacental circulation includes the uterine artery. Normal trophoblastic invasion of the maternal spiral arteries in the first half of pregnancy causes maximum vessel distention and increased blood flow to the pregnant uterus. So, the uterine artery waveform changes from a relatively high-resistance waveform in the nonpregnant state to a low-resistance waveform in pregnancy, with continuous forward flow throughout diastole. In the first trimester, Doppler ultrasound is used to detect aneuploidy and an increased risk for congenital heart disease with evaluation of the ductus venosus waveform, and screening for preeclampsia by evaluation of the uterine artery waveform.

In the second and third trimesters, Doppler ultrasound is mainly used for risk assessment in growth-restricted fetuses, in prediction and assessment of PIH, and in noninvasive detection of fetal anemia.

Discuss the role of obstetric Doppler USG in the first trimester.

- The ductus venosus is a small connection between the umbilical/portal system and the inferior vena cava. It has a characteristic waveform and sound. Color Doppler flow is used to localize the site of aliasing between the left portal vein and the inferior vena cava which is best seen in sagittal plane in the first trimester at the time of NT screening.
- The three components of the ductus venosus waveform are the S wave which reflects ventricular systole, the D wave which reflects ventricular diastole, and the A wave which reflects atrial contraction.
- Reversal of the A wave is always abnormal and shows an increased risk of aneuploidy and congenital heart disease; in twins, reversal of the A wave is a marker for an increased risk of the twin-to-twin transfusion syndrome.
- Doppler USG of the ductus venosus for aneuploidy screening is performed between 10 and 14 weeks' gestation, along with evaluation of NT and first-trimester anatomic structures. Doppler USG of the ductus venosus is also performed in the second and third trimesters to assess cardiac function in fetuses with high-output conditions and to assess cardiac strain in fetuses with fetal growth restriction due to abnormal placentation. During ductus venosus sampling, the fetus should be at rest.

What is the role of obstetric Doppler USG in the second and third trimesters?

- Doppler USG is done in the second and the third trimesters to monitor fetal well-being, the umbilical and the middle cerebral arteries (MCAs) being the important ones **(Fig. 3)**. The normal placental vascular bed is of low resistance, with continuous forward flow in the umbilical artery, throughout the cardiac cycle. As pregnancy progresses, the diastolic flow also increases, and so the systolic/diastolic (S/D) ratio decreases with advancing gestational age. The S/D ratio and the presence of absent or reversed end-diastolic flow are used to manage fetal growth restriction and to stage the twin-to-twin transfusion syndrome.
- The PI is used to study blood flow throughout the cardiac cycle. It is important to note that the resistance to flow in the umbilical arteries varies along the length of the umbilical cord, the highest being at the abdominal site of insertion of the umbilical cord, intermediate in free-floating loops of the umbilical cord, and lowest at the placental site of umbilical cord insertion.
- In multiple gestations, the sampling is done at or as close as possible to the

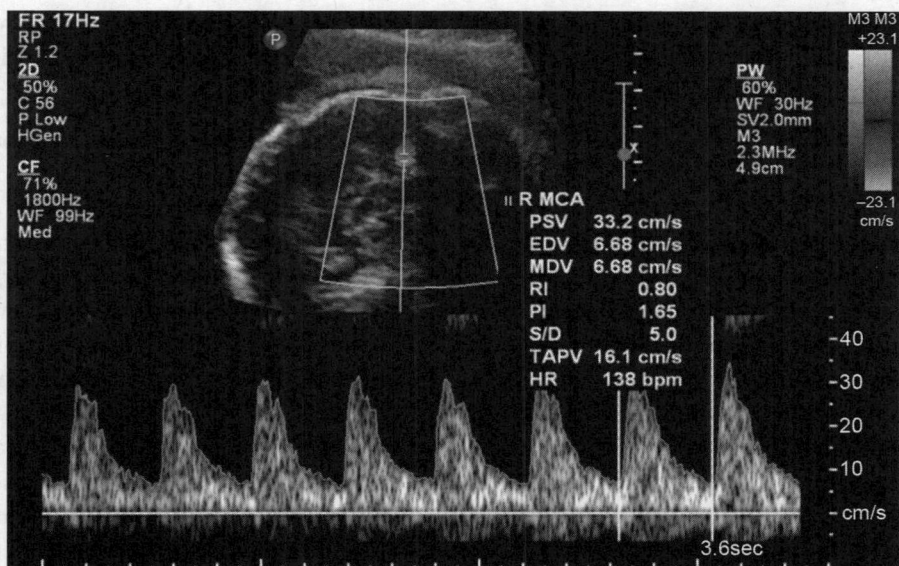

Fig. 3: Normal middle cerebral artery Doppler. *(For color version, see Plate 15)*
Courtesy: Radiopedia.

abdominal site of umbilical cord insertion of each fetus to ensure appropriate comparisons in the same fetus over time. In singleton pregnancy, the umbilical artery sampling is recommended in free-floating loops of umbilical cord.

What are the principles of management in abnormal Doppler?

- When the results of Doppler are abnormal, management is determined by the severity of the finding. With decreased umbilical diastolic flow (increased S/D ratio), the Doppler USG is performed weekly and delivery is considered soon after attainment of lung maturity.
- When absent end-diastolic umbilical artery flow is demonstrated, corticosteroid therapy is started and Doppler USG is performed two to three times per week. Delivery is considered if serial Doppler examinations reveal a worsening.
- Reversal of end-diastolic flow in the umbilical artery is usually a preterminal event and the fetus should be delivered as soon as possible.

What is the role of fetal Doppler USG of the middle cerebral artery?

- It is used for noninvasive assessment of fetal anemia and calculation of the cerebroplacental ratio (CPR) as a measure of fetal brain sparing. The assessment of fetal anemia by using Doppler USG of the MCA can be done as early as 18 weeks.
- The CPR is a ratio of the MCA PI to the umbilical artery PI. It compares fetal brain perfusion to that of the placenta. In normal circumstances, flow in the MCA is fairly high resistance, and flow in the umbilical artery should be low resistance, with continuous antegrade flow and a continuous increase in the diastolic flow as the pregnancy progresses. The S/D ratio and PI in the umbilical artery should always be lower than that in the MCA.
- In response to hypoxia, the fetus diverts blood flow to the brain, increasing the

MCA diastolic flow, thereby decreasing the PI and altering the ratio of the umbilical artery flow to the MCA flow. Also, whenever unexplained fetal hydrops is encountered, fetal anemia should be looked for as a cause.

What are the changes observed in Doppler USG of umbilical vein?
- Umbilical vein carries oxygenated blood from the placenta to the fetus and shows continuous flow.
- The changes in intrathoracic pressure due to fetal breathing alter flow dynamics in the vein to produce undulations in the umbilical vein waveform that are not linked to the cardiac cycle.
- Pulsatile flow in the umbilical vein is an ominous finding and when present, indicates abnormal placental pressures which compromise right heart function with back pressure through the right ventricle to the right atrium, back out the ductus venosus (which shows a decreased or reversed A wave) all the way into the umbilical vein, where forward flow decreases during diastole resulting in a pulsatile waveform with diminished forward flow in the umbilical vein during ventricular diastole.

Discuss ductus venosus Doppler.
Ductus venosus Doppler is used to screen aneuploidy and congenital heart disease in the first trimester, but it is used to assess cardiac strain in the second and third trimesters. When placental function is impaired, a larger portion of umbilical vein blood flow is shunted to the left side of the heart due to the head-sparing effect. This shunting decreases flow to the liver, impairing liver growth and restricting fetal weight gain. An absent or reversed A wave (i.e., decreased forward flow) in the ductus venosus is a strong predictor of stillbirth.

What is the importance of diastolic notching in uterine artery?
- The uterine artery is a branch of the internal iliac artery which runs anteriorly in the pelvis to enter the myometrium at the uterocervical junction. The waveform is high resistance with low diastolic flow and early diastolic notching in a nongravid uterus.
- In a gravid uterus, the early diastolic notching persists till the late second trimester, after which it disappears and coincides with the completion of the secondary wave of trophoblastic invasion.
- An abnormal waveform is characterized by increased resistance and persistence of a diastolic notch beyond the late second trimester. A diastolic notch is associated with adverse outcomes, including fetal growth restriction, maternal preeclampsia, increased risk of preterm delivery, and fetal distress in labor. Fetal activity does not alter the uterine artery waveform, unlike those of the umbilical artery, the umbilical vein, and the MCA.

What is the importance of performing color Doppler USG of cord insertion site?
- Doppler USG helps to localize the placental site of cord insertion (normal insertion being at the placental disc) and to rule out different abnormal cord insertion, e.g., marginal insertion, valementous insertion, vasa previa.
- The placental site of umbilical cord insertion should be documented in both longitudinal and transverse planes to avoid false-negative results.

SUGGESTED READING

1. International Society of Ultrasound in Obstetrics and Gynecology, Bilardo CM, Chaoui R, Hyett JA, Kagan KO, Karim JN, Papageorghiou AT. ISUOG Practice Guidelines (updated): performance of 11-14-week ultrasound scan. Ultrasound Obstet Gynecol. 2023;61:127-43.
2. Jones J, Yu Y, Yap J, et al. Failed early pregnancy. Radiopaedia.org. [online] Available from https://doi.org/10.53347/rID-9040 [Last accessed April, 2024].
3. Kennedy AM, Woodward PJ. A Radiologist's Guide to the Performance and Interpretation of Obstetric Doppler USG. MDRadioGraphics. 2019;39:893-910.
4. Levi CS, Lyons EA. The first trimester. In: Rumack CM, Wilson SR, Charboneau JW, Levine D (Eds), Diagnostic Ultrasound, 4th edition, vol 2. . New York: Mosby; pp. 1072-118.
5. Salomon LJ, Alfirevic Z, Berghella V, Bilardo CM, Chalouhi GE, Da Silva Costa F. ISUOG Practice Guidelines (updated): performance of the routine mid-trimester fetal ultrasound scan. Ultrasound Obstet Gynecol. 2022;59:840-56.

23 Drugs in Obstetrics and Gynecology

Sandhya Jain, Nazia Parveen, Astha Srivastava, Sumeet Singla

■ OBSTETRICS

What is oxytocin titration technique?
Oxytocin should be started with a low dose (because of variation in the response of the uterus to a particular dose) but escalated quickly when there is no response. Oxytocin has a half-life of 3–4 minutes and duration of action of approximately 20 minutes. It is prepared by diluting 1 mL vial containing 5U oxytocin in 4 mL saline resulting in 1 U/mL preparation. 2 mL of this is to be diluted in 500 mL Ringer lactate and started at a drip rate of 16 drops/min, which is equivalent to 2 mIU/min; it is escalated every 20 minutes; the maximum dose is 32–64 mIU/min. Conditions where fluid overload is to be avoided, e.g., heart disease hypertension, infusion with high concentration, and reduced drop rate, are preferred. When the optimal response is achieved (uterine contraction sustained for about 45 seconds and numbering three contractions in 10 minutes), the administration of the particular concentration in mIU/min is to be continued. The side effects of oxytocin are uterine hyperstimulation, uterine rupture, water intoxication, hyponatremia, hypotension, etc.

What is active management for third stage of labor? Mention contraindications of methergine.
World Health Organization (WHO) recommendations for active management of the third stage of labor (AMTSL), 2012:

- The use of uterotonics for the prevention of postpartum hemorrhage (PPH) during the third stage of labor is recommended for all births. Oxytocin [10 IU intramuscular (IM)] is the recommended uterotonic drug for the prevention of PPH.
- In settings where skilled birth attendants are available, controlled cord traction (CCT) is recommended for vaginal births, if the care provider and the parturient woman regard a small reduction in blood loss and a small reduction in the duration of the third stage of labor as important. In settings where skilled birth attendants are unavailable, CCT is not recommended. CCT is the recommended method for removal of the placenta in cesarean section.
- Sustained uterine massage is not recommended as an intervention to prevent PPH in women, who have received prophylactic oxytocin **(Fig. 1)**. Postpartum abdominal uterine tonus assessment for early identification of uterine atony is recommended for all women.

Contraindications of methergine:
- Chronic and gestational hypertension
- Rh-negative mother as there is more risk of fetomaternal hemorrhage
- In heart disease patient, as methergine increases preload by sudden uterine contraction, which squeezes blood in systemic circulation and increases afterload by causing vasoconstriction. Thus, it may cause congestive cardiac failure.

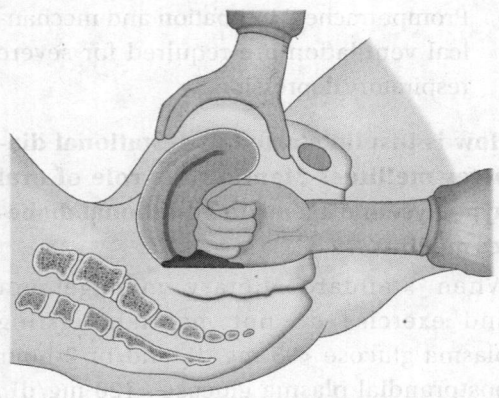

Fig. 1: Uterine massage.

- In multiple pregnancies, it is contraindicated after delivery of the first baby because it may cause fetal compromise in second twin due to tetanic uterine contraction.

What antihypertensives can be safely used in pregnancy? Mention their doses, schedule, and side effects.

The various antihypertensives that can be used in pregnancy are as follows:
- *Labetalol:* It is the drug of choice. It has alpha-1 antagonist and nonselective beta-antagonist action (1:3). Oral dose is 100 mg TDS and may be increased to 800 mg/day. It is very effective for emergency control of severe hypertension. The initial dose is 20 mg IV; if BP is not controlled, 40 mg is given in the next 10 minutes and then 80 mg every 10 minutes for two additional doses (maximum 220 mg). Side effects include orthostatic hypotension, headache, dry mouth, and tremulousness.
- *Methyldopa:* It has central sympatholytic action. In large doses, it inhibits the enzyme dopa-decarboxylase in brain and periphery and forms false transmitter methyl-noradrenaline. It is a drug of choice. It is safe for both mother and fetus. Dose: 250–500 mg, 2–3 times a day. Maximum dose 2 g/day. The onset of action is slow and full action comes in 6 hours. *Side effects:* Lethargy, dry mouth, sedation, thrombocytopenia, hepatitis, depression, postural hypotension, and hemolytic anemia.
- *Hydralazine:* It acts by peripheral vasodilatation, as it relaxes smooth muscles. It also increases cardiac output and renal blood flow. Oral dose is 100 mg/day, in five divided doses. In hypertensive emergencies, it can be used parenterally, the initial dose being 5 mg IV or 10 mg IM, which is repeated every 15–20 minutes, until satisfactory BP control is achieved. Side effects include late decelerations and hyperdynamic circulation.
- *Nifedipine:* It acts by direct arteriolar vasodilatation by inhibition of slow inward calcium channels. Action starts in 15 minutes; peak action at 30 minutes after ingestion. The dose is 10–20 mg, every 4–6 hourly. Side effects include hypotension, headache, tachycardia, coronary steal phenomenon, and inhibition of labor.
- *Nitroglycerin:* It relaxes mainly venous (also arterial) smooth muscles.
  Dose—5 µg/min IV to be increased every 3–5 minutes; up to 100 µg/min. Side effects include tachycardia, headache, and methemoglobinemia. It is used in hypertensive crisis for a short time only.
- *Prazosin:* It is a selective alpha-1 blocker. The usual dose is 1–4 mg BD or TDS. It may cause first-dose hypotension.

What are the various regimens of magnesium sulfate ($MgSO_4$) in eclampsia? Mention its toxic levels and precautions.

Magnesium sulfate is the drug of choice in eclampsia. Regimens used are:

Pritchard regimen:
- 4 g magnesium sulfate as 20% solution IV at the rate of 1 g/min, 10 g magnesium sulfate as 50% solution; one-half (5 g) is injected deeply in upper and outer quadrants of each buttock through a 3-inch long 20-G needle.
- 5 g of 50% solution IM into upper and outer quadrants of alternate buttocks 4 hourly.
- It is discontinued 24 hours after delivery.

Zuspan regimen:
- 4–6 g magnesium sulfate IV over 15–20 minutes followed by 1–2 g/hr IV infusion.
- Magnesium sulfate is discontinued 24 hours after delivery.

Monitoring:
- Patellar reflex present
- Respiratory rate >12 breaths/min
- Urine output >100 mL in 4 hours
- Oxygen saturation
- Blood pressure **(Table 1)**

Treatment of toxicity:
- For mild-to-moderate respiratory depression, magnesium sulfate should be withheld and 1 g of 10% calcium gluconate IV should be given.
- Prompt tracheal intubation and mechanical ventilation are required for severe respiratory depression.

How is insulin started in gestational diabetes mellitus? Mention the role of oral hypoglycemic agents in gestational diabetes mellitus.

When standard dietary management and exercise do not maintain fasting plasma glucose <95 mg/dL and/or 2-hour postprandial plasma glucose <120 mg/dL, then insulin therapy is recommended. The total insulin requirement in a day is calculated according to period of gestation: 0.7 U/kg/day from 1 to 18 weeks, 0.8 U/kg/day from 18 to 26 weeks, 0.9 U/kg/day from 26 to 36 weeks, and 1 U/kg/day from 36 to 40 weeks.

- *Basal–bolus regimen:* It is the most physiological regimen—purported to provide good and easily titrable blood sugar control. It comprises four injections—thrice-a-day premeal short-acting/regular insulin and bedtime intermediate-/long-acting insulin. The dose of insulin (as per week of gestation) is calculated. Half of this is given as bedtime insulin and the other half is divided into three equal premeal boluses of short-acting insulin.
- *Split-mix regimen:* Two-thirds of the total calculated dose of insulin is given subcutaneously (S/C), before breakfast, in the morning, and one-third is given S/C, before dinner, in the night. The insulin used is a mixture of 30% rapid acting/regular insulin and 70% intermediate acting/lente insulin. It may be in the form of commercially available premixed (30/70) insulin or self-mixed insulin (by drawing insulin from separate vials of regular and lente insulin).

TABLE 1: Correlation of $MgSO_4$ levels with signs and symptoms of toxicity.

Blood levels of magnesium (mg/dL)	Signs and symptoms
4–8	Therapeutic
9–12	Nausea, warmth, flashing, somnolence, diplopia, weakness, loss of patellar reflexes
15–17	Muscle paralysis, respiratory arrest
18–20	Cardiac arrest

Types of insulin
- *Rapid-acting insulin:* Insulin lispro and aspart are rapid-acting insulin. The advantage of rapid-acting insulin is that it can be given immediately before meal. Moreover, they have greater stability and consistency of action. These insulin analogs improve postprandial excursions compared with human regular insulin and are associated with lower risk of delayed postprandial hypoglycemia.
- *Short-acting insulin:* Regular insulin needs to be taken at least 30 minutes before taking meal.
- *Intermediate-acting insulin:* Neutral protamine Hagedorn (NPH) insulin has slow onset and long duration of action; hence it is suitable for providing basal requirement of insulin.
- *Long-acting insulin:* It includes analogs glargine and detemir. These long-acting analogs have a peakless action for 24 hours. In a meta-analysis (2011), eight cohort studies done in 702 women were reviewed to study the safety of insulin glargine in pregnancy. It was shown that insulin glargine does not cause an increase in adverse fetal outcome. In a randomized controlled trial (RCT) (2014), insulin detemir was found to be well tolerated and safe for use in pregnant women with type 1 diabetes.

Safety during pregnancy: Insulin lispro, regular, and NPH are Food and Drug Administration (FDA) category B drugs, while insulin aspart and insulin glargine are FDA category C drugs.

Oral hypoglycemic agents: Two oral hypoglycemic agents have been recommended for use in pregnancy at present—glyburide and metformin.

- *Sulfonylureas:* Studies using first-generation sulfonylureas in pregnancy showed high-placental transfer and prolonged neonatal hypoglycemia. Results of RCTs using glyburide have demonstrated that these oral hypoglycemics have the lowest rate of placental transfer and have been used to treat gestational diabetes mellitus (GDM). They were found to be comparable to insulin in improving glucose control, with similar incidence of macrosomia, cesarean section, and neonatal hypoglycemia. The safety of glyburide in the first trimester and in women with type 2 diabetes remains to be investigated.
  - *Glyburide/Glibenclamide* is second-generation sulfonylurea (category B). It does not cross placenta (fetal levels <1% of maternal levels). The onset of action of glyburide is 4 hours and the duration of action is 10 hours. Its main side effect is dose-related hypoglycemia. Dose is to start with 2.5 mg HS, which can be increased by 2.5 mg/wk and maximum up to 20 mg/day.
- *Metformin:* It is a pregnancy category B drug and its long-term effects of in utero exposure have not been well studied. It acts by decreasing gluconeogenesis and by increasing hepatic utilization of glucose. Side effects are gastrointestinal upset, weight loss, and lactic acidosis. Metformin is a second-generation biguanide. It crosses placenta but no teratogenic effect has been noted. A minimal amount of drug is transferred in breast milk, and there is no harmful effect on the baby. Metformin is given in divided doses with maximum of 2,500 mg/day. It is initiated at 500 mg twice daily, and increments of 500 mg/week can be done according to blood sugar levels.

- *Current evidence:* MiG Trial (2008), an RCT conducted on 751 patients with GDM, concluded that metformin does not cause any increase in perinatal complications; moreover, it was preferred by these women over insulin, but supplemental insulin was required in 46% cases. The same set of workers reviewed the babies of these women at the age of 2 years (MiG the offspring follow-up) and compared body composition of babies in these two groups. It was seen that babies in the metformin group had more subcutaneous fat, but total fat remained the same in both groups. There was less visceral fat in babies in the metformin group; hence, higher insulin sensitivity was expected.

What are the principles of anticonvulsant therapy in pregnancy?

The major pregnancy-related threats to women with epilepsy are an increased seizure frequency and risk of congenital malformations in the offspring. On an average, 7% of the offspring of epileptic women have major congenital malformations compared with 3% in general population. There is an increased incidence of preeclampsia, perinatal mortality, cesarean delivery, and preterm birth among epileptic women.

Preconceptional counseling includes the recommendation to switch to the least teratogenic drug regimen, or possibly even discontinue medication before conception. It is recommended to give 5 mg/day of folic acid to women of high-risk group. No change in therapy should be done during the first trimester.

Malformations are more prevalent with high-serum anticonvulsant levels; polytherapy imposes a higher risk than monotherapy. Thus, as far as possible, monotherapy in the lowest dose is preferred. Level 2 ultrasound determines anomalies, if any.

Benefits of breastfeeding outweigh the potential risk with antiepileptic drug (AED) in a neonate and they are mostly safe. Postpartum contraception should be discussed with the patient. Co-administration of oral contraceptives and anticonvulsants such as phenobarbital, primidone, phenytoin, and carbamazepine may cause breakthrough bleeding and contraception failure because all anticonvulsants induce the hepatic microsomal enzyme system, which in turn increases estrogen metabolism. Oral contraceptives with 50 mg of estrogen should be used in patients on anticonvulsants.

Phenytoin: Phenytoin, when used in the first trimester of pregnancy, causes the fetal hydantoin syndrome in 7–10% of offspring consisting of microcephaly, growth retardation, developmental delay, dysmorphic craniofacial features, and hypoplasia of nails and distal phalanges. Teratogenicity is strongly linked to inadequate production of the enzyme epoxide hydrolase by the fetus.

Carbamazepine: Though it is the preferred anticonvulsant in pregnancy, the teratogenic potential is unclear. Minor malformations like craniofacial defects, fingernail hypoplasia, and developmental delay have been associated with its use.

Valproic acid: Fetuses exposed to this drug in the first trimester have a 10% risk of major congenital malformations, and it is not to be used during pregnancy.

Levetiracetam: Levetiracetam has no adverse effect in fetus. Theoretically, bone abnormalities are suspected but no definite evidence is there. Folic acid should be added and screening of fetus is to be done (FDA category C).

Lamotrigine: Oral clefts have been reported in 1–4% cases. More studies are required to establish the safety (FDA category C). There is no adverse effect on infants of lactating mother (FDA category C).

Ethosuximide: Ethosuximide is safe regarding teratogenic potential, so it should be considered the drug of choice for absence seizures. It is safe for infants, who are on breastfeeding (FDA category C).

Enumerate various prostaglandins used in pregnancy. Mention their uses and contraindications.

Prostaglandins that are important during pregnancy, labor, delivery, and postpartum period are prostaglandins E and F (PGE and PGF). Unlike oxytocin receptors, which are active only in the later part of pregnancy, prostaglandin receptors are always present in myometrium. Gemeprost (methyl ester of PGE1), dinoprostone (PGE2 analog), carboprost (PGF2), and misoprostol (PGE1 analog) are the various prostaglandins that are available. Prostaglandins can act effectively on the cervix and uterus when:

- Placed as a suppository or pessary in the vagina, immediately adjacent to the cervix
- Administered intracervically
- Injected intramuscularly
- Taken orally

Use of prostaglandins in obstetrics

- *Medical termination of pregnancy:* Prostaglandins and their analogs are used extensively to terminate pregnancies.

    Misoprostol is used in conjunction with mifepristone as an option for medical abortion. Mifepristone acts as a progesterone antagonist and removes progesterone support for trophoblast attachment to decidua in early pregnancy, resulting in decidual necrosis, increased prostaglandin production, and uterine contraction. Misoprostol softens the cervix and causes strong uterine contraction. Misoprostol is teratogenic, if used in the first trimester, and anomalies reported include front-facial lesions (Mobius syndrome).

Contraindications are:
- Ectopic pregnancy (EP) or undiagnosed adnexal mass
- Chronic renal failure
- Chronic adrenal failure or concurrent corticosteroid therapy
- Asthma
- Cardiac failure
- Hemorrhagic disorder
- Drug allergy

Carboprost (250 mg) IM every 3 hourly (to a maximum of eight doses) can also be used for medical termination of pregnancy (MTP). Dinoprostone suppositories (20 mg), popular abroad, are not available in India.

- *Induction of labor:* Dinoprostone gel is administered 500 mg intracervically or 1–2 mg in the posterior fornix. It may be repeated after 6 hours, to a maximum of three doses. The woman should be in bed for 30 minutes and is monitored for uterine activity and fetal heart rate. Unpleasant side effects include nausea, vomiting, diarrhea, pyrexia, and bronchospasm.

    Misoprostol, 25 µg intravaginally every 4 hours, to a maximum of five doses or orally 50 µg, every 4 hourly, is an effective drug for induction of labor. It is cheap, thermostable, easily administered, has a long shelf-life, and least side effects.

- *Postpartum hemorrhage:* Carboprost is recommended in a dose of 250 µg IM and repeated to a maximum of eight doses at 15–19 minute intervals. Misoprostol 600–1,000 µg orally or rectally works as effectively as standard oxytocic drug.

What are the various indications of anticoagulant use in pregnancy? Mention their mechanism of action and dose.

Various anticoagulants used in pregnancy are as follows:
- Heparin
  - *Unfractionated heparin:* It acts by activating plasma antithrombin III (ATIII). The heparin–ATIII complex then binds to clotting factors of intrinsic and common pathways (Xa, II, IXa, XIa, XIIa, and XIIIa) and inactivates them.
  - *Low-molecular-weight heparin (LMWH):* It selectively inhibits factor Xa with little effect on IIa. The important advantages of LMWHs are better and more predictable subcutaneous availability, long and consistent half-life, no need for laboratory monitoring with activated partial thromboplastin time (aPTT), and dose calculation on weight basis. Commonly available LMWHs are: Enoxaparin (Clexane), Dalteparin (Fragmin), Reviparin, Nadroparin, Parnaparin, etc.
- *Warfarin:* It interferes with the synthesis of vitamin K-dependent clotting factors, i.e., II, VII, IX, and X. It behaves as a competitive antagonist of vitamin K and reduces the level of functional clotting factors.

Indications of anticoagulant use in pregnancy
- *Antiphospholipid antibody syndrome:* Low-dose aspirin (60–80 mg) blocks conversion of arachidonic acid to thromboxane and sparing prostacyclin production. It is started as soon as pregnancy is confirmed. Unfractionated heparin is used in the dose of 5,000–10,000 U S/C BD. LMWHs are more frequently used because of their unique advantages. They are started once fetal cardiac activity is seen on ultrasound.
- *Prophylaxis of deep vein thrombosis (DVT):* All pregnant women with prior history of DVT, pulmonary embolism (PE), or prolonged bed rest (because of medical and/or obstetrical reasons) and those immobilized after major abdominal/pelvic/orthopedic surgery must be anticoagulated prophylactically with either unfractionated heparin (5,000 U S/C BD) or LMWH (Enoxaparin 40 mg or Dalteparin 2,500 IU S/C OD). Prophylaxis is continued for the entire duration of pregnancy (for cases of prior DVT/PE), or till the postsurgical patient becomes ambulatory.
- *Treatment of DVT:* Intravenous unfractionated heparin is given as a 5,000 U loading dose, followed by continuous infusion at the rate of 1,000 U/hr. After 4 hours, aPTT is determined, and dose is adjusted to maintain it in the range of 1.5–2.5 times. Alternatively, LMWHs can be used to obviate frequent monitoring. Treatment is continued for 6–12 weeks postpartum.
- *Cardiac diseases* requiring anticoagulation are mechanical valve prostheses, mitral valve stenosis with atrial fibrillation, left atrial thrombus, primary pulmonary hypertension, Eisenmenger's syndrome, and peripartum cardiomyopathy.

In the first trimester, heparin is used in a dose of 5,000 U S/C 6 hourly or LMWH 40 mg S/C BD. Warfarin is avoided in the first trimester because of a high incidence of warfarin syndrome

(6–10%—hypoplasia of nose, eye socket, hand bones, and growth retardation). In the second trimester, warfarin is safe [start with 1–4 mg daily, titrating to an international normalized ratio (INR) of 2–3]. After 37 weeks, heparin is restarted. It is stopped prior to induction or when the patient goes into labor. Heparin is restarted 6 hours after normal delivery and 24 hours after cesarean section along with warfarin, overlapping the two for 4–5 days till therapeutic INR levels are regained, when heparin is stopped.

What is the role of tocolysis in modern obstetrics? Why are calcium channel blockers preferred over beta-agonists?

Tocolysis is supported but not recommended by the current Royal College of Obstetricians and Gynaecologists (RCOG) guidelines support, as there is no clear evidence regarding improvement in outcome. They may prolong gestation for 2–7 days, which can provide time for administration and effect of steroids and provide time for transport of the mother to a better equipped center for neonatal care.

Various tocolytics are as follows:

- *Calcium channel blockers (CCBs):* They are preferred over beta-agonists because maternal side effects are less frequent and less severe. There is no clear effect on perinatal death, but they seem to reduce the risk of neonatal respiratory distress syndrome and neonatal jaundice. For patients at >32 + 0 and ≤34 + 0 weeks of gestation, nifedipine is the choice for first-line therapy, given the potential for adverse fetal effects with use of indomethacin at this gestational age. Nifedipine 20–30 mg orally is given as the initial loading dose, followed by an additional 10–20 mg orally every 3–8 hours for up to 48 hours, with a maximum dose of 180 mg/day. The most common side effects are flushing, headache, dizziness, and nausea.
- *Beta-agonist (terbutaline):* Terbutaline causes myometrial relaxation by binding with beta-2-adrenergic receptors and increasing intracellular adenyl cyclase which leads to drop in intracellular free calcium.
  - *Dose:* 0.25 mg can be administered S/C every 20–30 minutes for up to four doses or until tocolysis is achieved. Once labor is inhibited, 0.25 mg can be administered S/C every 3–4 hours until the uterus is quiescent for 24 hours. *Continuous intravenous infusion* at 2.5–5 µg/min and increasing by 2.5–5 µg/min every 20–30 minutes to a max of 25 µg/min, or until the contractions have abated.
  - *Side effects:* Fever, headache, tachycardia, tremors, chest pain, pulmonary edema, and metabolic disturbances like hyperglycemia and hypokalemia
  - *Monitoring:* Monitor fluid intake, urine output, and maternal symptoms, especially shortness of breath, chest pain, or tachycardia. Glucose and potassium concentrations should be monitored every 4–6 hours during parenteral drug administration.
  - The FDA has warned that injectable terbutaline should not be used for prolonged (beyond 48–72 hours) treatment of preterm labor, and oral terbutaline should not be used for tocolysis.
  - *Contraindications:* Cardiac disease, poorly controlled hyperthyroidism or diabetes mellitus. We suggest withholding the drug if the maternal heart rate exceeds 120 beats/min.

- *Prostaglandin synthetase inhibitors:* Indomethacin is the most commonly used drug in this class. For most patients ≤ 32 + 0 weeks of gestation who are candidates for tocolysis, we use indomethacin for first-line therapy. There are the risks of premature closure of ductus, renal and cerebral vasoconstriction, necrotizing enterocolitis, and oligohydramnios with this drug; hence, it is not popular.
- *Nitric oxide donors:* Nitroglycerin may reduce perinatal morbidity and mortality by decreasing the risk of premature delivery. A 50-mg transdermal patch, applied on the abdomen releases drug at the rate of 10 mg/ day. If the contractions do not settle in 1 hour, an additional patch can be used. The patch is left in place for 12 hours.
- *Magnesium sulfate:* It is ineffective at delaying birth or preventing birth and its use is associated with increased infant mortality.
- *Atosiban:* It is a selective oxytocin-vasopressin receptor antagonist. It competes with oxytocin for binding to oxytocin receptors in the myometrium and decidua, thus preventing the increase in intracellular free calcium that occurs when oxytocin binds to its receptor. It also inhibits oxytocin-induced production of prostaglandin F2 alpha, but not prostaglandin E2. The half-life of atosiban is 18 minutes. It decreases contractions by 75% in 3 hours. It is safe and effective with minimal side effects. The RCOG guidelines recommend its use in preterm labor.
Dose: 6.75 mg IV stat over 1 minute followed by an infusion of 18 mg/hr for 3 hours and then 6 mg/hr for up to 45 hours. It can be given for up to 48 hours and total dosage should not be >330 mg.

Adverse effects: These include tachycardia, palpitations, hypotension, headache, and vomiting. It is contraindicated in hepatic and renal disorders.

What are the parenteral iron preparations to treat anemia in obstetrics?
Indications:
- Oral iron therapy fails or is not tolerated
- Patient is noncompliant
- *After 32 weeks of gestation:* Ensures compliance
- Failure to absorb oral iron in malabsorption syndrome, inflammatory bowel disease, and chronic inflammatory illness
- Along with erythropoietin.

Any one of the three formulae can be used to calculate the dose of parenteral iron:
1. 4.4 × body weight in kg × hemoglobin deficit (g/dL)
2. Body weight in kg × (desired hemoglobin—patient's hemoglobin) × 2.2 + 1,000 mg
3. 250 mg of elemental iron for each gram of hemoglobin deficit and add another 50% for iron store supplementation

Parenteral iron is administered either IM or IV.

Intramuscular preparations are:
- Iron–sorbitol–citrate complex
- Iron dextran

Intravenous preparations are:
- Iron sucrose
- Iron dextran
- Sodium ferric gluconate complex in sucrose

Iron–sorbitol–citric acid and iron dextran both are associated with multiple adverse drug reactions, both local and systemic; therefore, iron sucrose is now preferred.

Currently, iron sucrose is the most commonly used iron preparation. It has low molecular weight; hence, it is of better use in patients on hemodialysis. No test dose is required; sensitivity reactions are less common, although serious hypersensitivity and anaphylactic reactions have been noticed.

Contraindications: Hypersensitivity, hemosiderosis, hemochromatosis, etc.

Dosage: Single maximum dose is 200 mg and can be repeated up to three doses per week.

Adverse drug reaction:
- *Common:* Change in taste, nausea, vomiting, diarrhea, muscle cramps, pain in arms and legs, and burning sensation at the injection site
- *Less common:* Body ache, abdominal pain. Patient may develop hypotension or hypertension.

Preparation: Venofer, Xenofer, and Hemofer—available as 5 mL ampule and contains 20 mg elemental iron/mL.

Safety during pregnancy: FDA category B.

Newer injectable iron preparation for postpartum use:
- *Ferric carboxymaltose (FCM):* Injection FCM, a new-generation IV iron, comprises a macromolecular iron hydroxide complex tightly bound in a carbohydrate shell. It is a novel nondextran-containing type 1 complex designed to be administered in large doses by rapid (over 15 minutes) IV infusion. Its design allows for controlled delivery and minimal risk of acute toxicity and there is a much wider therapeutic window. FCM can be given as a dose of up to 20 mL (equivalent to 1,000 mg of elemental iron, based on a concentration of 50 mg of elemental iron per mL). It is administered over 15 minutes. Infusion should be started slowly and observation for any side effects should be done. A number of trials have shown efficacy and safety of this agent in iron-deficient patients in a number of different settings including heavy uterine bleeding, and postpartum women. Trials have proven safety of FCM in postpartum women.

Discuss the use of ursodeoxycholic acid in obstetrics.

Ursodeoxycholic acid (UDCA) is the preferred treatment of maternal pruritus due to intrahepatic cholestasis of pregnancy (IHCP) in a dose of 300 mg three times a day (or 15 mg/kg/day) until delivery. A decrease in pruritus is usually seen within 1–2 weeks, and biochemical improvement is usually seen within 3–4 weeks. Fetal/neonatal outcomes were not improved with UDCA treatment compared with placebo. The FDA does not list IHCP as an indication for UDCA treatment.

Mechanism of action: UDCA is a bile acid, improves biliary flow, enhances the protective bicarbonate environment on the surface of cholangiocytes, and protects the liver from bile acid-induced apoptosis. Furthermore, UDCA markedly decreases biliary cholesterol saturation by inhibiting the absorption of cholesterol in the intestine and its secretion into bile, demonstrated by reduced cholesterol fraction of biliary lipids. The use of UDCA is contraindicated in patients with obstructive cholestasis due to a potential risk of biliary integrity disruption.

What is the use of recombinant factor VIIa in postpartum hemorrhage?

One of the recent and novel advancements in the management of PPH has been the use of recombinant activated factor VII (rFVIIa) (NovoSeven). Recently, rFVIIa has been approved for use in Glanzmann thrombasthenia and factor VII deficiency. Outside these indications, any use is considered "off-label", and the responsibility for and decision to use rFVIIa rest with the prescribing clinician. Unlike most other clotting factor products, which are inactive precursor proteins, rFVIIa is an activated form of clotting factor.

Mechanism of action: It activates conversion of factor X to factor Xa, which initiates the common pathway of the coagulation cascade; prothrombin is activated to thrombin, which then converts fibrinogen to fibrin to form a hemostatic plug, thereby achieving clot formation at the site of hemorrhage (hemostasis). NovoSeven RT-half-life: 2.3 hours, administer as slow IV bolus over 2–5 minutes depending on the dose administered.

Use: rFVIIa may be used in the management of refractory PPH. For pregnant women with Glanzmann thrombasthenia, the use of rFVIIa may provide control of bleeding without exposure to allogeneic platelets.

Once all surgical and nonsurgical definitive hemostasis procedures to arrest active bleeding have been attempted and bleeding continues, the use of rFVIIa (NovoSeven) could be considered, prior to hysterectomy. The recommended dose is 60–90 µg/kg body weight administered by IV bolus injection. Peak coagulant action can be expected at 10 minutes. A second dose can be administered based on clinical response of the individual patient after 30 minutes of the first dose. If bleeding persists after two doses of rFVIIa, then consider hysterectomy. It should only be used where the clinician(s) considers that the benefits outweigh the risk of critical bleeding.

Describe antithyroid drugs which can be used in pregnancy. Mention their doses, schedule, and side effects.

Propylthiouracil (PTU) and methimazole are antithyroid medications which can be used in pregnancy. PTU is the drug of choice for hyperthyroidism during the first trimester of pregnancy and in women with methimazole allergy. Methimazole is not preferred in the first trimester of pregnancy, in view of methimazole embryopathy, characterized by aplasia cutis, esophageal atresia, choanal atresia, facial abnormalities, and developmental delay. In the second trimester, PTU is shifted over to methimazole because the risk of hepatotoxicity associated with PTU is high. PTU is the preferred antithyroid drug during lactation also as it is minimally secreted in breast milk. It is used in Graves disease, nodular goiter, and solitary toxic adenoma. It is not used for transient hyperthyroidism, e.g., in gestational trophoblastic disease (GTD), hyperemesis gravidarum, and gestational transient thyrotoxicosis. Free thyroxine (FT4) should be maintained near the upper normal range to prevent fetal hypothyroidism and fetal goiter. Main side effects include liver injury, agranulocytosis, and lupus-like syndrome. Methimazole is preferred in second and third trimesters of pregnancy. It is not preferred during lactation. Main side effects include skin rash, agranulocytosis, alopecia, and anaplastic anemia.

Drug dosages
- PTU:
  - Hyperthyroidism:
    - *Initial dose:* 300–450 mg/day to be administered orally in three divided doses
    - *Maintenance dose:* 100–150 mg/day to be administered orally in three divided doses
  - Graves disease in pregnancy:
    - *Initial dose:* 50–150 mg to be administered orally three times a day
    - *Maintenance dose:* 50 mg to be administered orally twice or three times a day

- *Methimazole:*
  - Hyperthyroidism
    - *Initial dose:* 15–40 mg/day to be administered orally in divided doses in mild and moderate cases. Dosages of 60 mg/day can be used in severe cases.
    - *Maintenance dose:* 5–30 mg/day to be administered orally in three divided doses.
  - Graves' disease in pregnancy
    - *Initial dose:* 10–20 mg/day to be administered orally once a day
    - *Maintenance dose:* To be changed as per the reduction in thyroid function tests

Describe a drug which can be used for hypothyroidism in pregnancy.

Levothyroxine (LT4) is safe during pregnancy and lactation and FDA category A drug. It is used in subclinical hypothyroidism, overt hypothyroidism, and myxedema coma. The recommended initial dose is 12.5–25 μg/day. The dose can be titrated by an increase of 25 μg/day every 2–4 weeks, until thyroid-stimulating hormone (TSH) is normalized. During pregnancy, all patients with overt hypothyroidism with TSH >2.5 mIU/L should be treated with LT4. Patients with preexisting hypothyroid must increase their dose by 25% as soon as pregnancy is confirmed, due to increased requirement during pregnancy. The goal of treatment is to maintain serum TSH <2.5 mIU/L.

Discuss the management of subclinical hypothyroidism in pregnancy.

Levothyroxine therapy is recommended for women with a TSH > 10.0 mIU/L and TPOAb positive women with a TSH between 4 and 10.0 mIU/L.

Levothyroxine therapy can be considered for women with TPOAb negative with a TSH between 4 and 10.0 mU/L and TPOAb positive women with a TSH between 2.5 and 4 mU/L.

Describe the role of corticosteroids in preterm labor.

Corticosteroids stimulate the pulmonary beta receptors and help in synthesis and release of surfactants into the alveolar spaces.

Uses: For patients with gestation <34 weeks in active labor, in patients with fetal growth restriction between 24 and 35 + 6 weeks, in all elective cesarean sections done before 38 + 6 weeks

Dosage: Inj. Dexamethasone 6 mg IM per dosage, a total of four dosages is given 12 hours apart; injection Betamethasone 12 mg per dosage, a total of two dosages is given 24 hours apart.

Both steroids have similar efficacy and safety and no significant difference in reducing perinatal morbidity and mortality; however, dexamethasone shows less incidence of intraventricular hemorrhage and shorter neonatal intensive care unit (NICU) stay. The recommended formulation of betamethasone should be a mixture of long-acting betamethasone acetate and fast-acting betamethasone phosphate which is not available in India. The available salt in India is betamethasone phosphate which is only short-acting, and this salt of betamethasone has no added advantage over dexamethasone sodium phosphate.

■ GYNECOLOGY

What is the mechanism of action of clomiphene?

Clomiphene acts as a selective estrogen receptor modulator (SERM). It competitively inhibits estrogen binding to estrogen receptors (ERs) and has mixed agonist and antagonist activity, depending upon the target tissue. Clomiphene exerts its major effects on the hypothalamus, pituitary, ovary, and uterus. Unlike estrogen, clomiphene citrate (CC) binds nuclear ERs for a prolonged period and depletes them. By binding to ERs in the hypothalamus, it prevents negative feedback of estrogens. Consequently, there is an increase in the pulsatile secretion of gonadotropin-releasing hormone (GnRH), which results in a rise of luteinizing hormone (LH) and FSH. It acts best when a certain amount of estrogen is present in the body. Clomiphene is an estrogen agonist in the absence of estrogen, thereby enhancing FSH stimulation of LH receptors in granulosa cells. Clomiphene acts primarily as an antiestrogen in the uterus, cervix, and vagina. The following findings may explain why pregnancy rates are relatively low when ovulatory rates are so high in women administered clomiphene cycles:

- The normal increase in endometrial thickening that occurs during spontaneous menstrual cycles is largely absent during clomiphene-induced cycles, despite higher estradiol levels.
- Abnormal luteal phase endometrial morphology

Dosage: Clomiphene 50 or 100 mg is prescribed daily for 5 days between days 2 and days 6 of periods. Stepping up the dose by 50 mg/cycle have been prescribed but doses >150 mg daily are not recommended due to increased antiestrogenic effect and ovarian hyperstimulation syndrome (OHSS) risk. CC is now considered to be a second-line agent for women with polycystic ovary syndrome (PCOS) as letrozole therapy results in higher birth rates.

- *Maximum:* 4–6 cycles
- *Maximum dose:* 750 mg/cycle

Clomiphene resistance: When CC stimulation fails to induce ovulation in six consecutive cycles in spite of stepping up the dose to 150 mg, it is categorized as clomiphene resistance. This occurs in 15–20% of patients. *Causes:* Obese women and hyperandrogenism.

Treatment options:
- *Extended course treatment (7–10 days):* 50% may ovulate by this
- Adding adjuvants like metformin, myo-inositol, and D-chiro-inositol in obese polycystic ovarian (PCO) patients
- Combination with gonadotropins
- CC stimulation after laparoscopy and ovarian drilling
- Changing to other oral ovulation-inducing agents like tamoxifen

Clomiphene failure: Failure to conceive even after three ovulatory cycles following CC stimulation. In this case, other causes of infertility other than anovulation need to be reconsidered.

What are the newer therapies for endometriosis?

Conventionally, the drugs used to treat endometriosis have been oral contraceptives, nonsteroidal anti-inflammatory drugs (NSAIDs), progestins, danazol, and GnRH agonists. It must be noted that medical interventions do not improve fertility, diminish endometriomas, or treat complications of deep endometriosis such as ureteral obstruction.

Newer therapies include the following:
- *Letrozole:* It is a third-generation aromatase inhibitor. Aromatase is the key enzyme in the synthesis of estrogen and mediates conversion of androstenedione and testosterone to estrone and estradiol. Letrozole is a highly potent and specific suppressor of estrogen production, locally and systemically. The drug is used along with progesterone, calcium, and vitamin

D supplements in endometriosis as add-back therapy to prevent the potential risk of bone loss and osteopenia. The dose given is 2.5 mg daily for 3 months.
- *Levonorgestrel intrauterine device (LNG-IUD):* Locally administered levonorgestrel has a profound effect on the endometrium. It induces endometrial gland atrophy and decidualization of stroma, reduces endometrial cell proliferation, and increases apoptotic activity. It relieves menstrual pain associated with recurrent endometriosis.
- *Dienogest:* It is a progestogen-only hormone preparation. Its mechanism of action is suppressing estradiol production and thus preventing the growth of the endometrium. It does not have glucocorticoid or antimineralocorticoid activity. Dose is 2 mg daily. It can be started on any day of the menstrual cycle and is to be taken every day without interruption. It is as effective as GnRH agonists in the treatment of endometriosis, has a lower incidence of hypoestrogenic side effects (e.g., hot flashes and reduced libido), and causes significantly smaller bone-mineral density reductions. Adverse effects are breast discomfort, nausea, and irritability. Weight gain, depressed mood, headache, migraine, and menorrhagia are among the other side effects.
- *Danazol-loaded IUD:* Promising data has been reported for a danazol-loaded IUD in women with adenomyosis.
- *Gestrinone:* It is a 19-nortestosterone derivative, similar in action to danazol but long lasting. It has progestogenic and mild androgenic activity, induces regression of endometriotic implants, and is efficacious in reducing pain.
- *Antiangiogenic drug:* Angiogenesis has been claimed as one of the mechanisms involved in pain production. A correlation between ovarian endometriomal vascularization and symptoms could be possible. Antiangiogenic drugs, e.g., endostatin, antivascular endothelial growth factor (anti-VEGF), and angiostatin, are under trial in animal models and may emerge as new therapies for the endometriosis-associated pain.

Classify progestogens and enumerate their uses.

Natural form—progesterone

Synthetic progesterone:
- Progesterone derivatives such as 17-alpha hydroxyprogesterone caproate, medroxyprogesterone acetate, and megestrol acetate
- Stereoisomers of progesterone such as dydrogesterone
- *Testosterone derivatives:* Ethisterone and dimethisterone
- *19-nor-steroids (nortestosterone derivatives):* Norethisterone acetate, norethynodrel, allylestrenol, ethynodiol diacetate, and newer progestogens such as desogestrel, gestodene, and norgestimate, which are lipid soluble

Newer preparations with dose and indications:
- *Natural micronized progesterone and dydrogesterone:* Endogenous progesterone is synthesized from cholesterol steroids in a two-step enzymatic process and produced mainly by the corpus luteum and the placenta, with some contribution from the adrenal glands. The half-life of endogenous progesterone is about 5 minutes, and it is metabolized mainly by the liver to pregnanediol. In the bloodstream, progesterone is bound mostly to albumin. Exogenous progesterone when taken orally is absorbed rapidly, but almost the

entire dose is metabolized completely in first pass through the gut and liver. Hence, exogenous progesterone is given preferably by vaginal or injectable route. Micronization is the process of reducing the average diameter of particles such that the particles that are produced are only a few micrometers in diameter.

- Dydrogesterone is a progestogen that has chemical structure and pharmacological action similar to endogenous progesterone. Unlike other synthetic progesterone, it has high-specific affinity for progesterone receptors and no affinity for androgen, mineralocorticoid, glucocorticoid, and estrogenic receptors. Both micronized progesterone and dydrogesterone are closely related to endogenous progesterone.
- Progesterone is currently used in early pregnancy for various indications by oral, vaginal, and IM route and as tablets, capsules, vaginal pessaries, injections, and gels.

Progesterone supplementation for luteal support in assisted reproductive techniques (ART): To improve implantation and pregnancy rates in ART cycles (both in GnRH agonist and in antagonist protocols), adequate luteal phase support is required. This can be achieved by hCG or by using progesterone. Deficiency of endogenous progesterone causes implantation failure and early miscarriages; hence, progesterone supplementation is given. It is started just after oocyte retrieval/embryo transfer. The duration of exogenous progesterone therapy generally varies up to 10–12 weeks of gestation. In ART cycles, progesterone can be used as:
- *IM progesterone:* 50–100 mg/day
- *Vaginal micronized progesterone:* 600–800 mg/day
- *Oral dydrogesterone:* 20–30 mg/day

Progesterone support in recurrent pregnancy loss and threatened miscarriage: Recurrent spontaneous miscarriage is spontaneous loss of three or more consecutive pregnancies before 20 weeks of gestation. One of the causes of recurrent pregnancy loss is deficiency of endogenous progesterone in early pregnancy. Progesterone induces secretory changes in the endometrium, which is necessary for endometrial maturation, endometrial stabilization, and embryo implantation, thus preventing pregnancy loss.

Various progesterones used in recurrent pregnancy loss are as follows:
- *Recurrent miscarriage:*
  - Oral dydrogesterone 10 mg BD till 20 weeks of pregnancy
  - *Micronized progesterone:* 400 mg/day vaginally till 20 weeks of pregnancy
- *Threatened miscarriage:*
  - *Micronized progesterone:* 400 mg/day vaginal till bleeding stops
  - *Dydrogesterone:* 40 mg loading dose followed by 20–30 mg daily till 7 days after bleeding stops

Candidates for progesterone supplementation: The American College of Obstetricians and Gynecologists (ACOG 2023) recommends vaginal progesterone for the following indications:
- For patients with singleton pregnancies and no history of prior pulmonary tuberculosis (PTB) who have a short cervix (≤25 mm) on transvaginal ultrasound examination at 18–24 weeks. Daily vaginal progesterone is better than oral to reduce the risk for PTB.
- For patients with singleton pregnancies and a positive history of prior PTB, offer vaginal progesterone to those with a

short cervix (≤25 mm) on transvaginal ultrasound examination at 16–24 weeks

Pregnancies where the benefit of progesterone supplementation is unproven:
- Singleton pregnancy with prior preterm birth
- Positive fetal fibronectin test
- Uterine anomaly or assisted reproductive technology
- Unselected twin pregnancies
- After preterm prelabor rupture of membranes
- Threatened or established preterm labor
- Maintenance therapy after threatened preterm labor

Doses of micronized progesterone: 90–400 mg beginning as early as 18 weeks of gestation.

Hydroxyprogesterone caproate (17-OHPC) is a synthetic progestogen with minimal to no androgenic activity. 17-OHPC preparation was approved in 2011 by the FDA to reduce the risk of recurrent preterm birth in pregnant females with a singleton pregnancy who have a history of a prior spontaneous preterm delivery. However, in 2023, the US FDA concluded that use of 17-OHPC is not supported by available evidence and withdrew its approval.

What are the estrogen preparations used in gynecology?

Oral preparations are as follows:
- *Conjugated equine estrogen (CEE):* This is a preparation containing natural estrogens and is considered safe to use in postmenopausal women as compared to the synthetic estrogen like ethinylestradiol. Systemic estrogens are used mainly to treat vasomotor symptoms, i.e., hot flashes in postmenopausal women. Estrogens prevent postmenopausal osteoporosis; however, their use is not indicated solely for this purpose. It contains conjugated estrogens, which are sodium salts of the sulfate esters of natural estrogen. Sodium estrone sulfate is the main component of this preparation that gets converted to the active forms—estrone (by action of enzyme estrone sulfatase) and estradiol. The commonly used daily doses are 0.625 mg of CEE.
- *Ethinyl estradiol (EE):* It is a derivative of estradiol 10–20 µg/day.
- *Estradiol valerate:* It is the valeric-acid ester of estradiol and is chemically and biologically similar to endogenous human estradiol. Dose: 1–2 mg/day. It is used to treat menopausal symptoms and also for growth of endometrium in conditions like Asherman's syndrome and ART.
- *Continuous-release skin patch* is available that contains estradiol as hemihydrates preparation.
- *Low-dose preparations for local application:* Vaginal estrogenic creams, rings, and tablets are used for management of urogenital atrophy in postmenopausal women. These local preparations may contain estriol, estradiol, or CEE. Systemic absorption is very less, so progesterone administration is not required. Estriol succinate cream (Evalon cream 1%) is a short-term hormone replacement therapy (HRT) used to treat atrophic vaginitis. It comes in the pack of 15 g/tube. One application contains 0.5 g cream, which corresponds to 0.5 mg estriol. One tube lasts for a month.

What are the causes of galactorrhea? What are the drugs used to treat hyperprolactinemia?

Galactorrhea is inappropriate discharge of milk-containing fluid from the breast. It is considered abnormal, if it persists for longer than 6 months after childbirth or discontinuation of breastfeeding. The various causes of galactorrhea are all due to a state of hyperprolactinemia and include the following:

Physiological factors:
- Pregnancy, lactation, sleep, emotional stress, and coitus

Hypothalamic–pituitary stalk damage (loss of inhibitory effect of dopamine):
- *Tumors*—craniopharyngioma, meningioma, and metastases
- Empty sella syndrome, granulomas, trauma, and irradiation

Pituitary prolactin hypersecretion: Prolactinoma and acromegaly

Systemic disorders: Chronic renal failure, hypothyroidism, cirrhosis, and epileptic seizures

Drugs: Chlorpromazine, haloperidol, metoclopramide, methyldopa, reserpine, opiates, ranitidine, cimetidine, tricyclic antidepressants, fluoxetine, verapamil, estrogens, and antiandrogens

Miscellaneous: Chiari–Frommel syndrome, Forbes–Albright syndrome, and ectopic production by tumors such as carcinoma of lung

Cabergoline is an ergoline derivative with high affinity and selectivity for the D2 receptor. It has an extremely long plasma half-life of about 65 hours, allowing once- or twice-weekly administration. It normalizes serum prolactin levels in 85–86% and normal gonadal function in 90%.

Side effects: Constipation, nasal stuffiness, dry mouth, nightmares, insomnia, and vertigo.

Bromocriptine is a dopamine receptor agonist that suppresses prolactin secretion. It is started in the dose of 0.625–1.25 mg HS and gradually increased every week. Most patients respond to a dose of 5–7.5 mg daily in divided doses, but doses up to 30 mg have been used. Nausea, vomiting, and postural hypotension may occur in ~25% of patients after the initial dose. Bromocriptine is also available as IM injection (Parlodel-LAR) used in an initial dose of 50 mg, increasing to 100 mg; it produces an acute reduction in the prolactin level by 30–80%.

Cabergoline is more effective and causes fewer adverse effects than bromocriptine. Therapy should be continued for approximately 12–24 months (depending on the degree of symptoms or tumor size) and then withdrawn if prolactin levels have returned to the normal range. After withdrawal, approximately one sixth of patients maintain normal prolactin levels. Response to therapy should be monitored by checking fasting serum prolactin levels and checking tumor size with MRI. Most women (approximately 90%) regain cyclic menstruation and achieve resolution of galactorrhea.

Dosage: 0.25 mg twice a week

Increased by 0.25 mg, maximum 1 mg twice a week according to the patient's serum prolactin level. Increase slowly every 4 weeks. Duration 12–24 months.
- Cardiovascular evaluation and echocardiography before initiating treatment are advisable
- Routine echocardiographic monitoring every 6–12 months or as clinically indicated

Other uses of cabergoline:
- OHSS
- Lactation suppression
- Uterine myomas
- Endometriosis

Contraindications of cabergoline:
- Uncontrolled hypertension or known hypersensitivity to ergot derivatives
- History of cardiac valvular disorders, echocardiographic demonstration of valve leaflet thickening, valve restriction, or mixed valve restriction-stenosis, history of pulmonary, pericardial, or retroperitoneal fibrotic disorders

Describe the medical management of fibroids.

- Correction of iron deficiency anemia.
- *Control of menorrhagia:* Tranexamic acid 500–1,000 mg three times a day, norethisterone acetate, and combined oral contraceptive (COC) pills
- Levonorgestrel-releasing intrauterine system (Mirena); it is a T-shaped IUD with a reservoir of 52 mg of levonorgestrel released daily at the rate of 20 µg. It has been proven to reduce the duration of bleeding and amount of menstrual loss due to inhibition of endometrial proliferation. It is a therapeutic modality for myoma-associated menorrhagia and anemia. IUDs also provide highly effective long-acting contraception. First, identifying patients with significant submucosal fibroids is important since the risk of expulsion of the IUD is greater in patients with fibroids that distort the endometrial cavity.
- GnRH analogs produce a hypogonadotropic hypogonadism state. GnRH analogs, including antagonists and agonists, can reduce heavy menstrual bleeding (HMB). Agonists also significantly reduce fibroid volume but have potential adverse effects that limit use. When used for 6 months, they cause reduction in fibroid size by 50–80%, e.g., Leuprolide acetate 3.75 mg IM once a month, Goserelin 3.6 mg S/C every 28 days, Triptorelin 3.75 mg IM every 3 weeks, Nafarelin 800 µg intranasally twice daily.
- *GnRH antagonists:* Oral GnRH antagonists are a relatively new generation of medical therapy. Elagolix, Relugolix, and Linzagolix, oral GnRH analogs which are FDA approved, are being used in USA and Europe.
- *GnRH agonists:* They are primarily used as either preoperative therapy (typically 3–6 months in duration) or as transitional therapy for patients in late perimenopause as they move to menopause. For patients with fibroids and anemia who are planning surgery for fibroids but have not responded adequately to iron-only therapy, a short course of preoperative GnRH agonist treatment plus iron is an established option.
- *Ulipristal acetate (UPA):* It is a selective progesterone receptor modulator. Two recent clinical trials (PEARL 1 and PEARL 2, 2012) have revealed that UPA brings about 42% reduction in the size of fibroid and improvement in heavy menstrual bleeding (98% reduction in heavy periods and 89% achieved amenorrhea) at a daily dose of 10 mg; the effect is comparable to GnRH analogs. In addition, there is no initial steroid flare with UPA as seen with leuprolide acetate. The side effect is much lesser than GnRH analogs; there is only 10% risk of hot flashes as compared to 40% risk of hot flashes with GnRH analog. Ulipristal acetate is not typically used for the treatment of uterine fibroids as cases of serious liver toxicity, liver transplantation, and fatalities have been reported.

Contraindications: Liver disorders (severe), genital bleeding of unknown etiology, uterine, cervical, ovary, and breast cancers

Dosage: 5 mg orally daily for only 3 months

Adverse drug reaction: Headache, nausea, abdominal pain, etc.

Ulipristal is also available worldwide for emergency contraception. It can be used for emergency contraception up to 120 hours after intercourse. An advantage of ulipristal over hormonal oral agents is that it appears to maintain high efficacy for 120 hours after intercourse. It is the only oral emergency contraception licensed for use between 72 and 120 hours. No significant side effects have been reported. It is marketed as a single 30 mg tablet under the brand name Ella or EllaOne for use as an emergency contraceptive.

Safety during pregnancy: Pregnancy category X

- *Mifepristone:* Mifepristone at doses of 5–50 mg for 3–6 months has been reported to decrease heavy menstrual bleeding and, in some studies, fibroid volume. However, some studies reported abnormal endometrial histology at the conclusion of therapy. Mifepristone 50 mg/day for 3–6 months produces amenorrhea and shrinkage of tumor by 50%.
- Danazol 400–800 mg daily for 3–6 months reduces the size of the tumor and is often used prior to myomectomy to reduce uterine vascularity.
- Gestrinone, also known as ethyl-norgestrienone, is a synthetic steroid of the 19-nortestosterone, which has androgenic, antiestrogenic, and anti-progestogenic properties and is used primarily in the treatment of endometriosis.

It is used in 2.5 mg twice weekly. Treatment is limited to a single course of 6 months duration per lifetime.

What are the therapeutic uses of gonadotropins in gynecology?

Most commonly available pituitary gonadotropins for commercial use are as follows:

- Human menopausal gonadotropin (hMG), which contains 75 IU of LH and 75 IU of FSH
- Pure FSH, which is especially useful for ovulation induction in women who have elevated levels of endogenous LH as in PCOS
- *Recombinant gonadotropins:* They have the advantage of higher purity and specific activity, batch-to-batch consistency, and complete absence of contamination by other gonadotropins. Purified uFSH has some LH activity, but rhFSH does not.
- *hCG:* It is used to trigger ovulation when the ovarian follicles are mature. Both urinary and recombinant hCG preparations are available. A dose of 250 µg of recombinant hCG appears to be equivalent to the standard doses of urinary hCG (5,000–10,000 units)

Uses:

- Anovulatory infertility where other factors are excluded; the dose is adjusted according to ultrasonographic monitoring of follicular growth and serum estradiol level. Treatment is started on the second day of menstrual cycle and continued until ovulation occurs.
- Induction of superovulation using hyperstimulation protocols in women undergoing assisted reproduction therapy
- Primary and secondary amenorrhea caused by pituitary failure
- hCG is administered for luteal phase support in infertility and early abortions

- Male infertility (hypogonadotropic hypogonadism)
- Cryptorchidism

Describe various antiandrogens used in the treatment of hirsutism.
- Any pharmacologic therapy for hirsutism should be given a trial of at least 6 months, before making any changes in dose, adding a medication, or switching to a new medication. This is because the growth phase of a hair follicle is approximately 6 months; a significant reduction in hair growth may not occur before then.
- For most of the females, COCs are the first-line drug; an antiandrogen can then be added if the clinical response is suboptimal after 6 months of therapy.
- The COCs and antiandrogens do not have US FDA approval for the indication of hirsutism. Therefore, these therapies represent "off-label" use.
- These preparations also provide additional nonhirsutism benefits such as contraception, cycle management, and reduction of other hyperandrogenic symptoms such as acne. For females with PCOS, COCs also provide the additional benefits of preventing the development of endometrial hyperplasia and restoring regular menstrual cyclicity.
- The COC which contains a progestin with low or neutral androgenicity, such as norethindrone or norgestimate, is best for this purpose. It is better to avoid COC preparations containing the most androgenic progestin, levonorgestrel.
- When hormonally evaluating females who have been on a COC, it is best to discontinue the medications for at least 8 weeks, as it takes at least this length of time for measured androgens and sex hormone binding globulin (SHBG) levels to return to basal values.
- *Spironolactone:* It is the first choice of antiandrogen. It is an aldosterone and androgen receptor antagonist that is structurally similar to progestin. It competes with dihydrotestosterone (DHT) for binding to the androgen receptor and inhibits enzymes involved in androgen biosynthesis. The beneficial effect also starts by 4th month of treatment. The drug reduces androgen level. Spironolactone is considered safest among all antiandrogens. The starting dose is 50 mg twice daily and increased to 100 mg twice daily as needed. The side effects of spironolactone include hyperkalemia (a rare problem in females with normal renal function and aldosterone secretion). The serum potassium level is measured in all patients after 1 month. Females with renal insufficiency should not be prescribed spironolactone, because of the high risk of hyperkalemia.
  - *Daily dose:* 100–200 mg with cyclical EE produces relief in 60% of cases.
  - *Side effects:* Transient diuresis, gynecomastia, hyperkalemia, etc
- *Finasteride:* It inhibits 5-alpha-reductase type 2, the enzyme that converts testosterone to DHT. Only a partial inhibitory effect occurs when used for excess hair growth because the enhanced 5-alpha-reductase activity in hirsutism involves both type 1 and type 2 enzymes. It is used by some clinicians at doses of 1–5 mg/day, but there are concerns about its inadvertent use in early pregnancy, given the essential role of DHT in the development of male external genitalia.
- *Flutamide:* It is a nonsteroidal androgen receptor antagonist. It is used primarily in the management of prostate cancer, but it has been used off-label for managing hirsutism. The efficacy of flutamide

(250–750 mg/day) is similar to that of spironolactone (100–200 mg/day) and finasteride (5 mg/day). However, the use of flutamide for hirsutism is discouraged since it has been associated with hepatotoxicity, even at doses as low as 62.5 mg (a dose that has not been shown to be effective for hirsutism in randomized clinical trials).
- *Side effects:* Hepatotoxicity, dry skin, and oligomenorrhea
- *Cimetidine:* It is a histamine receptor antagonist and blocks androgen action at the receptor site.
- *Glucocorticoids:* Dexamethasone and prednisolone reduce adrenocorticotropic hormone (ACTH) and thereby androgen secretion in the adrenal gland.
- *Others*: Two weak antiandrogens, CPA (a 17-hydroxyprogesterone derivative) and drospirenone, are the progestin component in some COCs:
  - *Drospirenone,* a progestin used in some COCs, is a very weak antiandrogen. The dose used with EE in COCs (3 mg) is equivalent to approximately 25 mg of spironolactone. Drospirenone-containing COCs have been associated with a higher risk of VTE than COCs containing second-generation progestins. A progestin-only contraceptive pill containing drospirenone is available, but no data are available for its possible efficacy for treating hirsutism.
  - *Cyproterone acetate (CPA):* It competes with DHT for binding to the androgen receptor and reduces serum LH and ovarian androgen concentrations. It is used in a low dose (2 mg) as the progestin component of COCs or as a higher dose (12.5–100 mg) as monotherapy or with estrogen.

The effect starts by 4th month. Combination with EE is necessary to prevent pregnancy, avoid teratogenic effects, regularize the menstrual cycle, and increase the SHBG level. Drug regulatory agencies in Europe have recommended limiting its use to "second-line" therapy because of a perceived increase in the risk of hepatotoxicity compared with other available progestins.

What is RU 486? What are its therapeutic applications?

RU 486 (mifepristone) is an antiprogestin that competitively blocks both progesterone and glucocorticoid receptors. By opposing the activity of progesterone, mifepristone elicits a variety of effects that make the uterus more susceptible to abortion. These effects include cervical dilation, decidual necrosis, increased endogenous PG production, and increasing uterine sensitivity to exogenously administered PG. Mifepristone administration gradually elicits a fivefold increase in sensitivity to PG 24–48 hours after its administration. The synergy between mifepristone and PG permits greater efficacy of PG at lower doses, potentially minimizing side effects. Mifepristone and misoprostol have been found to be safe and effective in first- and second-trimester induction abortion.

Uses:
- *Therapeutic abortion:* It is used for the medical induction of abortion in combination with misoprostol. It increases the sensitivity of the uterus to prostaglandins. A dose of 200 mg of mifepristone followed by 400 µg misoprostol induces abortion in more than 95% of cases with up to 7 weeks of amenorrhea. It is also useful in ripening

of the cervix in midtrimester abortions. Mifepristone 200–600 mg augments the action of prostaglandins when given 24–48 hours prior and reduces the dose and side effects of prostaglandins. A shorter induction–abortion interval is noted.
- *Postcoital contraception:* It blocks the action of progesterone on endometrium, causes sloughing and shedding of the decidua, and causes abortion. It can also be used as a monthly contraceptive or as a "morning after pill" to induce menstruation.
- Missed abortion
- Uterine fibroid
- *EP:* In unruptured ectopic gestation, it is injected locally as medical therapy.
- *Cushing syndrome:* Because of its antiglucocorticoid activity.

Describe the use of gonadotropin-releasing hormone agonist in gynecology.
Gonadotropin-releasing hormone agonists are used for 3 months in monthly dose to reduce fibroid volume. It causes reduction in fibroid volume by 30% and total uterine volume by 35%. Reduction of uterine size occurs in the first 3 months. Following discontinuation of GnRH analog, menses return in 4–8 weeks' time and uterus returns to pretreatment levels in 4–6 months. It causes atrophy of the endometriotic implants in the same dose.

Adverse drug reaction: Osteoporosis, hot flashes, dry vagina, headache, depression, loss of libido, night sweats, breast atrophy, etc.

Dosage of GnRH agonists in fibroid and endometriosis:
- *Leuprolide:* 3.75 mg IM monthly or 11.5 mg IM every 3 months
- *Goserelin:* 3.6 mg S/C monthly
- *Nafarelin:* 200 µg intranasal twice daily

Add-back therapy: Side effects of GnRH agonists can be minimized by addition of low-dose progestin or estrogen–progestin in add-back regimens.

One of the following can be given:
- *Progestin only:* Norethisterone 1.2 mg or norethisterone acetate 5 mg/day
- *Combined estrogen and progestogen:*
  - Conjugated estrogen 0.625 mg plus medroxyprogesterone acetate—2.5 mg or norethisterone acetate—5 mg or norethisterone acetate—5 mg daily
  - Estradiol 2 mg plus norethisterone acetate—1 mg daily
- Raloxifene (SERM)—60 mg orally daily

What is the role of myoinositol in polycystic ovary syndrome?
Myoinositol and D-chiroinositol are two main inositol stereoisomers present in our body. In PCOS patients, administration of myoinositol and D-chiroinositol (40:1 ratio) has been shown to improve insulin sensitivity, restore regular menstrual cycles, induce ovulation, and improve hyperandrogenism. Currently available formulation (tablet Normoz) contains 13.8 mg of D-chiro-inositol and 550 mg of myoinositol.

What is the role of methotrexate in gynecology?
Mechanism of action: Methotrexate (MTX) is a folic acid antagonist. It inhibits deoxynucleic acid (DNA) synthesis and cell reproduction, primarily in actively proliferating cells such as malignant cells, trophoblasts, and fetal cells.

Methotrexate is the primary pharmaceutical agent that is used for the management of disorders arising from trophoblastic tissue. Its widespread international use is mostly attributable to its noninvasive, safe, and effective

TABLE 2: Methods of IM methotrexate administration.

Protocols	Evaluation
Single-dose methotrexate 50 mg/m² IM	• Measure β-hCG on days 4 and 7 • If difference <15%, repeat weekly until undetectable • If difference >15%, repeat and begin on new day 1
Multiple doses Methotrexate 1 mg/kg IM, days 1, 3, 5, 7 Leucovorin 0.1 mg/kg IM, days 2, 4, 6, 8	Continue alternate-day injection until β-hCG level falls 15% in 48 hours or 4 doses of methotrexate given; then weekly β-hCG until undetectable

characteristics as a treatment option for EP and GTD, with the large added benefit of fertility preservation. *Dosing and administration*: Treatment of EP uses an intermediate MTX dose [50 mg/m² body surface area (BSA) or 1 mg/kg body weight] **(Table 2)**.

Adverse reactions: Adverse reactions to MTX are usually mild and self-limited. The most common are stomatitis and conjunctivitis. Rare side effects include gastritis, enteritis, dermatitis, pneumonitis, alopecia, elevated liver enzymes, and bone marrow suppression.

Describe the use of vasopressin in gynecology.

Vasopressin is a nanopeptide, secreted from the posterior pituitary gland. It causes vasoconstriction by acting through the vasopressin (V1) receptor and exerts its antidiuretic action through the V2 receptors in the kidney. The synthetic vasopressin injection has been used as a hemostatic agent for over 50 years in various gynecological surgeries such as cervical conization, hysterectomy, and myomectomy, to reduce blood loss. Vasopressin is used as an off-label drug during myomectomy.

Dose: It has concentration of 20 units in one ampule. Dilute 20 units of vasopressin in 100 mL of saline (0.2 U/mL); 4–6 units of vasopressin equals 20–30 mL of this solution. The half-life of IM vasopressin is 10–20 minutes and the duration of action is 2–8 hours. Avoid concentrations > 1 U/mL. Do not exceed a total dosage of injection approximately 5 U. Always alert the anesthesiologist before the injection of vasopressin, so they are vigilant for changes in vital signs. Avoid intravenous injection.

Side effects: Although vasopressin induces uterine contraction and thereby decreased blood loss, transfusion, and operative time, it can cause general hypotension and severe vasoconstriction within 2 or 3 minutes when vasopressin is injected into the muscular layer of the uterus. Typically, these changes return to normal after 15–25 minutes, but they can also have a fatal effect on the patient. Their severe complications could be sudden cardiac arrest starting with bradycardia, pulmonary edema, and myocardial infarction.

Describe the use of topical 5-fluorouracil in gynecology.

Topical 5-fluorouracil (5-FU) is used for the treatment of skin cancers and lesions caused by human papillomavirus (HPV), including genital warts, vulvar intraepithelial neoplasia, and vaginal intraepithelial neoplasia. The 5-FU treatment of genital disease is an off-label use of the medication because it has not been approved by the FDA or recommended by the ACOG for this use. Topical therapy is suitable if invasive disease is not suspected based on findings from cytology, vaginoscopy, or histology. Persistent VaIN 2 and selected VaIN 3 lesions may be medically treated using

5% 5-FU cream. Response rates as high as 75% have been reported.

Side effects: Burning, pain, inflammation, edema, or painful ulcerations. For this reason, topical 5-FU has a limited role in the primary therapy of high grade squamous intraepithelial lesion (HSIL).

Dose: 3 mL of cream should be applied to vaginal vault by a plastic vaginal applicator every other day bedtime during the first week of treatment and once weekly, thereafter for up to 10 weeks. Additionally, an occlusive, water-resistant ointment can be spread on the vulva for protection. Protective gloves are worn when handling 5-FU cream and measures are taken to avoid 5-FU contact by sexual partners.

Patients to be counseled for contraception and consent for off-label medication use. Close monitoring is required for excessive inflammation and ulceration, which can lead to vaginal or vulvar scarring.

Describe the use of topical imiquimod cream in gynecology.

Imiquimod cream is a topical immune response modifier and is often the preferred initial treatment for recurrent vulvar HSIL. It can also be used as initial therapy for carefully selected patients (e.g., patients with clitoral lesions) who prefer to avoid excision and ablation, provided that they are able to comply with a long treatment course (4–6 months).

Imiquimod is applied topically to individual lesions, not to the entire vulva. A typical course involves applying a thin layer of cream three to five times per week (alternating days) for a total duration of 16 weeks.

Side effects: Inflammation at the application site, including mild-to-moderate erythema or erosions. Up to two-thirds of patients reduce the number of applications due to local side effects.

CHAPTER 24

Prescription Writing

Neerja Goel, Anshuja Singla, Ankita Jain

■ INTRODUCTION

Definition: Prescription is a written, verbal, or electronic order of a registered medical practitioner for one or more medicines together with the directions to the pharmacists for their preparations and to the patient for their use.

■ CONTENTS OF A PRESCRIPTION

- Date of the order
- Patient's name and address
- Name of the drug
- Strength of the drug
- Quantity of the drug
- Directions for the use
- Practitioner's name, address, telephone number, and registration number

■ PRINCIPLES FOR WRITING PRESCRIPTION

- Always write legibly.
- Use metric system (gram, liter).
- Always sign and put the date.
- Be precise.
- Be accurate.
- Use precautions.
- Never abbreviate drug names.
- Prefix zero before decimals, for example, 0.25 mg Digoxin.
- Not to use bid or tid; instead, use twice or thrice a day.
- Write mL instead of cc.
- Write microgram.
- Write units instead of IU or U.
- Write time 8 AM or 8 PM instead of twice daily.

■ PARTS OF PRESCRIPTION

- *Superscription:* More commonly, Rx is thought to be an abbreviation or a Latin word that is "Receipe" meaning "take thou" or "you take please", an order to the pharmacists or dispensers for preparing medicines.
  - Rx may be derived from Egyptian word "Eye of the honus", a symbol denoting health or may be a symbolic appeal by a physician to the God Jupiter (God of knowledge, learning, and healing) for the prescription's success.
- *Inscription:* Body of the prescription consisting of the official names and amounts of drug
  - Basis—chief ingredient
  - Adjuvants—secondary active drug to assist the action of the basis
  - Corrigents/corrective (if any) to correct the undesirable quality or action of the basis
  - Solvent/vehicle—to give a suitable form of administration
- *Subscription:* This provides direction to the pharmacist/dispenser.
- *Transcription:* Direction to the patient; contains instructions about the amount of drug and time and frequency of doses to be taken.

- Signature of the treating physician which should be legibly signed with seal and date.

ABBREVIATIONS WHICH ARE UNIVERSALLY ACCEPTED AND SHOULD BE USED

Abbreviation	Full words	Meaning
Rx	recipe	Take thou
sig	signature	
a.c.	ante cibos	Before meals
p.c.	post cibos	After meals
b.i.d.	bis in die	Twice a day
t.i.d.	ter in die	Thrice a day
q.i.d.	quarter in die	Four times a day
stat	statum	Immediately
s.o.s	si opus sit	If necessary
o.d.	omni die	Daily
o.m.	omni mane	Every morning
o.n.	omni necte	Every night
p.o.	per os	By mouth
q.s.	quantum sufficient	A sufficient quantity
h.s.	horasomni	At bedtime

MODEL PRESCRIPTION

Date: 00/00/0000
Dr. Neerja Goel
MD, MS, FICOG, FIMSA & FAMS
Obstetrician and Gynecologist
Reg. No. DMC-6919

Pvt. OPD: Sharda Hospital
10 AM to 1 PM, Monday to Saturday
Mobile: 0000000
Email: XXXXXXXXXX

Patient's Name: XXXXXXXX, 32 y/f a case of primary infertility resident of Greater NOIDA
Planned for ovulation induction

Ovulation Induction in Unexplained Infertility

Prerequisites
- Sonography on day 2 for baseline parameters:
  - Endometrial thickness (ET)
  - Antral follicular count.
- Serum estradiol should be more than 200 pg/mL.
- Anti-Müllerian hormone (AMH) more than 3

Rx
Tablet Letrozole 2.5 mg once a day from 2nd to 6th day of menstrual cycle.

Ultrasonography for follicle monitoring from day 9 of last menstrual period to be continued till follicle matures to 18–20 mm size.

Injection human chorionic gonadotropin 10,000 IU intramuscularly to be given for rupture of follicle. Micronized progesterone 200 mg twice a day till pregnancy is achieved or till next period comes.

Ovulation induction in letrozole-resistant cases
- Injection human menopausal gonadotropin (hMG) 1 amp [75 IU follicle-stimulating hormone (FSH) and 75 IU luteinizing hormone (LH)] intramuscularly (IM) from D3
- Follicular monitoring till follicle size of 18 mm, serum estradiol >200 pg/mL (indicate adequate response of gonadotropin)
- Injection human chorionic gonadotropin (hCG) 10,000 IU IM with timed intercourse/IUI

Ovulation induction in hyperprolactinemia:
- Tablet cabergoline 0.25 mg biweekly, can be increased to 1.5 mg biweekly Or
- When prolactin levels normalize (<20 mIU); tablet clomiphene citrate 50 mg/100 mg or tablet letrozole (D2–D6) with timed intercourse/IUI

Ovulation induction in polycystic ovary syndrome:
- Tablet metformin 500 mg 1 BD with meals to be increased up to 500–850 mg TDS with induction by ovulating-inducing drug on D2–D6 with follicular monitoring from day 9 of menses
- If no response with tablet metformin and clomiphene citrate, gonadotropin-releasing hormone (GnRH) protocol:
  - Short protocol—GnRH (0.1 mg) IM from D1 till follicle matures with recombinant follicle-stimulating hormone (rFSH) from D3
  - Long protocol—GnRH (0.1 mg) IM from D21 of previous menstrual cycle for downregulation followed by injection FSH/hMG 75 IU IM till follicle matures
  - Fixed-dose regimen—constant daily dose of 75–150 IU
  - Chronic low-dose step-up regimen—37.5–75 IU/day, increment of 37.5 IU till the estradiol level increases >200 pg/mL, follicle >10 mm size; the same dose to be continued

POLYCYSTIC OVARY SYNDROME IN ADOLESCENCE

- *General measures:*
  - Weight reduction
  - Lifestyle modification
  - Local depilatory methods for hirsutism associated with polycystic ovarian disease (PCOD)
- *Drugs:*
  - Oral contraceptive pill × 21 days for 6 cycles (third-generation progestins preferred due to less androgenic effect)
  - Tablet metformin 1,500–2,000 mg in divided doses × 3–6 months if required

HIRSUTISM

- *Physical measures for hair removal:*
  - Depilation (removal of hair from surface)—chemical depilation in form of gel, cream, lotion, aerosol, bleaching, shaving, depilating agents, waxing, electrolysis, laser treatment, eflornithine hydrochloride 13.9% cream locally
  - Epilation (removal of entire hair shaft and root)—temporary mechanical methods like plucking, threading, and waxing and permanent methods like thermal destruction by electrolysis or laser therapy
- *Hormonal treatment:*
  - Estrogen–progestin (progestin with low androgenic property), oral contraceptives 1 OD × 21 days for 6 cycles Or
  - Tablet cyproterone acetate 2 mg daily with tablet ethinylestradiol 30 µg D5–D25
- *Antiandrogens (used alone):*
  - Tablet spironolactone 50–100 mg twice daily from D5 to D25 × 6 months Or
  - Tablet cyproterone acetate 12.5–100 mg × 10 days during the follicular phase of menstrual cycle Or
  - Tablet finasteride—5 mg/day
- *Weight reduction*

HYPERPROLACTINEMIA

- *Medical management:* Tablet cabergoline 0.25 mg biweekly, can be increased to 1.5 mg biweekly
  Or
- Surgical treatment (for macro-adenomas)

ENDOMETRIOSIS

- Nonsteroidal anti-inflammatory drugs (NSAIDs)

- *Progestogen:*
  - Tablet medroxyprogesterone acetate 30 mg OD × 3–6 months Or
  - Tablet megestrol acetate 40 mg OD Or
  - Tablet lynestrenol 10 mg OD Or
  - Tablet dydrogesterone 20–30 mg OD Or
  - Tablet dienogest 2 mg orally once daily Or
  - Mirena as intrauterine contraceptive device (IUCD)
- *Antiprogestins:*
  - Tablet gestrinone—1.25–2.5 mg twice weekly × 6–9 months
  - Tablet danazol 400–800 mg orally in four divided doses × 6–9 months (not used now)
- *GnRH analogs (medical oophorectomy):*
  - Injection leuprolide—3.75 mg IM monthly or 11.25 mg IM/subcutaneously (SC) once in 3 months
  - Injection goserelin 3.6 mg SC monthly
  - Injection nafarelin 200 mg twice daily as intranasal spray.

EMERGENCY CONTRACEPTION

- Yuzpe regimen—oral contraceptive pill 50 µg of ethenyl estradiol and 0.5 mg of levonorgestrel to be repeated after 12 hours
- Tablet levonorgestrel—1.5 mg single dose orally within 72 hours Or
- Ulipristal acetate 30 mg orally single dose within 120 hours of intercourse
- Tablet ethinylestradiol 0.2 mg + Tablet levonorgestrel 2 mg orally 2 tablets and repeated after 12 hours Or
- Tablet ethinylestradiol (50 µg) + Tablet norgestrel (0.25 mg) orally 2 tablets and repeated after 12 hours
- Cu-T insertion, within 5 days—most effective method Or
- Tablet mifepristone 25–50 mg single dose within 120 hours of exposure.

PREMENSTRUAL SYNDROME

- *Primary strategy:*
  - Lifestyle modification
    - Caffeine restriction
    - Exercise daily
    - High-carbohydrate diet
    - Salt restriction
  - Counseling
  - Exercise
  - Stress reduction/relaxation techniques
  - Cognitive behavioral therapy
- *Secondary strategy:*
  - Calcium 1,200–1,600 mg daily
  - Magnesium 300–400 mg daily
  - Vitamin B_6 50 mg daily
  - Vitamin E 400 IU daily
  - Primrose oil 500 mg 3 times a day for a maximum of 7 days
  - Omega-3 fatty acid 2,000 mg daily
- *Tertiary strategy:*
  - Antidepressant and serotonin reuptake inhibitor antidepressant (SSRI)
  - Hormone therapy, contraceptive and progesterone
  - GnRH analogs
  - NSAIDs
  - Diuretics
  - Dopamine agonist
  - Antianxiety agents
- *Follow-up:* If the initial therapy is effective over the first three cycles, the patient should be evaluated every 3–6 months.

PROPHYLACTIC MEDICATION FOLLOWING SEXUAL ASSAULT

- Tablet azithromycin 1 g PO stat single dose
- Injection ceftriaxone 250 mg IM stat single dose
- Tablet tinidazole 2 g PO stat single dose

- Injection Hep-B 1 mL IM stat to be repeated at 1 month and 6 months (not necessary if previously vaccinated with documented immunity)
- Injection tetanus toxoid (TT) 0.5 mL IM stat
- Tablet zidovudine 300 mg BD × 28 days + Tablet lamivudine 150 mg × 28 days
- Emergency contraception within 72 hours or copper T within 5 days
- Human papillomavirus (HPV) immunization in female survivors between 9 and 26 years and male survivors aged 9–21 years
  - First vaccination dose stat, second dose at 1–2 months, and last dose at 6 months.

MANAGEMENT OF ACUTE PELVIC INFLAMMATORY DISEASE

Oral/intramuscular regimen:
- Injection ceftriaxone 250 mg IM single dose Plus
  Tablet doxycycline 100 mg orally twice daily × 14 days With or without
  Tablet metronidazole 500 mg orally twice daily × 14 days Or
- Injection cefoxitin 2 g IM single dose and tablet probenecid 1 g orally concurrently in a single dose Plus
  Tablet doxycycline 100 mg orally twice daily × 14 days With or without
  Tablet metronidazole 500 mg orally twice daily × 14 days Or
- Any other third-generation cephalosporin parenteral (ceftizoxime or cefotaxime) Plus
  Tablet doxycycline 100 mg orally twice daily × 14 days With or without
  Tablet metronidazole 500 mg orally twice daily × 14 days

Parenteral regimen:
- Injection cefotetan 2 g intravenously (IV) every 12 hours Plus
  Doxycycline 100 mg orally or IV every 12 hours Or
- Injection cefoxitin 2 g IV every 6 hours Plus
  Doxycycline 100 mg orally or IV every 12 hours Or
- Injection clindamycin 900 mg IV 8 hours Plus
  Gentamicin with loading dose IV or IM (2 mg/kg)
  Note: It is followed by a maintenance dose (1.5 mg/kg) every 8 hours.

Alternate parenteral regimen:
- Injection ampicillin/sulbactam 3 g IV every 6 hours Plus
  Tablet doxycycline 100 mg orally or IV every 12 hours

BACTERIAL VAGINOSIS

Recommended regimens:
- Tablet metronidazole 500 mg every 12 hourly × 7 days Or
- Metronidazole gel 0.75%, one full applicator (5 g) intravaginally, once daily × 5 days Or
- Clindamycin cream 2%, one full applicator (5 g) intravaginally, at bedtime × 7 days

Alternative regimens:
- Tablet tinidazole 2 g once daily × 2 days Or
- Tablet tinidazole 1 g once daily × 5 days Or
- Tablet clindamycin 300 mg 12 hourly × 7 days Or
- Clindamycin ovules 100 mg intravaginally, once at bedtime × 3 days

TRICHOMONAS VAGINALIS

- Tablet metronidazole 2 g orally single dose Or
- Tablet tinidazole 2 g orally single dose

Alternatively: Tablet metronidazole 500 mg orally 12 hourly × 7 days

VULVOVAGINAL CANDIDIASIS

- *Uncomplicated vulvovaginal candidiasis (VVC):*
  Most commonly and effective available treatment of VVC is locally applied azole drugs. Symptoms will usually resolve within 2–3 days. Tablet fluconazole (150 mg) orally single dose is equally effective.
- *Complicated VVC:*
  Tablet fluconazole (150 mg) stat followed by the same dose after 72 hours Or
  A prolonged topical regimen for 10–14 days
  For local irritative symptoms, weak topical steroid 1% hydrocortisone cream may be helpful.
  - *Topical antifungal preparations*:
    - 1% clotrimazole cream, 5 g intravaginally for 7–14 days
    - 2% clotrimazole cream, 5 g intravaginally for 3 days
    - 2% butoconazole cream, 5 g intravaginally for 3 days
    - 2% miconazole cream, 5 g intravaginally for 7 days
    - Miconazole (200 mg) vaginal suppository for 3 days
    - Miconazole (100 mg) vaginal suppository for 7 days
    - Nystatin (100,000 U) vaginal tablet, 1 tablet for 14 days
- *Recurrent VVC:*
  - Tablet fluconazole (150 mg) for every 3 days for three doses (induces remission of chronic symptoms)
  - Tablet fluconazole (150 mg) one tablet/week for 6 months (suppressive therapy)

ABNORMAL UTERINE BLEEDING

- Tablet tranexamic acid 500–1,000 mg three to four times a day × 5 days
- Tablet mefenamic acid 500 mg three times a day × 5 days
- Tablet norethisterone 10 mg three times a day till bleeding stops
  - Followed by 10 mg two times a day × 7 days
  - Followed by 10 mg once daily × 14 days for first cycle
  - Followed by tablet norethisterone 10 mg once daily D5–D26 for 3–6 cycles Or
  - Tablet medroxyprogesterone 10 mg 1 once daily from D16 to D25 (3–6 months)
- Oral contraceptive pills (containing ethinylestradiol 35 µg) BD to QID × 5 days
  - Tapering to 1 BD × 28 days for three to six cycles
- Intrauterine progesterone [levonorgestrel-releasing intrauterine system (LNG-IUS)] over 5 years
- Depot medroxyprogesterone acetate (DMPA) IM
- Danazol 200–800 mg daily into two or four divided doses (Not used now)
- Surgical management (nonresponder to medical management or family completed).

FIBROID UTERUS

- Tablet tranexamic acid 500–1,000 mg three to four times a day × 5 days (during menstruation)
- Leuprolide acetate depot (3.75 mg/month or 11.25 mg/3 months IM) Or
- Injection goserelin (3.6 mg every 28 days for 3–6 months SC) Or
- Nafarelin 800 µg intranasal in two to three divided doses

- Tablet ulipristal acetate 5 or 10 mg/day orally × 3–6 months
- Tablet mifepristone 5–50 mg/day orally 3–6 months
- Intrauterine progesterone (LNG-IUS) over 5 years
- Tablet danazol 200–800 mg daily into two or four divided doses for 6–12 months
- Focused ultrasound treatment/surgical management under MRI guided (nonresponder to medical management).

HORMONE THERAPY FOR MENOPAUSE

- *In hysterectomized with oophorectomized patients:*
  - Tablet conjugated equine estrogen (CEE) 0.625 mg OD or estradiol valerate 1–2 mg OD along with calcium carbonate 1,000 mg and bisphosphonate 35 mg weekly on empty stomach except in a patient when hysterectomy is done for endometriosis, progestins have to be added to estrogen to avoid recurrence.
- *In natural menopause:*
  - CEE 0.625 mg and medroxyprogesterone acetate 2.5 mg daily. Or 1 mg of estradiol valerate + 5 mg of dydrogesterone (Femoston Conti) daily for 5 months with a gap of 1 month every 6 monthly
- *Turner syndrome:* After the closure of forearm epiphysis, one should give natural estrogen for 2–3 years followed by cyclic sequential hormone replacement therapy (HRT) till the natural age of menopause
- *Asherman syndrome:* After the correction of intrauterine adhesions by hysteroscopic adhesiolysis, one should give a cyclic sequential regimen for at least 6 months to 1 year with insertion of a postoperative inert intrauterine device.
- *Premature ovarian insufficiency (POI):* In these patients, a cyclic sequential regimen with natural estrogen and metabolically friendly progestin should be given from 1 to 25 days where the progestin is added from D14 to D25 of cycle for the endometrium to be shed.

OBSTETRICS

Iron Deficiency Anemia in Pregnancy

- Indian Council of Medical Research (ICMR)/World Health Organization (WHO) recommendations:
  - *Drugs used in iron deficiency anemia (IDA):*
    - Iron
    - Folic acid
    - Vitamin C
    - Anthelmintic
- Recommendations by the WHO and the Ministry of Health and Family Welfare (MoHFW) in IDA have been shown in **Table 1**.
- *Deworming:* Single-dose tablet albendazole 400 mg stat between 14 and 16 weeks

Indications for Blood Transfusion

Indications for blood transfusion have been shown in **Box 1**.

Pregnancy with Preterm Labor

WHO guidelines (2015; published in Lancet 2016):

- Antenatal steroids 24–34 weeks (injection dexamethasone 6 mg 12 hourly for four doses or injection betamethasone 12 mg 24 hours apart two doses)
- Tocolysis; 24–26 weeks with intact membranes with suspicion of preterm labor

TABLE 1: Recommendations by the WHO and the Ministry of Health and Family Welfare (MoHFW) in iron deficiency anemia.

	During pregnancy		Postpartum
	Prophylaxis	**Treatment**	
WHO	Daily 60 mg iron + 400 µg folic acid till term	Daily 120 mg iron + 400 µg folic acid till term	Daily 60 mg iron + 400 µg folic acid—3 months
MoHFW	Daily 100 mg iron + 500 µg folic acid—6 months	• Mild anemia—two iron and folic acid tablets/day—100 days • Moderate anemia—intramuscular (IM) iron therapy + oral folic acid • Severe anemia—intravenous (IV) sucrose	Daily 100 mg iron + 500 µg folic acid—6 months

BOX 1: Indications for blood transfusion (BT).

Antepartum period
- Pregnancy <34 weeks:
  – Hemoglobin (Hb) <5 g/dL with or without signs of cardiac failure or hypoxia
  – 5–7 g/dL—in presence of impending heart failure
- Pregnancy >34 weeks:
  – Hb <7 g/dL even without signs of cardiac failure or hypoxia
  – Severe anemia with decompensation
- *Anemia not due to hematinic deficiency:*
  – Hemoglobinopathy or bone marrow failure syndromes
  – Hematologist should always be consulted
- Acute hemorrhage:
  – Always indicated if Hb <6 g/dL
  – If the patient becomes hemodynamically unstable due to ongoing hemorrhage
- Intrapartum period
  – Hb <7 g/dL (in labor)
  – Decision of BT depends on medical history or symptoms
- *Postpartum period*
  – Anemia with signs of shock/acute hemorrhage with signs of hemodynamic instability
  – *Hb <7 g% (postpartum):* Decision of BT depends on medical history or symptoms

- Nifedipine (20–30 mg stat orally repeated after 30 minutes followed by 10–20 mg 6 hourly for 48–72 hours) (maximum dosage is 160 mg in 24 hours) Or
- Atosiban (6.75 mg IV start over a minute followed by infusion of 18 mg/hr for 3 hours and then 6 mg/hr for up to 45 hours. Total duration not more than 48 hours and total dose not more than 330 mg). Or
- Magnesium sulfate for a period of gestation <32 weeks (4 g bolus IV followed by 2 g/hr infusion for 24 hours). It also has a role in neuroprotection of the baby who is in established preterm labor or has a planned preterm birth within 24 hours.
- Antibiotics only if preterm prelabor rupture of the membranes (PPROM), antenatal erythromycin 250–500 mg IV 6 hourly for 48 hours and then 250 mg orally 6 hourly for 10 days or till woman enters established labor, whichever is sooner. Or
- If allergic to erythromycin, vaginal swab culture of group B *streptococci*, penicillin (ampicillin—0.5–2 g IV every 6 hourly for 48 hours and then 0.5–2 mg orally for 10 days) and not amoxicillin–clavulanate combination should be given. Or
- Injection clindamycin 600–900 mg three times a day IV for 48 hours followed by tablet clindamycin 150–300 mg four times a day for 10 days.
- If there is prior history of preterm birth or mid-trimester loss or cervical length

<25 mm, prophylactic vaginal progesterone or prophylactic cerclage for 16–34 weeks can be advised.

RCOG 2019 (Royal College of Obstetricians and Gynaecologists) and NICE 2015 (National Institute for Health and Care Excellence) suggest:
- Antibiotics only if PPROM, antenatal erythromycin 250 mg orally 6 hourly for 10 days or till woman enters established labor, whichever is sooner.
- Antenatal steroids 24–34 weeks (injection dexamethasone 6 mg 12 hourly for four doses or injection betamethasone 12 mg 24 hours apart two doses). It can be offered to women between 34 and 35 + 6 weeks of pregnancy who are in suspected, diagnosed, or established preterm labor.
- Tocolyis can be considered in women between 24 and 25 + 6 weeks of gestation with intact membranes and are in suspected preterm labor. It can be offered to women between 26 and 33 + 6 weeks.

ACOG 2016 (American College of Obstetricians and Gynecologists; preterm labor) and 2018 (PROM):
- Antenatal steroids 24–34 weeks (injection dexamethasone 6 mg 12 hourly for four doses or injection betamethasone 12 mg 24 hours apart two doses). It can also be given between 34 and 36 + 6 weeks gestation as it decreases newborn respiratory morbidity. A single repeat course of antenatal corticosteroids can be considered in women less than 34 weeks' gestation and are at risk of delivery within the next 7 days, and whose prior course of steroid was given 14 days prior.
- Role of tocolysis is only to enable administration of corticosteroids and magnesium sulfate for neuroprotection as well as transport to a tertiary care center.
- Antibiotics only if preterm PPROM, antenatal intravenous ampicillin 2 g every 6 hours and erythromycin 250 mg 6 hourly for 48 hours and then oral amoxicillin 250 mg orally 8 hourly and erythromycin base 333 mg every 8 hours for a total of 7 days.

Pregnancy with Heart Disease

RCOG 2011 guidelines:
- *Antepartum*:
  - A woman with murmur in heart or history of cardiac problem should be attended by a team of consultant obstetrician, cardiologist, and anesthetist.
  - Women at low risk should receive routine care.
  - Women with high risk of adverse events, to be attended on a regular basis preferably by the same obstetrician (who has appropriate competencies) in the antenatal clinic.
  - Blood pressure should be measured manually with a sphygmomanometer.
  - Pulse rate and its rhythm should be measured as it may indicate the first sign of volume overload.
  - Any change in murmur or any lung changes associated with pulmonary edema should be auscultated as it is recommended in all cases of significant cardiac compromise.
  - Oxygen saturations should be checked periodically in women with cyanotic heart disease (preferably in each trimester or more frequently in case of any clinical signs of deterioration).
  - A fetal echocardiogram during the second trimester should be offered to women with a structural congenital heart disease. It is carried out by an accredited pediatric/fetal cardiologist.

- Multidisciplinary meeting at 32–34 weeks for the plan of delivery management regarding supervising the labor, cesarean section requirement, second-stage management, and appropriate prophylaxis postpartum hemorrhage management (a low-dose syntocinon infusion is probably the safest option, and at cesarean section prophylactic uterine compression sutures can be considered).
- *Intrapartum:*
  - The principle of management is to minimize cardiovascular stress. It can be achieved by the use of epidural anesthesia and assisted vaginal delivery. Cesarean section can be done only for obstetric indications.
  - Care of pregnant women with significant heart disease should be done in appropriate tertiary units which have high-dependency and intensive care units.
- *Postpartum:*
  - The length of recommended stay in hospital and any suggested special measures (such as anticoagulation or observation in a high-dependency area). The follow-up should be at done at a joint clinic.
  - Appropriate contraception should be advised.
- *Labor:* ACOG 2011 is the latest which says:
  - Ampicillin 2 g IV or cefazolin 1 g or ceftriaxone 1 g IV
  - Allergic to ampicillin; ceftriaxone 1 g IV or oral clindamycin 600 mg or azithromycin 500 mg orally
  - These are administered 30–60 minutes before the anticipated delivery time as is feasible.

Obstetric Cholestasis

- Tablet ursodeoxycholic acid 13–15 mg/kg/day in two divided doses
- Lotion calamine locally
- Tablet chlorpheniramine 4 mg 4–6 hourly
- Tablet dexamethasone 12 mg × 7 days—tapered in the next 3 days (should not be used as first-line therapy—RCOG 2011)
- Tablet menadiol sodium phosphate (vitamin K) 10 mg 1 OD (if prothrombin time is prolonged)

Human Immunodeficiency Virus in Pregnancy

Recommended Regimen (Lifelong)

- Triple-drug antiretroviral therapy (ART)—Tenofovir (TDF) 300 mg + Lamivudine (3TC) 300 mg single fixed-dose combination (FDC) pill (one pill/day) + Efavirenz (EFV) 600 mg (one pill/day)
- Triple-drug ART—Tenofovir (TDF) 300 mg + Lamivudine (3TC) 300 mg single FDC pill (one pill/day) + Dolutegravir (DTG) 50 mg (one pill/day)
- Co-trimoxazole should be started if CD4 count is ≤250 cells/mm^3 and continued through pregnancy, delivery, and breastfeeding as per national guidelines (*Dose:* Double strength tablet—1 tab daily)

Chorioamnionitis and Postpartum Endometritis

- Injection ampicillin 1–2 g IV 6 hourly
- Injection gentamicin 1.5 mg/kg IM or IV 8 hourly
- Injection metronidazole 500 IV 8 hourly

Or

If allergic to penicillin:
- Injection cefotaxime 1–2 g IV/IM 8 hourly

Or

- Injection ceftriaxone 1–2 g IV/IM 8–12 hourly Plus
- Injection metronidazole 500 mg IV 8 hourly Or
- Injection clindamycin 600–900 IV 8 hourly
- Injection gentamicin 1.5 mg/kg IM 8 hourly
  (Treatment continued till 24 hours after the patient becomes afebrile.) (WHO 2015: A combination of clindamycin and gentamicin is recommended for the treatment of postpartum endometritis.)

Toxoplasmosis

- *Tablet spiramycin:* 1 g/day tablet 8 hourly daily till delivery (if infection acquired at <18 weeks of gestation)
  Or
  After 18 weeks of gestation:
- *Tablet pyrimethamine:* 50 mg every 12 hours for 2 days followed by 50 mg daily (after the first trimester of pregnancy)
- *Tablet sulfadiazine:* 75 mg/kg, followed by 50 mg/kg every 12 hourly (maximum 4 g/day)
- *Tablet folinic acid:* 10–20 mg/day (during and 1 week after completion of pyrimethamine)

Chlamydia Trachomatis in Pregnancy

United States Centers for Disease Control and Prevention (CDC) 2015 guidelines:

Recommended regimen: Azithromycin 1 g orally in a single dose

Alternative regimens:
- Amoxicillin 500 mg orally three times a day for 7 days Or
- Erythromycin base 500 mg orally four times a day for 7 days Or
- Erythromycin base 250 mg orally four times a day for 14 days Or
- Erythromycin ethylsuccinate 800 mg orally four times a day for 7 days Or
- Erythromycin ethylsuccinate 400 mg orally four times a day for 14 days.

Malaria

- *Plasmodium vivax malaria:*
  - *P. vivax* malaria can be treated with chloroquine.
  - Tablet chloroquine 600 mg stat; 300 mg after 6–8 hours followed by 150 mg BD × 2 days
- *Plasmodium falciparum malaria:*
  - The artemisinin combination therapy should be given in second and third trimesters of pregnancy, while quinine is recommended in the first trimester.
  - *Dose:* Injection artesunate IM/IV—2.4 mg/kg on 0, 12, and 24 hours followed by daily for 4 days
- *Uncomplicated malaria:*
  - Oral quinine 600 mg 8 hourly and oral clindamycin 450 mg 8 hourly for 7 days
  - Avoid starting treatment on empty stomach
  - First dose to be given under observation
  - Repeat dose if vomiting within 30 minutes
  - Ask to report back if no improvement/deteriorate
- *Severe or complicated malaria:*
  - In the first trimester of pregnancy, parenteral quinine is the drug of choice (quinine 20 mg/kg intravenously in D5% over 4 hours followed by 10 mg/kg 8 hourly) (maximum dose of quinine: 1.4 g) plus clindamycin IV 450 mg 8 hourly
    When patient is able to take orally, tablet quinine 600 mg TDS for 5–7 days with oral clindamycin 450 mg 8 hourly for 5–7 days

- In second and third trimesters, parenteral artesunate derivatives are preferred (IV 2.4 mg/kg at 0, 12, 24 hours followed by daily, when the patient is able to take orally artesunate 2 mg/kg daily for 7 days)
- *Primaquine* is contraindicated in pregnant women.

Pregnancy with Genital Herpes

- *First or second trimester (until 27 + 6 weeks of gestation):*
  - Tablet acyclovir 400 mg three times a day for 5 days
  - For symptomatic relief, tablet paracetamol and topical lidocaine 2% gel can be offered.
- *Third trimester (from 28 weeks of gestation):*
  - Tablet acyclovir 400 mg thrice a day for 5 days and continue with daily suppressive acyclovir 400 mg three times daily until delivery
- *Recurrent genital herpes:*
  - Analgesia with standard doses of paracetamol can be used as supportive treatment.
  - Daily suppressive acyclovir 400 mg thrice a day should be considered from 36 weeks of gestation.
- *Primary or recurrent genital lesions at the onset of labor:*
  Primary episode:
  - In all women presenting with primary episode of genital herpes lesions at the time of delivery or within 6 weeks of the expected date of delivery, cesarean section should be recommended.
  - Vaginal delivery can be offered with IV acyclovir given intrapartum to the mother (5 mg/kg every 8 hours) and also to the neonate (IV acyclovir 20 mg/kg every 8 hours).

Recurrent genital herpes:
- In women with recurrent genital herpes lesions at the onset of labor, vaginal delivery should be offered.
- *Genital herpes in PPROM (before 37 + 0 weeks of gestation):*
  Primary genital herpes in PPROM:
  - The mother should be recommended to receive IV acyclovir 5 mg/kg every 8 hourly even if she was on conservative management initially.
  - To reduce the implications of preterm delivery upon the infant, prophylactic corticosteroids should be considered.

Recurrent genital herpes in PPROM:
- Tablet acyclovir 400 mg three times daily for the mother.

Chickenpox in Pregnancy

RCOG guidelines:
- Contact of suspected individual should be avoided.
- Treatment should be symptomatic and hygiene to be maintained.
- Tablet acyclovir is considered if the woman presents less than 24 hours of appearance of rashes.
- Delivery is to be avoided until 5–7 days after the onset of maternal rash.
- Tablet acyclovir 800 mg five times a day for 7 days.
- Intravenous acyclovir in case of severe infection.
- If a pregnant woman is not immune to VZV and she had significant exposure, she should be offered varicella zoster immunoglobulin (VZIG) as soon as possible; it is effective when given up to 10 days after contact.

Urinary Tract Infection in Pregnancy

- No clear recommendation on the antibiotic or duration of treatment

- Before starting any treatment, urine routine and culture should be sent.
- *Single-dose treatment:*
  - Capsule ampicillin 2 g stat Or
  - Capsule amoxicillin 3 g stat Or
  - Tablet cephalosporin 2 g stat Or
  - Tablet nitrofurantoin 200 mg Or
  - Tablet sulfamethoxazole/trimethoprim 1,600/320 mg in a day in divided doses
- *3-day course:*
  - Capsule ampicillin 250 mg 8 hourly × 3 days Or
  - Capsule amoxicillin 500 mg 6 hourly × 3 days Or
  - Tablet cephalosporin 250 mg 6 hourly × 3 days Or
  - Tablet ciprofloxacin 250 mg 12 hourly × 3 days Or
  - Tablet levofloxacin 250 or 500 mg once a day × 3 days Or
  - Tablet nitrofurantoin 100 mg 12 hourly × 3 days Or
  - Tablet sulfamethoxazole/trimethoprim 800/160 mg 12 hourly × 3 days
- *Other:*
  - Tablet nitrofurantoin 100 mg 6 hourly × 10 days
  - Tablet nitrofurantoin 100 mg 12 hourly × 5–7 days
  - Tablet nitrofurantoin 100 mg at night × 10 days
- *For suppression of bacterial persistence or recurrent urinary tract infection (UTI) in pregnancy:*
  - Tablet nitrofurantoin 100 mg at night for till remaining pregnancy.
- *Treatment failure:*
  - Tablet nitrofurantoin 100 mg 6 hourly × 21 days.

Syphilis

- *Primary/second/early latent of <1 year of duration:*
  - Injection benzathine penicillin G 2.4 MU IM (by some school of thought, there is recommendation of second dose after 1 week of 1st dose.)
- *Latent syphilis of unknown or >1 year duration/tertiary syphilis:*
  - Injection benzathine penicillin G 2.4 MU weekly IM for 3 weeks
- *Neurosyphilis:* Injection aqueous procaine penicillin 2.4 MU IM + Tablet probenecid 500 mg 6 hourly for 10–14 days. Or
- Injection aqueous crystalline penicillin G 3–4 MU IV 4 hourly for 10–14 days.

Gonorrhea

- Injection ceftriaxone 250 mg single dose IM Or
- Tablet azithromycin 1 g single dose orally

Patients with Normal Vaginal Delivery with Episiotomy

- Capsule amoxicillin 500 mg TDS × 5 days Or
- Capsule cephalexin 500 mg QID × 5 days (Not required in a clear wound of episiotomy)
- Tablet ibuprofen 400 mg TDS × 3 days
- Exclusive breastfeeding till 6 months
- Contraception after 6 weeks in exclusively breastfeeding patients
- Abstinence for 2 weeks (after that as per desire)
- Avoid squatting for 6 weeks if episiotomy was given.
- Avoid heavy workload for 6 weeks.
- Maintain proper hygiene.

Puerperal Sepsis

- Plenty of oral fluids Or
  Intravenous fluids (Ringer lactate, DNS) to maintain hydration

- Injection clindamycin 900 mg IV 8 hourly plus injection gentamicin 1.5 mg/kg IM 8 hourly. 1 g injection ampicillin IV 6 hourly should be added if no response within 48 hours. Or
- Injection amoxicillin plus clavulanic acid plus injection gentamicin plus metronidazole
- Tablet/IV infusion of paracetamol if fever
- Temperature, input–output charting

ICMR 2019 suggests injection piperacillin-tazobactam 4.5 g IV 6 hourly for 7–14 days. Clindamycin and gentamicin can be considered as second-line therapy. If the patient is in shock, consider imipenem/meropenem with or without amikacin plus vancomycin to cover methicillin-resistant *Staphylococcus aureus* (MRSA).

Thromboprophylaxis for Moderate- and High-risk Patients for Deep Vein Thrombosis

- *Unfractionated heparin (UFH):* 5,000–7,500 units, 7,500–10,000 units, and 10,000 units in first, second, and third trimesters of pregnancy, respectively, administered SC unless activated partial thromboplastin time (aPTT) is elevated
- *Low-molecular-weight heparin (LMWH):* Enoxaparin 40 mg, dalteparin 5,000 IU SC OD before surgery and once a day postoperatively.

Management of Venous Thromboembolism in Pregnancy and Puerperium

- Heparin 10,000 IU IV followed by 10,000 IU every 12 hourly. The dose is adjusted according to aPTT with a therapeutic range of 1.5–2.5 and it should be 6 hours after injection. It is continued for 5–7 days.
- LMWH—enoxaparin 1 mg/kg every 12 hourly; dalteparin 200 units/kg once daily; dalteparin 100 units/kg twice a day. (The target anti-Xa level to be maintained with therapeutic range 0.6–1.0 units/mL for 12 hourly dose but a bit higher for once-daily dose.)
- Warfarin (postpartum)—initial dose 5–10 mg for the first 2 days; then a daily maintenance dose of 5 mg which usually results in an international normalized ratio (INR) of 2–3.

25 Contraception

Rashmi Malik, Annu Kumari

What are the different methods for contraception?
- *Temporary contraception*
  - Natural behavioral family planning methods
    - Total abstinence
    - Coitus interruptus
    - Fertility awareness-based methods
    - Lactational amenorrhea method
  - Barrier contraceptive
    - Mechanical
      - Male condom
      - Female condom
      - Diaphragm
      - Cervical cap
    - Chemical
      - Spermicidal substances
      - Foam tab
      - Creams, jellies
    - Combined
  - Intrauterine contraceptive device (IUCD)
  - Steroidal (hormonal) contraceptives
    - Oral hormonal contraceptives (pills)
      - Combined low-dose or standard dose pills
      - Multiphasic pills (biphasic or triphasic)
      - Very low-dose pills
      - Combined pills with newer progestogens
      - Progestogen-only pills (mini-pill)
      - Emergency contraceptive pill (ECP)
    - Nonoral hormonal contraceptives
      - Levonorgestrel (LNG)-releasing intrauterine devices (LNG-IUD)
      - Injectable
      - *Only progestogen:* Depot medroxyprogesterone acetate (DMPA) and norethisterone enanthate (NET-EN)
      - Combined injectable contraceptive
      - Implants
      - *Vaginal ring:* NuvaRing
      - Transdermal patches
  - Emergency contraception
  - Uterotubal junction devices
    - Silastic/ceramic plugs
  - Miscellaneous
    - Male pill
    - Centchroman
- *Permanent contraception*
  - Male—vasectomy
  - Female—sterilization operation

What are different WHO Medical Eligibility Categories for contraceptive methods?
The World Health Organization (WHO) has given four categories to determine the eligibility of a candidate for any contraceptive method:
1. *Category 1:* There is no restriction and the contraceptive method can be used.
2. *Category 2:* The method can be used as the advantages are much more than the risks.

3. *Category 3:* The method should be avoided in these cases as the potential risks are more than the contraceptive advantages offered by the method.
4. *Category 4:* The contraceptive method is not to be used in these conditions as the risks are unacceptable.

Are there any devices which can help to check Medical Eligibility Categories for different medical conditions in the outpatient department?

The WHO contraceptive wheel **(Fig. 1)** is a device which can be used easily to check Medical Eligibility Categories (MEC) for any contraceptive method for any given condition.

The wheel aligns contraceptive methods, displayed on the inner disk, with specific medical conditions or characteristics depicted around the outer rim. The numbers visible in the viewing slot indicate whether a woman with a known condition or characteristic can initiate the use of the contraceptive method.

The WHO has also launched an easy-to-use application in 2019 to check for eligibility of nine common contraceptive methods for various medical conditions. It is available for both Android and Apple devices.

What is GATHER approach?

The steps of good counseling can be remembered with the acronym GATHER.

- *G*—Greet clients and give them full attention.
- *A*—Ask the client so as to understand their contraceptive requirements, how much knowledge they have, and what are their concerns or misconceptions.
- *T*—Tell the clients about the contraceptive methods they can choose from as per their requirements.
- *H*—Help them to choose the most appropriate method for them.
- *E*—Explain them about the chosen method in details.
- *R*—Return visits should be encouraged for follow-up, in case of any side effects or concerns. This helps in the successful continuation of the method.

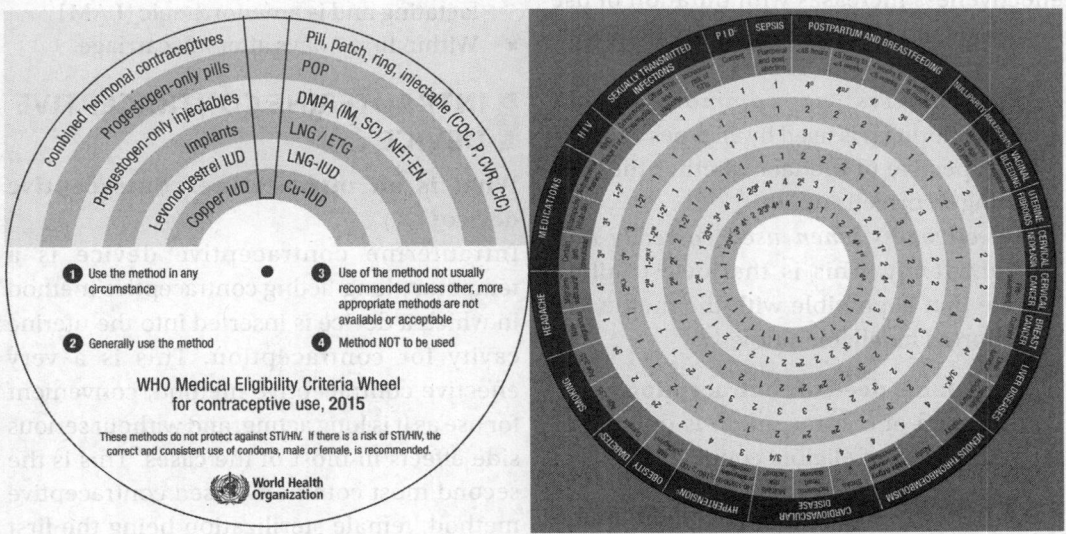

Fig. 1: Medical Eligibility Categories (MEC) wheel. *(For color version, see Plate 16)*

How do you describe contraceptive effectiveness of a method? What are the failure rates of different methods?

Failure rate per hundred-woman years of exposure (HWY)

This (Pearl index) is calculated by multiplying total accidental pregnancies during use of a method with 1,200 and dividing with the total months of use of the method. Total months of use are calculated by the multiplication of number of women using method and the months for which it was used. The effectiveness of a contraceptive method is determined not only by the inherent effectiveness of the method but also by the fact as to how consistently and correctly the method is used. This can vary as per age of the client, duration of use, education level, socioeconomic factors, etc. Therefore, the methods whose success is dependent on the correct and consistent use by the clients have a wide range of effectiveness in different populations. Therefore, effectiveness is usually described as likelihood of pregnancy in the first year of contraceptive use as the effectiveness increases with duration of use in user-dependent methods. Effectiveness is reported in two ways **(Table 1)**:

1. *Effectiveness as commonly used:* Considering it is used by all types of users, irrespective of the fact whether they are using it correctly or not
2. *Effectiveness when used correctly and consistently:* This is the lowest failure rate that is possible with the method as reported in reliable studies.

What is unmet need of contraception?

Unmet need of contraception is defined as the percentage of eligible couples who want to delay pregnancy by more than 2 years but are not using contraception. Unmet need is an important measure pointing to the drawbacks and limitations of the family welfare program implementation. The current unmet need of contraception in India is 9.0% [National Family Health Survey (NFHS) 5]. High unmet needs are due to the unavailability of quality services which are easily accessible; there are only few methods to choose from, concerns and misconceptions about the potential side effects, and partners not approving the contraceptive use.

How can a healthcare provider be reasonably certain that a woman is not pregnant?

In a reproductive age woman, one can be sure that a woman is not pregnant if she does not have any signs or symptoms of pregnancy and has any one of the following criteria:
- Maintain abstinence since the last normal periods
- Using a reliable contraceptive method properly
- Within 7 days since the last normal periods, i.e., first 7 days of a cycle
- Within 4 weeks of last childbirth if she is not lactating
- Within 6 months postpartum, if she is fully lactating and is amenorrhoeic (LAM)
- Within first 7 days after miscarriage.

INTRAUTERINE CONTRACEPTIVE DEVICE

What is an intrauterine contraceptive device?

Intrauterine contraceptive device is a temporary long-acting contraceptive method in which a device is inserted into the uterine cavity for contraception. This is a very effective contraceptive method, convenient for use as it is long acting, and without serious side effects in most of the cases. This is the second most commonly used contraceptive method, female sterilization being the first one (WHO).

TABLE 1: Contraceptive effectiveness of different methods.

Method	Effectiveness: Pregnancies per 100 women per year with consistent and correct use	Effectiveness: Pregnancies per 100 women per year as commonly used
Combined oral contraceptives (COCs) or "the pill"	0.3	7
Progestogen-only pills (POPs) or "the minipill"	0.3	7
Implants	0.1	0.1
Progestogen-only injectables	0.2	4
Monthly injectables or combined injectable contraceptives (CIC)	0.05	3
Combined contraceptive patch and combined contraceptive vaginal ring (CVR)	0.3	7
Intrauterine device (IUD): Copper containing	0.6	0.8
Intrauterine device (IUD) Levonorgestrel	0.5	0.7
Male condoms	2	13
Female condoms	5	21
Male sterilization (vasectomy)	0.1	0.15
Female sterilization (tubal ligation)	0.5	0.5
Lactational amenorrhea method (LAM)	0.9 (in 6 months)	2 (in 6 months)
Standard days method (SDM)	5	12
Basal body temperature (BBT) method	NA	
Two-day method	4	14
Symptothermal method	<1	2
Emergency contraception pills (ulipristal acetate 30 mg or levonorgestrel 1.5 mg)	• <1 for ulipristal acetate emergency contraceptive pills (ECPs) 1 for progestin-only ECPs • 2 for combined estrogen and progestin ECPs	
Calendar method or rhythm method	Reliable effectiveness rates are not available	15
Withdrawal (coitus interruptus)	4	20

Source: www.who.int>health-topics

Which are the different intrauterine contraceptive devices you know?

First generation: These were unmedicated, inert devices. They are not available now.
- Lippes loop

Second generation: These are medicated devices containing copper with improved contraceptive effectiveness. Earlier devices like copper-T (CuT) 200 are no longer available. The ones available now are:

- Copper-T (CuT) 380A (effective for 10 years)
- Multiload 375 (effective for 5 years)
- Multiload 250 (effective for 3 years)

Third generation: These are hormone-releasing devices which release progestin.
- Mirena (LNG releasing, effective for 5 years).

Fourth generation: Frameless contraception
- *Gynefix:* It consists of six 5-mm copper sleeves threaded onto monofilament polypropylene thread. At the proximal end of thread, a knot is present which is anchored into myometrium at the fundus thus securing device in the uterine cavity.

What are the different copper intrauterine contraceptive devices?
- *Cu-7:*
  - Polypropylene impregnated with barium sulfate
  - Has transcervical thread tails
  - 200 mm^2 of copper
  - *Life span:* 3 years
- *CuT 200:*
  - Polypropylene impregnated with barium sulfate
  - 200 mm^2 of copper
  - *Life span:* 4 years
- *Multiload Cu 250/multiload Cu 375* **(Fig. 2A):**
  - Polypropylene with 250 mm^2 or 375 mm^2 of Cu
  - Arms are flexible serrated
  - Available in preloaded inserters
  - *Life span:* 3 and 5 years, respectively
  - Available in sterilized packs
- *CuT 380A* **(Fig. 2B):**
  - Polyethylene impregnated with barium sulfate
  - 314 mm^2 of copper wire on vertical stem and 33 mm^2 on either sleeve
  - *Life span:* 10 years
  - Free supply in India.
- Nova CuT 200
- Modified CuT 200 with a silver core; life span is 5 years.

Identify and describe the contraceptive device shown in Figure 3. What are its advantages and disadvantages?
The contraceptive device is Mirena (LNG-IUCD). It is a T-shaped polyethylene frame with a steroid reservoir. It has 52 mg of LNG

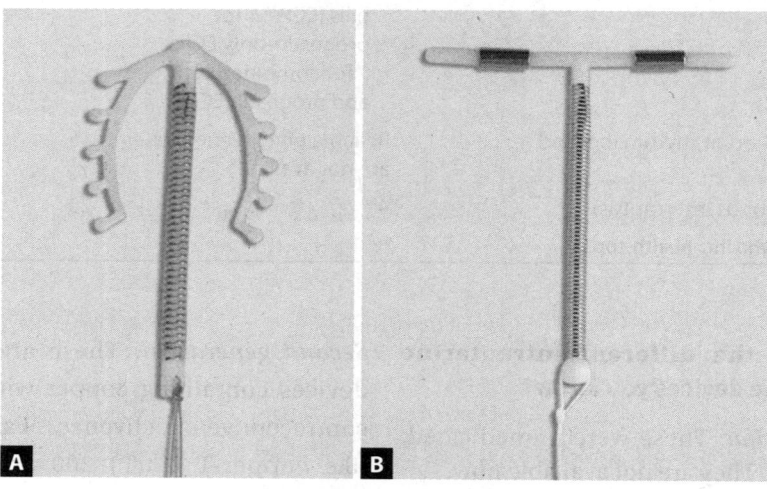

Figs. 2A and B: (A) Multiload 250; (B) CuT 380A.

which is released at the rate of 20 μg/day and has a life span of 5 years. There is evidence that Mirena remains effective up to 7 years.

Advantages:
- Reduction of blood loss
- Reduction of dysmenorrhea in endometriosis
- Beneficial effects on fibroids

Disadvantages:
- Irregular bleeding
- Oligomenorrhea and amenorrhea

What is the mechanism of action of an intrauterine contraceptive device?
- There are biochemical and histological changes in the endometrium.
- It causes increased tubal motility.
- There may be impaired sperm ascent.
- Copper ions are toxic to the sperm.

What are the contradictions for intrauterine contraceptive devices (Table 2)?
WHO risk categories for LNG-IUD are the same as for Cu-IUD except for few added conditions in higher categories as follows:

Category 2: Diabetes, migraine, history of hypertension (HT) where BP cannot be evaluated, severe HT, vascular disease, gallbladder disease, cervical intraepithelial neoplasia (CIN), high risk for human immunodeficiency virus (HIV), history of deep vein thrombosis/pulmonary embolism

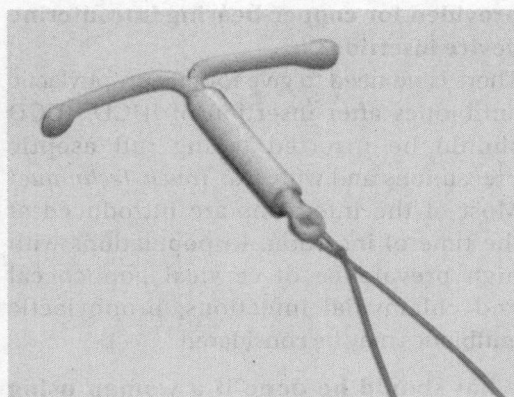

Fig. 3: Mirena.

TABLE 2: Contraindications for intrauterine device insertion (WHO Medical Eligibility Criteria 2015).

WHO risk category 4 (absolute contraindication)	WHO risk category 3 (relative contraindication)	WHO risk category 2 (use with caution)
• Pregnancy • Puerperal sepsis • Immediate after septic abortion • Unexplained vaginal bleeding • Malignant trophoblastic disease • Cervical cancer • Endometrial cancer • Ovarian cancer • Uterine fibroids with distortion of uterine cavity • Current PID • Current purulent cervicitis • Pelvic tuberculosis	• Postpartum 48 hours to 4 weeks • SLE with severe thrombocytopenia • Benign trophoblastic disease • High risk for STIs • HIV (WHO stage 3 or 4)	• Age <20 years • Nulliparous • Postpartum <48 hours (breastfeeding) • Second-trimester abortion • Valvular heart disease (complicated) • Severe dysmenorrhea • Endometriosis • Past PID with no subsequent pregnancy • Vaginitis • HIV (WHO stage 1 or 2) • Anemia

(HIV: human immunodeficiency virus; PID: pelvic inflammatory disease; SLE: systemic lupus erythematosus; STI: sexually transmitted infections)

(DVT/PE), major surgery with prolonged immobilization, immunosuppressive therapy, dyslipidemia, multiple risk factors for cardiovascular disease (CVD), antiretroviral (ARV) therapy, and postpartum IUCD (PPIUCD).

Category 3: Less than 48 hours postpartum, past history of carcinoma breast, severe cirrhosis, systemic lupus erythematosus (SLE), current or history of ischemic heart disease (IHD)

Category 4: Current breast cancer

On the other hand, conditions such as menorrhagia, dysmenorrhea, endometriosis, past pelvic inflammatory disease (PID) are category 1 for LNG-IUD as due to hormonal action LNG-IUD causes improvement in these conditions.

When can an intrauterine contraceptive device be inserted in a postpartum woman?

Postpartum (including postcesarean section)
- After delivery, IUCD can be inserted immediately after delivery of the placenta or anytime within the first 48 hours. This is known as postpartum IUCD.
- If not inserted within 48 hours after delivery, IUCD can be inserted after 6 weeks. If she is amenorrhoeic, IUCD can be inserted if it is sure that she is not pregnant.

  If she has resumed menses after delivery, IUCD can be inserted as advised for other women having menstrual cycles.
- Puerperal sepsis is a contraindication for PPIUCD insertion.

Postabortion
- After first-trimester abortion, IUCD can be inserted immediately after abortion.
- After second-trimester abortion also, IUCD can be inserted immediately postabortion.
- Septic abortion is a contraindication for IUCD.
- After the medical method of abortion in the first trimester, IUCD can be inserted once the abortion is complete (around day 15th) and presence of infection is ruled out. Ensure completion of abortion by pelvic examination or by ultrasonography (USG).

Should prophylactic antibiotics be provided for copper-bearing intrauterine device insertion?

There is no need to give routine prophylactic antibiotics after insertion of IUCD. IUCD should be inserted taking full aseptic precautions and with *"No Touch Technique".* Most of the infections are introduced at the time of insertion. In populations with high prevalence of cervical gonococcal and chlamydial infections, prophylactic antibiotics may be considered.

What should be done if a woman using a copper-bearing intrauterine device is diagnosed with pelvic inflammatory disease?

If a woman has PID with IUCD in situ, she should be given full course of antibiotics. There is no need to remove the IUCD unless she wants to get it removed. If she wishes IUCD removal, it should be removed after starting antibiotic treatment. If symptoms do not improve and IUCD is in situ, then it should be removed while continuing antibiotics. Counseling about condom use should be done.

What should be done if a woman using a copper-bearing intrauterine device is found to be pregnant?

If a woman is pregnant with IUCD in situ, the following needs to be done:
- Do clinical examination to check for threads (ensuring IUCD is in situ) and rule out ectopic pregnancy.

- Do USG to rule out ectopic pregnancy.
- If it is intrauterine pregnancy, discuss with the woman whether she wants to continue pregnancy or wants medical termination. If she wants to keep the pregnancy, explain to her that it is better to remove the CuT though this has a small risk of causing miscarriage. But if she continues pregnancy with IUCD, she is at an increased risk of first- and second-trimester abortion including septic abortion and preterm delivery.
- If threads are visible or are curled up in the canal, remove the IUCD after informing the patient.
- If IUCD threads are not visible, do USG for localization of the IUCD. There is a possibility that IUCD has been expelled out, that is why she has conceived.
- But if IUCD is in situ and she wants to continue pregnancy, tell her about the risks. She should be counseled to report immediately if she has heavy bleeding, pain, vaginal discharge or fever.
- If she opts for MTP (medical termination of pregnancy), IUCD is removed at the time of surgical evacuation.

How can you use an intrauterine contraceptive device for emergency contraception?

After unprotected intercourse, IUCD can be inserted within 5 days and it acts as emergency contraception. This has the advantage as this will provide continuous contraception after insertion. The contraindications for IUCD should be ruled out.

What is PPIUCD?

PPIUCD is postpartum insertion of IUCD. Taking advantage of the immediate postpartum period for counseling on family planning and IUCD insertion, PPIUCD insertion is being promoted under national program. The increased institutional deliveries are the opportunity to provide women easy access to immediate PPIUCD services. The salient features are as follows:

- Any of the devices, CuT 380 A, Multiload, or Mirena can be inserted as PPIUCD.
- Counseling is very important. Ideally, counseling should be done in the antenatal period. If done during labor, it should be done only in the latent phase. During the active phase of labor and immediate postpartum period, women are too stressed to make an informed decision, which leads on to less tolerance to side effects and lower continuation rates.
- The PPIUCD can be inserted postplacental, i.e., immediately after delivery of placenta, at the time of cesarean section, or anytime within the first 48 hours after delivery.
- PPIUCD can be inserted only by a service provider who has undergone appropriate training for the same. This is to avoid complications.
- Full aseptic precautions should be taken while PPIUCD insertion.

Are there any contraindications for PPIUCD insertion?

PPIUCD should not be inserted in the following cases:
- After 48 hours till 6 weeks after delivery
- In cases of chorioamnionitis
- If during labor there was prolonged rupture of membrane, i.e., >18 hours
- Cases of puerperal sepsis
- Postpartum hemorrhage which is uncontrolled or severe.

Identify the barrier method shown in Figure 4 and describe it.

This is female condom. It is a barrier contraceptive to be used by the female partner. It has a long 15 cm polyurethane sheath that fits loosely in the vagina. On both the ends of the sheath, there are two rings which are flexible. The inner ring is to be placed high up inside the vagina. The outer ring covers the labia and perineum. This condom comes prelubricated with silicone-based lubricant. So basically, female condom has features of both diaphragm and condom.

What is the contraceptive method shown in Figure 5?

This contraceptive is vaginal sponge named commercially as Today. It is made of polyurethane and it contains 1 g of Nonoxynol-9 which is a spermicidal agent. So, basically this is a chemical barrier method. This has the shape of a mushroom. The concave side covers the cervix. Dimensions of sponge are 2 inches in diameter and 1.25 inches in thickness. On the bottom, a loop is attached for easy removal. This acts as a contraceptive by three actions:
1. During coitus, it releases a spermicidal agent which kills the sperms.
2. Due to sponge action, it absorbs the ejaculate.
3. It blocks the entrance of sperms in the cervical canal.

It is effective for 24 hours. Failure rate is 9–27 per 100 women years.

Identify the images shown in Figures 6A and B.

These are female barrier contraceptive methods—cervical cap and diaphragm.

What do you know about combined oral pill?

Combined oral contraceptive (COC) pills are contraceptive pills containing both estrogen

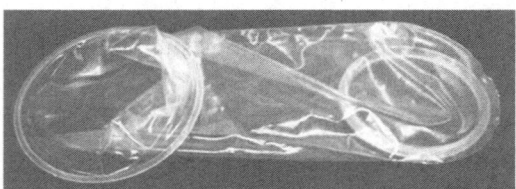

Fig. 4: Female condom.

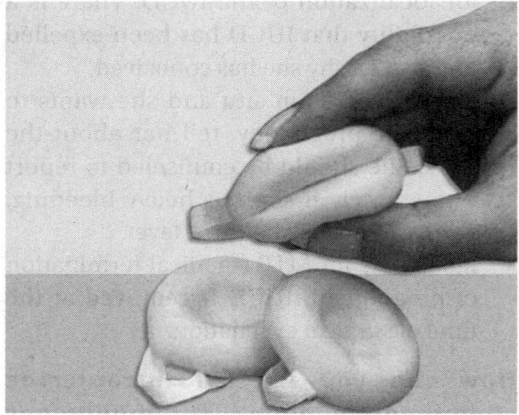

Fig. 5: Vaginal sponge (Today).

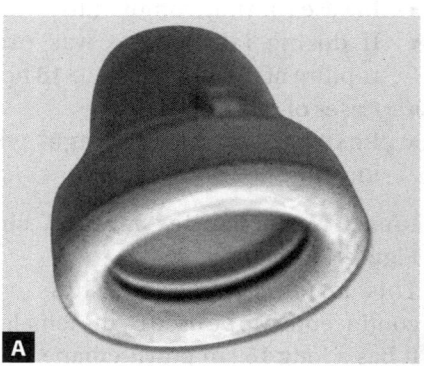
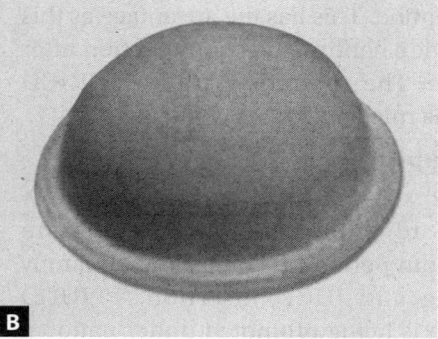

Figs. 6A and B: (A) Cervical cap; (B) Diaphragm.

TABLE 3: Contraceptive pills containing both estrogen and progesterone hormones.

Preparation	Estrogen	Progestogens
Mala D	30 µg	Norgestrel 0.3 mg
Mala N	30 µg	Norethisterone 1.0 mg
Ovral	50 µg	Levonorgestrel 0.25 mg
Ovral L	30 mg	Levonorgestrel 0.15 mg
Duoluton-L	50 µg	Levonorgestrel 0.15 mg
Novelon	30 µg	Desogestrel 0.25 mg
Femilon	20 µg	Desogestrel 0.15 mg

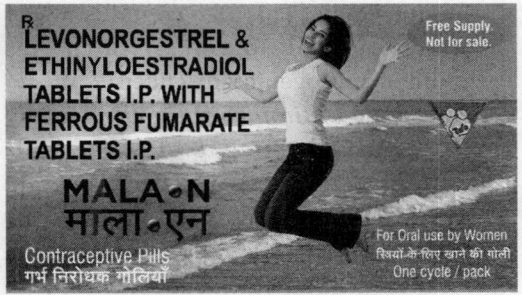

Fig. 7: Mala N. *(For color version, see Plate 16)*

and progesterone hormones **(Table 3)**. Estrogen is ethinylestradiol (EE), while progestogen varies in different formulations. Pills come in the monthly pack containing 21 active hormonal tablets with or without seven placebo tablets containing iron and vitamins. Twenty-eight pills are taken continuously and after the last placebo pill, the next pack is started immediately without a break. While in packs with 21 pills, a break of 7 days is given for menstruation to occur. Mala N **(Fig. 7)** is the COC which is available free from the government of India.

What do you know about mini-pill?

- Mini-pills are progesterone-only pills. These are for situations where estrogens are contraindicated. They are known as POPs (progestogen-only pills). Earlier pills contained norgestrel 75 µg or norethisterone 350 µg or LNG 30 µg. These were known as mini-pills.
- POP available in India is Cerazette which contains 75 µg desogestrel.
- POPs are to be taken once a day, continuously throughout the cycle without any break.
- POPs are to be taken at the same time every day (not later than 4 hours of the previous time).
- Failure rate is higher than combined pills.
- These do not have estrogen-related side effects and can be taken where estrogens are contraindicated, so they are useful for lactating mothers and perimenopausal females.
- Menstrual abnormalities are common with these pills.
- Progestogen-related side effects can occur, such as mood changes, loss of libido, and weight gain, though with newer pills androgenic side effects are not seen.
- *Mechanism of action of these pills:*
  - Thickens the mucous plug and makes it impermeable to sperms: Peak action 2–4 hours and lasts for 20–24 hours
  - *Desogestrel-containing POP:* Inhibits ovulation
  - Renders endometrium unsuitable and unreceptive to implantation
  - Accelerates tubal motility: Thereby accelerates ovum transport before its maturity for implantation
  - Disturbs normal corpus luteal function.

Which newer pills are now available?

- *Pills with very low-dose estrogen:* The dose of estrogen in low-dose pills is 35 µg while in very low-dose pill it is 20 µg. This has very less incidence of estrogen-related side effects like nausea, breast tenderness,

and headache. This also contains newer progestogen desogestrel which has minimal androgenic side effects.
- *Pills with antiandrogenic effects:* The progestin component of these pills contains either cyproterone acetate (CPA; antiandrogenic action) or drospirenone (DSP; antiandrogenic plus antimineralocorticoid action). These pills are very useful in patients with acne and hirsutism. DSP also decreases weight and BP in the users.
- *Postcoital pill:* Also known are emergency contraception (discussed later).
- *Pills with extended cycle length:* These are low-dose combined contraceptive pills with the same composition as standard COC. Only the pack contains 84 active pills to be taken continuously followed by 7 pill-free days.

What is the mechanism of action of oral contraceptive pills?

Mechanism of action
- Combined pills' main contraceptive action is due to inhibition of ovulation. The hormones released from pills act on the hypothalamus and by negative feedback they inhibit the release of gonadotropin-releasing hormone (GnRH). Due to low GnRH, release of follicle-stimulating hormone (FSH) and luteinizing hormone (LH) from the anterior pituitary gets suppressed. It is also suggested that estrogen and progesterone directly act on pituitary, also inhibiting the release of FSH and LH. Due to low FSH, follicular growth does not occur. As LH surge is inhibited, therefore ovulation does not occur.
- There is effect on the endometrium altering the maturation of the endometrium. So, endometrium becomes unsuitable for implantation.
- Progesterone acts on the cervical mucus making it thick, viscid, and scanty, thus impermeable to sperms.
- Progesterone also acts on the tubes, altering the motility.

What are the contraindications to combined oral contraceptive pills (Table 4)?

What is the difference between various progestins used in contraceptive preparations?

The various progestogens differ in their affinity and action on various steroid receptors **(Table 5)**.

How do you manage breakthrough bleeding on oral pills?

Breakthrough bleeding occurs in almost half of all patients at some time. It may be due to failure to take the pill at the same time each day. It is more common with low-dose pill. However, with newer pills cycle control is good. It diminishes after the first 3–4-pill cycles.

Management
Double-up daily dose of pills in an attempt to stop the bleeding and discontinuing the pills to restart them on the fifth day of bleeding are now considered ill-advisable. The following measures should be taken:
- Switching to another low-dose compound
- Increase in the estrogen dose of the pill temporarily or taking a short course of additional estrogen temporarily
- A search for pathological cause of bleeding must be made.

What is pill amenorrhea?

After stopping the combined pills, around 20% of the women do not get withdrawal bleeding. This is known as pill amenorrhea. When this happens, first, one should rule out pregnancy. Once pregnancy is ruled out, the woman should be reassured that there is nothing

TABLE 4: Contraindications for use of oral contraceptive pills: Medical eligibility criteria for initiation of low-dose combined oral contraceptive pills.

WHO risk category 4 (absolute contraindication)	WHO risk category 3 (method of last choice)	WHO risk category 2 (use with caution)
• Breastfeeding <6 weeks postpartum • Smoking age >35 years, >15 cigarettes/day • Multiple risk factors for cardiovascular disease (older age, smoking, diabetes, HT) • Major surgery with prolonged immobilization • BP >160/100 mm Hg • HT with vascular disease • History or current deep vein thrombosis, pulmonary embolism • Known thrombogenic mutations • Current and history of ischemic heart disease • History of cerebrovascular accidents • Complicated valvular heart disease (pulmonary HT, atrial fibrillation, history of SABE) • Migraine with aura • Migraine without aura, age >35 years • Current breast cancer • DM >20 years • DM with nephropathy/retinopathy/neuropathy or other vascular disease • Active viral hepatitis (<3 months since asymptomatic or abnormal liver functions) • Severe cirrhosis • Liver tumors (benign/malignant)	• Breastfeeding 6 weeks to 6 months postpartum • Postpartum nonbreastfeeding <21 days • Smoking age >35 years, <15 cigarettes/day • Systolic 140–150 mm Hg, diastolic 90–99 mm Hg • Adequately controlled BP • Known hyperlipidemias • Migraine without aura, age <35 years • Past history of carcinoma breast with no evidence of disease for 5 years • Current gallbladder disease or history of medically treated • Past history of COC-induced cholestasis • Mild compensated cirrhosis • Rifampicin, certain anticonvulsants • ARV therapy using Ritonavir-boosted protease inhibitors	• Age >40 years • Breastfeeding >6 months postpartum • Smoking age <35 years • Obesity (BMI >30 kg/m^2) • Past history of pregnancy induced hypertension (PIH) • Major surgery without prolonged immobilization • Superficial thrombophlebitis • Uncomplicated valvular heart disease • Unexplained vaginal bleeding before evaluation • CIN, cervical cancer • DM <20 years duration with no vascular disease • GB disease treated by cholecystectomy • Asymptomatic GB disease • History of pregnancy-induced cholestasis • Breast disease—undiagnosed mass • Sickle cell disease • Griseofulvin • Antiretroviral therapy using NNRTIs

(DM: diabetes mellitus; ARV: antiretroviral; BMI: body mass index; CIN: cervical intraepithelial neoplasia; COC: combined oral contraceptive; GB: gallbladder; HT: hypertension; PIH: pregnancy-induced hypertension; NNRTI: non-nucleoside reverse transcriptase inhibitors)

wrong and she will resume periods after she stops this contraceptive method. Therefore, for continued contraceptive action, she should start a new pack on the scheduled day (after 7 days of pill-free interval). But if she is really disturbed and wants periods every

TABLE 5: A comparison of various progestins.

Progestin	Estrogenic	Antiestrogenic	Androgenic	Antiandrogenic	Antimineralo-corticosteroid
Progesterone	–	–	–	+	+
Older progestins:					
• MPA	–	–	+	–	–
• Norethisterone	–	+	+	–	–
• Levonorgestrel	–	+	+	–	–
Newer progestins:					
• Desogestrel	–	–	–	–	–
• Cyproterone acetate	–	–	–	+	–
Drospirenone	–	–	–	+	+

(MPA: medroxyprogesterone acetate)

cycle, she can be switched over to higher estrogen-containing pills or EE 0.02 mg tablet can be taken for the last 7 days of the 21-day pack for few months. The other option is to switch over to triphasic pills which have less amenorrhea.

What are serious cardiovascular side effects of combined pills?

Combined pills can have serious cardiovascular side effects:

- *Venous thromboembolism:* It is dependent on the dose of estrogen used in the pill. As compared to nonusers, COC users have 5–6 times more risk of DVT and 2–3 times more risk for superficial thrombosis. Therefore, combined pills are avoided if there are other risk factors for thromboembolism.
- *Myocardial infarction:* With earlier pills, the risk was increased to 2–3 times more than nonusers. Both estrogen and progestogen components are responsible. But with proper selection of patients, low-dose pills, and newer progestogens, the incidence is decreasing.
- *Cerebrovascular stroke:* Again due to estrogenic action, cerebral thrombosis can occur. This is more common than cerebral hemorrhage as a cause of stroke in pill users. As this is not dose dependent, it cannot be avoided by decreasing the dose of estrogens.

What is the effect of contraceptive combined pills on genital malignancies?

Cervix: Combined oral contraceptive pill use increases the incidence of cervical dysplasia and carcinoma in situ. There is a 2–3 times increase in the risk of invasive cervical cancer after pill use for more than 5 years. But all these cancers are seen in women infected with persistent high-risk oncogenic HPV strains. This is the primary cause and association with pills may be indirect.

Breast cancer: Epidemiological evidence suggests that there is little increased risk of developing breast cancer among current or recent users. The risk is more in women who started using COCs in adolescent periods as breasts are developing at that stage. But after stopping pills for more than 10 years, the risk is the same as in nonusers. The studies have also found increased risk mainly in the users of triphasic pills.

Liver: Oral contraceptive use is associated with an *increase in the risk of benign "liver"* tumors, such as *hepatocellular adenomas. The risk is small, but this can be fatal due to severe intraperitoneal hemorrhage.* However, association with malignant hepatocellular carcinoma is less clear with studies reporting contradictory findings.

What are the beneficial side effects of pills?
Combined hormonal pills have may other beneficial effects apart from the contraceptive action. These include the following:
- *Better menstrual cycles:* With combined pill usage, cycles become regular and blood flow decreases resulting in improved hemoglobin. There is also reduction in dysmenorrhea and premenstrual syndrome.
- *Prevention of PID:* There is prevention of ascending infection from the lower genital tract due to thickening of the cervical mucus and inhibition of uterine contractions. Also, by preventing pregnancy and abortion, the resultant sepsis is avoided.
- *Prevention of ectopic pregnancy:* Suppression of ovulation prevents all pregnancies including ectopic also. Prevention of tubal damage due to PID results in less incidence of future ectopic pregnancy also.
- *Genital malignancy:* Due to progesterone action on the endometrium, endometrial carcinoma risk is decreased up to 50% and the protection continues long after discontinuation of pills. Similarly, there is a decrease in the ovarian cancer risk by 40–80% due to inhibition of ovulation. This protection also continues for 15–20 years after stopping the pills.
- *Breast disease:* Current and long-term uses cause 30–50% reduction in the benign breast diseases.
- *Functional ovarian cysts:* Due to suppression of ovulation, combined pills protect against all the functional cysts.
- Some studies have suggested reduced risk of fibroids, colorectal carcinoma, rheumatoid arthritis, and benign thyroiditis, but the evidence is not conclusive.
- Improvement in bone mineral density also occurs.

What do you know about Chhaya (Fig. 8)?
Chhaya is Centchroman, a nonsteroidal oral contraceptive pill supplied free under family planning program by the government of India. It is also popularly known as Saheli in market. This comes in the dosage of 30 mg tablet. The first tablet is taken on the first day of the cycle. After that it is to be taken twice a week for the first 3 months, followed by weekly. Usually, it is suggested to fix the days of the week like Sunday and Thursday, for the pill intake.

Centchroman binds to estrogen receptors and has weak estrogenic and strong anti-estrogenic action. It does not inhibit ovulation. Contraceptive action is due to local effects on the genital tract causing abnormal

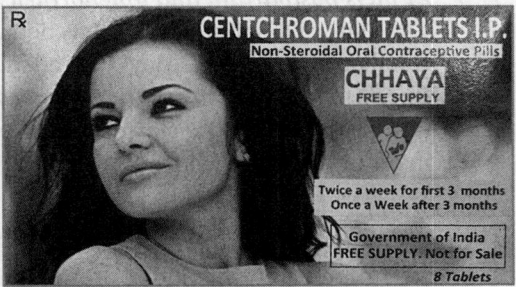

Fig. 8: Centchroman. *(For color version, see Plate 16)*

decidualization leading to defective implantation. Due to antiestrogenic action, tubal motility gets altered and also cervical mucus becomes hostile for the sperms. After stopping the pills, fertility returns within 6 months.

The advantage is that it avoids all the major side effects of steroidal contraceptive. Common side effects are menstrual disturbances like oligo or amenorrhea.

It is also used in the treatment of abnormal uterine bleeding (AUB). Clinical trials are undergoing for its use in the treatment of breast cancer and hormone replacement therapy (HRT).

When can a postpartum woman start use of oral combined contraceptives?
Postpartum (breastfeeding)
- *<6 weeks postpartum:* COCs are totally contraindicated.
- *6 weeks to 6 months:* COCs are contraindicated (MEC 3) unless other methods are not available or not acceptable. This is as COCs decrease the milk production.
- *>6 months and still amenorrheic:* Can start COCs if pregnancy has been ruled out. Backup for 7 days is needed.
- *>6 months and having normal menstruation:* COCs to be started just like in other women.

Postpartum (nonbreastfeeding)
- *<21 days postpartum:* COCs are contraindicated.
  - *21 days postpartum and amenorrheic:* Can start COCs if pregnancy has been ruled out. Backup for 7 days is needed.
  - *21 days postpartum and menses resumed:* COCs to be started just like in other women.

Postabortion
- Combined oral contraceptives can be started immediately. No added protection is needed if started within 7 days.

What can a woman do if she misses combined oral contraceptives?
- *For 30–35 µg EE pills:*
  - Missed one or two active (hormonal) pills:
    - She should take one pill as soon as she remembers and continue rest of the pack as usual. There is no need for added protection.
  - Missed three or more active (hormonal) pills:
    - She should take one pill as soon as she remembers and continue rest of the pack as usual. Backup method should be used for 7 days.
    - If pills are missed in the third week, she should finish the pack and then start the new pack immediately discarding the inactive 7 pills.
    - If pills are missed in the first week and there is unprotected sex, ECP should be taken.
- *For 20 µg EE pills:*
  - If she misses one pill, the advice is same as above for one or two missed pills.
  - If she misses two or more pills, the advice is same as above for missed three or more pills.
- *In any COCs if inactive pills are missed:*
  - Discard the inactive pills and start a new pack.

Identify the contraceptive method shown in Figure 9 and what is its advantage?
Extended-use COC pills (a pack of Seasonale): It contains 30 µg EE with 150 µg of LNG in each active pill. A pack contains 91 pills **(Fig. 8)**. A woman has to take active pill for 84 days and then placebo pills for 7 days. These extended regimens result in fewer bleeding days. Seasonale reduces the frequency of menstrual periods from 13 per year to 4 per year. With continuous use of pills for 1 year, more than 50% women

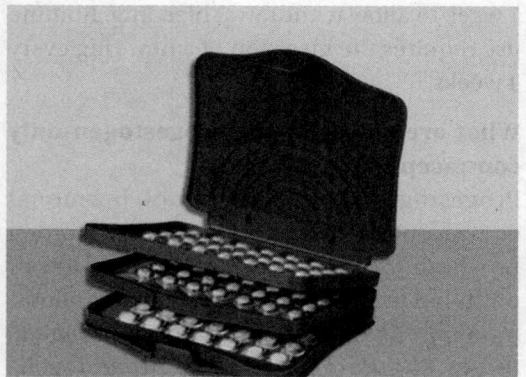

Fig. 9: Seasonale.

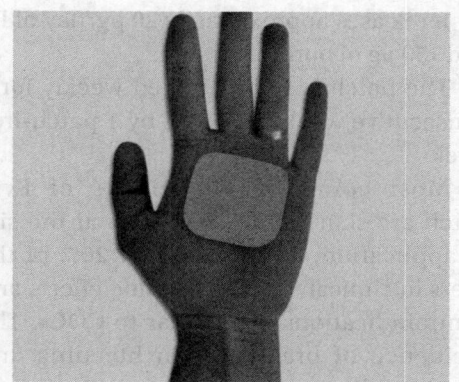

Fig. 10: Combined contraceptive patch (Evra).

become amenorrheic. Continuous use of oral contraceptives also significantly reduces side effects associated with hormone withdrawal, including migraine, headaches, premenstrual syndrome, mood changes, and heavy or painful monthly bleeding. All monophasic pills can be used like this. If taken without any break at all, it is known as *continuous use*. The main disadvantage with these regimens is irregular bleeding.

What is drospirenone? What is the advantage of using it in combined pill?

Drospirenone is a progestin that is an analog of spironolactone. It is essentially an antimineralocorticoid progestin. In addition, DSP has some antiandrogenic action; its potency is about 30% of CPA, the most potent antiandrogenic progestin. It has pharmacodynamic properties very similar to progesterone and has been used with EE in a COC Yasmin (EE 30 μg plus DSP 3 mg). Yasmin received the US Food and Drug Administration (FDA) approval in 2001 and is now available in many countries. Contraceptive efficacy equals to the other combined OCs in the first year of use. Yaz is very low-dose COC which contains 20 μg EE plus 3 mg of DSP with 24/4 regimen.

Advantages:
- Reduces acne and hirsutism
- Improved sense of well-being
- Effective for treating premenstrual syndrome/premenstrual dystrophic syndrome. Use of DSP-containing OCP is associated with less water retention and thus less weight gain than traditional COCs.

What contraceptive method is shown in Figure 10?

This is the transdermal combined contraceptive patch. It is available in market as Ortho Evra/Evra. It was approved by the US FDA in 2002 and is available in Europe, Canada, Hong Kong, Singapore, South Korea, and the US.

This is a 20 cm^2 (4 cm × 5 cm) patch containing 750 μg of EE and 6,000 μg of norelgestromin (a biologically active metabolite of norgestimate) **(Fig. 10)**.

The patch consists of three layers in a matrix-type arrangement. The backing outer polyester layer provides support for the middle layer that contains the adhesive and hormones and the inner layer is a polyester layer that is removed from the adhesive layer just before application.

It releases approximately 20 μg/day of EE and 150 μg of norelgestromin.

The patch is to be applied weekly for 3 consecutive weeks followed by 1 patch-free week.

Most common side effects of Evra patch are skin irritation or rash at the site of application, affecting about 20% of the users in clinical trials. Other side effects and contraindications are similar to COCs. The incidence of breakthrough bleeding and spotting is low among users of the Ortho Evra patch and decreases with longer use.

Identify the hormonal contraceptive method shown in Figure 11.

This is the vaginal combined contraceptive ring called *NuvaRing*. It is a flexible, soft, transparent ring made of ethylene vinyl acetate copolymer within silicone tubing. The ring is available in only one size, 4 mm in thickness and 54 mm in diameter **(Fig. 10)**.

It releases 15 μg EE and 120 μg etonogestrel per day. The larger progestin-containing segment is separated from the estrogen-containing segment by impermeable glass barriers.

The ring is self-inserted by the woman and worn for 3 weeks followed by removal for 1 week to allow withdrawal bleeding. Routine use requires the insertion of a new ring every 4 weeks.

What are the different progestogen-only contraceptives?

Progestogen-only methods of hormonal contraception provide options for women in whom estrogens are contraindicated or not tolerated. There are oral, subcutaneous, intramuscular, intrauterine, and intravaginal routes of administration for progestogen-only contraceptives **(Table 6)**.

Identify the contraceptive method shown in Figure 12.

This is injectable progestin-only contraceptive available under the family welfare program of the government of India. This is depot preparation containing 150 mg of medroxyprogesterone acetate.

What is the mechanism of action of progestin-only contraceptives?

The mechanism of action of progestogen-only contraceptives depends on the progestogen activity and dose **(Table 7)**. There are three important actions of progestogens leading to contraceptive effect:
1. Suppression of ovulation

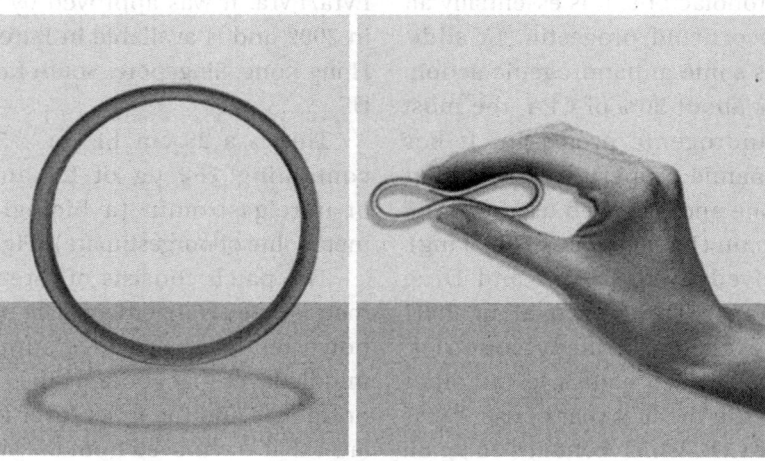

Fig. 11: NuvaRing.

Contraception

TABLE 6: Progestogen-only contraceptives.

Route of administration	Contraceptive methods	Progestin
Oral	Mini-pill	Levonorgestrel, norethisterone, ethynodiol diacetate, norgestrel, lynestrenol, desogestrel
Injectable	Depo-Provera (DMPA)	Medroxyprogesterone acetate
	NET-EN	Norethisterone
Subcutaneous implants	Norplant	Levonorgestrel
	Jadelle	Levonorgestrel
	Implanon	Desogestrel
Intrauterine device	Mirena	Levonorgestrel

(DMPA: depot medroxyprogesterone acetate; NET-EN: norethisterone enanthate).

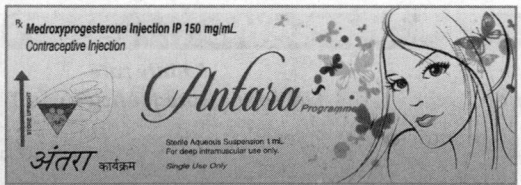

Fig. 12: Progestin-only contraceptive. *(For color version, see Plate 16)*

2. Thickening of cervical mucus
3. Involution of endometrium making it hostile for implantation

When can a woman have repeat progestogen-only injectables—depot medroxyprogesterone acetate or norethisterone enanthate?

Injection DMPA is repeated every 3 months and injection NET-EN is repeated every 2 months. Repeat injections can be given 2 weeks early or late from the scheduled date. If late by >2 weeks, injection can be given if she is surely not pregnant and back-up method is to be used for 7 days.

What can be done if a woman has menstrual abnormalities when using progestogen-only injectables?

Amenorrhea: She should be reassured as amenorrhea is expected on injectable contraceptives. Nothing needs to be done. But if this is unacceptable, the method should be discontinued.

Irregular spotting: Irregular spotting is common especially in the first cycle. If it persists, rule out other gynecological problems and treat accordingly. If no cause is found and it is bothersome, the method should be discontinued.

Heavy or prolonged bleeding: This is also common in the first cycle. But if it persists, rule out other causes and change the method if it is unacceptable.

What are different types of contraceptive implants?

Various contraceptive implants available or under development are mentioned in **Table 8**.

What is Implanon NXT (Fig. 13)?

Implanon NXT has been recently launched by the government of India. It contains barium sulfate which is radio-opaque and this makes it different from Implanon. It contains a total of 68 mg of etonogestrel. It is effective for 3 years.

When to insert Implanon NXT?

Implanon NXT should be inserted on day 1–5 of menstrual cycle.

TABLE 7: Contraindications to progestogen-only pills (WHO Medical Eligibility Criteria).

WHO 4: Absolute contraindication	Current carcinoma, breast
WHO 3: Method of last choice	Breastfeeding <6 weeks; current deep vein thrombosis, pulmonary embolism, history of carcinoma breast with disease free for >5 years; severe liver cirrhosis; liver tumors; IHD or CVA patients; women on Rifampicin and certain anti convulsants; SLE with antiphospholipid antibodies
WHO 2	History of ectopic pregnancy, multiple risk factors for arterial cardiovascular disease, severe HT, history of thromboembolism; major surgery with prolonged immobilization; hyperlipidemia; migraine with aura; unexplained vaginal bleeding; diabetes; gallbladder disease; mild liver cirrhosis

(CVA: cerebrovascular accidents; HT: hypertension; IHD: ischemic heart disease; SLE: systemic lupus erythematosus)

TABLE 8: Contraceptive implants.

Implant	Distinctive components	Dose	Registration	Life span	Failure rate (pregnancies/year)
Norplant	Six silicone capsules releasing LNG	216 mg	In about 60 countries	7 years*	<1
Jadelle	Two silicone rods releasing LNG	140 mg	In some European countries, USA, Thailand, and Indonesia	5 years	<1
Implanon	One polymer (resin) rod releasing etonogestrel	68 mg	Australia, Indonesia, India, and many European countries	3 years	<1
Nestorone	One silicone rod releasing nestorone	150 mg	Brazil	2 years	<1
Uniplant (Nomegestrel)	1 silicon rod	55 mg	Egypt	1 year	

(LNG: levonorgestrel)
*Approved for 5 years.

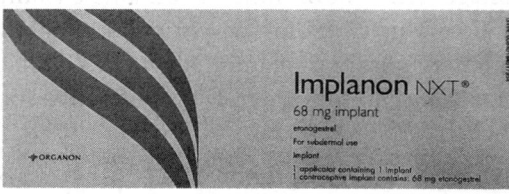

Fig. 13: Implanon NXT.
(For color version, see Plate 16)

Following abortion or miscarriage: Within 5 days of the first trimester and between 21 and 28 days following second-trimester abortion

Postpartum: If not breast feeding, between 21 and 28 days postpartum

Breastfeeding: After fourth postpartum week.

Insertion of Implanon is done under aseptic conditions in correct measurable anatomical position, i.e., overlying triceps muscle about 8–10 cm from the medial epicondyle of humerus and 3–5 cm between triceps and biceps.

What are the contraindications for Implanon NXT?
- Known or suspected pregnancy
- Active thromboembolic disorder
- Severe hepatic disease or presence or history of liver tumors
- Sex steroid-sensitive malignancies
- Known or suspected cancer of breast
- Undiagnosed vaginal bleeding
- Hypersensitivity to active substance or any of excipients of Implanon NXT

How can a woman take emergency contraceptive pills?
There are three types of pills which can be taken for emergency contraception:
1. Ulipristal acetate ECPs (UPAECPs)
2. LNG-only ECPs (LNG-ECPs)
3. Combined estrogen–progestogen ECPs (combined ECPs)

Emergency contraceptive regimens are:

Ulipristal ECP: Taken as a single dose of 30 mg tablet.

LNG-ECP: Taken as either single dose of 1.5 mg tablet or two tablets of 0.75 mg taken 12 hours apart.

Combined pills: Four tablets of low-dose contraceptive pills (EE 30 µg to be taken and repeated after 12 hours. If using very low dose pill (EE 20 µg), 5 tablets or if high dose pill (50 µg). Because of severe side effects of nausea and vomiting, this regimen is not preferred.

All the emergency pills are to be taken as soon as possible after the unprotected sexual intercourse within 120 hours. They are more effective if taken early. After 72 hours, ulipristal is more effective than LNG-ECP.

When can one start hormonal contraception after taking emergency contraceptive pill?
After taking progestogen-only contraceptive pill, hormonal contraception can be immediately started. After Ulipristal, hormonal contraception is started on 6th day due to hormonal interactions. Backup plan for 7 or 2 days is to be used in both cases as per the method used.

What are the male contraceptives under trial?
Male contraceptives have been under trial for many decades. Various combination preparations have been tried. Male hormonal contraception consists of administration of testosterone or a derivative androgen so as to suppress the pituitary release of gonadotropins, thus suppressing the spermatogenesis. At the same time, androgens thus administered ensure physiological androgen action, thus maintaining virilization and avoiding significant antiandrogenic side effects. Also, a progestin or GnRH antagonist is added to this to augment spermatogenesis suppression. Various agents have been used in numerous trials with varying results. Current combinations of testosterone with progestins completely suppress spermatogenesis without severe side effects in 80–90% of men, with significant suppression in the remainder of individuals. Recent trials with new longer acting forms of injectable testosterone, which can be administered every 8 weeks, combined with progestogens, administered either orally or by long-acting implant, have yielded promising results and may soon result in the marketing of a safe, reversible, and effective hormonal contraceptive for men.

A nonhormonal pill derived from Justicia gendarussa plant is also under trial and has been approved in Indonesia.

What is RISUG?

RISUG is a male contraceptive method which has been developed in India, and clinical trials are undergoing for the method and has completed phase 3 clinical trial. This is a long-acting but reversible method. RISUG stands for reversible inhibition of sperm under guidance. In this procedure, styrene maleic anhydride (SMA) complexed with solvent dimethyl sulfoxide (DMS) is injected into vas deferens. This causes partial blockage of the vas and also disrupts the sperms that pass through it, resulting in contraceptive effect. In clinical trials, it has been found to be effective for more than 15 years.

What are the different procedures for female sterilization?

Surgical procedures, timing of procedure, and related occlusion techniques are given in **Table 9**.

What are the eligibility criteria for sterilization?

Eligibility criteria for sterilization (government of India) are as follows:
- The client must have been married.
- Male clients should preferably be below the age of 60 years.
- Female client should be below the age of 45 years and above 22 years.
- Although the number of children is not a necessary criterion, the couple should have at least one child whose age is above 1 year.
- Clients or their spouses must not have undergone sterilization in the past (not applicable in cases of failure of sterilization).
- Clients must be in a perfectly normal state of mind so as to understand the full implication of sterilization.

TABLE 9: Procedures for female sterilization.

Approach	Surgical procedure and timing	Occlusion techniques
Abdominal	Minilaparotomy (postpartum, postabortion, or interval)	• Ligation and excision • Mechanical devices (clips, rings)
	Laparoscopy (interval, first-trimester MTP)	• Mechanical devices (clips, rings) • Electrocoagulation
	Laparotomy (in conjunction with other surgeries, e.g., cesarean section, salpingectomy, ovarian cystectomy)	• Ligation and excision • Mechanical devices (clips, rings) • Silastic band
Transvaginal (*no longer recommended*)	Colpotomy	• Ligation and excision • Mechanical devices (clips, rings)
	Culdoscopy	• Mechanical devices (clips, rings) • Electrocoagulation
Transcervical (experimental)	Hysteroscopy (interval only)	• Physical occlusion (plug, silicon) • Chemical agents (e.g., quinacrine) • Electrosurgery or YAG laser • Mechanical (Essure)

(MTP: medical termination of pregnancy)
Note: Transcervical approaches for tubal occlusion have been studied for several years, but to date none of these methods have been found to be completely safe and effective enough for implementation into routine service.

- Mentally ill clients must be certified by a psychiatrist, and consent in such cases should be given by legal guardian/spouse.
- The client must be informed of all the available methods of family planning and must make an informed decision for sterilization voluntarily.
- The written consent of spouse is not required for sterilization procedures.
- A relevant medical history, physical examination, and laboratory investigations need to be completed to ascertain eligibility for surgery.

What are the contraindications for female sterilization?

There is no medical condition that would absolutely restrict a person's eligibility for sterilization, although some conditions and circumstances will require that certain precautions are taken, including those where the recommendation is C (Caution), D (Delay), or S (Special). Where the risks of sterilization outweigh the benefits, long-term, highly effective contraceptive methods are a preferable alternative, considering the risks and benefits of sterilization versus the risks of pregnancy, and the availability and acceptability of highly effective, alternative methods. **Table 10** details the various categories for female sterilization as per Government Reference Manual for Female Sterilization 2014.

TABLE 10: Categories for female sterilization.

Caution	Delay	Special
- Previous abdominal or pelvic surgery - Obesity - Controlled BP - Uncomplicated heart disease - History of ischemic heart disease - Stroke - History of CVA - History of DVT or PE - Epilepsy - Depressive disorder - Current breast cancer - Uterine fibroids - PID without subsequent pregnancy - Uncomplicated diabetes - Mild cirrhosis - Hypothyroidism - Liver tumors - Kidney disease - Thalassemia and sickle cell disease - HIV	- Severe anemia (Hb <7 g%) - Current pregnancy - 8–42 days postpartum - Pregnancy with severe pre-eclampsia or eclampsia - Postpartum or postabortal complications (infection, hemorrhage, trauma) - Current DVT/PE - Major surgery with prolonged immobilization - Abdominal skin infection - Current ischemic heart disease - Lung disease like pneumonia - Systemic infection - Unexplained vaginal bleeding - Large blood collection in uterus - Malignant trophoblastic disease - Current PID - Genital tract cancers - Current purulent cervicitis - Current gallbladder disease - Uncontrolled diabetes	- Conditions that increase chances of heart disease or stroke, i.e., older age, smoking, high BP, or diabetes - Hypertension (BP >160/100 mm Hg) - Complicated heart disease - Coagulation disorder - Chronic lung disease - Endometriosis - Pelvic tuberculosis - Fixed uterus due to previous surgery or infection - Abdominal wall or umbilical hernia - Postpartum or postabortion uterine rupture or perforation - Diabetes of 20 years or more/with organ damage - Hyperthyroidism - Severe cirrhosis of liver - AIDS

(AIDS: acquired immunodeficiency syndrome; CVA: cerebrovascular accidents; DVT: deep vein thrombosis; HIV: human immunodeficiency virus; PE: pulmonary embolism; PID: pelvic inflammatory disease)
Note: Client should be offered some other contraceptive till the procedure can be done.

What are the common causes of female sterilization failure?

Common cases of failure of female sterilization are:
- Doing sterilization while she had already conceived.
- If surgery is performed wrongly, i.e., rather than fallopian tubes some other structures, most commonly round ligaments, are ligated.
- If tubes are partially occluded.
- If tuboperitoneal fistula forms later on.

What are two simple but important precautions to prevent failure?

1. Sterilization should be done after ruling out pregnancy. Ideal is to perform the procedure within the first 7 days of the periods.
2. Second important thing is to properly identify the tubes while ligating. The best is to trace the tube till fimbrial end before ligation.

CHAPTER 26

Medical Termination of Pregnancy Act with Amendments

Richa Sharma

Medical termination of pregnancy is governed by the Medical Termination of Pregnancy (MTP) Act, which was first enacted in 1971. The new MTP (Amendment) Act 2021 expands the access to safe and legal abortion services on therapeutic, eugenic, humanitarian, and social grounds to ensure universal access to comprehensive care. The main purpose of this chapter is to provide a comprehensive overview of amended MTP Act 2021.

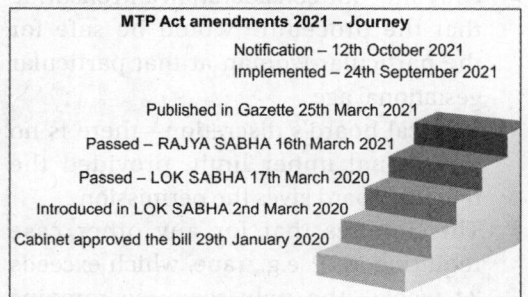

Who should do medical termination of pregnancy—person eligibility?

A RMP meaning a practitioner with a recognized MBBS/PG degree or diploma (as defined in the Indian Medical Council Act, 1956) and whose name has been entered in a state medical register can do MTP.

1.1. *RMP with PG degree or diploma in obstetrics and gynecology [can do MTP at any period of gestation (POG)]*

1.2. *RMP—MBBS (can do MTP after specific training)*

1.2.1. *MTP up to 9 weeks by medical method only*—if having an experience of at least 3 months at any hospital in obstetrics and gynecology OR has independently performed 10 cases of MTP by medical method of abortion under the supervision of RMP, in a hospital established or maintained by government or government-approved training center

1.2.2. *MTP up to 12 weeks by medical and surgical methods*—if they have assisted 25 cases of MTP out of which at least 5 have been done independently in a hospital established or maintained by government or government-approved training center

1.2.3. *MTP up to and beyond 24 weeks*—1 year experience in obstetrics and gynecology or 6 months' house job in obstetrics and gynecology

1.3. *Who should give the opinion for MTP:*
- MTP < 20 weeks—1 RMP opinion
- MTP between 20 and 24 weeks—not less than 2 RMP opinion
- Beyond 24 weeks—medical board decision (*Note:* After 24 weeks, 2 RMPs should perform the MTP)
- In order to save the life of mother, MTP can be done at any place and the opinion of two RMPs is not applicable.

Who can constitute the Medical Board?

Members—gynecologist, pediatrician, radiologist, any other member as notified by the government

Functions:
- To examine the woman and her reports
- Provide the opinion of Medical Board in Form D (rejection or approval) *within 3 days* of receiving the request for MTP
- To ensure that MTP, when advised by the Medical Board, is carried out with all safety precautions along with appropriate counseling *within 5 days* of the receipt of the request

Powers of Medical Board:
- To allow or deny MTP beyond 24 weeks of gestation
  Only after due consideration and ensuring that the procedure would be safe for woman at that POG and whether fetal malformation has a substantial risk of it being incompatible with life or if the child is born it may suffer from such physical or mental abnormalities to be seriously handicapped
- Co-opt other specialists in the Board and ask for any additional investigations if required, for deciding on the termination of pregnancy.

What are the indications for medical termination of pregnancy?

2.1. *Up to 20 weeks*
- To save the life of mother
- To prevent grave physical or mental injury to mother
- If there is a risk of physical or mental congenital abnormalities in the baby
- Humanitarian ground: Rape
- Contraception failure (both married and unmarried)

2.2. *Between 20 and 24 weeks*
- Survivors of sexual assault or rape or incest
- Minors
- Change of marital status during the ongoing pregnancy (widowhood and divorce)
- Women with physical disabilities
  - *[major disability as per criteria laid down under the Rights of Persons with Disabilities Act, 2016 (49 of 2016)]*
- Mentally ill women including mental retardation
- Fetal malformation that has substantial risk of being incompatible with life or if the child is born it may suffer from such physical or mental abnormalities to be seriously handicapped
- Women with pregnancy in humanitarian settings or disaster or emergency situations as declared by government

2.3. *Beyond 24 weeks*
For fetal malformations only
- Malformations that are incompatible with life or risk of physical/mental abnormalities, which can lead to serious handicap after birth
- Only after due consideration and ensuring that the procedure would be safe for the particular woman at that particular gestational age
- Medical board's discretion—there is no gestational upper limit, provided the medical board gives the permission
- This implies that for any other case requiring MTP, e.g., rape, which exceeds 24 weeks, the only recourse remains through a *Writ Petition*.

Where can medical termination of pregnancy be done?
Hospital established or maintained by the government (no separate registration needed)
- Primary health center (PHC)—up to 8 weeks
- Community health center (CHC)—up to 12 weeks
- District hospital—up to 20 weeks
- Medical college—any POG (up to 24 weeks and beyond)

Private health facility which is approved by government, i.e., district-level committee (DLC).

For MTP up to 9 weeks, medical methods of abortion (MMA) drugs can be prescribed by a RMP at their clinic, provided such a RMP has access to a place which is approved for MTP (under Section 4 of the MTP Act, 1971; read with MTP Amendment Act, 2002 and Rules 5 of the MTP Rules) and should display a certificate to this effect from the owner of the approved place.

Center approval by district-level committee: Government health facilities are approved for MTP; no separate approval is needed by DLC but all private health facilities need to get their centers approved for MTP. Approval depends upon the infrastructures. Form A has to be filled and necessary documents must be attached—hospital registration certificate, owner's photo, RMP degree/diploma/MBBS degree with specified training certificate and MCI or state medical registration certificate, anesthetist's degree and registration certificates, affidavit undertaking specifying that RMP and anesthetists are consultants in a particular health facility. Approval is given in form B; this form should be displayed in the area where MTP services are scheduled. [Form A, B—**Annexures 1, 2**]

What is the infrastructure requirement up to 12 weeks (category A)?
- Gynecology examination/labor table
- Resuscitation and sterilization equipment
- Drugs and parenteral fluids for emergency use, notified by the government of India from time to time
- Backup facilities for treatment of shock
- Facilities for transportation.

What is the infrastructure requirement up to 24 weeks and beyond (category B)?
- Operation table
- Instruments for performing abdominal or gynecological surgery
- Anesthetic equipment
- Resuscitation and sterilization equipment
- Drugs and parenteral fluids for emergency use
- Facilities for transportation

Infrastructure requirement beyond 24 weeks
- Operation table and instruments for performing abdominal or gynecological surgery
- Anesthesia equipment, resuscitation, and sterilization equipment
- Availability of drugs, parenteral fluids, and blood for emergency use, as may be notified by the central government from time to time
- Facilities for procedure under ultrasound guidance.

Once approval is given, it is permanent and renewal is not required, but periodic inspections will be there. CMO can recommend cancel/suspending the approval, based upon the inspections.

Report to the DLC and they may suspend or cancel the approval after hearing from the owner.

Reasons for cancellation of registration:
- If the place is not maintained properly and MTPs are not done under safe and hygienic condition
- If there was death or injury to a pregnant woman due to unsafe and unhygienic conditions, can seek any information or seize any article, medicine, admission register, or other documents

What documentation is required for MTP? (Annexures 3–8)
It is mandatory to fill all four forms, whenever MTP of a normally localized and live pregnancy is done. Forms need not be filled in the cases of ectopic pregnancy, missed or incomplete abortion, etc. Record all the information in the following forms, irrespective of the technique of abortion, i.e.,

MMA or surgical, and also irrespective of any trimester.

Consent Form: Form C (Consent of a woman is sufficient provided she is more than 18 years and mentally sound; consent of husband or male partner is desirable but not mandatory. If she is <18 years or mentally ill, then a guardian must give the consent. The guardian need not be blood related but can be anyone taking care of that patient.)

Opinion Form
For MTP <20 weeks' gestation—Form 1

For MTP between 20 and 24 weeks' gestation—Form E

For MTP >24 weeks' gestation—Form D by medical board

(Form I and Form E should be filled within 3 hours of MTP.)

Form II—Monthly Reporting Form (previous month data must be sent to the district CMO, within the first week of every month)

Form III—Admission Register for case records
It is a secret document, so do not open to all, but open under authority of law. Confidentiality has to be maintained. Keep under custody of owner/head of hospital and *preserve for a period of 5 years.*

How should the forms be stored?
Duly filled Form C and Form I/E must be placed in an envelope and sealed by a RMP, to be kept in safe custody until it is sent to the head of the hospital or the owner of the approved place.

Significance: The new law will contribute toward ending preventable maternal mortality to help meet the Sustainable Development Goals (SDGs) 3.1, 3.7, and 5.6. SDG 3.1 pertains to reducing maternal mortality ratio whereas SDGs 3.7 and 5.6 pertain to universal access to sexual and reproductive health and rights.

The amendments will increase the ambit and access of women to safe abortion services and will ensure dignity, autonomy, confidentiality, and justice for women who need to terminate pregnancy.

■ SUGGESTED READING

1. NHM Ministry of Health & Family Welfare, Government of India. Comprehensive Abortion Care, 2023. [online] Available from https://nhm.gov.in/images/pdf/programmes/maternal-health/guidelines/CAC_Training_&_Service_Guidelines_2023.pdf [Last accessed April, 2024]
2. The gazette of India CG-DL-E-26032021-226130, published by Ministry of law and Justice (Legislative Department) New Delhi, the 25th March, 2021/Chaitra 4, 1943 (Saka).
3. [online] Available from https://www.who.int/publications/i/item/9789240039483 [Last accessed April, 2024].

Annexure 1

FORM A
[See sub-rule (2) of rule 5]
FORM OF APPLICATION FOR THE APPROVAL OF A PLACE UNDER CLAUSE (b)
OF SECTION 4 OF THE ACT

Category of approved place:
(A) Pregnancy can be terminated up to twelve weeks
(B) Pregnancy can be terminated up to twenty-four weeks
 (i) Name of the place (in capital letters): _____
 (ii) Address in full: _____
 (iii) Nongovernment or Private or Nursing Home or Other Institutions:
 (iv) State, if the following facilities arc available at the place:

CATEGORY A
(i) Gynecological examination or labor table.
(ii) Resuscitation equipment.
(iii) Sterilization equipment.
(iv) Facilities for treatment of shock, including emergency drags.
(v) Facilities for transportations, if required.

CATEGORY H
(i) An operation table and instruments for performing abdominal or gynecological surgery.
(ii) Drugs and parental fluids in sufficient supply for emergency cases.
(iii) Anesthetic equipment, resuscitation equipment and sterilization equipment.

Place: _____
Date: _____   Signature of the owner for the place

Annexure 2

FORM B
[See sub-rule (6) of rule 5]
CERTIFICATE OF APPROVAL

The place described below is hereby approved for the purpose of the Medical Termination of Pregnancy Act. 1971 (34 of 1971).

As read within up to: _____ weeks

Name of the Place: _____

Address and other descriptions: _____

Name of the owner: _____

Place :

Date :   To the Government of the_____

CHAPTER 27

Consent in Family Planning: Medicolegal Aspects

Rashmi Gupta

INTRODUCTION

Consent is defined under Indian Contract Act (because doctor–patient relationship is a contract) as "two or more persons are said to consent when they agree to the same thing in the same sense".

The Supreme Court of India has stated that "it is important to recognize that reproductive choices can be exercised to procreate as well as to abstain from procreating". This means that there should be no restriction, whatsoever on exercise of reproductive choices such as women's right on insistence on use of contraceptive methods or not to use them.

In order to make an informed decision about safe and reliable contraceptive measures, comprehensive information, counseling and support should be accessible for all people, including people with disabilities, ethnic minorities, people living with HIV or any other reproductive tract infection, minors, sexual assault survivors, mentally challenged people, etc. It is a general legal and ethical principle that one must get the valid consent before starting any family planning methods.

What are the various types of informed consent?

- Implied
- Verbal
- Written

Implied consent: Implied consent refers to when a patient passively cooperates in a process without discussion for formal consent. The principles of good communication apply in these circumstances, and health professionals need to provide the patient with enough information to understand the procedure and why it is being done. Implied consent does not need to be documented in the clinical record. Example: In a family planning setting, when a patient comes for clinical examination, it is considered implied consent.

Verbal consent: A verbal consent is where a patient states their consent to a procedure verbally but does not sign any written form. This is adequate for routine treatment such as for diagnostic procedure and prophylaxis, provided that full records are documented. Example: When a patient comes in family planning OPD setting for intrauterine contraceptive device (IUCD) insertion, injection DMPA (depot medroxyprogesterone acetate), oral contraceptive pills (OCP) (temporary methods of contraception).

Written consent: A written consent is necessary in case of extensive intervention involving risks where anesthesia or sedation, restorative procedures, any invasive or surgical procedures, administering of medications with known high risks, and so on are sued. Example: Male and female sterilization process as it is a permanent method.

What are the principles of decision-making and consent?

There are seven principles of decision-making and consent. These are as follows:
1. All clients have the right to be involved in decisions about their treatment and care and be supported to make an informed decision if they are able.
2. It is an ongoing process focused on meaningful dialogue, the exchange of relevant information specific to the individual client.
3. All the clients have the right to be listened to, and to be given the information they need to make a decision, and time and support they need to understand it.
4. Healthcare providers must try to understand what matters to the client, so they can share relevant information about the benefits and harms of proposed option. Alternative options should also be offered to the client.
5. Healthcare providers must start with a presumption that all adult clients have the capacity to make decision about their treatment and care.
6. The choice of treatment or care for clients who lack capacity to make decision (minors and mentally challenged) is to be made by guardians of the client.
7. Client whose right to consent is affected by law should be supported to be involved in the decision-making process and to exercise choice if possible.

What is the significance of an informed written consent?

Before the procedure, the client and the doctor must complete and sign the consent form. This form is a legal document that shows a client's participation in the decision and a doctor's agreement to have the procedure done, despite being told about the alternative reversible method.

Signing of document means:
- Client received all relevant information about the procedure from healthcare professional.
- Client understands the information.
- Client uses this information to determine whether or not he/she wants the procedure.
- Client agrees or consented to get the treatment option.
- Client can choose to opt out anytime (even from the OT table), if he/she does not want the procedure and may opt for an alternative method of contraception.
- Client knows that the permanent method may fail although the chances are low.
- Client knows about the indemnity scheme in case of failure of method and knows when to reach the hospital in case of experiencing the failure.

What are the conditions where informed consent is required in Family Planning in India?
- Sterilization (both male and female)
- Medical termination of pregnancy (MTP)

When was MTP Amendment Act passed? What is the period of gestation admissible for medical termination of pregnancy?
- MTP Act was passed in 1971 and MTP Amendment Act was passed in 2021.
- There is no limit of gestation for termination.

Is the husband's consent required for women to undergo medical termination of pregnancy?

No, husband's consent is not required for women to undergo MTP.

Is the consent of husband necessary for sterilization?

No, the consent of husband is not necessary for sterilization.

What is section 88 in the Indian Penal Code?

Section 88 provides protection to the doctor if the patient dies after implied or expressed (informed) consent and the doctor has given treatment in good faith (has to be proved).

If cesarean section concurrent with sterilization has been performed or any other sterilization procedure has been performed with the consent of the client but later the spouse of the client alleges that sterilization has been performed without her/his consent, how such case should be dealt with?

As per the guidelines, consent of spouse is not required for sterilization and the signed consent of client suffices. The same may be communicated to the spouse. However, the Government of India encourages joint counseling of couples, although it is not mandatory.

Why is the word "partner" mentioned in the consent form?

A client can be married, divorced, or separated. The word "partner" in the consent form includes the spouse or the current partner.

Who can provide "consent" in case of a mentally unsound "ever married" client?

For a mentally unsound "ever married" client, a certificate from a psychiatrist indicating their unsound mental status is required. Thereafter, the legal guardian can provide consent, if the client is otherwise fit to undergo surgery.

In a situation where the client does not turn up for a sterilization procedure even after giving a written "consent", can the provider be held responsible for not providing services?

No, the provider would not be held responsible and in such cases LAMA (Left Against Medical Advice) should be documented in the case sheets to avoid any litigation in future.

If a client refuses to undergo sterilization operation in the operation theater even after signing the "Consent Form", can the client be forced to undergo sterilization?

No, in such cases the client cannot be forced to undergo sterilization at that juncture and instead should be counseled to come later for the same.

Is it mandatory to take signature/thumb impression of the client in case she/he refuses to undergo the procedure on the operating table after signing the "informed consent" form?

No, signature/thumb impression of the client is not mandatory if she/he refuses the procedure. Documentation of the refusal should mandatorily be done in the case sheet with a witness. However, it is preferable to have the client's signature/thumb impression too in these cases.

Can postpartum sterilization procedure be performed in a situation where the client has given a "conditional consent" before C-section? (Sterilization procedure depending on the sex of the baby born)

No, there is no scope for "conditional consent" in the sterilization program. The client has to decide in advance whether she wants to get the procedure done or not, irrespective of the sex of the baby born and give a clear "consent".

What is the documentation required for the sterilization procedure?

*Ligation Consent Form (**Annexure 1**) must be filled for both male and female sterilization* before the procedure. The consent form modified over the years by the Government of India has the phrase "all information has been explained and read out to me in my own language". Moreover, since some clients are unable to read and write, a signature or thumb impression has a legal sanctity whereas verbal communications cannot be admissible as evidence in a court of law. Therefore, in order to avoid any litigation/allegation of coercion or lack of understanding of conditions elaborated in the consent form, there is a provision of signature of witness along with the client's signature/thumb impression. Manuals published by the government of India are in the English language only. However, states are free to translate them in their local language provided the contents translated are verbatim and convey the same meanings, intents, and legal connotations.

What documentation is required for medical termination of pregnancy?
The following documents are required for both medical and surgical termination of pregnancy; however, as per MTP Amendment Act 2021, there are different forms to be filled and signed by the client and Registered Medical Practitioner for different periods of gestation.

Give the list of medical termination of pregnancy records.
- Form "C" **(Annexure 2)**
- Form "D" **(Annexure 3)**
- Form "E" **(Annexure 4)**
- Form "I" **(Annexure 5)**
- Form "II" **(Annexure 6)**
- Form "III" **(Annexure 7)**

Form "C": Client must fill and sign consent form "C" before the procedure. If the client is a minor, the guardian should sign the consent form. If the client is a mentally ill person, a certificate from a psychiatrist indicating their unsound mental status is required. Therefore, the legal guardian can provide the consent.

Form "D": A medical board should be constituted for termination beyond 24 weeks. Form "D" should be signed by authorized medical board (for congenital malformations incompatible to life).

Form "E": It should be filled and signed by two Registered Medical Practitioners for 20–24 weeks of gestation. The categories may be prescribed by rules made under MTP Amendment Act 2021.

Form "I": It should be filled and signed by one Registered Medical Practitioner for up to 20 weeks of gestation.

Form "II": It is a monthly reporting form (to be sent to the district authorities).

Form "III": Every head of the hospital or owner of the approved center shall maintain a register in the format of form III for recording details of the admissions or women for the termination of their pregnancies. Admission register shall be a secret document and the information contained there like the name and other particulars of the pregnant woman shall not be disclosed to any person. All columns mentioned by the MTP Act should be included in the admission register.

Consent should be sealed after the procedure; information cannot be divulged to anyone unless asked by court of law.

SUGGESTED READING

1. Comprehensive Abortion Care, Training and Services Delivery Guidelines, Ministry of Health and Family Welfare, Government of India, 2018. [online] Available from https://nhm.gov.in/New_Updates_2018/NHM_Components/RMNCHA/MH/Guidelines/CAC_Training_and_Service_Delivery_Guideline.pdf. May 2024.
2. J Fam Med Primary Care. (Official Journal of the Academy of Family Physicians of India). 2014;3(1):68-71.
3. Standards & Quality Assurance in Sterilization FAQs: Frequently asked Question, Family Planning Division, Ministry of Health and Family Welfare, Government of India, March 2016.

Annexure 1

Application cum Consent Form for Sterilization Operation

An informed consent is to be taken from all clients of sterilization before the performance of the surgery as per the consent form placed below

Name of Health Facility:_____

Client Hospital Registration Number:_____

Date:____/____/20____

1. Name of the Client: Shri/Smt._____
2. Name of Husband/Wife: Shri/Smt_____
3. Address_____
4. Contact No:_____
5. Names of all living, unmarried dependent children_____
    (i)_____ Age_____
    (ii)_____ Age_____
    (iii)_____ Age_____
    (iv)_____ Age_____
6. Father's name of beneficiary: Shri_____
7. Address:_____
8. Religion/Nationality:_____
9. Caste—SC/ST/General_____
10. Status—APL/BPL_____
11. Educational Qualifications_____
12. Business/Occupation:_____
13. Operating Center:_____

I, Smt/Shri_____(client) hereby give consent for my sterilization operation. I am ever married. My age is ...... years and my husband/wife's age is ...... years. I have ...... (Nos.) male and ...... (Nos.) female living children. The age of my youngest living child is ...... years.

a. I have decided to undergo the sterilization/re-sterilization operation on my own without any outside pressure, inducement or force. I declare that I/my spouse have/has not been sterilized previously (not applicable in case of re-sterilization).
b. I am aware that other methods of contraception are available to me. I know that for all practical purposes this operation is permanent and I also know that there are still some chances of failure of the operation for which the operating doctor and health facility will not be held responsible by me or by my relatives or any other person whomsoever.
c. I am aware that I am undergoing an operation, which carries an element of risk.
d. The eligibility criteria for the operation have been explained to me and I affirm that I am eligible to undergo the operation according to the criteria.
e. I agree to undergo the operation under any type of anesthesia, which the doctor/health facility thinks suitable for me and to be given other medicines as considered appropriate by the doctor/health facility concerned. I also give consent for any additional life-saving procedure, if required.
f. I agree to come for follow-up visits to the Hospital/Institution/Doctor/health facility as instructed, failing which I shall be responsible for the consequences, if any.
g. If, after the sterilization operation, I experience a missed menstrual cycle, then I shall report within 2 weeks of the missed menstrual cycle to the doctor/health facility and may avail of the facility to get an MTP done free of cost. I shall be responsible for the consequences, if any.
h. I understand that Vasectomy does not result in immediate sterilization. *I agree to come for semen examination 3 months after the operation to confirm the success of sterilization surgery (Azoospermia) failing which I shall be responsible for the consequences, if any. (*Applicable for male sterilization cases).
i. In case of complications, failures and the unlikely event of death attributable to sterilization, I/my spouse and dependent unmarried children will accept the compensation as per the existing provisions of the Government of India "Family Planning Indemnity Scheme" as full and final settlement and will not be entitled to claim any other compensation including compensation for upbringing of the child, if any, born on account of failure of sterilization, over and above the one offered, from any court of law in this regard.

I have read the above information or the above information has been read out and explained to me in my own language and that this form has the authority of a legal document.
    I am aware that I have the option of deciding against the sterilization procedure at any time without sacrificing my rights to other reproductive health services.

Date:_____   Signature or Thumb Impression of the Client

Name of Client:_____

Signature of Witness (Clients side):_____

Full Name:_____

I am aware that client is ever married and has one living child over one year of age.
Signature of ASHA/Counselor/Motivator:_____
Full Name:_____
FullAddress:_____

I certify that I have satisfied myself that:
a. Shri/Smt.....................is within the eligible age-group and is medically fit for the sterilization operation.
b. I have explained all clauses to the client and that this form has the authority of a legal document.
c. I have filled the medical record-cum-checklist and followed the standards for sterilization procedures laid down by the Government of India.

Signature of Operating Doctor   Signature of Medical Officer in-charge of the Facility

(Name of Operating Doctor)   (Name of Medical Officer in-charge of the Facility)

Date:.....................   Date: ....

Seal: Seal:

DENIAL OF STERILIZATION
I certify that Shri/Smt_____is not a suitable client for_____
sterilization/re-sterilization for the following reasons:
1. _____
2. _____

He/She has been advised the following alternative methods of contraception.
1. _____
2. _____

Signature of the Doctor making the decision

Date:_____

Name and full Address:_____

Annexure 2

FORM C
(Consent Form)

I_____daughter/wife of_____
aged about_____years of_____
(here state the permanent address)
at present residing at_____do hereby give my consent to
be termination of my pregnancy at_____
(State the name of place where the pregnancy is to be terminated).

Place:_____
Date:_____

Signature

(To be filled in by guardian where the woman is a lunatic or minor).

I_____son/daughter/wife of_____
aged about_____years of_____at present residing
at_____(permanent address)
_____do hereby give my consent to the termination of my
pregnancy of my ward_____who is a minor/lunatic at_____
_____

(Place of termination of pregnancy).

Place:_____

Date:_____

Signature

Annexure 3

FORM D

[See sub-clause (ii) of clause (b) of rule 3A]
Report of the Medical Board for Pregnancy Termination Beyond 24 weeks

Details of the woman seeking termination of pregnancy:
1. Name of the woman:_____
2. Age:_____
3. Registration/Case Number:_____
4. Available reports and investigations:_____

S.No.	Report	Opinion on the findings

5. Additional investigations (if done):

S.No.	Investigations done	Key findings

6. Opinion by Medical Board for termination of pregnancy:
   a. Allowed
   b. Denied

Justification for the decision:
7. Physical fitness of the woman for the termination of pregnancy:
   a. Yes
   b. No

Members of the Medical Board who reviewed the case:

S.No.	Name	Signature

Date and Time:_____

Annexure 4

FORM E
Opinion Form of Registered Medical Practitioners
(For gestation age beyond twenty weeks till twenty-four weeks)
[See sub-rule (2) of rule 4A]

I_____

(Name and qualifications of the Registered Medical Practitioner in block letters)

_____

(Full address of the Registered Medical Practitioner)

I_____

(Name and qualifications of the Registered Medical Practitioner in block letters)

_____

(Full address of the Registered Medical Practitioner) hereby certify that we are of opinion, formed in good faith, that it is necessary to terminate the pregnancy of

_____

(Full name of pregnant woman in block letters)

resident of_____

(Full address of pregnant woman in block letters)

which is beyond twenty weeks but till twenty-four weeks under special circumstances as given below*.

*Specify the circumstance(s) from (a) to (g) appropriate for termination of pregnancy beyond twenty weeks till twenty-four weeks:

(a) Survivors of sexual assault or rape or incest
(b) Minors
(c) Change of marital status during the ongoing pregnancy (widowhood and divorce)
(d) Women with physical disabilities [major disability as per criteria laid down under the Rights of Persons with Disabilities Act., 2016 (49 of 2016)]
(e) Mentally ill women including mental retardation
(f) The foetal malformation that has substantial risk of being incompatible with life or if the child is born it may suffer from such physical or mental abnormalities to be seriously handicapped
(g) Women with pregnancy in humanitarian settings or disaster or emergency situations as declared by Government

We hear by give intimation that we terminated the pregnancy of the woman referred to above who bears the Serial No. in the Admission Register of the hospital/approved place.

Signature of the Registered Medical Practitioner

Place:_____

Date:_____

Note: Account may be taken of the pregnant woman's actual or reasonably foreseeable environment in determining whether the continuance of her pregnancy would involve a grave injury to her physical or mental health.

Annexure 5

FORM I
RMP Opinion Form
(For gestation age upto twenty weeks)
[See Regulation 3]

I_____

(Name and qualifications of the Registered Medical Practitioner in block letters)

_____

(Full address of the Registered Medical Practitioner)

_____

hereby certify that I am of opinion, formed in good faith, that it is necessary to terminate the pregnancy of

_____

(Full name of pregnant woman in block letters)

_____

resident of_____

(Full address of pregnant woman in block letters)

_____

for the reasons given below*.

I hereby give intimation that I terminated the pregnancy of the woman referred to above who bears the Serial No. _____ in the Admission Register of the hospital/approved place.

Place:_____

Date:_____

Signature of the Registered Medical Practitioner

*of the reasons specified items (a) to (e) write the one which is appropriate:
a. in order to save the life of the pregnant woman
b. in order to prevent grave injury to the physical and mental health of the pregnant woman,
c. in view of the substantial risk that if the child was born it would suffer from such physical or mental abnormalities as to be seriously handicapped
d. as the pregnancy is alleged by pregnant woman to have been caused by rape
e. as the pregnancy has occurred as a result of failure of any contraceptive device or methods used by a woman or her partner for the purpose of limiting the number of children or preventing pregnancy.

Note: Account may be taken of the pregnant woman's actual or reasonably foreseeable environment in determining whether the continuance of her pregnancy would involve a grave injury to her physical or mental health.

Place: _____
Date: _____

Signature of the Registered Medical Practitioner

Annexure 6

FORM II

[Refer Regulation 4(5)]

Month & Year:_____

1. **Name of the State:**
2. **Name of Hospital/approved place:**
3. **Duration of pregnancy:** *(Give total number only under each sub-head)*
   (a) Up to 9 weeks (Medical Methods of Abortion Only):
   (b) Up to 12 weeks (Surgical Methods of Abortion Only):
   (c) Between 12–20 weeks:
   (d) Between 20–24 weeks:
   (e) Beyond 24 weeks:
4. **Religion of woman**: *(Give total number under each sub-head)*
   (a) Hindu:
   (b) Muslim:
   (c) Christian:
   (d) Others:
5. **Termination with acceptance of contraception:** *(Give total number under each sub-head)*
   (a) Sterilization:
   (b) IUCD:
   (c) OCP/Injectable Contraceptive:
   (d) Others:
6. **Reasons for termination**: *(Give total number under each sub-head)*
A. **Up to 20 weeks of gestation**
   (a) Danger to the life of the pregnant woman:
   (b) Grave injury to the physical and mental health of the pregnant woman:
   (c) Pregnancy caused by rape:
   (d) Substantial risk that if the child was born, it would suffer from such physical or mental abnormalities as to be seriously handicapped:
   (e) Failure of any contraceptive device or method:
B. **Between 20–24 weeks of gestation**
   (a) Survivors of Sexual Assault/Rape/Incest:
   (b) Minors:
   (c) Change of marital status during the ongoing pregnancy (widowhood and divorce):
   (d) Women with physical disabilities [major disability as per criteria laid down under the Rights of Persons with Disabilities Act, 2016 (49 of 2016)]:
   (e) Mentally ill women including mental retardation:
   (f) The foetal malformation that has substantial risk of being incompatible with life or if the child is born it may suffer from such physical or mental abnormalities to be seriously handicapped:

(g) Women with pregnancy in humanitarian settings or disasters or emergency situations as declared by Government:

C. **Beyond 24 weeks of gestation**
   (a) The foetal malformation that has substantial risk of being incompatible with life or if the child is born it may suffer from such physical or mental abnormalities to be seriously handicapped:

Signature of the Officer In-charge with Date

Annexure 7

FORM III

[Refer Regulation 5]

Admission Register

(To be destroyed on the expiry of five years from the date of the last entry in the Register)

Name of Facility: _____

Month _____ Year _____

S. No.	Date of Admission	Name of the Patient	Wife/Daughter of	Age	Religion	Address	Duration of Pregnancy	Reasons on which Pregnancy is terminated	Date of termination of Pregnancy	Date of discharge of patient	Results Remarks	Name of Registered Medical Practitioner(s) by whom the opinion is formed (For pregnancy beyond 24 weeks mention the names of Medical Board members)	Name of Registered Medical Practitioner(s) by whom Pregnancy is terminated	Method of MTP (MVA/EVA/MMA/D&C/Others)	Post-Abortion Contraception (Tubal Ligation (TL)/IUCD/OCP/Injectables/Others/None)
1	2	3	4	5	6	7	8	9	10	11	12	13	14	15	16

CHAPTER 28

Definitions

Archana Mehta, Shivangini Sahay, Neerja Goel, Anshuja Singla

■ GYNECOLOGY

- *Puberty:* It is the period during which secondary sexual characteristics develop and capability of sexual reproduction is attained or a child develops physically and mentally into adulthood. The physiological changes follow an orderly sequence with an initial acceleration of growth followed by breast budding (thelarche) occurring at a median age of 11 years. This is followed by the growth of pubic hair at 10.5 years and axillary hair at 12.5 years (adrenarche). Menarche is a late event occurring at 12.8 years. Peak height velocity approximately 8 cm/year occurs just prior to the onset of menses. Estrogen promotes closure of epiphysis so final height is usually attained about 2 years after menarche. The process of puberty usually starts at 8 years of age and is completed by the age of 16 years.
- *Precocious puberty:* It is defined as pubertal development occurring more than 2.5 standard deviation earlier than the average age. Traditionally, it has been defined as appearance of secondary sexual characteristics before the age of 8 years in female and 9 years in male. It has been classified according to the underlying pathophysiology into three types:
  1. Gonadotropin-dependent precocious puberty (true precocious puberty/central precocious puberty)
  2. Gonadotropin-intendent puberty (pseudoprecocious puberty/peripheral precocious puberty)
  3. Incomplete precocious puberty (premature thelarche, premature adrenarche)
- *Delayed puberty:* It exists in girls who failed to develop any secondary sexual characteristics by the age of 13 years, have not had menarche by age 15 years, or in whom 5 or more years have passed since the onset of pubertal development without attainment of menarche.
- *Heterosexual puberty:* It is characterized by development that is characteristic of the opposite sex occurring at the expected age of normal puberty.
- *Primary amenorrhea:* Absence of menses by 15 years of age in the presence of secondary sexual characteristics or by 13 years of age when there is no visible secondary sexual characteristic development. The World Health Organization (WHO) has described three classes of amenorrhea.
- *Secondary amenorrhea:* It is defined as absence of menstruation for three normal cycles or 6 months.
- *Intersex:* It is a general term used for a variety of conditions in which a person is born with a reproductive/sexual anatomy that does not seem to fit the typical definition of a male or female. An estimate for intersex prevalence is 1 in 2,000.

- *Hirsutism:* It is excessive growth of terminal hair in a male distribution. It is change in quality, size, length of hair as well as pigmentation and not the number of hairs. Ferriman–Gallwey scoring is done for the severity of hirsutism. It must be differentiated from hypertrichosis, which is nonandrogen-dependent excessive hair growth anywhere in the body (vellus type). About 10% of young female population in the United States of America (USA) is found to be hirsute and in 60–70% of cases, it is due to polycystic ovarian syndrome (PCOS).
- *Virilization:* It is defined as the presence of signs of masculinization in woman. These include, in addition to hirsutism, breast atrophy, deepening of voice, temporal balding, clitoromegaly, increased libido, and increased muscle mass.
- *Polycystic ovarian syndrome:* Using the Rotterdam PCOS diagnostic criteria, presence of two out of the following three criteria:
  1. Oligo and/or anovulation
  2. Hyperandrogenism (clinical and/or biochemical)
  3. Polycystic ovaries with the exclusion of other etiologies

  The morphology of polycystic ovary has been defined as an ovary with 20 or more follicles measuring 2–9 mm in diameter and/or increased ovarian volume (>10 cm^3) on transvaginal ultrasonography with a transducer frequency ≥8 MHz. Even a single ovary is sufficient for the diagnosis. It is the most common endocrine disorder in women (prevalence 5–10%).
- *Premature ovarian insufficiency (POI):* It is a clinical syndrome defined by loss of ovarian activity before the age of 40 years. The diagnostic criteria include:
  i. Oligo/amenorrhea for at least 4 months
  ii. An elevated follicle-stimulating hormone (FSH) level >25 IU on two occasions more than 4 weeks apart. Prevalence is 1 in 100 by age 40 years, 1 in 1,000 by age 30 years, and 1 in 250 by age 35 years

  Genetic factors are thought to have a strong relationship with POI.
- *Infertility:* It is defined as 1 year of unprotected intercourse without pregnancy. 90% of healthy young couples conceive in 1 year.
- *Fecundability:* It is probability of pregnancy per cycle. About 20% of healthy couples conceive in a single cycle.
- *Fecundity:* It is the probability of achieving a live birth in a single cycle.
- *Clomiphene failure:* If ovulation occurs with clomiphene but the patient fails to conceive, it is labeled as clomiphene failure.
- *Clomiphene resistance:* If ovulation fails to occur with 3 months therapy of clomiphene at 150 mg/day for 5 days, it is labeled clomiphene resistance.
- *Luteal phase defect:* It is characterized by inadequate endometrial maturation due to a qualitative or quantitative disorder of corpus luteum functions. For diagnosis, there should be at least two endometrial biopsies out of phase (lagging behind) in two consecutive cycles. It accounts for 4% of infertility.
- *Ovarian hyperstimulation syndrome (OHSS):* It is a syndrome with a wide spectrum of clinical and laboratory symptoms and signs, ovarian enlargement, and a fluid shift from the intravascular to extravascular space manifesting as ascites, pleural effusion, hemoconcentration, oliguria, electrolyte

imbalance, and hypercoagulability. It can be mild (13.5%), moderate (3–6%), and severe (0.1–0.2%).
- *Assisted reproductive technology:* It involves all techniques involving direct manipulation of oocytes outside the body.
- *In vitro fertilization (IVF):* It involves a sequence of highly coordinated steps beginning with controlled ovarian hyperstimulation with exogenous gonadotropins, followed by oocyte retrieval transvaginally under ultrasound guidance, fertilization in laboratory, and transcervical transfer of embryos into the uterus.
- *Intracytoplasmic sperm injection (ICSI):* It involves the injection of a single sperm within the ooplasm of the oocyte. It is the only option for severe male infertility due to oligoasthenospermia, obstructive azoospermia, and repeated fertilization failures with conventional IVF due to any reason.
- *In vitro maturation (IVM) of oocyte:* It is a promising new technique where cumulus-oocyte complex (COC) is collected from antral follicles with or without prior mild FSH stimulation. The COC is then cultured in maturation media containing 75 mL of FSH/luteinizing hormone (LH) and human serum albumin (HSA) at 37°C in an atmosphere of 5% carbon dioxide (CO_2) and 95% air with high humidity. They are checked at 24 and 48 hours for maturity followed by ICSI of mature oocytes. Standard IVF is then carried out. Embryo transfer is performed after laser-assisted hatching to avoid reduced implantation due to hardened zona pellucida followed by prolonged culture. The process of IVM circumvents the need for inconvenient, costly, and at times dangerous gonadotropins stimulation of ovaries.
- *Gamete intrafallopian transfer:* Placing retrieved oocyte and sperm into the fallopian tube via laparoscopic/laparotomy where fertilization takes place
- *Zygote intrafallopian transfer:* Placing zygotes created by IVF, at a stage prior to cleavage into the fallopian tube
- *Aspermia:* It means failure of formation or emission of semen.
- *Azoospermia:* It means there is no sperm in semen.
- *Severe oligospermia:* <2–10 × 10^6 sperms/mL
- *Asthenospermia:* <5–10% motile sperms
- *Poor morphology:* <4% normal forms
- *Oligoasthenoteratozoospermia (OAT):* It is the most common finding in semen analysis of an infertile male. According to WHO, the OAT syndrome refers to individual semen samples with abnormalities in sperm numbers, motility, and morphology. OAT is present if there is:
  - An ejaculate volume <1.4 mL
  - A sperm concentration <16 × 10^6/mL
  - A total sperm number <39 × 10^6
  - A sperm motility <42% of total motility or 30% of progressive motility
  - A sperm morphology <4% normal forms
- *Intrauterine insemination (IUI):* IUI with a washed sperm concentrate (devoid of seminal plasma)
- *Abnormal uterine bleeding (AUB):* It is defined as any bleeding from the genital tract that is a deviation from the normal in frequency, regularity, duration, or quantity. It may be acute or chronic.
  - *Acute AUB is defined as an episode of uterine bleeding in a woman of reproductive age who is not pregnant, which is of sufficient quantity to require immediate intervention to prevent further blood loss.*

- *Chronic AUB is defined as bleeding from the uterine body that is abnormal in frequency, regularity, duration, and/or volume and has been present for at least the majority of the past 6 months.*
- **Heavy menstrual bleeding:** It is defined as excessive menstrual blood loss which interferes with a woman's physical, social, emotional, and/or mental quality of life.

  The International Federation of Gynecology and Obstetrics (FIGO) classification of AUB

PALM	COEIN
P: Polyp	C: Coagulopathy
A: Adenomyosis	O: Ovulatory dysfunction
L: Leiomyoma	E: Endometrial
M: Malignancy and hyperplasia	I: Iatrogenic
	N: Not yet classified

- *Frequent and infrequent menstruation:*
  - *Frequent uterine bleeding*: Cycles <24 days
  - *Infrequent uterine bleeding*: Cycles >38 days
- *Dysmenorrhea:* It is pain with menstruation usually cramping in nature and centered in lower abdomen, affecting 60% of menstruating women.
  - *Primary (spasmodic) dysmenorrhea:* It is menstrual pain without pelvic pathology. It is confined to adolescent girls and appears within 2 years of menarche. The pain begins a few hours before or just with the onset of menstruation. The severity of pain lasts usually for few hours but may extend up to 48–72 hours. Pain is spasmodic and confined to lower abdomen and may radiate to the medial aspect of thighs. Systemic discomforts like nausea, vomiting, fatigue, diarrhea, headache, and vasomotor changes may be present.
  - *Secondary (congestive) dysmenorrhea:* Painful menses associated with underlying pelvic pathology. The pain is dull and situated in back and in front without radiation. It usually begins 1–2 weeks prior to the period and persists until a few days after cessation of bleeding. The onset and duration of pain depend upon the pathology producing the pain. There is no systemic discomfort unlike primary dysmenorrhea. The most common cause of secondary dysmenorrhea is endometriosis followed by adenomyosis and an intrauterine device.
- *Premenstrual syndrome:* Cyclic recurrence in the luteal phase of menstrual cycle of a combination of distressing physical, psychological, and/or behavioral changes of sufficient severity to result in deterioration of interpersonal relationship and/or interference with normal activities. Diagnosis is made by using the Daily Record of Severity of Problems (DRSP) questionnaire. The incidence is around 40%.
- *Endometriosis:* It is defined as the presence of endometrial tissue (glands and stroma) outside the uterus. The most frequent site of implantation is the pelvic viscera and the peritoneum. Though endometriosis is found in 10% of women in reproductive age group, it is thought to be responsible for a much higher percentage (20–50%) of infertility and chronic pelvic pain. Some of the common associated symptoms are progressively worsening dysmenorrhea, acquired dyspareunia, and premenstrual spotting.

- *Adenomyosis:* It is characterized by the presence of endometrial gland and stroma in the myometrium, at least one low-power field from the basis of endometrium. The incidence is unknown.
- *Obesity:* It is defined as the accumulation of excess body fat that leads to pathology or body mass index (BMI) >25 kg/m^2 or increase in waist-to-hip ratio >0.82 for females (ideal ratio for Indian men 0.88 and for women 0.8).

$$BMI = \frac{Weight\ in\ kilogram}{Height\ in\ square\ meter}$$

WHO Asian BMI classification:
Normal = 18.5–22.9 kg/m^2
Underweight = <18.5 kg/m^2
Overweight = 23.0–24.9 kg/m^2
Obese I = 25.0–29.9 kg/m^2
Obese II = >30 kg/m^2

- *Metabolic syndrome:* It is defined as presence of any three of following:
  - Female waist >35 inches
  - High triglyceride levels (>150 mg/dL)
  - Low level of high-density lipoprotein (HDL) (<40 mg/dL in males and <50 mg/dL in females)
  - High blood pressure (BP) >130/85 mm Hg
  - Fasting blood glucose level 100 mg/dL or higher

    Metabolic syndrome predisposes an individual to diabetes and cardiovascular disease. This is of interest because a child exposed to maternal obesity is at an increased risk of developed metabolic syndrome.

- *Chronic pelvic pain:* It is intermittent or constant pain in lower abdomen or pelvis of a woman of at least 6 months; duration not occurring exclusively with menstruation or intercourse and not associated with pregnancy.

- *Vulvodynia or vulvar pain syndrome:* This term was introduced by Friedrich in 1987. Vulvodynia, most often described as burning pain, occurs in the absence of relevant visible findings or specific clinically identifiable neurologic disorder. Prevalence is about 8%. Several causes include embryologic abnormalities, increased urinary oxalates, genetic or immune factors, hormonal factors, inflammation, infection, and neuropathic changes. The current International Societies for the Study of Vulvovaginal Disease (ISSVD) definition of vulvodynia is vulvar pain of at least 3 months' duration, without a clear, identifiable cause, which may have a potential associated factor. It is diagnosis of exclusion and is an idiopathic pain disorder.

The classification of vulvodynia is based on the site of pain, whether it is generalized or localized and whether is provoked or unprovoked or mixed.

Three important diagnostic criteria are:
1. Entry dyspareunia
2. Vestibular erythema
3. Positive swab test (light pressure with a cotton-tipped swab induces severe pain)

- *Vaginismus:* It is involuntary spasm of pubococcygeal and associated muscles causing painful and difficult penetration of vagina, during sex, tampon insertion, or clinical examination.
- *Dyspareunia:* It is a recurrent genital pain that occurs just before, during, or after intercourse.
- *Urinary incontinence:* It is defined as a complaint of any involuntary leakage of urine.
- *Urgency:* It is sudden and compelling desire to pass urine which is difficult to defer.

- *Urge incontinence:* It is involuntary leakage of urine accompanied by or immediately preceded by urgency.
- *Stress incontinence:* It is involuntary leakage of urine on effort, exertion, sneezing, or coughing.
- *Genuine stress incontinence:* It is a urodynamic diagnosis and refers to involuntary leakage of urine with sudden rise of intra-abdominal pressure in absence of detrusor activity.
- *Painful bladder syndrome:* It is the complaint of suprapubic pain related to bladder filling, accompanied by other symptoms, such as increased day time and night time frequency, in the absence of previous urinary infection or other obvious pathology.
- *Interstitial cystitis:* It is painful bladder syndrome with typical cystoscopic and/or histological features in the absence of infection or other pathology.
- *Overactive bladder syndrome (OAB):* Urinary urgency with or without urge incontinence usually with frequency and nocturia, if there is no infection or proven pathology. It is a diagnosis based on symptoms alone, rather than urodynamic findings. OAB can be further classified as OAB wet (with incontinence) or OAB dry (without incontinence).

  16.6% of population aged over 40 years have OAB symptoms.
- *Detrusor overactivity:* It is defined as a urodynamic observation characterized by involuntary detrusor contractions during the bladder filling phase which may spontaneous or provoked.

  So, detrusor overactivity is a urodynamic diagnosis whereas OAB is a clinical diagnosis.
- *Pelvic organ prolapse:* It is defined as the protrusion or herniation of pelvic organs into or out of the vagina that occurs due to failure of the anatomical supports.
- *Radical trachelectomy:* It is fertility-sparing treatment for early stage carcinoma cervix where cervix is removed at the lower uterine segment leaving the upper isthmus and uterine corpus intact to allow for pregnancy. Along with this, laparoscopic pelvic lymph node sampling is done. A permanent prophylactic cerclage is placed for prevention of premature delivery.
- *Emergency contraception:* It is the contraception provided after the act of unprotected sexual intercourse.

OBSTETRICS

- *Fertility rate:* This is the number of live births per 1,000 females in the reproductive age group (15–44 years).
- *Stillbirth:* It means a baby born with absence of signs of life at or after 28 weeks.
- *Stillbirth rate:* It is the number of stillborn neonates per 1,000 neonates born including live birth and stillbirths.
- *Perinatal mortality rate:* It is the number of stillbirths plus neonatal deaths per 1,000 total births.
- *Infant death:* All deaths of live born infants from birth through 12 months of age
- *Infant mortality rate:* The number of infant deaths per 1,000 live births
- *Term neonate:* A neonate born any time after 37 completed weeks of gestation and up to 42 completed weeks is considered to be a term infant.
- *Early term neonate:* It refers to a neonate born at 37 completed weeks up to $38^{6/7}$ weeks.
- *Full-term neonate:* It denotes a neonate born at 39 completed weeks up to $40^{6/7}$ weeks.

- *Late-term neonate:* It describes a neonate born at 41 completed weeks up to $41^{6/7}$ weeks.
- *Preterm neonate:* It describes a neonate born before 37 completed weeks and after 20 weeks. A neonate born before 34 completed weeks is early preterm, whereas a neonate born between 34 and 36 completed weeks is late preterm.
- *Post-term neonate:* It means a neonate born any time after completed 42nd week beginning with day 295.
- *Abortus:* It means a fetus or an embryo removed or expelled from the uterus during the first half of gestation (20 weeks or less) or in the absence of accurate dating criteria, born weighing <500 g.
- *Maternal mortality ratio:* It is the number of maternal deaths that result from the reproductive process per 100,000 live births. Used more commonly but less accurately are the terms maternal mortality rate and maternal death rate. The term ratio is more accurate because it includes in the numerator the number of deaths regardless of pregnancy outcome, e.g., live births, stillbirths, ectopic pregnancies, while the denominator includes the number of live births.
- *Bad obstetric history:* Any disappointment or disaster in the reproductive carrier of a woman in the form of abortion, preterm births, stillbirth, neonatal death, or third-stage complication that has influence on the current pregnancy outcome is defined as bad obstetric history.
- *Recurrent pregnancy loss (RPL):* It is classically defined as three or more consecutive first-trimester losses at <20 weeks of gestation or with fetal weight <500 g. American Society for Reproductive Medicine (ASRM) (2020) defines RPL two or more failed pregnancies confirmed by sonographic or histopathological examination.
- *Hyperemesis gravidarum:* It is defined as severe unrelenting nausea and vomiting that produces weight loss, dehydration, ketosis, alkalosis from loss of hydrochloric acid, and hypokalemia. Acidosis develops from partial starvation.
- *Gestational hypertension:* It indicates BP that reaches 140/90 mm Hg or greater for the first time after mid-pregnancy (20 weeks) but lack proteinuria and resolves by 12 weeks postpartum.
- *Pre-eclampsia:* It is multisystem inflammatory disorder beyond 20 weeks of gestation characterized by de novo onset of hypertension (BP ≥ 140/90 mm Hg) taken on two occasions 4 hours apart.
  - *With proteinuria*:
    - ≥300 mg in 24 hours or
    - Urine protein creatinine ratio ≥0.3 or
    - Dipstick 1+ persistent
  - *Or hypertension without proteinuria characterized by*:
    - *Thrombocytopenia:* Platelet <100,000/μL
    - *Renal insufficiency:* Creatinine >1.1 mg/dL or doubling of baseline
    - *Liver involvement:* Serum transaminase levels twice normal
    - *Cerebral symptoms:* Headache, visual disturbances, convulsions
    - Pulmonary edema
- *Eclampsia:* It is defined as seizures that cannot be attributed to any other cause in a woman with pre-eclampsia.
- *Chronic hypertension:* It is a known case of hypertension or a case of hypertension detected before 20 weeks of gestation in the absence of neoplastic trophoblastic disease and multiple pregnancies.

- *Pre-eclampsia superimposed upon chronic hypertension:* It is occurrence of pre-eclampsia in women with chronic hypertension.
- *HELLP syndrome:* It is pre-eclampsia in association with hemolysis, elevated liver enzymes levels and low platelet counts (HELLP). It is found in 10% of pregnancies complicated by severe pre-eclampsia.
  Criteria:
  - *Hemolysis:*
    - Abnormal peripheral smear
    - Lactate dehydrogenase (LDH) >600 U/mL
    - Bilirubin >1.2 mg/dL
  - *Elevated liver enzyme level:*
    - Serum glutamic-oxaloacetic transaminase (SGOT) >70 IU/mL
    - Lactate dehydrogenase >600 U/mL
  - *Low platelet counts:* <100,000/mm^2
- *Antiphospholipid antibody syndrome:* Diagnosed if a single clinical and a laboratory criterion is present.
  Clinical criteria:
  - One or more episodes of arterial, venous, or small-vessel thrombosis, occurring in any tissue or organ
  - *Complications of pregnancy:* One or more unexplained deaths of a morphologically normal fetus >10 weeks of gestation documented by ultrasound or by direct examination
  Or
  - One or more preterm births of a morphologically normal neonate at or before 34 weeks of gestation due to severe pre-eclampsia or placental insufficiency
  Or
  - Three or more consecutive abortions before 10 weeks' gestation with no maternal hormonal or anatomic abnormalities, normal maternal and paternal chromosomes, and other causes of recurrent losses being ruled out.
  Laboratory criteria:
  - *Anticardiolipin (aCL) antibodies:* aCL immunoglobulin M (IgM) antibodies present in moderate or high titers on two or more occasions at least 12 weeks apart
  OR
  - *Lupus anticoagulant (LA):* Detection of LA using phospholipids-dependent tests for coagulation such as dilute Russell viper venom test (dRVVT), kaolin clotting time (KCT), and activated partial thromboplastin time (aPTT)
  OR
  - Anti-β_2 glycoprotein IgG or IgM
- *Antepartum hemorrhage:* Bleeding from or into the genital tract.
  - *Placenta previa:* The bleeding may be the consequence of some separation of a placenta in the vicinity of cervical canal after 20 weeks of gestation.
  - *Abruptio placentae:* It may be separation of placenta elsewhere in the uterine cavity.
  - *Vasa previa:* When the bleeding is due to velamentous insertion of umbilical cord with rupture and hemorrhage from a fetal blood vessel at the time of rupture of membranes
- *Small for gestational age:* In clinical practices, it is defined as the one with estimated fetal weight (EFW) or abdominal circumference <10th percentile.
- *Fetal growth restriction (FGR):* According to American College of Obstetricians and Gynecologists (ACOG), it is either an EFW <10th percentile for gestational age or an abdominal circumference (AC) <10th percentile of gestational age. According

to Society for Maternal–Fetal Medicine (SMFM) Delphi criteria consensus is used for classification of FGR.

Early FGR	Late FGR
(Gestational age <32 weeks) in absence of congenital anomalies	(Gestational age ≥32 weeks) in absence of congenital anomalies
AC/EFW <3rd centile or UA-AEDF OR 1. AC/EFW <10th centile combined with 2. Ut A PI >95th centile and/or 3. UAPI >95th centile	AC/EFW <3rd centile Or at least two out of three of following: 1. AC/EFW <10th centile 2. AC/EFW crossing centiles >2 quartiles on growth centiles 3. CPR <5th centile or UA PI >95th centile
(AC: abdominal circumference; CPR: cerebroplacental ratio; EFW: estimated fetal weight; FGR: fetal growth restriction; PI: pulsatility index; UA: umbilical artery; Ut A: uterine artery)	

- *Dizygotic twins (fraternal):* Twin fetuses resulting from fertilization of two separate ova
- *Monozygotic twins:* Twins resulting from the division of a single ovum

If division occurs before inner cell mass (morula) and the outer layer of blastocyst is not yet committed to become chorion that is within the first 72 hours after fertilization, two embryos, two amnions, and two chorions will develop. There will evolve a diamniotic, dichorionic, and monozygotic twin pregnancy. There will be two distinct placenta or a single fused placenta.

If division occurs between 4th and 8th day after the inner cell mass is formed, there will be diamniotic, monochorionic, and monozygotic twin pregnancy.

If the amnion has already become established (after 8 days of fertilization), there will be monochorionic, monoamniotic, and monozygotic twin pregnancy.

If diversion is initiated even later, that is, after the embryogenic disk is formed, cleavage is complete and conjoined twins are formed.

- *Superfetation:* In superfetation, an interval as long as or longer than an ovulatory cycle intervenes between fertilizations. Superfetation requires ovulation during the course of pregnancy. It is unproved in humans.
- *Superfecundation:* It refers to the fertilization of two ova within a short period of time but not at the same coitus nor necessarily by sperm from the same male. It may be that twin ova are not fertilized by sperm from the same ejaculate.
- *Chimerism:* A chimera is an individual whose cells originated from more than one fertilized ovum.
- *Anemia in pregnancy:* The WHO defines anemia as hemoglobin <11 g% in first and third trimesters and <10.5 g% in the second trimester.
- *Asymptomatic bacteriuria:* This refers to persistent, actively multiplying bacteria within the urinary tract without symptoms. A clean voided specimen containing more than 100,000 organisms per microliter is considered evidence of infection.
- *Preterm labor:* It is onset of labor after period of viability but before 37 completed weeks or 259 days of pregnancy.
- *Threatened preterm labor:* When there are documented uterine contractions but no evidence of cervical change.
- *Premature rupture of membranes:* It is rupture of fetal membranes occurring prior to the onset of labor. The incidence is 3–18.5%.
- *Preterm premature rupture of membranes:* It is rupture of membranes occur ring

before 37 weeks and responsible for 30% of preterm deliveries.
- *Prolonged pregnancy:* Commonly called post-term pregnancy, it lasts longer than 42 weeks or 294 days beyond the first day of last menstrual period (LMP).
- *Postdatism:* It implies pregnancy lasting beyond the estimated due date at 40 weeks. It occurs in 3–12% of pregnancies.

  Prolonged pregnancies are at an increased risk for macrosomia resulting in shoulder dystocia and fetal injury, oligohydramnios, meconium aspiration, intrapartum fetal distress, and stillbirth. Maternal risk includes trauma, hemorrhage, and labor abnormalities.

  The most common cause of prolonged pregnancy is inaccurate dating.
- *Scalp stimulation test:* It is an alternative to scalp blood sampling to note the fetal heart acceleration in response to fetal scalp pinching.
- *Vibroacoustic stimulation test:* Electronic artificial larynx is placed over maternal abdomen. A normal response is a fetal heart rate (FHR) acceleration of 15 beats/min for at least 15 seconds occurring within 15 seconds after the stimulation.
- *Fetal pulse oximetry:* It is a method to assess fetal oxyhemoglobin saturation after rupture of membranes in labor. A pad-like sensor is inserted through cervix and positioned against fetal face. Fetal oxygen <30% for 2 minutes is associated with fetal distress.
- *Fetal electrocardiography:* It is internal monitoring of FHR and a special equipment to process the fetal electrocardiogram (ECG). In fetal ECG, hypoxia typically causes an elevation of the ST segment and T wave which are changes due to catecholamine surge, adrenoreceptor activation, and myocardial glycogenolysis. There may be ST segment depression or biphasic ST.
- *Tachysystole:* More than five contractions in 10 minutes averaged over a 30-minute window
- *Hyperstimulation:* Tachysystole accompanied by an abnormal FHR pattern
- *Uterine hypertonus:* Single contraction lasting for >2 minutes
- *Lie:* Refers to longitudinal axis of the fetus relative to longitudinal axis of uterus. Fetal lie can be longitudinal, transverse, or oblique.
- *Presentation:* Refers to fetal part that directly overlies the pelvic inlet. In longitudinal lie, the presentation can be cephalic or breech.
- *Malpresentation:* Any presentation other than vertex. It is seen approximately in 5% of all term labors.
- *Attitude:* Refers to position of head with regard to fetal spine (degree of flexion and/or extension of the fetal head)
- *Position:* Refers to relationship of the fetal presenting part to maternal pelvis. It can be assessed accurately on vaginal examination. For cephalic presentation, if the occiput is directly anterior, the position is occipitoanterior; if the occiput is toward the mother's right side, the position is right occiput anterior (ROA). In breech presentation, sacrum is the reference point and positions are left sacrum anterior (LSA), left sacrum posterior (LSP), right sacrum anterior (RSA), and right sacrum posterior (RSP).

  In vertex presentation, the position can be determined by palpation of fetal sutures. Sagittal suture is easiest to palpate. Epidural analgesia is associated with an increased risk of occipitoposterior presentation (12.9%).

- *Station:* It is a measure of descent of bony presenting part of the fetus through birth canal. The current standard classification (−5 to +5) is based on a quantitative measure in centimeter of the distance of the leading bony edge from the ischial spine. Midpoint (0 station) is defined as the plane of maternal ischial spines. The ischial spine can be palpated on vaginal examination at approximately 8 and 4 o'clock positions.
- *Engagement:* It is passage of the widest diameter of the presenting part to a level below the plane of pelvic inlet
- *Molding:* The change in the shape of fetal head to allow it to pass through the birth canal during childbirth. It has four grades.
- *Caput succedaneum:* The portion of fetal scalp immediately over the cervical os which becomes edematous from prolonged pressure from the dilated cervical os or vaginal walls during delivery.
- *Cephalhematoma:* It is the hemorrhage between skull and the periosteum of newborn secondary to rupture of blood vessels crossing the periosteum.
- *Induction of labor:* It involves methods to initiate uterine contractions in pregnant women to bring about cervical dilation with the aim of vaginal delivery prior to the onset of spontaneous labor.
- *Programmed labor:* It is an indigenously developed protocol of labor management which not only reduces duration of labor but also reduces maternal and fetal morbidity and mortality. It provides adequate pain relief, optimizes labor, and reduces the incidence of difficult vaginal delivery and cesarean section. It also helps planning intervention in time. It is maintained on a simple partograph.
- *Partogram:* It is a composite graphic record of key data (maternal and fetal) during labor entered against time on a single sheet of paper.
- *Dysfunctional labor:* It is defined as those labors which fail to progress due to either nondilatation of the cervix or nondescent of the presenting part.

Shoulder dystocia: It is difficulty in delivery of shoulder after head has been delivered. It usually requires additional obstetrics maneuvers to deliver the fetal body after routine axial traction on fetal head has been unsuccessful. The head to body delivery time is of >60 seconds.

- *Postpartum hemorrhage (PPH):*
  - *Primary PPH:* It is defined as *blood* loss of ≥500 mL from the genital tract within 24 hours after birth of baby or 10% change of hematocrit value following delivery or any amount of blood loss making the patient hemodynamically unstable.
  - *Severe PPH:* A cumulative blood loss of ≥1,000 mL or blood loss with signs or symptoms of hypovolemia within 24 hours during or after vaginal delivery/cesarean section.
  - *Secondary PPH:* It is defined as an excessive vaginal bleeding in the period from 24 hours after delivery to 12 weeks postpartum.
- *Puerperal fever:* Temperature 38°C (100.4°F) or higher, on two occasions within the first 10 days of puerperium, exclusive of the first 24 hours and to be taken orally by a standard technique at least four times daily
- *Postpartum blues:* It is a temporary condition beginning in the first 2–4 days after giving birth, peaks between postpartum days 5–7, and dissipates by

the end of the second postpartum week. It is characterized by an unfamiliar episode of crying, irritability, depression, emotional lability, feeling separate and distant from the baby, insomnia, and poor concentration.
- *Postpartum psychosis:* The most serious postpartum illness, postpartum psychosis occurs in 1–2 per 1,000 births. It is characterized by mood lability, agitation, confusion, thought disorganization, hallucinations, and disrupted sleep.
- *Down syndrome:* It is defined as trisomy 21 and is screened by triple test comprising human chorionic gonadotropin (hCG), urinary estriol, and alpha-fetoprotein.
- *Stem cells:* These are undifferentiated cells and can differentiate into any type of specialized cell including trophoblastic cells. These can be pluripotent, multipotent, or unipotent type.
- *Cloning:* It is a procedure whereby an adult donor nucleus is introduced into an enucleated recipient egg. With appropriate stimulus, such a cell grows into an embryo containing exactly the same genetic material as the donor.

■ TYPES OF BIRTH DEFECTS
- *Anomaly:* It is a structural feature that departs from the normal.
- *Syndrome:* It is a recognizable pattern of structure defect often with a predictable history that can be identified on several patients, thus allowing diagnosis and classification.
- *Sequence:* It is a pattern of defects that results from a single event early in pregnancy.
- *Association:* It means grouping of anomalies that frequently occur together but are not actual syndromes.
- *Malformation:* It is a morphologic defect resulting from abnormal development.
- *Disruption:* It is a morphological defect resulting from extrinsic breakdown or interference with normal development.
- *Deformation:* It is an abnormal form, shape, or position caused by mechanical forces.

29 Anesthetic Techniques

Manpreet Singh, Namita Grover

■ INTRODUCTION

Various anesthesia techniques are used for operations in both obstetrics and gynecology. Usually, these operations are in lower abdomen or pelvis. Most often, spinal anesthesia (SA), epidural anesthesia (EA), or combined spinal–epidural anesthesia (CSEA) is used for such procedures. When the patients have some contraindications to regional anesthesia, then general anesthesia (GA) is administered. Central neuraxial analgesia is the most versatile method of labor analgesia and the gold standard technique for pain control in obstetrics that is currently available.

What are procedures which can be conducted under spinal anesthesia?

Spinal anesthesia can be given for cerclage operation, nonobstetric surgery, forceps delivery, cesarean section, or removal of retained placenta. The most frequent indication for SA in pregnancy is cesarean section.

What are the drugs that can be used for spinal anesthesia/epidural anesthesia? Why lignocaine is not a preferred drug?

These are lidocaine, tetracaine, ropivacaine, and bupivacaine. The hyperbaric solution of 0.5% bupivacaine (with dextrose) is commonly used in India. This provides early onset, dense block and longer duration of anesthesia.

Lignocaine provides a short-to-intermediate duration of action. It may cause neurotoxicity that limits its use.

What is patient-controlled epidural analgesia?

Patient-controlled epidural analgesia (PCEA) is a novel method of the drug delivery system, providing several advantages, including the ability to reduce the drug dosage. Self-control and self-esteem may be vital for a positive experience in childbirth, and PCEA achieves both. Thus, it is a useful alternative for the maintenance regimen. The ideal PCEA regimen is controversial. The demand-only PCEA (5-mL bolus, 15-min lockout interval) results in less local anesthetic (LA) consumption but an increased incidence of breakthrough pain, higher pain scores, shorter duration of effective analgesia, and lower maternal satisfaction when compared with PCEA with background infusion (5-mL bolus, 10–12-min lockout interval, and 5–10 mL/h infusion). So background infusion is used in PCEA.

What are newer local anesthetics and adjuncts that are useful for decreasing pain?

The availability of newer LAs like ropivacaine and levo-bupivacaine have contributed toward the increased maternal safety in terms of being less cardiotoxic after an inadvertent intravenous injection. However, for the dosage used for labor analgesia, cardiotoxicity is not a major issue.

α-2 agonist, clonidine and cholinesterase inhibitors, and neostigmine have been used as adjuvants for labor analgesia. Both the drugs possess a common mechanism of action that can be beneficial. They can be administered either epidurally or via the intrathecal route. Spinal clonidine, in doses of 100–200 µg, produces excellent labor analgesia of short duration but at the cost of more sedation and hypotension. Spinal clonidine in doses of 50 µg administered with bupivacaine and sufentanil mixture significantly prolonged the labor analgesia without producing serious adverse effects.

What are various techniques that can be used for obstetric surgeries?

Various anesthetic techniques are:
- SA
- EA
- Caudal epidural anesthesia
- CSEA

How ultrasound is helpful in neuraxial block?

Ultrasound is used in the detection of neurospinal anatomy for administration of the central neuraxial blockade. Ultrasound imaging of the spine has recently been proposed to facilitate identification of the epidural space and predict difficult spine score, especially in women with abnormal lumbosacral anatomy (scoliosis) and those who are obese. The ultrasound-determined insertion point and very good agreement between ultrasound depth (UD) and needle depth (ND) has been found. The proposed ultrasound single-screen method, using the transverse approach, can be a reliable guide to facilitate labor epidural insertion. Thus, the epidural failure rate can be minimized in patients with difficult backs.

What are the methods to provide analgesia in vaginal delivery?

Various methods are used to provide analgesia in vaginal delivery. These are:
- Nonpharmacological methods
- Pharmacological methods.

Nonpharmacological methods
- *Natural childbirth*: Patients are taught the art of relaxation and a measure of pain control through learned breathing patterns and concentration.
- *Transcutaneous electrical nerve stimulation:* It is beneficial in patients who have moderate-to-severe contraction pains in an otherwise reasonably normal labor. It is a very easy technique and effective in most of patients.

Transcutaneous electrical nerve stimulation delivers painless electrical current to specific nerves intermittently. The mild electrical current generates heat which helps in relieving of stiffness. It improves mobility and relieves pain. The treatment is believed to stimulate the body's production of endorphins or natural pain killers (NPKs). Some authors believe that it works on Melzack and Wall gate theory of pain (1965).

Pharmacological methods
- *Nitrous oxide:* It does not interfere with uterine contractions nor has it any effect on the fetus.

  Premixed 50% nitrous oxide (N_2O)/oxygen (O_2) (Entonox) is very acceptable to patients. Inhalation is started at the onset of contraction. The other combination for this purpose is isoxan (Entonox with 0.2% isoflurane).
- *Opioids:*
  - Pethidine is an excellent strong analgesic which relaxes spasm of cervix and has a wide margin of safety. It is very useful in cases with rigid, slowly dilating cervical os. It can, however, depress fetal respiration, which can be reversed by naloxone 3 µg/kg intravenous (IV) (to be given slowly).
  - *Tramadol:* It is a synthetic opioid, which acts centrally and may decrease pain.

- *Morphine:* Small doses of morphine can be used sometimes. It may increase the intervals between contractions and may depress them.
- Pentazocine
- Fentanyl
- Sufentanil
- Alfentanil
- Remifentanil

Remifentanil is an ultra-short-acting synthetic potent opioid. It has a rapid onset of action and is readily metabolized by plasma and tissue esterases to an inactive metabolite. The effective analgesia half-life is 6 minutes, thus allowing effective analgesia for consecutive uterine contractions. It readily crosses the placenta but is extensively metabolized by the fetus. Because of its pharmacokinetic profile, this agent has an advantage over other opioids.

What is "walking epidural" or "ambulatory analgesia"?

Combined spinal–epidural anesthesia technique of rapid intrathecal analgesia, with combination of flexible epidural analgesia using low-dose opioids and LAs, can provide a selective sensory block with minimal motor blockade, allowing parturient to ambulate. This term is called "ambulatory analgesia". Truly selective sensory blockade with preservation of dorsal column (proprioceptive) function is the chief characteristic of ambulatory analgesia.

What are characteristics of "safe ambulation"?

Safe ambulation with low-dose CSEA is characterized by:
- No postural hypotension or any such symptoms
- Minimal or no motor block
- Minimal or no proprioceptive block
- Maternal and fetal monitoring is required
- Cooperative and understanding parturient is essential
- Presenting part of fetus should be engaged and well applied to cervix
- Suitable conditions are to be provided (good epidural catheter fixation, disconnecting of IV line, clear floor for easy and comfortable walking).

What should be the protocol for labor analgesia units for conduction of a successful block and for better results?

The following protocol should be followed for a successful *ambulatory analgesia*:
- No obstetric contraindication to the patient ambulating or to intermittent fetal monitoring
- Informed written consent from patient and preload the patient with 500 mL of Ringer lactate
- After the anesthesia is injected, monitor
- After 30 minutes, check the motor power of the patient by straight leg raising test and Breen modified Bromage score.
- If normal, make her sit on side of bed and reassess her blood pressure for orthostatic hypotension. If not, make her stand by bedside and recheck orthostatic vital signs and ask her to slightly bend her knees.
- Then make her walk and check her ability to walk without support by "trial walk" and Romberg's sign. At this moment, the patient can walk around, sit, and go to bathroom.
- Instruction to pass urine every hour should be given. No barefoot walking is allowed.
- Follow each top-up doses by checking on the patient's vital parameters, fetal monitoring, and motor power grade.

What are the advantages of "walking epidurals" during labor?

The advantages of "walking" epidurals are as follows:
- Gravity helps in the rate of cervical dilatation

- Movement of pelvis may encourage correct position of fetal head and it may increase the spontaneous delivery rate.
- Upright posture may decrease tendency to aortocaval compression and result in better neonatal status.
- It produces complete relief of pain in most parturients.
- Risk of aspiration is diminished as compared to GA.
- If properly conducted, no serious maternal/fetal complications
- Can be extended for operative delivery
- Mother is awake and can actively participate in delivery process without pain.

What is "paracervical block" and explain the procedure?

The pain transmission from uterus may be blocked at the base of broad ligament lateral to cervix. Local anesthetic is injected in the submucosa of fornix by a guarded needle. It is introduced into lateral fornix and is advanced 2–3 mm through vaginal mucosa, where 10 mL of diluted LA solution is injected bilaterally.

This technique is effective only in the first stage of labor. The Frankenhauser ganglion, which contains all visceral sensory nerve fibers from the uterus, cervix, and upper vagina, is anesthetized. The somatosensory fibers from peritoneum are not blocked.

What are the adverse effects of paracervical block?

A major adverse effect associated with paracervical block (PCB) is development of fetal bradycardia which occurs within 2–10 minutes of injection and lasts for 3–30 minutes. Various theories for the bradycardia have been proposed:
- Direct LA toxicity due to intravascular absorption in fetus
- Reflex bradycardia from manipulation of fetal head
- Decreased uterine blood flow caused by constriction of uterine artery when LA is closely applied

Bradycardia and fetal acidosis decreased oxygenation and increased chances of neonatal depression.

What are precautions and contraindications of paracervical block?

Paracervical block should be avoided in high-risk patients with suspected uteroplacental insufficiency, in complicated deliveries (breech and multiple gestation) and in premature births.

The following precautions should be taken while giving PCB:
- It should not be placed when cervix is >8 cm dilated.
- Adrenalin should not be used with LAs.
- PCB needs continuous fetal monitoring.
- Needs full preparedness for fetal resuscitation and immediate delivery.

What is "pudendal nerve block" and how is it given?

"Pudendal nerve block" is given in patients where simple instrumental delivery is required, and there is no availability of spinal or epidural blockade or when these are contraindicated.

This block can be given by the transvaginal or transperitoneal approach. The pudendal nerves are derived from lower sacral nerve roots (S2–S3–S4) and it supplies vaginal vault, perineum, rectum, and parts of bladder.

Transvaginal approach: With the patient in lithotomy position, a guarded needle is introduced through the side wall of vagina and into the sacrospinous ligament, medial and posterior to the ischial spine. The needle is advanced until it emerges from the ligament, and 10 mL of 1% lignocaine is injected **(Fig. 1)**.

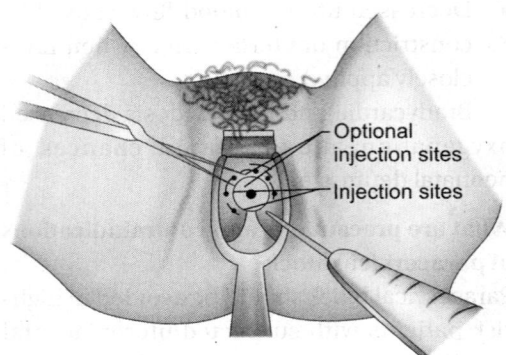

Fig. 1: Pudendal nerve block.

Transperitoneal approach: The needle is inserted through perineum at a point halfway between the fourchette and ischial tuberosity and advanced until the tip lies behind ischial spine where 10 mL of 1% lignocaine is deposited.

Complications:
- Intravascular injection
- Vaginal and ischiorectal hematoma
- Retropsoas and subgluteal abscess

What are the recent advances in neuraxial analgesia?

The recent advances include the following:
- *Technical advances:*
  - CSEA
  - Continuous spinal analgesia using microcatheters
  - Ambulatory epidurals, concepts of minimum local anesthetic volume (MLAV) and minimum local anesthetic dose (MLAD), low-dose and ultra-low-dose epidurals
- *Pharmacological advances:*
  - Ropivacaine, levobupivacaine
  - *Newer opioids:* Sufentanil, remifentanil
  - *Adjuvants:* Clonidine and neostigmine
- *Technological advances:*
  - Availability of ultrasound to facilitate localization of epidural space, minimizing failures
  - Patient-controlled epidural analgesia regimens
- Newer insights into the myths and controversies associated with neuraxial techniques
- Effect and timing of epidural on cesarean section, maternal and neonatal outcomes, breast feeding
- With-holding the dose in the second stage of labor
- Intrathecal placement of epidural catheter for reducing the incidence of postdural puncture headache (PDPH) in the event of inadvertent dural puncture
- Role of CT scans and MRI in detecting complications associated with neuraxial blocks

What is "postdural puncture headache"?

A headache after a spinal block may be a "postspinal headache" if:
- It is different from any headache previously experienced by the patient.
- It is initiated or made worse by adoption of the sitting or erect posture.
- It has occipital and nuchal components.
- It is relieved by abdominal compression, which raises the venous pressure. It mostly occurs in *younger* patients and occurs much less when *fine pencil-point* needles are employed. Onset is within 3 days and usually worse when the patient sits or stands. It is often occipital and associated with pain and stiffness in neck—may be vertical or frontal or can cause pain in orbit.

It occurs due to increased cerebrospinal fluid (CSF) leak after dural puncture. Headache may last days, weeks, or months, but usually 1–2 weeks. It may be due to low CSF pressure; there occur changes in hydrodynamics of the fluid, with loss of cushioning of brain and pressure on vessels and sensitive brain structures like basal dura, tentorium, etc.

How can postdural puncture headache be prevented and treated?

The problem of PDPH is better avoided than treated. The factors that have been implicated in influencing the development of PDPH are:
- *Needle size:* Increasing incidence with larger diameter of needle
- *Needle bevel orientation:* Higher incidence with perpendicular insertion to longitudinal orientation of dural fibers
- *Angle of needle approach to dura mater:* Decreased incidence with more acute angle of approach
- *Needle tip design:* Lower incidence with pencil-point or conical-point needles
- *Number of dural punctures:* Higher incidence with an increased number of dural punctures
- *Gender:* Higher incidence in women
- *Age:* Higher incidence in younger patients
- *Prior history of postdural puncture headache:* Higher incidence in these patients

Treatment of postdural puncture headache
Often *self-limiting* and disappears *within 1 week*. Treatment—pharmacological and nonpharmacological methods.

Nonpharmacological methods:
- Bed rest
- *Increased fluids:* Intravenous fluids initially and later oral
- Abdominal binders
- Increased tea or coffee intake

Pharmacological methods:
- *Analgesia*: Acetaminophen and codeine
- *Caffeine, theophylline, and sumatriptan*: Cerebral vasoconstrictor activity of caffeine. Regimen is 500 mg caffeine and sodium benzoate over 4 hours by IV infusion or 300 mg caffeine given orally.
- *Long-acting steroids (adrenocorticotropic hormone preparation)*: Intramuscularly (20 U or 60 U) or 1.5 U/kg over 1 hour in 1–2 L of Ringer lactate.
- *Methylergometrine*: Some people have used it as it causes vasoconstriction.

What is "water birth" method?

During "water birth", the mother gives birth to her child in a pool or tub full of water. Water improves the chances of a normal delivery without the use of painkillers or drugs, which may be required in a conventional method. Water helps to provide relief from pain and offers great benefits to the parturient. There is no chance of the baby's death due to asphyxiation or drowning. Immersion in warm water raises the body's temperature and causes the blood vessels to dilate, resulting in increased blood circulation. Thus, larger quantities of blood and oxygen are able to reach the uterine muscles.

A water birth allows a mother to maneuver her body during the labor process with the water offsetting the pressure experienced during childbirth. The hydrostatic pressure of the water relieves the discomfort of contractions and relaxes the body, which in turn stimulates the release of endorphins (body's NPKs).

What are the advantages of this method and what monitoring is required during childbirth process?

Advantages
- Water immersion for labor and delivery is a safe option with low-risk pregnancies.
- No increase in infection for the mother or baby
- No increase in hemorrhage for the mother
- No increase in aspiration of fluid by the baby

Monitoring during childbirth process
The babies are monitored with *Doppler every 15–30 minutes* during the first stage of

labor. During the second stage of labor, *the fetal heart rate is monitored every 5 minutes.* Water-proof Dopplers are available so the mother does not have to get out of the water for fetal monitoring.

CARDIOPULMONARY RESUSCITATION IN PREGNANT PATIENT

What is the overall maternal mortality rate?
- *13.95* deaths per *100,000* maternities.
- Cardiac arrest in pregnancy—*1:20,000* in 2007, and *1:30,000* in 2002.

What is the survival rate?
6.9% (poorer than others)

What are common etiological causes of cardiac arrest in pregnant patients?
The common etiological causes are:
- *Cardiac disease:*
  - Acute myocardial infarction (MI)
  - Aortic dissection
  - Congenital heart disease and pulmonary hypertension (HTN)
- Magnesium (Mg) toxicity
- Preeclampsia/eclampsia
- Pulmonary thromboembolism
- Amniotic fluid embolism
- Anesthetic complications

Why periarrest period is important in cardiac arrest in pregnancy?
Periarrest period is important because:
- We face two patients at one time.
- Best hope of fetal survival is maternal survival.
- Certain physiological changes due to pregnancy are to be understood.
- Critical patients are to be identified at an earliest and try to prevent cardiac arrest.

How can it be prevented at that moment?
It can be prevented as follows:
- Place the patient in the full left-lateral position.
- Give 100% O_2.
- Intravenous access above the diaphragm
- Assess for hypotension.
- Consider reversible cause of critical illness.

What are the steps for resuscitation of a pregnant patient?
The following are the steps of resuscitation:
1. Call for help and activate maternal cardiac arrest team immediately.
2. Do not forget to document event onset time.
3. *Patient positioning:* Place patient in supine position.
4. With manual left uterine displacement for obviously gravid uterus **(Figs. 2A and B)**

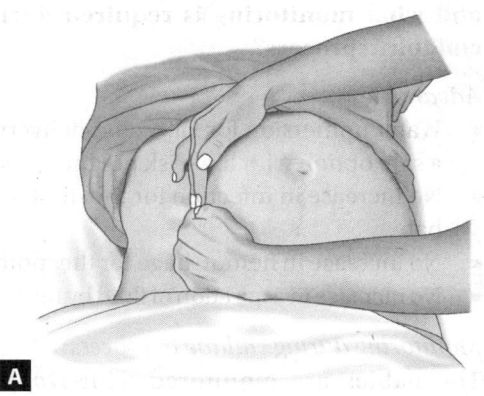
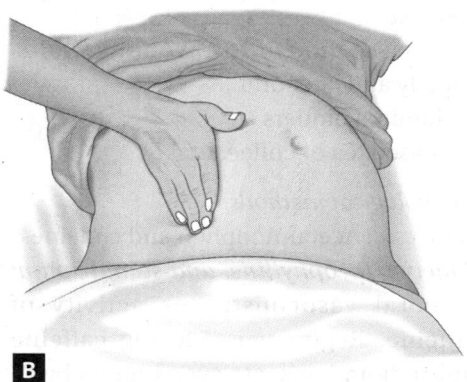

Figs. 2A and B: Manual left uterine displacement for gravid uterus.

Anesthetic Techniques

Flowchart 1: Algorithm of advanced cardiac life support.

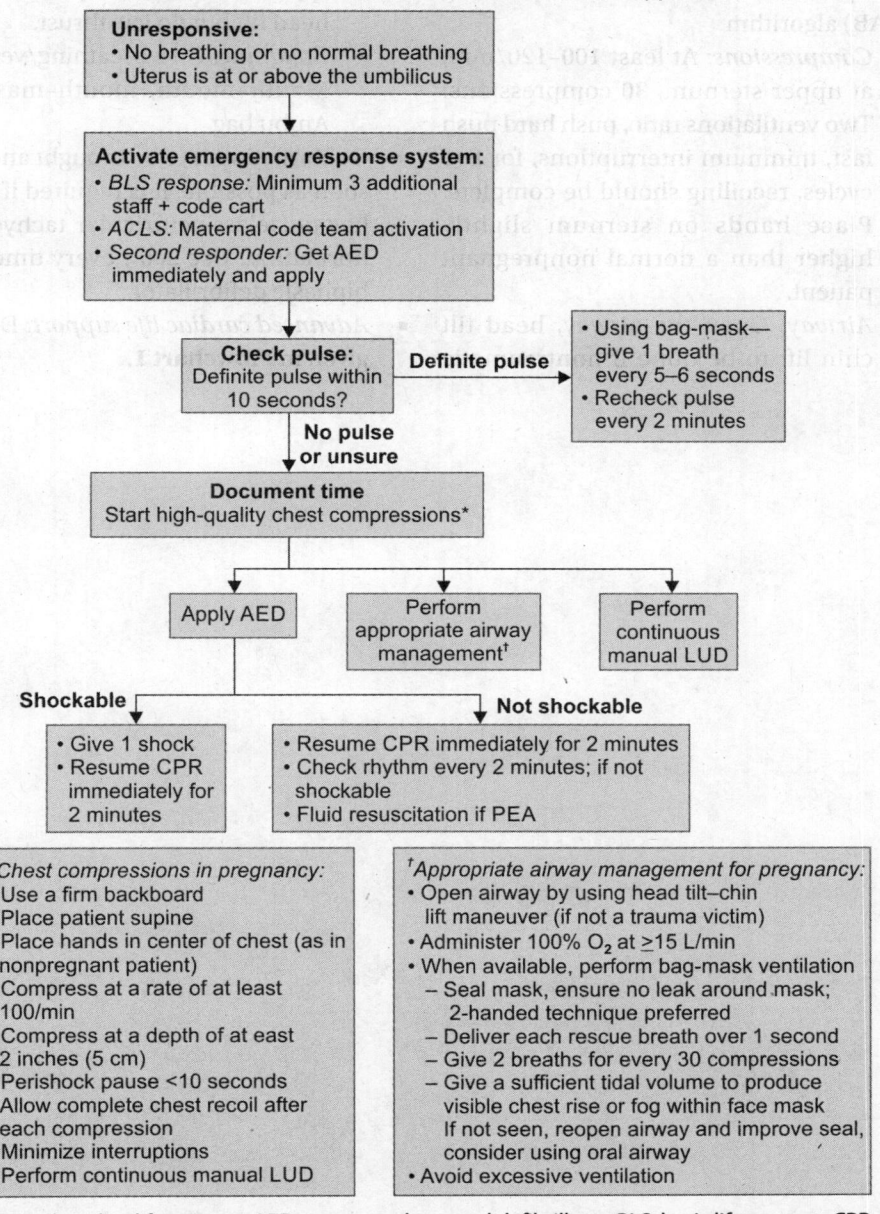

(ACLS: advanced cardiac life support; AED: automated external defibrillator; BLS: basic life support; CPR: cardiopulmonary resuscitation; LUD: left uterine displacement; O_2: oxygen; PEA: pulseless electrical activity).

5. Compressions, airway, and breathing (CAB) algorithm
   - *Compressions:* At least 100–120/min, at upper sternum, 30 compressions: Two ventilations ratio, push hard push fast, minimum interruptions, for five cycles, recoiling should be complete. Place hands on sternum slightly higher than a normal nonpregnant patient.
   - *Airway:* Open the airway, head tilt chin lift to be done if nontraumatic spine, if trauma in spine then avoid head tilt but do jaw thrust.
   - *Breathing:* Give breathing/ventilation: Mouth–mouth, mouth–mask, or by Ambu bag
- Defibrillation is to be brought and used as soon as possible. It is required if a patient has pulseless ventricular tachycardia or fibrillation. Use 200 J every time if it is a biphasic defibrillator.
- *Advanced cardiac life support:* Details are given in **Flowchart 1**.

CHAPTER 30

Fluids and Electrolytes

Manpreet Singh, Namita Grover

■ INTRODUCTION

The administration of intravenous (IV) fluid is a core expertise for anesthesia providers and an area in which we have an important role in advising clinical colleagues. Alongside the traditional triad of maintenance of unconsciousness, pain relief, and neuromuscular relaxation, IV fluid therapy is a core element of the perioperative practice of anesthesia. The aims of perioperative fluid administration should be to avoid dehydration, maintain an effective circulating volume, and prevent inadequate tissue perfusion during a period when the patient is unable to achieve these goals through normal oral fluid intake. The choice of fluid type in a variety of clinical situations can be rationally guided by an understanding of the physicochemical and biologic properties of the various crystalloid and colloid solutions available in combination with the available clinical trial data.

Each clinical decision about fluid therapy has two key elements: Which fluid to use and how much fluid to give. This chapter will review all the types of fluids required in obstetrics and gynecology in different indications.

What is the purpose of administration of fluids during perioperative practice?

The purpose of fluids' administration is to:
- Replace insensible fluid losses (evaporation, diffusion) during the anesthetic period.
- Replace sensible fluid losses (blood loss, sweating) during the anesthetic period.
- Maintain an adequate and effective blood volume.
- Maintain cardiac output and tissue perfusion.
- Maintain patency of an IV route of drug administration.

■ EVALUATION OF FLUID LOSS

How can you evaluate fluid loss clinically or on examination?

Intravascular volume can be assessed using physical or laboratory examinations or with advanced hemodynamic monitoring techniques.

Various signs of hypovolemia and dehydration are shown in **Table 1**.

Laboratory signs of dehydration:
- Rising hematocrit (HCT)
- Progressive metabolic acidosis
- Urinary specific gravity >1.010
- Urinary sodium <10 mEq/L
- Urinary osmolality >450 mOsm/kg
- Hypernatremia
- *Blood urea nitrogen (BUN):* Creatinine = 10:1
- *Radiologically:* Signs of increased pulmonary vascular and interstitial markings (Kerley "B" lines) or diffuse alveolar infiltrates
- *Central venous pressure (CVP):* A good guide to diagnose and treat hypovolemia

TABLE 1: Signs of hypovolemia.			
Sign	Fluid loss (percentage of body weight)		
	5%	10%	15%
Mucus membranes	Dry	Very dry	Parched
Sensorium	Normal	Lethargic	Obtunded
Orthostatic changes	None	Present	Marked
Heart rate			>15 bpm increase
Blood pressure			>10 mm Hg decrease
Urinary flow rate	Mildly decreased	Decreased	
Pulse rate	Normal or Increased	Increased >100 bpm	Markedly increased >120 bpm
Blood pressure	Normal	Mild decrease with respiratory variation	Decreased

▪ INTRAVENOUS FLUIDS

What are crystalloids? Give the detailed composition of common crystalloids that are used in various clinical scenarios.

Crystalloid solutions
- Contain a similar concentration of sodium to plasma
- Are excluded from the intracellular compartment because the cell membrane is generally impermeable to sodium
- Cross the capillary membrane from the vascular compartment to the interstitial compartment
- Are distributed through the whole extracellular compartment
- Normally, only a quarter of the volume of crystalloid infused remains in the vascular compartment.

Various crystalloid solutions are described in **Table 2**.

To restore circulating blood volume (intravascular volume), crystalloid solutions should be infused in a volume at least three times the volume lost.

What are colloids? Describe the detailed composition of commonly used colloids.

Colloid solutions
- Initially tend to remain within the vascular compartment
- Mimic plasma proteins, thereby maintaining or raising the colloid osmotic pressure of blood
- Provide longer duration of plasma volume expansion than crystalloid solutions
- Require smaller infusion volumes

Various colloid solutions are described in **Table 3**.

What are advantages and disadvantages of crystalloids and colloids?

The advantages and disadvantages are given in **Table 4**.

There is no evidence that colloid solutions are superior to normal saline (sodium chloride 0.9%) or balanced salt solution (BSS) for resuscitation. Literature still fails to conclude the superiority of one type over other.

How will you measure the perioperative fluid requirement of a patient undergoing surgery?

Perioperative fluid therapy includes replacement of preexisting fluid deficits, of normal losses (maintenance requirements), and/or of surgical wound losses (including blood loss).

TABLE 2: Composition of crystalloid replacement solutions.

Composition of several crystalloid fluids

Solution	Type	Na	Cl	K	Ca	Mg	Lact	Acet	Gluc	% Dex	pH	Osm
Plasma	–	144	107	5	5	1.5	–	–	–	–	7.5	290
2.5% Dextrose, 0.45% NaCl	M	77	77	–	–	–	–	–	–	2.5	4.0	280
2.5% Dextrose, 1/2 strength LRS	M	65.5	55	2	1.5	–	14	–	–	2.5	5.0	263
5% Dextrose	–	–	–	–	–	–	–	–	–	5	4.0	252
10% Dextrose	–	–	–	–	–	–	–	–	–	10	4.0	505
0.9% NaCl	R	154	154	–	–	–	–	–	–	–	5.0	308
Ringer's solution	R	148	156	4	4.5	–	–	–	–	–	6.0	309
LRS	R	130	109	4	3	–	28	–	–	–	6.5	273
PlasmaLyte A	R	140	98	5	–	3	–	27	23	–	7.4	294
PlasmaLyte 148	R	140	98	5	–	3	–	27	23	–	5.5	294
PlasmaLyte 56 + 5% Dextrose	M	40	40	16	–	3	–	16	–	5	5.0	362
PlasmaLyte 56	M	40	40	13	–	3	–	16	–	–	5.5	110
7.5% Hypertonic NaCl	R	1,283	1,283								5.0 5.7	2,567

(LRS: lactated Ringer's solution)

Maintenance fluid is measured using the following formula:

Weight	Rate
For first 10 kg	4 mL/kg/hr
For next 10–20 kg	Add 2 mL/kg/hr
For each kg above 20 kg	Add 1 mL/kg/hr
For example, for maintenance fluid requirements for a 50-kg female = 4 × 10 kg (40 mL/hr) + 2 × 10 kg (20 mL/hr) + 1 × 30 kg (30 mL/hr) = 90 mL/hr	

How do you calculate the surgical fluid loss?
The most commonly used method for estimating blood loss is measurement of blood in the surgical suction container and visually estimating the blood on surgical sponges and laparotomy pads (laps). A fully soaked sponge (4 × 4) is said to hold 10 mL of blood, whereas "soaked lap" holds 100–150 mL. A medium-sized sponge is said to hold 80 mL of blood when fully soaked. Serial HCTs or hemoglobin concentrations reflect the ratio

TABLE 3: Composition of commonly used colloids.

Fluid	Na⁺ (mmol/L)	K⁺ (mmol/L)	Ca²⁺ (mmol/L)	Cl⁻ (mmol/L)	Base (mEq/L)	Colloidosmotic pressure (mm Hg)
Gelatin (urea linked): E.g., hemaccel	145	5.1	6.25	145	Trace amounts	27
Gelatin (succinylated): E.g., Gelofusine	154	<0.4	<0.4	125	Trace amounts	34
Dextran 70 (6%)	154	0	0	154	0	58
Dextran 60 (3%)	130	4	2	110	30	22
Hydroxyethyl starch 450/0.7 (6%)	154	0	0	154	0	28
Albumin 5%	130–160	<1	V	V	V	27
Ionic composition of normal plasma	135–145	3.5–5.5	2.2–2.6	97–110	38–44	27

(V: varies between different brands)

TABLE 4: Advantages and disadvantages of crystalloids and colloids.

	Advantages	Disadvantages
Crystalloids	• Few side effects	• Short duration of action
	• Low cost	• May cause edema
	• Wide availability	• Weighty and bulky
Colloids	• Longer duration of action	• No evidence that they are more clinically effective
	• Less fluid required to correct hypovolemia	• Higher cost
		• May cause volume overload
	• Less weighty and bulky	• May interfere with clotting
		• Risk of anaphylactic reactions

of blood cells to plasma, not necessarily blood loss during long procedures or when estimates are difficult.

What is "third space" and other fluid losses?

Some surgical procedures are associated with obligatory losses of fluids other than blood, e.g., evaporation and internal redistribution of body fluids. Internal redistribution of body fluids—often called "third spacing"—causes massive fluid shifts and severe intravascular depletion. Traumatic, inflamed, or infected tissue can sequester large amounts of fluid in its interstitial space and can translocate fluid across serosal surfaces or into bowel lumen. Thus, the result is an obligatory increase in a nonfunctional component of the extracellular compartment, as this fluid does not readily equilibrate with the rest of the compartments. This fluid shift cannot be prevented by fluid restriction and is at the expense of both the functional extracellular compartments, as this fluid does not readily equilibrate with the rest of the compartments.

How will you replace blood loss?
Blood loss should be replaced with crystalloid or colloid solutions to maintain intravascular volume until the danger of anemia outweighs the risk of transfusion. Blood loss at that time is replaced by red blood cells (RBCs) to maintain hemoglobin concentration (or HCT).

Some key points regarding fluid replacement are:
- HCT of 21–24% corresponds to hemoglobin 7–8 g%.
- Practically, lactated Ringer's solution is used approximately three times volume of blood lost or colloid in a 1:1 ratio, until transfusion point replaces one unit of blood lost during surgery.
- The transfusion point can be determined preoperatively from HCT and by estimating blood volume.

How do you replace redistributed fluid and evaporative losses?
These losses are primarily related to wound size and extent of surgical dissections and manipulations. Procedures can be classified based on whether tissue trauma is minimal, moderate, or severe **(Table 5)**.

What is the fluid choice perioperatively?
The volume of fluid administered and fluid choice is thought to alter the movement of fluid between the body compartments. Generally, either 0.9% saline or a balanced solution such as Hartmann's solution is used. The 0.9% saline has a chloride concentration of 154 mmol which is significantly higher than serum chloride. It is well recognized that its use can lead to a hyperchloremic acidosis. Balanced solutions, which include Hartmann's solution or PlasmaLyte®, are considered more physiological and generally preferred for perioperative fluid management.

TABLE 5: Fluid requirement depending on tissue trauma.

Degree of tissue trauma	Additional fluid requirement (mL/kg)
Minimal	0–2
Moderate	2–4
Severe	4–8

What do you know about liberal versus restricted fluid administration strategies?
Estimating perioperative fluid losses can be challenging. The period of fasting preoperatively, intraoperative surgical time, surgical losses, and insensible losses all need to be considered. Replacement based on these estimated values alone incorporates significant assumptions. The value in replacing this volume has therefore been questioned. Similarly, evidence for insensible losses, or third space losses, requiring liberal replacement, is inconsistent. The definition of what constitutes a liberal versus a restrictive fluid strategy varies but can be in the region of >5 L for a liberal strategy and <3 L for a conservative strategy. Studies comparing these two groups have shown differing results, but the trend is toward increased morbidity and mortality in the liberal fluid groups, particularly those undergoing high risk or major surgery. A positive fluid balance has been shown to be associated with increased mortality. However, as one strategy did not appear to fit all patient groups, some of these earlier studies commented on a need for individualized goal-directed therapy (GDT).

What is goal-directed therapy?

Goal-directed therapy aims to meet the patient's increased oxygen demand incurred in the perioperative period. The targets of GDT are cardiac output >4.5 L/min/m^2 and an oxygen delivery >600 mL/min/m^2. The management of perioperative fluid administration is a different entity to fluid management in the setting of a patient presenting acutely unwell, for example with sepsis intervention, guided by hemodynamic monitoring.

Perioperative GDT describes fluid administration, with the aim of optimizing a patient's cardiac function and ultimately oxygen delivery. It is used for a time-limited period, both during and after a surgical intervention. The fluid is given with the aim of increasing preload and therefore stroke volume and cardiac output to potentially supranormal targets.

How do you use advanced assessment of fluid status?

Echocardiography is an increasingly useful bedside tool for the assessment of a patient's fluid status. It is becoming readily available, in intensive care, and is moving toward being as commonplace at the bedside as a stethoscope. Echocardiography can be used to assess preload, contractility, and afterload and changes in these parameters in response to a fluid challenge.

What are the advanced cardiac output monitors that can be useful in fluid administration?

Significant developments have been made in methods of assessing cardiac output and oxygen delivery. A pulmonary artery catheter is still considered the gold standard method; however, it is now used less in clinical practice. The esophageal Doppler is placed at the midthoracic level in the esophagus and measures the velocity of flow in the descending aorta which is used to calculate cardiac output and change in stroke volume. Currently, the most commonly used method of cardiac output measurement in intensive care or high dependency unit is pulse contour analysis to indirectly calculate cardiac output. This requires an arterial catheter, classically placed in either the radial or the femoral artery, and uses computer-based algorithms to calculate stroke volume from pulse pressure and compliance. There are five main commercially available devices; the PiCCO (Pulsion medical systems, Munich, Germany), LiDCOplus (LiDCO, Cambridge, UK), LiDCOrapid (LiDCO, Cambridge, UK), VolumeView/EV1000 (Edwards Lifesciences, Irvine CA, USA), and FloTrac (Edwards LifeSciences, Irvine CA, USA). All of these devices, except the FloTrac, require calibration. *Use of these techniques assists assessment of a patient's cardiac output and intravascular volume status*. This often involves assessment of whether a patient's preload can be augmented to increase stroke volume with fluid administration. Perioperative fluid therapy can be guided by whether a patient is fluid responsive or not.

What is fluid expansion, fluid responsiveness, and its prediction?

Venous return is equal to cardiac output. The Frank–Starling mechanism describes the process by which the heart is able to accommodate and then eject all blood returned to it, despite variations in venous return. An increased venous return or increased preload increases ventricular filling and the end-diastolic volume. This increases stretch of the cardiac myocyte, which increases sarcomere length with resultant increased force of contraction leading to an increase in volume of blood ejected from the heart. In order for a fluid challenge to be effective, it therefore needs to be of sufficient volume to cause stretch of the cardiac myocytes and test the Frank–Starling principle. If the heart is able to accommodate the increased volume, then stroke volume will increase; otherwise, the volume will remain within the venous system. The total blood volume can theoretically be divided into unstressed and stressed volumes. The unstressed volume is the volume that fills the blood vessels, without causing a rise in pressure. The stressed volume is any additional volume, which will cause both a pressure rise and elastic distension of the vessel wall.

When a fluid challenge is given, the aim is to expand the stressed volume. The elastic properties, or compliance of the vessel, determine the resultant degree of distension in response to the fluid challenge. Assessing fluid responsiveness is important every time fluids are given. If possible, the response to fluids should be predicted before their administration. *The prediction of a patient's fluid responsiveness aims to identify those who may benefit from an increase in IV volume with an increase in stroke volume and cardiac output.* Predictors of fluid responsiveness include high pulse pressure variation, stroke volume variation, vena cava collapsibility index, dynamic passive leg raising test, and end occlusion expiratory test. These assess beat-to-beat variations in either pulse pressure or stroke volume; however, they are only validated in ventilated patients with tidal volumes of >8 mL/kg and no arrhythmias. When the decision to administer fluids has been made, the best way to do it is with a fluid challenge. A fluid challenge can be used to assess for fluid responsiveness without the limitations associated with pulse pressure variation or stroke volume variation and it can be both diagnostic and therapeutic. The aim of using a small volume of fluid is to reduce the risk associated with fluid overload if additional resuscitation is not required. However, if the volume of fluid given is not adequate to stress the system, then the response of patients who could be fluid responsive may be misinterpreted. A patient is deemed fluid responsive if stroke volume or cardiac output increases by at least 10% following a fluid challenge. These all help to find the significance of fluid responsiveness.

What is fluid challenge test? How it is helpful in the management of hypotension?

The following guideline is useful for a "fluid challenge" test with CVP:

Step 1: Obtain general history and laboratory baseline values and measure CVP.

Step 2: Give IV 200 mL of appropriate solution (normal saline) over 10 minutes.

Step 3: Observe systemic circulation for an improvement in blood pressure, peripheral perfusion, and urine output. Reexamine (auscultate) chest for presence of crepitations, rhonchi, or other adventitious rounds.

Step 4: Measure CVP:
- If <2 mm Hg, repeat process until there is either improvement in systemic circulatory function or emergence of adverse chest physical findings.
- If >5 mm Hg, continued volume expansion is unlikely to improve venous return, hence administer more fluid only when the clinical situation demands.
- If between 2 and 5 mm Hg, wait for 10 minutes and again measure CVP to compare with "baseline" measurement.
- If increase is >2 mm Hg, repeat the entire process.

- If rise in CVP remains between 2 and 5 mm Hg, repeat the entire process but reduce the quantity of fluid challenge.
- If increase in CVP does not occur and the patient has clinical findings of lower systemic circulatory function, start vasopressors according to requirement and indication.

What are complications of fluid administration?

Overly rapid infusion of any type of fluid may precipitate:
- Pulmonary edema
- Acute respiratory distress syndrome
- Compartment syndrome (e.g., abdominal compartment syndrome, extremity compartment syndrome)
- Hemodilution resulting from crystalloid infusion is not injurious by itself, although HCT must be monitored to note whether threshold values for transfusion are met.

RBC transfusion has a low risk of directly transmitting infection, but in critically ill patients, it seems to cause a slightly higher rate of hospital-acquired infection. This risk may be minimized by using blood <12 days old; such RBCs are more plastic and are less likely to cause sludging in the microvasculature.

■ ELECTROLYTES

How much total potassium is present in an adult?

Total body potassium in a 50 kg patient is 2,500 mEq and it is at the rate of 50 mEq/kg body weight. 2% is present in extracellular fluid (ECF) and 98% intracellular fluid (ICF).

What is the concentration of potassium in intra- and extracellular fluids and in what ratio?

Potassium concentration is 5 mEq/L in ECF and 150 mEq/L in ICF and net ratio is 1:30 and serum potassium is 3.5–5.5 mEq/L.

What are the factors affecting serum potassium level?

Various factors that affect the potassium levels in body are:
- Blood pH: Acidosis   Alkalosis
  - pH ± 0.1   K ± 0.6 mEq/L
  - pH 7.4   K 4.0 mEq/L
  - pH 7.3   K 4.6 mEq/L
- Glucose and insulin decrease K^+.
- Adrenaline and beta agonist decrease K^+.
- Aldosterone increases potassium excretion.
- Diuretics cause loss of potassium.
- *Ventilation:* Hyperventilation decreases K; hypoventilation increases K.

What is hypokalemia and what are its causes?

Whenever serum K^+ is <3.0 mEq/L, it is called hypokalemia. It can be classified as:
- *Hypokalemia (without potassium loss)*
  - Alkalosis
  - Hyperventilation
  - Insulin excess
  - Beta-2 agonist salbutamol
- *Hypokalemia (with potassium loss)*
  - *GI system:* Vomiting, diarrhea, gastric aspiration, biliary and fecal fistula
  - *Renal system:* Diuretics, loop furosemide, hyperosmolar mannitol
  - Decrease in intake of potassium

What are the clinical features of hypokalemia?

Various signs and symptoms of hypokalemia are as follows:
- *Neuromuscular function:* In potassium deficiency, the extracellular potassium concentration usually decreases more than the intracellular concentration, thereby altering this ratio. This ratio change is presumably at least partially responsible for skeletal muscle weakness, intestinal ileus, and abnormalities of cardiac electrical conduction that may

accompany hypokalemia. Skeletal muscle weakness is most prominent in the legs and rarely affects muscles innervated by cranial *nerves*.
- *Renal system*: Decrease in concentrating ability, often resulting in polyuria. Metabolic alkalosis is common, and extreme potassium deficiency may result in hypoventilation.
- *Orthostatic hypotension*: Autonomic nervous system dysfunction.
- *Changes on the ECG*: Initially, a U wave appears immediately after the T wave, prolonged QT interval, prolonged PR interval, ST segment depression, T wave inversion, and a prominent U wave. Ventricular fibrillation (VF) is a common terminal dysrhythmia in the presence of hypokalemia.

How will you treat a patient with hypokalemia?
The steps that are to be followed while treating hypokalemia are:
- *Oxygen therapy:* By face mask (mild), intermittent positive pressure ventilation (IPPV, severe)
- *Potassium therapy*
- Mild infusion of <10 mEq/hr
- *Moderate to severe:* Bolus 20–40 mEq (in 15 minutes)
- If it is given through infusion, then it should be done under ECG monitoring.
- In no case should the rate of potassium infusion be more than 40 mEq/hr.
- *Correct the cause*: Alkalosis, vomiting.
- Serial estimation of serum potassium 4 hourly

What are the contraindications of potassium therapy?
The contraindications are:
- Renal failure
- Hyperkalemia
- Metabolic acidosis
- Extensive soft-tissue injury
- Extensive burn injury
- Massive blood transfusion

What is hyperkalemia?
Hyperkalemia means an abnormally elevated level of potassium in the blood. The normal potassium level in the blood is 3.5–5.0 (mEq/L).

Potassium levels
- *5.1–6.0 mEq/L:* Mild hyperkalemia
- *6.1–7.0 mEq/L:* Moderate hyperkalemia
- *7 mEq/L:* Severe hyperkalemia

What are the signs/symptoms of hyperkalemia?
- *Asymptomatic:* Sometimes, patients report vague symptoms including nausea, fatigue, muscle weakness, or tingling sensations.
- *More serious symptoms:* Slow heartbeat and weak pulse. Severe hyperkalemia can result in cardiac arrest.
- Slowly rising potassium level (such as with chronic kidney failure) is better tolerated than an abrupt rise in potassium levels. Unless the rise in potassium has been very rapid, symptoms of hyperkalemia are usually not apparent until potassium levels are very high (typically 7.0 mEq/L or higher).

Other causes: Kidney dysfunction, diseases of the adrenal gland, potassium shifting out of cells into the blood circulation, and medications such as angiotensin-converting enzyme (ACE) inhibitors, nonsteroidal anti-inflammatory drugs (NSAIDs), angiotensin II receptor blockers (ARBs), and potassium-sparing diuretics.

In tissue destruction, dying cells release potassium into the blood circulation. Examples of tissue destruction causing hyperkalemia include trauma, burns, surgery, hemolysis (disintegration of RBCs), massive lysis of tumor cells, and rhabdomyolysis (a condition involving destruction of muscle cells that is sometimes associated with muscle injury, alcoholism, or drug abuse).

There is no definite correlation between any ECG changes and the serum potassium. The relationship depends on individual patient sensitivity and the rapidity of development of the hyperkalemia.

What are the treatment measures for hyperkalemia?

Treatment measures include:
- *Potassium removal:* Kayexalate—oral administration is 15–30 g in 50–100 mL of 20% sorbitol
- Rectal administration is 50 g in 200 mL 20% sorbitol
- *Shift potassium:* Glucose 1 ampule of D50 and regular insulin 5–10 units IV
- Bicarbonate 1 ampoule IV
- Nebulized albuterol (10–20 mg)
- Goal is to decrease body K^+ and shift K from ECF to ICF
- Discontinue exogenous K^+ intake
- Calcium gluconate (5–10 mL of 10%) or calcium chloride to counter myocardial effects of hyperkalemia
- Dialysis if conservative measures fail

Discuss hyponatremia. What are its clinical effects?

- Normal value of sodium in serum is 135–145 mEq/L.
- Hyponatremia occurs when Na^+ is <135 mEq/L.
- *Concentration changes:* Changes in serum Na^+ are inversely proportional to total body water (TBW).

Etiology (Flowchart 1):
To differentiate the etiology: Systemic review of the causes is done:
- Exclude hyperosmolar causes (hyperglycemia/mannitol)
- Consider depletional/dilutional causes
- *Extrarenal [gastrointestinal tract (GIT)] loss:* Urine Na (<20 mEq/L)
- *Renal loss:* Urine Na (>20 mEq/L)

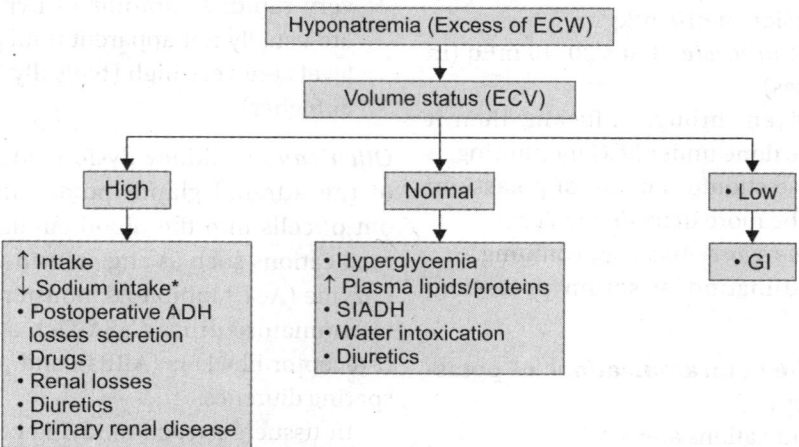

Flowchart 1: Etiology of hyponatremia.

*Low serum sodium level can be due to Na^+ depletion, dilution, intentional or iatrogenic.

(ADH: antidiuretic hormone; ECV: extracellular volume; ECW: extracellular water; GI: gastrointestinal; SIADH: syndrome of inappropriate antidiuretic hormone secretion)

How will you treat hyponatremia?
Most cases treated by free water restriction. If severe: Restrict Na^+. Symptomatic hyponatremia (<120 mEq/L)
- *If neurological signs and symptoms present:* Give 3% NS
- Increase Na^+ level no more than 1 mEq/L/hr until serum level is 130 mEq/L or s/s improve.

Asymptomatic hyponatremia: Increase Na^+ level by no more than 0.5 mEq/L to a maximum of 12 mEq/L/day. It should be slower in chronic states.

Rapid correction may cause pontine myelinolysis with seizures, weakness/paresis, akinesia and unresponsiveness and further permanent brain damage and death.

Briefly discuss hypernatremia.
Hypernatremia (>145 mEq/L) can be due to loss of free water or gain of Na^+ in excess of water **(Flowchart 2)**.

How will you treat hypernatremia?
When hypernatremia alone is present, then treat associated water deficit and if it is associated with hypovolemia then treat with normal saline, followed by hypotonic fluid (D5 or D5 in ¼ NS) after restoration of adequate volume status.

Water deficit is calculated as follows:

$$\text{Water deficit (L)} = \frac{\text{Serum} - 140 \times \text{TBW}}{140}$$

- Decrease in Serum Na^+ no more than 1 mEq/hr and 12 mEq/day
- *Chronic hypernatremia:* Sodium correction (0.7 mEq/L/hr)
- Overly rapid correction may cause cerebral edema and herniation.
- Assess neurological status and serum Na^+ frequently.

What are the causes of hypercalcemia?
Hypercalcemia is defined as serum Ca > 8.5–10.5 mEq or increase in ionized calcium level > 4.2–4.8 mg/dL.

Causes
- Increased intake or absorption
- Milk-alkali syndrome
- Vitamin D or vitamin A excess
- Endocrine disorders
- Primary hyperparathyroidism (adenoma, hyperplasia, carcinoma)
- Secondary hyperparathyroidism (renal insufficiency, malabsorption)

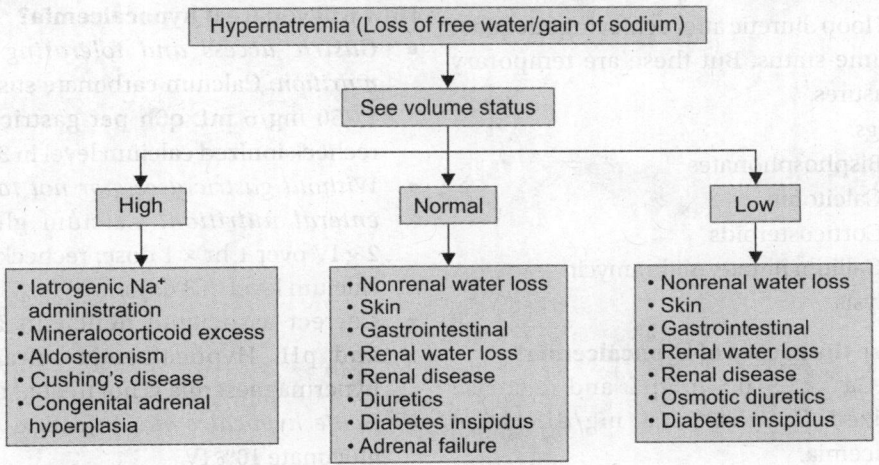

Flowchart 2: Causes of hypernatremia.

- Acromegaly
- Adrenal insufficiency
- Neoplastic diseases
- Miscellaneous causes
- Thiazide diuretic induced
- Paget's disease of bone
- Immobilization
- Familial hypocalciuric hypercalcemia
- Complications of renal transplantation
- Iatrogenic

What are the signs and symptoms of hypercalcemia?

Signs and symptoms are:
- *GIT:* Anorexia, nausea/vomiting, abdominal pain
- *Neuromuscular:* Weakness, confusion, coma, bone pain
- *Renal:* Polydipsia
- *Cardiovascular system (CVS):* Hypertension, arrhythmia, polyuria
- *ECG:* Short QT interval, prolonged PR and QRS interval, QRS voltage, T wave flattening and widening, AV block, cardiac arrest

How will you treat hypercalcemia?

Symptomatic hypercalcemia (>12 g/dL) requires treatment.
- Start with saline volume expansion—this decreases renal resorption of Ca.
- Add loop diuretic after achieving adequate volume status. But these are temporary measures.
- *Drugs:*
  - Bisphosphonates
  - Calcitonin
  - Corticosteroids
  - Gallium nitrate, mithramycin
- Dialysis

What are the causes of hypocalcemia?

Serum Ca^{2+} <8.5-0.5 mEq/L and decrease in ionized Ca^{2+} <4.2-4.8 mg/dL cause hypocalcemia.

Causes of hypocalcemia are:
- *Decreased intake or absorption*
- Malabsorption
- Small bowel bypass, short bowel
- Vitamin D deficit
- *Increased loss*
  - Alcoholism
  - Chronic renal insufficiency
  - Diuretic therapy
- *Endocrine disease*
  - Hypoparathyroidism (genetic, acquired, including hypo- and hypermagnesemia)
  - Sepsis
  - Pseudohypoparathyroidism
  - Calcitonin secretion with medullary carcinoma of the thyroid
  - Familial hypocalcemia

What are the signs and symptoms of hypocalcemia?

Hypocalcemia is characterized by:
- *Neuromuscular:* Hyperactive reflexes, paresthesia, carpopedal spasm seizures, Chvostek sign, Trousseau sign
- *CVS:* Heart failure, cardiac contractility.
- *ECG:* Prolonged QT interval, T wave inversion, heart block, VF

How will you treat hypocalcemia?
- *Gastric access and tolerating enteral nutrition:* Calcium carbonate suspension 1,250 mg/5 mL q6h per gastric access; recheck ionized calcium level in 3 days.
- *Without gastric access or not tolerating enteral nutrition:* Calcium gluconate 2 g IV over 1 hr × 1 dose; recheck ionized calcium level in 3 days.
- Correct associated deficit in Mg, K^+, and pH. Hypocalcemia refractory if hypermagnesemia is not treated first.
- *Acute hypocalcemia:* Injection calcium gluconate 10% IV.

Briefly describe magnesium as electrolyte.
Magnesium is the second most abundant intracellular cation in the human body. Magnesium plays an important role in the activity of electrically excitable tissues. It also regulates the movement of calcium into smooth muscle cells, which gives it a pivotal role in the maintenance of cardiac contractile strength and peripheral vascular tone.

Describe hypomagnesemia.
Causes
- Antibiotic therapy—aminoglycosides, amphotericin B, pentamidine, digitalis, cisplatin, cyclosporine
- Alcohol-related illnesses, secretory diarrhea, diabetes mellitus, acute myocardial infarction (MI)

Clinical manifestations: According to serum magnesium levels
- 3–5 mEq/L—hypotension, vasodilatation
- 5–7 mEq/L—drowsiness, hypotonia, absent deep tendon reflex (DTR)
- >10 mEq/L—respiratory depression
- 12–15 mEq/L—unconscious
- >15 mEq/L—cardiac arrest

Describe the symptoms and treatment of hypomagnesemia.
Symptoms
- *Increased neuromuscular irritability:* Hyperreflexia, positive Chvostek or Trousseau sign, tremor, tetany, convulsions, muscle weakness
- *Cardiovascular:* Heart failure, dysrhythmias, hypotension
- *ECG changes:* Prolonged PR and QT intervals, widened QRS complexes, ST segment depression and T-wave inversion

Treatment
- *Chronic deficiency:* 6 g oral $MgSO_4$ per day
- Severe hypomagnesemia
- 1.5–2 g IV $MgSO_4$ over 1–2 hours, up to 8–12 g on the first day, followed by 4–6 g/day
- Correct coexisting hypokalemia, hypocalcemia, and hypophosphatemia.

What precautions should be taken during magnesium therapy?
The following parameters are to be taken care of:
- *Renal functions monitoring:* Prior and during therapy
- Serial estimation of serum magnesium levels
- Clinical monitoring for DTRs
- Look for hourly urine output.

Describe hypomagnesemia.
- Rarely seen, most commonly in *renal failure,* or in *patients being treated for preeclampsia or eclampsia*
- *Mg:* Central nervous system (CNS) depressant, decreases neuromuscular activity
- *Other signs:* Depressed DTRs, respiratory depression, hypotension, heart block, cardiac arrest
- Consider hypermagnesemia in patients with hyperkalemia and hypercalcemia.

Treatment
- Stop Mg administration, IV fluids followed by IV furosemide, 5 mL 10% $CaCl_2$ over 5 minutes (directly antagonizes effect of Mg^+)
- *Oxygen therapy:* Face mask (IPPV)
- *CVS support:* Hypotension; arrhythmias—IV fluids, inotropes, antiarrhythmic drugs.
- Dialysis (renal failure)

What is the dose schedule of magnesium for eclampsia, ventricular tachycardia, and ventricular fibrillation?
- *Eclampsia:* 2–4 g (16–32 mEq) IV 5–10 minutes followed by IV infusion 1 g/hr.
- *Ventricular tachycardia (VT) and VF:* 2 g (16 mEq) IV 10–15 minutes (E)

CHAPTER 31

Assisted Reproductive Technologies and Surrogacy

Vikas Yadav, Neerja Goel

INTRODUCTION

Infertility causes immense mental exhaustion and trauma, best described by infertile couples themselves. Around 6–8% of infertile couples need medical intervention involving the use of advanced assisted reproductive technology (ART) procedures such as in vitro fertilization (IVF) or intracytoplasmic sperm injection (ICSI). Assisted reproductive technologies involve a range of fertility treatments to aid in reproduction for couples suffering from infertility. These include IVF, gamete donation—sperm and donor egg, intrauterine insemination (IUI), and surrogacy.

As per an estimate, around 2.8–3.2 crore couples in the reproductive age group in India are infertile and only 1–2% seek medical help. The first IVF baby, Louise Brown, was born at Oldham and district general hospital in Manchester on July 25, 1978, in the United Kingdom through the efforts of Dr Robert G Edwards and Dr Patrick Steptoe. India's first IVF baby, Kanupriya, alias Durga, was born 67 days later on October 3, 1978, through the efforts of Dr Subhas Mukherjee in Kolkata.

One in six couples will encounter problems related to fertility, defined as failure to achieve a clinical pregnancy even after 12 months of regular intercourse. Couples are turning to ART for help. Fertility treatments are complex, and each ART cycle consists of several steps; the stakes are high as conception may not occur. With this in mind, it is important that each step of the ART cycle is supported by good evidence from well-designed studies.

A brief overview of various ART procedures that have been described in the literature is given in the following text.

What is intrauterine insemination (self with husband or donor semen)?

Intrauterine procedure involves placing the husband's processed semen or donor semen inside the uterine cavity.

Intrauterine insemination is commonly done in cases of: Hostile uterine cervix, oligozoospermia, and unexplained infertility.

There is a general agreement in the literature that chances of success are better with IUI to the tune of 8–12%. IUI is preferred in mild stimulation cycles with maturation of two or three follicles that can be monitored by ultrasound starting from day 8/9 of cycle. The majority of pregnancies occur in the first six cycles.

What is the procedure of in vitro fertilization?

In vitro is a procedure done in the laboratory-restricted and highly controlled conditions. IVF involves controlled ovarian stimulation to obtain multiple mature oocytes which is usually done by starting patients on injectable gonadotropins, either pure human menopausal gonadotropin (hMG) or recombinant follicle-stimulating hormone (FSH). Based on the protocol of IVF, the follicles are monitored by transvaginal sonography (TVS). At the appropriate moment of follicular growth, usually when at least more than three lead follicles cross 16–18 mm follicle size, a trigger agent, either human chorionic gonadotropin (hCG) or agonist trigger, is given and after 34–36 hours of the trigger, the follicles are aspirated to obtain the oocytes. The oocytes are mixed with appropriately capacitated spermatozoa from the husband (or the donor semen) and kept in an incubator for fertilization which is observed microscopically after 15–18 hours. Embryos are transferred into the uterine cavity between days 3 and 6 after oocyte aspiration.

What are the indications for in vitro fertilization?
Common indications in today's practice include: Bilateral blocked tubes, endometriosis, semen abnormalities, and failure of pregnancy with repeated ovulation induction cycles.

What is gamete intrafallopian tube transfer or tubal embryo transfer?
Gamete intrafallopian tube transfer (GIFT) is done in infertile couples with healthy fallopian tubes. Tubes are accessed by laparoscopy or by retrograde catheterization through the cervix.

What is meant by oocyte donation or embryo donation?
Oocyte donation involves fertilizing the oocytes of an anonymous oocyte donor with the husband's sperm and transferring the resultant embryo into the infertile female. Common indications for which OD is commonly warranted are: Gonadal dysgenesis; premature ovarian failure or insufficiency; ovarian failure due to ovarian surgery such as extensive endometriosis surgery, radiation exposure, or chemotherapy exposure; women who have resistant ovary syndrome or who are poor responders to ovulation induction; women who are carriers of recessive autosomal disorders and who have attained premature menopause; menopausal females who due to some familial tragedy like loss of living issue at later age of life seeks to revive fertility options.

Embryo donation means transferring of an embryo produced using anonymous oocyte and donor's semen into the female partner of the couple seeking fertility option. It is usually done in cases where a male has azoospermia with failed testicular sperm extraction (TESE) and female partner has low serum anti-Müllerian hormone (AMH) values.

Describe surrogacy.
The surrogate does not use her own egg and has no DNA or genetic relation to the child she is carrying. There are four types of surrogacy: (1) Gestational surrogacy where the surrogate mother carries a child for another person who cannot. The surrogate does not share DNA with the child and is not the genetic mother. (2) Altruistic surrogacy where the surrogate agrees to be a surrogate without being compensated. Altruistic surrogates are typically helping someone they know, such as a close friend or family member and will likely only receive reimbursement for medical costs. (3) Independent or agency-assisted surrogacy. (4) Domestic or international surrogacy. According to a new law, only altruistic surrogacy is legal to practice in India.

What is intracytoplasmic sperm injection?
Intracytoplasmic sperm injection is a procedure where a motile spermatozoon is directly injected inside a mature M2 grade oocyte using a very fine and magnified microscope and should be considered in the presence of severe sperm abnormalities. ICSI can also be considered in couples with history of fertilization failure in normal conventional IVF cycles.

What are the surgical sperm extraction procedures?

Common indications of the procedure are congenital bilateral absence of the vas deferens (CBAVD), obstructive azoospermia, nonobstructive azoospermia, anejaculation, and retrograde ejaculation.

Microsurgical epididymal sperm aspiration (MESA) involves aspiration of sperm from epididymis under magnification.

Percutaneous epididymal sperm aspiration (PESA) and testicular sperm aspiration/extraction (TESA/TESE): These are simplified, minimally invasive outpatient procedures allowing the physicians to recover the sperm in patients with obstruction in the outlet tract or vas deferens. PESA involves a needle to be introduced percutaneously into the epididymis and the contents aspirated. The aspirate is observed under the microscope to see if motile sperm are present or not. In *TESA*, the needle is introduced in the testicle itself. In *TESE*, the seminiferous tubules along with the sperm are recovered surgically and observed under a microscope to retrieve sperms.

Discuss the role of cryopreservation.

Excess embryos are usually obtained in IVF/ICSI treatment. Cryopreservation of embryos is routinely done to increase cumulative live birth rates. It allows embryos to be available for future use by the couple; cryopreservation is also useful in avoiding the risk of ovarian hyperstimulation.

Evaluation of couples who present with infertility always starts with detailed history taking from both male and female or the partner. Individual counseling as well as basic knowledge to couples about the fertility period during the menstrual cycle can be provided during the same session.

What are the important points in history taking and evaluation of infertile couple?

Infertility is always approached with both husband and wife being evaluated simultaneously and counseled regarding the various options available to treat depending upon the cause of infertility. Patient selection for referral and, finally, for ART should be based on the findings of basic investigations done to find out the cause of infertility.

Husband:
- Physical examination, both systemic and local, needs to be done to detect any problem that might be the cause of infertility.
- Detailed semen analysis with morphology and if required functional tests may be done.
- Semen analysis with DNA fragmentation is done in cases of recurrent pregnancy loss (RPL) or recurrent implantation failure.
- Screening for infections including syphilis by doing serum VDRL, hepatitis B virus (HBV), hepatitis C virus (HCV), and human immunodeficiency virus (HIV), and if any positive case it should be treated accordingly.

Wife:
- *Physical examination*: Check thyroid and galactorrhea in breast; local examination should be done to look for vaginal septum or cervical problem that might be the cause of infertility.
- *Testing ovulatory function/reserve*: Hormone assays are usually done between day 2 and day 5 of menses on empty stomach. Tests include serum FSH, luteinizing hormone (LH), AMH, prolactin, and thyroid-stimulating hormone (TSH). Patients with low AMH values are often correlated with days

2–5 antral follicle counts by TVS. Tests like cervical mucus studies, endometrial biopsy in the premenstrual phase to rule out tuberculosis (TB), histopathological examination, and serum progesterone estimation in the mid-luteal phase are now rarely performed and are done only when infectious pathology is suspected.

- Assessment of tubal patency includes hysterosalpingography (HSG), sonosalpingography, or laparoscopy.
- Screening for local factors including cervical mucus-related problems and lower genital tract infections, and if there is cervicitis or pelvic inflammatory disease (PID) it should be treated in accordance with Centers for Disease Control and Prevention (CDC) guidelines.
- Assessment of uterine cavity by hysteroscopy or 3D ultrasonography
- Screening for reproductive tract infections including syphilis, chlamydia, tuberculosis, HBV, HCV, and HIV
- Endocrinological investigations like TSH and serum prolactin

What should be the treatment approach to infertile couples?

It has been seen that 84% of couples conceive within 1 year of unprotected sexual intercourse.

- Couples with unexplained infertility are often given the option of diagnostic laparoscopy followed by three to four cycles of IUI.
- Couples with severe male factor infertility are counseled for IVF with ICSI.
- Couples with tubal factor infertility or low ovarian reserves are often given the option of IVF.
- In females with polycystic ovary syndrome (PCOS), ovulation induction along with insulin-sensitizing drugs are used.
- In azoospermia in males, options of PESA, TESA, and micro-TESE are available in cases of obstructive pathology, but many patients may require donor sperm for IUI or IVF.
- Couples with AMH <0.6 or premature ovarian failure related to either genetic problems such as Turner syndrome or prior chemo/radiotherapy will get benefitted by donor oocyte IVF.
- In females with multiple implantation failures, Asherman syndrome, or uterine hypoplasia, surrogacy is a reasonable option.

How is ovulation induction done?

Ovulation induction (OI) is a management option in women who have anovulatory cycles. Before starting OI, semen analysis should be done. Tubal status should also be checked in cases where history is suggestive of TB or any infectious pathology in pelvis. However, in cases of no prior history of TB or history suggestive of PID, patients can be started initially on three cycles of ovulation induction before checking tubal patency.

- Letrozole and clomiphene citrate are the first-line ovulation-inducing drugs and can be given for up to six to nine cycles. Women with polycystic ovaries and with high body mass index (BMI) may be offered metformin and other insulin sensitizer drugs in addition.
- Gonadotropin therapy is used in combination with either letrozole or clomiphene and is also used in females with hypogonadotropic hypogonadism.
- Women with hyperprolactinemia should be offered treatment with dopamine agonists such as cabergoline and can be continued along with ovulation induction drugs.

- Once couples have been prepared for treatment, the following steps make up an ART cycle:
  - Drugs/injectable gonadotropins are initiated to stimulate the growth of multiple ovarian follicles, while in agonist cycle, medications are given to suppress the natural menstrual cycle and downregulate the pituitary gland.
  - After ovarian stimulatory drugs/injectables are initiated, monitoring is undertaken at intervals to assess the growth of follicles.
  - When the follicles have reached an appropriate size, the next step involves giving a drug to bring about final maturation of the eggs (known as ovulation triggering, which is usually recombinant hCG or agonist trigger or sometimes dual trigger).
  - The next step involves egg collection (usually with a TVS probe to guide the pickup using 17G needle) and, in some cases of male infertility, sperm retrieval.
  - Next is the fertilization process, which is usually completed by IVF or ICSI.
  - Laboratory procedures follow for embryo culture: Culture media, oxygen concentration, coculture, assisted hatching, etc.
  - Embryos are then placed into the uterus. Issues of importance here include endometrial preparation, the best timing for embryo transfer, how many embryos to transfer, what type of catheter to use, the use of ultrasound guidance, need for bed rest, etc.
  - Then comes luteal phase support, for which several options are available, including administration of progesterone, estrogen (E2), and hCG.

What are pre-ART and adjuvant strategies?
Effective interventions include the following:
- Endometrial injury performed in the month before ovulation induction for ART appeared to increase both the live birth or ongoing pregnancy rate and the clinical pregnancy rate (moderate-quality evidence).
- Growth hormone in poor responders was associated with significant improvement in live birth rates.
- *Metformin treatment during IVF:* There was no clear evidence that metformin treatment before or during ART cycles improved live birth rates (low-quality evidence). However, use of this insulin-sensitizing agent increased clinical pregnancy rates and decreased the risk of ovarian hyperstimulation syndrome (OHSS).
- Laparoscopic tubal clipping was suggested for improving IVF pregnancy rates among women with hydrosalpinx
- Use of antioxidants like carnitine and coenzyme Q has shown promising results in male subfertility.

Discuss the ovarian stimulation protocols in in vitro fertilization (IVF).
Ovarian stimulation is a very complex process. Many different stimulation regimens have been developed and evaluated, and it is therefore very important for you to discuss your options in detail with your physician for choosing the absolute best protocol for individual circumstances in order to optimize the number of retrieved eggs, maximize the fertilization rate, and provide with the greatest possible chance for a healthy pregnancy.

Majorly, there are three types of stimulation protocols: Agonist, antagonist, and low-dose/short flare protocols for poor responders

1. *Agonist protocol:* In this regimen, a patient will take an agonist, either leuprolide or buserelin, starting from day 21 of the previous cycle. As soon as the patient has her periods, the dose of the agonist is reduced and the patient will then start taking FSH or hMG daily until her largest follicles are mature. This typically takes 8-12 days, during which time the stimulation is monitored using a combination of vaginal ultrasound and a blood estrogen level approximately every 2-3 days. When the largest follicle(s) reach 18-20 mm in average diameter, the eggs are ready to undergo the last step in their maturation process, and a single injection of hCG is given. If nothing else is done, the patient would ovulate approximately 36-42 hours after her hCG injection. The basic concept is that the pituitary gland is suppressed, the ovaries are stimulated, and the uterine lining is supported, in that order. While some practices make a big deal over the choice of gonadotropin (some use only "recombinant FSH", such as Gonal F or Follistim, while others primarily use urinary hMG drugs, such as Bravelle or Menopur), most studies suggest that there is very little, if any, difference in pregnancy rates between the different medications.

2. *Antagonist protocol:* Rather than slowly suppress the pituitary like an agonist does, an antagonist, most commonly cetrorelix acetate, rapidly suppresses the pituitary within few hours. Gonadotropin hormone-releasing hormone (GnRH) antagonist protocols have several advantages over GnRH agonist protocols. The number of daily injections is fewer (4-5 days) with antagonist protocol than the agonist protocol in which injections are required for 3-4 weeks. Also, the duration of time required to stimulate the follicles to maturity is lesser with the antagonists. In addition, your chance of developing ovarian hyperstimulation syndrome is less with GnRH antagonist protocols. Multiple research studies have compared IVF agonist and antagonist protocols with most showing similar pregnancy rates.

3. *Microdose flare protocol:* In patients with diminished ovarian reserve, or who had previous ovarian surgery, we can use our "poor responder protocol" called the "flare", the "microdose flare", or the "low dose Lupron" protocol. This regimen uses the same medications as the "Lupron overlap" protocol. The major difference is that by cutting the dose of Lupron down to one sixth of the routine dose, and by giving it twice daily, the Lupron actually turns the pituitary gland "on" rather than "off", producing major release of FSH. This "endogenous" or internal FSH acts directly on the patient's ovaries and it is then reinforced with very high doses of "exogenous" (injections) FSH to cause the ovaries to respond as much as they can.

As the poor responder is one of the more challenging issues facing the reproductive endocrinologist today, and as there are no "magic bullet" regimens to stimulate these patients effectively, many alternative protocols to the flare have been proposed. Some of these involve the use of oral medications, such as clomiphene or letrozole in addition to gonadotropins. Others involve newer supplements such as dehydroepiandrosterone (DHEA) while others still involve the use of injectable medications such as growth hormone. While many studies to evaluate the effectiveness of these additional medications have been conducted, there are unfortunately very few definitive conclusions that have been reached.

What is unexplained infertility?

Approximately 30% of infertile couples are considered to experience "unexplained infertility". This controversial diagnosis is made when no abnormalities of the female and male reproductive systems are identified. Unexplained infertility is inevitably a diagnosis by exclusion, following otherwise "standard" investigations.

India has become one of the new health tourism destinations, with commercial gestational surrogacy as an expanding market. So, to regulate the ART practices across the nation, a new bill was introduced by the Ministry of Health, Government of India, to regulate and follow ethical practices.

Discuss ART Bill 2022

The key features of the bill include the following:

- *ART clinic:* There shall be two levels of clinics, namely Level 1 ART clinics, where only IUI procedure is carried out, and Level 2 ART clinics, where the procedures or, as the case may be, techniques that attempt to obtain a pregnancy shall be carried out.
- *ART banks:* These will be responsible for screening, collection, and registration of the semen donor and cryopreservation of sperms; performing screening and registration of oocyte donor; and maintaining the records or data of all the donors and shall regularly update the National Registry.
- *Staff requirements for all ART clinics/banks*:
  - *Level 1 ART clinic:* Minimum staff requirement: 1 gynecologist with 1 counselor
  - *Level 2 ART clinic:* 1 director, 2 gynecologists, 2 embryologists (one senior and one junior embryologist), 1 andrologist, 1 anesthetist, 1 counselor
- *Registration of ART clinics and banks:* Every ART clinic and bank must be registered under the National Assisted Reproductive Technology and Surrogacy Registry. The registration will be valid for 5 years and may be renewed.
- *Eligibility criteria for infertile couples:* ART services may be commissioned by married couple where a woman is between 21 and 50 years of age and a man is between 21 and 55 years.
- *Eligibility criteria for donors:* A bank may obtain semen from a male between 21 and 55 years of age and eggs for female between 23 and 35 years of age. A woman donor can donate only once in her life, and not more than seven eggs may be retrieved from her. A bank must not supply gamete of a single donor to more than one commissioning party.
- An *insurance coverage* for a period of 12 months is given in favor of the oocyte donor by the commissioning couple or an agent recognized by the Insurance Regulatory and Development Authority established under the provisions of the Insurance Regulatory and Development Authority Act, 1999.
- *Tests done for donors:* Sperm/oocyte donor is tested for the following diseases: HIV, types 1 and 2; HBV; HCV; *Treponema pallidum* (syphilis) through VDRL; Chlamydia.
- *Case records*, forms of consent, laboratory results, microscopic pictures, sonographic plates or slides, and recommendations and letters shall be preserved by the ART clinic/bank, for a period of 10 years from the date of completion of ART procedures.

- The collection of sperms posthumously shall be done only if prior consent of the commissioning couple is available.

What are the Surrogacy Rules, March 2022?
- Application for registration shall be made by the surrogacy clinics to the appropriate authority in Form 3, accompanied by an application fee of ₹ 500,000 for the surrogacy clinic.
- Staff requirement is similar to level 2 ART clinic.
- The Act has prohibited and penalized commercial surrogacy, and also brought about an array of regulations in terms of qualifications for the intending couple, intending woman, and surrogate mother, and documents to be submitted for commencement of the process, etc.

When can a woman opt for surrogacy?
- When a woman has no uterus, missing uterus, abnormal uterus, or the uterus has been surgically removed due to any disease
- Failed to conceive even after multiple IVF or ICSI attempts
- In case of multiple pregnancy losses where the medical reason is unexplained
- If pregnancy is impossible due to some illness

Discuss the key points for Surrogacy (Regulation) Rules, 2022.
- The central government by issuing a notification declared the eligibility criteria and number of persons required at a registered surrogacy clinic. Further, the details for the minimum equipment required at such clinics are also specifically mentioned.
- The composition of such clinics as per the notification is that any such clinic shall have at least one gynecologist, anesthetist, embryologist, and counselor and the clinic may employ additional staff similar to the ART level 2 clinics.
- Gynecologist at surrogacy clinics shall be a medical postgraduate in gynecology and obstetrics and should have a record of performing 50 ovum pickup procedures and at least 3 years of working experience in an ART clinic under the supervision of a trained ART specialist.
- *Form 1* in the notification specifies the application form for Couple of Indian Origin, which means "The couple where both husband (male) and wife (female) are Overseas Citizens of India cardholders in accordance with the Acts, Rules, Instructions, or Guidelines being followed by the Ministry of Home Affairs from time to time subject to fulfilment of various criteria as per the Surrogacy (Regulation) Act, 2021" as introduced in the Surrogacy (Regulation) Amendment Rules, 2023, or an intending woman for availing surrogacy to receive a certificate of recommendation from the board.
- To safeguard the rights of the surrogate mother, the provision for insurance coverage has been introduced, which mandates the intending couple or woman to purchase a health insurance for the surrogate mother for 36 months.
- An affidavit before a Metropolitan Magistrate or a Judicial Magistrate of the first class shall be signed by the woman or couple with the intention of giving guarantee under section 2 of the Surrogacy (Regulation) Act, 2021.
- The maximum number of attempts of the surrogacy procedure shall not be more than three times.
- The surrogate mother shall give her free consent as per the specifications provided in Form.

- It has been decided that the gynecologist shall implant only one embryo, with an exception of three embryos in special cases.
- In case where a surrogate mother wants to abort the child, the abortion process is to be followed as per Medical Termination of Pregnancy Act, 1971.

What are the amendments to the surrogacy rules?

Since the inception of the Indian surrogacy law, there have been two amendments to the Rules. The *first amendment* to the Rules was vide notification dated October 10, 2022 ("2022 Amendment"). Rule 5(2) requires the intending couple to purchase insurance coverage for 36 (thirty-six) months and that such insurance coverage should be guaranteed by signing an affidavit. Earlier, the provision stated that this affidavit needs to be sworn by signing an affidavit before the Metropolitan Magistrate or Judicial Magistrate of the first class. The 2022 Amendment allowed it to be sworn before either of the additional two classes of authorities, i.e., Executive Magistrate or Notary Public. Thus, the 2022 Amendment allowed flexibility to the intending couple and made way for a quicker process of surrogacy application. The *second amendment* to the Rules has come in recently vide notification dated March 14, 2023 ("2023 Amendment"). In the earlier provision, it could have been implied that the surrogacy by donor gametes was permitted. However, through the 2023 Amendment, this provision has been substituted with a restrictive clause which states the following: "(d)(I) Couple undergoing Surrogacy must have both gamete from the intending couple and donor gametes is not allowed and (II) Single woman (widow/divorcee) undergoing surrogacy must use self-eggs and donor sperms to avail the surrogacy procedure."

SUGGESTED READING

1. Bahceci M, Sismanoglu A, Ulug U. Comparison of cabergoline and bromocriptine in patients with asymptomatic incidental hyperprolactinemia undergoing ICSI-ET. Gynecol Endocrinol. 2010;26(7):505-8.
2. Baranwal A, Chattopadhyay A. Proposition of Belief and Practice Theory for Men Undergoing Infertility Treatment: A Hospital Based Study in Mumbai, India. Front Sociol. 2020;5:43.
3. Bosch E, De Vos M, Humaidan P. The Future of Cryopreservation in Assisted Reproductive Technologies. Front Endocrinol (Lausanne). 2020;11:67.
4. Coward RM, Mills JN. A step-by-step guide to office-based sperm retrieval for obstructive azoospermia. Transl Androl Urol. 2017;6(4):730-44.
5. Darwish AM, El Saman AM. Is there a role for hysteroscopic tubal occlusion of functionless hydrosalpinges prior to IVF/ICSI in modern practice? Acta Obstet Gynecol Scand. 2007; 86(12):1484-9.
6. De Silva PM, Chu JJ, Gallos ID, Vidyasagar AT, Robinson L, Coomarasamy A. Fallopian tube catheterization in the treatment of proximal tubal obstruction: a systematic review and meta-analysis. Hum Reprod. 2017;32(4): 836-52.
7. Edinoff AN, Silverblatt NS, Vervaeke HE, Horton CC, Girma E, Kaye AD, et al. Hyperprolactinemia, Clinical Considerations, and Infertility in Women on Antipsychotic Medications. Psychopharmacol Bull. 2021;51(2):131-48.
8. Hibino Y. The advantages and disadvantages of altruistic and commercial surrogacy in India. Philos Ethics Humanit Med. 2023; 18(1):8.
9. Klitzman R. Buying and selling human eggs: infertility providers' ethical and other concerns regarding egg donor agencies. BMC Med Ethics. 2016;17(1):71.
10. Mizrachi Y, Weissman A, Rozen G, Rogers PAW, Stern C, Polyakov A. Timing of progesterone luteal support in natural cryopreserved embryo transfer cycles: back to basics. Reprod Biomed Online. 2022; 45(1):63-8.

11. Mol BW, Hart RJ. Unexplained Infertility. Semin Reprod Med. 2020;38(1):1-2.
12. Narayan G, Mishra HP, Suvvari TK, Mahajan I, Patnaik M, Kumar S, et al. The Surrogacy Regulation Act of 2021: A Right Step Towards an Egalitarian and Inclusive Society? Cureus. 2023;15(4):e37864.
13. Osmanlıoğlu Ş, Şükür YE, Tokgöz VY, Özmen B, Sönmezer M, Berker B, et al. Intrauterine insemination with ovarian stimulation is a successful step prior to assisted reproductive technology for couples with unexplained infertility. J Obstet Gynaecol. 2022;42(3): 472-7.
14. Pacchiarotti A, Selman H, Valeri C, Napoletano S, Sbracia M, Antonini G, Biagiotti G, Pacchiarotti A. Ovarian Stimulation Protocol in IVF: An Up-to-Date Review of the Literature. Curr Pharm Biotechnol. 2016;17(4):303-15.
15. Sadecki E, Weaver A, Zhao Y, Stewart EA, Ainsworth AJ. Fertility trends and comparisons in a historical cohort of US women with primary infertility. Reprod Health. 2022;19(1):13.
16. Shah A, Parisaei M, Garner J. Obstetric Complications of Donor Egg Conception Pregnancies. J Obstet Gynaecol India. 2019; 69(5):395-8.
17. Sharma RS, Saxena R, Singh R. Infertility and assisted reproduction: A historical and modern scientific perspective. Indian J Med Res. 2018;148(Suppl):S10-4.
18. Torres-Arce E, Vizmanos B, Babio N, Márquez-Sandoval F, Salas-Huetos A. Dietary Antioxidants in the Treatment of Male Infertility: Counteracting Oxidative Stress. Biology (Basel). 2021;10(3):241.
19. Von Schondorf-Gleicher A, Mochizuki L, Orvieto R, Patrizio P, Caplan AS, Gleicher N. Revisiting selected ethical aspects of current clinical in vitro fertilization (IVF) practice. J Assist Reprod Genet. 2022;39(3):591-604.
20. Zheng D, Zeng L, Yang R, Lian Y, Zhu YM, Liang X, et al. Intracytoplasmic sperm injection (ICSI) versus conventional in vitro fertilisation (IVF) in couples with non-severe male infertility (NSMI-ICSI): protocol for a multicentre randomised controlled trial. BMJ Open. 2019;9(9):e030366.

32 Principles of Counseling in Obstetrics and Gynecology

Surinder Singh Gulati

What is counseling?
The word counseling is derived from the Latin root "consilium" meaning advice. Many people remain perplexed about its true meaning, purpose, and intention. However, it is generally agreed that communication skills are fundamental to all interactions with people, whether they are seeking help or working with colleagues. In the medical practice, such skills in healthcare workers include *listening, exploring and clarifying problems, giving advice and information as well as support. In contrast, formal counseling is carried out by especially trained and supervised professional counselors.*

The British Association of Counselling defines counseling as follows:

"An interaction in which one person offers another person time, attention and respect, with the intention of helping that person explore and discover ways of living more successfully and towards greater wellbeing."

Such counseling is of seminal importance to the effectiveness of care and women's satisfaction with their consultations. People suffering from any disease or disability are confronted by problems which are as much psychological as physical and involve all members of their family and wider social network. Health care, whether preventive or treatment oriented, must include the psychosocial aspects of illness as well as the physical aspects, at all phases of the life cycle and at all stages of the disease. Everyone, from the student to the experienced practitioner, can benefit from appropriate training in this area where the social skills required are complex and uncertain.

Dealing with women who have problems associated with fertility, birth, and parts of the body relating to reproduction and sexuality, is an emotional process, yet all too often these matters are dealt with in a mechanistic way, leading to unfulfilled expectations of patients.

Describe the biopsychosocial model of counseling.
Theories, medical treatments, and popular traditions surrounding reproduction and menstruation have varied appreciably across time and differ across cultures. A dominant theme in the past and in present, friends and families, attitudes and beliefs about health and illness is for reproduction to be seen as a cause of psychological problems. Theories also tend to be one dimensional, emphasizing either biological or social factors, and this has led to an inadequate and an unhelpful understanding and treatment of women's problems. Existing models of reproductive problems such as the biological/medical or the sociocultural model fail to adequately address the influence of psychological factors in obstetric and gynecological patients.

The *biopsychosocial model* described in **Flowchart 1** represents the many influences (cultural, social, psychological, and biological) which a person experiences and reacts to in the context of reproductive

Principles of Counseling in Obstetrics and Gynecology

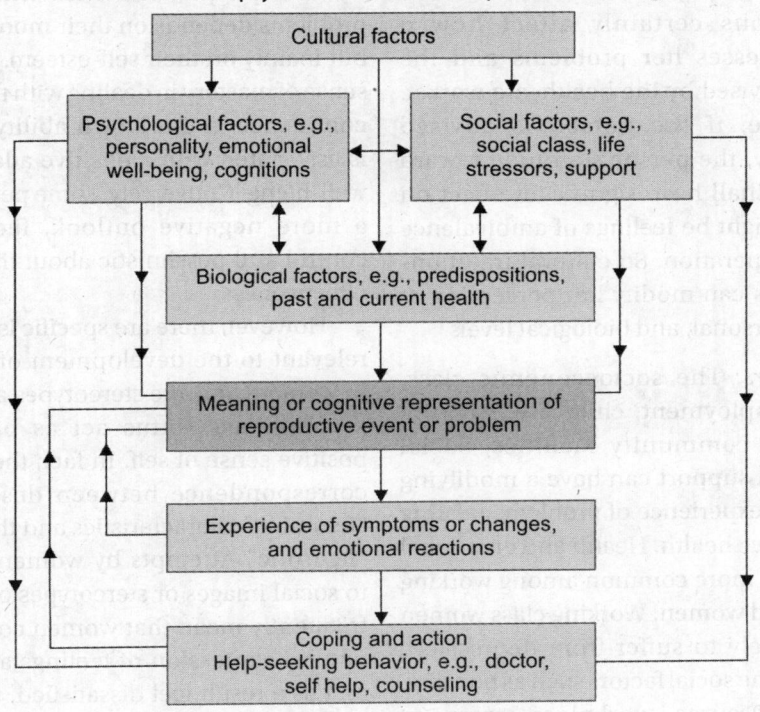

Flowchart 1: Biopsychosocial model of reproductive changes.

changes and problems. The main aim of this model is to attempt to understand the meaning that the problem or reproductive event has for a woman in context of her life.

Cognitive factors: These include women's internal thoughts, knowledge, attitude beliefs, expectations, and predictions when trying to understand and explain their symptoms. People develop internal representations of their illnesses, what it means to them, its causes, its duration, and prognosis. Women's expectations of their symptoms are based on available information and represent most women's experiences. The health worker should try to perceive the individual's representations of her problem as these will have a key influence in the resulting emotional reactions and due to which a person seeks medical or other kinds of help.

The following cognitive factors have been found to influence the experience of various health problems as well as help-seeking behavior:

- Level of knowledge of the person about her problem
- Explanations of its cause
- Expectations about the duration of the problem
- Memories of similar previous experiences
- Is the problem curable/controllable by herself, as well as by the others
- The value placed on health or reproductive changes compared with other aspects of her life
- Beliefs about her personal ability to overcome the problem
- Attitudes toward doctors and medical help

Cultural factors: A person's cultural beliefs and traditions certainly affect how a person expresses her problems and the treatment advised by the healthcare worker. For example, if the person is advised hysterectomy, the person's attitude toward her fertility shall have significant effect on her. There might be feelings of ambivalence toward the operation. So cultural traditions and practices can modify her perception at the social, personal, and biological levels.

Social factors: The socioeconomic class, access to employment, childcare, stressful life change, community facilities, social network, and support can have a modifying effect on the experience of problems relating to reproductive health. Health and emotional problems are more common among working class men and women. Working class women are more likely to suffer from depression, likely due to the social factors such as housing, financial pressures, workplace stress, or stressful life events, especially bereavements or losses. Looking after the family only makes the problem further complex. On the contrary, rewarding work and close supporting relationships significantly act as buffers against stress.

Psychological factors: Personality and mood affect how changes are regarded and how problems are dealt with. Here, personality means the tendencies a woman has to think, feel, and react in certain ways, the way in which she tends to view herself and the world, and the way she tends to relate to others. Most people think, feel, and act in a variety of ways according to the situation they are in, but particular characteristics can be identified, especially when repeated over time. Genetic predispositions also play a role in some cases like severe depression and psychotic conditions, such as maniac depression.

How people deal with challenges and problems depends on their mood at the time but mainly on their self-esteem. Optimism, a sense of mastery in dealing with the world and confidence in one's own ability, or efficacy is associated with a positive adaptation and well-being. Conversely, some people develop a more negative outlook, feeling out of control and pessimistic about their personal effectiveness.

However, there are specific issues that are relevant to the development of self-esteem in women. Sex role stereotypes and women's second-class status act as barriers to a positive sense of self. In fact, there is a close correspondence between descriptions of "feminine" characteristics and those deemed "neurotic". Attempts by women to conform to social images or stereotypes of femaleness frequently mean that women constrain their natural expression of feelings and thoughts and as a result feel dissatisfied, unauthentic, or depressed. In general, women tend to be judged against "male" concepts of normality. They are expected to be emotionally stable, meaning in control and consistent, rather than to moods which are variable, including both highs and lows which are related to the menstrual cycle.

Biological factors: These include the present ailment and symptoms, genetic predispositions to health problems, hormonal productions, and past history of ill health. These can influence how women experience reproductive events or problems. For example, genetically transmitted diseases such as thalassemia and hemophilia can influence the women's experience. Physical disabilities, tendency to miscarry, poorly controlled diabetes, hypertensive disorders, or other chronic diseases may mean that much of pregnancy is spent in hospital and is compounded by other related roles (wife and mother) which may lead to emotional distress.

Hormonal makeup is significantly seen as a significant factor in "women's" problems. However, some women appear to be more prone to menstrual problems than others. Hormonal basis alone does not explain the premenstrual symptoms or emotional problems experienced during midlife; cultural, social, and psychological factors are also relevant. In addition environmental changes, such as diet or stress, can modify hormonal factors that cause emotional turmoil. However, more studies are needed in this field.

Emotional problems and help-seeking behavior: Here we return to the center of the model—the woman's understanding or cognition of her reproductive event or problem. This will largely determine her emotional reactions, the way she copes, and the type of help she seeks.

Her coping strategies, such as whether to take time off work or whether to ignore a symptom, will depend in part on the expectations about the duration and severity of the problem as well on her ability to tolerate discomfort. Decisions to seek medical help are also determined by the woman's view of the problem, knowledge, beliefs and expectations, and faith in the medical system. Social factors (such as social support and type and availability of medical and other services) are also relevant. It is important to mention that this model is fluid in that perceptions of problems are constantly changing, depending upon the input from the various influences described.

What are the types of experiences of reproductive changes and problems in women?

Women's experiences of reproductive changes and problems come in several varieties. Their effect on the individual depends on the significance of the change or illness, its nature, and the psychosocial concept. *Studies have found that women attending gynecological clinics report high levels of emotional distress, higher than those in the general population or women attending other outpatient clinics. Counseling skills are essential if healthcare workers are to understand the reasons for seeking help.*

Some of the common problems in obstetrics and gynecology which may influence the women's emotions are summarized as follows:

Perception of symptoms
- The most common symptoms or first sign of reproductive changes are menstrual changes (menarche, heavier or irregular periods, spotting in between periods, or no periods), pain, and vaginal discharge. Problems become evident when expected changes do not occur or may be detected by screening programs, such as prenatal care and cervical screening services.
- Some problems may occur gradually and the patient gets insights from social comparisons or assessments of what is felt to be normal, how tolerable the symptom is, how day-to-day life is disrupted, and how long it is likely to last.
- On the contrary, in some cases, e.g., if a cancer comes as a sudden diagnosis without prior warning signs, this can lead to a radical change in her self-concept.
- A woman's perceptions and meanings (or cognitive representation) of a problem will influence how she feels and how she copes with it. People can have varied emotional reactions to their problems such as depression, anxiety, or irritability. They may deal with their feelings by crying, complaining, or showing irritability. Others hold their feelings

or bottle them up, leading to tiredness, physical tension, sexual disinterest, and sleeplessness. Some may obtain relief via smoking, alcohol, or drugs. Some people feel that it is more acceptable to talk about pain, hormonal changes, or physical symptoms than emotional problems.

Consultation
- A woman's experiences during a gynecologic consultation can distress her due to many factors like unmet expectations, problems in communication, anxiety about vaginal examinations, being examined vaginally without their legs being covered, and temperature of the speculum (too hot or too cold). Their need for equality, warmth, and respect may not be met. The gender of the gynecologist makes a difference. A study in Europe found that only 4% of women surveyed preferred a male doctor, 42% female doctor, while 54% said that they did not mind either sex. They had particular difficulty relating to young male doctors, while older men received relatively greater acceptance because there were less likely sex connotations.
- Doctor–patient relationships are by nature unequal, since the doctor or healthcare worker has advantages of medical knowledge and professional status. However, if symptoms, diagnosis, and treatment are discussed during internal examinations or when the patient is lying down or partially clothed, the power relation is further tipped toward the professional. In this situation, the women feel powerless and might consent to treatments and not express their real feelings and views. The presence of extraneous people in the room causes a sense of unease, especially when the woman's permission is not sought or their purpose explained.
- Hospital practices and procedures such as long waiting times, block bookings, cramped changing cubicle, being asked to undress before seeing the doctor, and lack of privacy also add to women's dissatisfaction and have a dehumanizing effect.

Investigations and minor operations, e.g., abortion or termination of pregnancy, dilatation and curettage, cervical cancer screening, sterilization, and other procedures.

How an investigation or minor operation shall impact the patient depends on several factors such as reasons for the intervention, how the decision to undergo the investigation is made, expectations of the procedure involved, experience of hospital/clinical staff, problems occurring during or after the intervention, past ability to cope with stressful situations, stage of the reproductive cycle, availability of social support, outcome of the investigation or operation, and implications for future health.

It is now observed that few problems result from abortions or terminations of pregnancy and many women feel relieved afterward. However, 5–10% of women do have stronger long-lasting reactions including feelings of anger, loss, or regret. But if a woman is refused termination, the outcome is unlikely to be satisfactory for the woman or child.

Cervical screening: Cervical malignancy is a common cancer in developing countries. India carries a quarter of the world's burden of cervical cancer. Large number of women are likely to have cervical smear tests, and a proportion will undergo more complex investigations such as human papillomavirus (HPV) DNA, colposcopy, cervical punch biopsy, and cone biopsy.

Some patients are mistakenly assured that the cervix is insensitive to pain and are not given analgesics, thus causing distress. Waiting for the results of the cervical smear, colposcopy, cone biopsy, and HPV DNA has been identified as the most difficult time by a majority of women undergoing the procedures. For many, the main concern understandably was whether they had cancer and what could be done about it.

Major surgery: Studies of women both before and after hysterectomy suggest that a woman's emotional state before the surgery is the best predictor of postoperative distress. Many women feel better after the operation, possibly because distressing symptoms, such as bleeding and prolapsed genitalia, are eliminated. However, women attending gynecological clinics and those who have hysterectomies do on an average experience high levels of distress. It is possible that in some cases, surgery is resorted to before other emotional or social problems are explored and managed appropriately.

Factors affecting the impact of hysterectomy:
- Severity of preoperative symptoms
- Age and whether the woman has had children or not
- Circumstances surrounding the decision
- Expectations and beliefs about hysterectomy and its consequences
- Past emotional problems and preoperative state
- Knowledge about and preparation for the operation
- Current relationships and social support
- Surgical approach, e.g., vaginal/abdominal/laparoscopic/robotic
- Cesarean hysterectomy, usually done in younger patients, will result in infertility. This is more likely to cause distress.
- Whether ovaries were retained or removed
- Sexual life after the operation, whether it will be normal or painful
- Length of time it would take for life to return to normal

Experience of childbirth
- Women's hopes, expectations, and experiences of childbirth are very variable. However, most would not deny the significance of the event and its immediate emotional impact. It brings about a major change in life, and anxieties about the pain are common, especially for first-time mothers. The amount of pain experienced during childbirth varies considerably but is described by many as the most intense pain they have felt in their life.
- The common concerns among the women are the unfamiliarity of the hospital, the procedures, unexpected events, how one will cope, and the baby's health. A major factor causing anxiety is about losing control. Other factors are the frequency of epidurals, drips to speed labor, monitors, episiotomies, instrumental delivery, and cesarean section. Personal satisfaction about labor was strongly related to personal control over it, the ability to control panic, and use of breathing exercises.
- There is now good evidence that shows that women who are socially supported during pregnancy and labor benefit in terms of improved health, both of themselves and their babies. Studies have shown that women who were socially supported during pregnancy and labor, comforted, encouraged, and praised by a volunteer companion felt that they coped better, had less pain and anxiety, and were most likely to be breastfeeding 6 weeks after birth. There is a widespread desire

- for continuity of care by the same person in maternity care and midwives are regarded the best placed to provide this.
- Women also require a greater choice in the type of maternity care. Many women complain lack of information, which would enable them to make a choice. Bad news is often conveyed in an unsympathetic manner. Too often, they experience an unwillingness on the part of professionals, to treat them as equal partners in making decisions about the birth of their child. It is concluded that women need to be given a choice on the basis of existing intervention rather than having to undergo such interventions as a routine.

Infertility: Investigations and treatment
Infertility affects about 10–15% of couples and can result in considerable emotional distress. Women have varying responses to infertility, with no particular pattern but can deeply affect a woman's feeling of self-worth. It can represent a major crisis that may dislodge a couple's long- and short-term plans. Feelings of guilt and failure are common. It is possible that stress may make a conception less likely, but more research is needed in this area. The need for sex at specified times can lead to sexual difficulties, and this can easily make affection and intimacy take a second place to the need to perform. An unmet need in the practice of infertility is the inadequate provision for emotional aspects of infertility, not enough information, and long waiting time between appointments. The patients experience prolonged treatment, and this has been described as a series of hopes and disappointments, joy to sadness and uncertainty. Such feelings are at a higher level in couples seeking treatment through new technologies such as in vitro fertilization, ovum or semen donation, intracytoplasmic sperm injection, etc. The facilities are not widely available, and they are expensive thus increasing stress. The patients require great motivation to persist with treatment, despite the expense and the failure to guarantee a successful result of carrying home a child. Couples tend to overestimate the likelihood of success and experience profound disappointment if pregnancy does not result. Donor insemination can highlight the male partner's disappointment or guilt about his infertility and bring up particular social and ethical issues as only the biological identity of the female partner is known. Another dilemma is whether or not to inform the child.

What are the women's experiences associated with the reproductive cycle?

Experiences of the different stages of the reproductive cycle vary considerably. For many women, menarche, menstruation, pregnancy, childbirth, and menopause present no particular problems. For those who feel tense, anxious, or depressed, it can be all too easy to attribute distress to hormonal changes. Although hormonal changes do occur, the bulk of evidence suggests that in the majority of women, psychosocial factors (i.e., what is going on in their lives) are the most likely causes of distress.

Premenstrual tension or syndrome
This refers to a wide range of symptoms including tension, depression, irritability, abdominal bloating, and breast tenderness. When asked generally about their menstrual cycles, 70% women acknowledge their symptoms. However, *when premenstrual syndrome (PMS) is carefully defined in terms of a definite increase in emotional and physical symptoms in the premenstrual phase with absence of symptoms in the follicular phase of the cycle, then severe PMS is relatively rare—about 5%.* True PMS can be accurately

diagnosed by keeping a diary. For others, the emotional problems can be more difficult to deal with during the premenstrual phase.

Premenstrual syndrome is not a simple biological phenomenon. No consistently abnormal patterns have been found, but this does not rule out the possibility of hormonal problems in some women. Various remedies have been tried, but there is no conclusive evidence available in their favor from clinical trials.

Postnatal depression: Postnatal depression (PND) requires to be differentiated from "postpartum blues" and puerperal psychosis. The former is a transient emotional disorder occurring in the first 3-5 days of childbirth and may last up to 2 weeks. It occurs in 75% of mothers and is self-limiting. Puerperal psychosis is a serious disorder usually requiring treatment by a psychiatrist in hospital; it affects about 2 per 1,000 mothers.

Severe PND affects about 10-15% mothers in varying degrees. The main symptoms of moderate-to-severe depression (PND) are feeling miserable and sad, lacking energy, lacking interest and pleasure in doing things, excessive anxiety, self-doubt, self-blame, and guilt as well as physical symptoms such as loss of appetite and early morning wakening (when not caused by the baby).

Causes of postnatal depression:
- Psychological changes consequent on childbirth, stresses, and demands of motherhood as well as exacerbation of existing emotional problems appear to be the main reasons. The experiences of motherhood include sleepless nights, tiredness, worry about mothering skills, feeding difficulties, a dramatic change in lifestyle, unable to cope, and feel out of control, thus leading to depression.
- A lack of social supportive network, especially in the early months of mothering, can make the depression chronic and can affect the mother-child relationship. This can affect the child's well-being and behavior. For a single parent, the financial and emotional burden can be still greater and self-neglect in the interest of child can increase the likelihood of depression.
- An increased risk of PND is observed in women who are unduly anxious in the antenatal period, have a family history of psychiatric disorder, or who have had a PND or a psychiatric disorder themselves.
- Previous experience of early loss or of a parent or baby dying during pregnancy also increases the likelihood of PND.

Menopausal problems: A common belief about the menopause that that it leads to a host of emotional and physical problems, but this is not supported by research findings. For most women, menopause is not a major crisis. 50-60% feel hot flushes and 10-20% perceive it as a problem. Two out of five women feel vaginal dryness, which can cause painful intercourse after the menopause. Depression in the average woman is not associated with menopause. Psychosocial factors such as having negative beliefs about menopause, being under stress, bereavement, being unemployed, and having social problems are the most common predictors of depressed mood as well as ill health. However, the variety of experiences and women's reactions to the menopause vary appreciably. Relaxation can be helpful in relieving hot flushes. Bodily changes because of their unpredictability can be difficult to deal with. There can be feelings of bereavement for the first time during midlife, and the emotional and physical reactions to grief can be misunderstood and can be attributed to menopausal changes. The woman should be enabled by the healthcare worker or professional counselor to clarify and reach appropriate attributions of distress, and this can be very helpful for the woman to deal with this stage of life. Premature menopause (stopping of periods before 40 years) can be a problem for some women. Hormone replacement therapy (HRT) is often recommended for women who have an early menopause to prevent osteoporosis.

Chronic reproductive problems
Pelvic pain: Pelvic pain is a common problem in gynecological patients and is often difficult to diagnose. Laparoscopy is usually needed to diagnose endometriosis and pelvic inflammatory disease, with which only two-thirds cases are diagnosed. Women also have difficulty in communicating with the health workers; for example, sexual problems like dyspareunia require gentle exploration. If no abnormality was found, the symptoms were seen as psychological or "it is all in your head".

In recent years, it has been recognized that in chronic pelvic pain the influences of attitudes and behavioral reactions to pain become relevant. All pain is seen as real, and factors maintaining pain may wary. Even when physical factors are identified, a person's mood and reactions will affect the way in which it is experienced. Despite these recent changes in conceptual understanding, women with chronic pelvic pain are sometimes described as having conflicts about sexuality or femininity, or as "hysterical" personalities.

Severe chronic pain usually leads to tiredness and depression, impacts sexual relations and fertility, can put strains on relations, and limit future life plans.

Gynecological cancer: Gynecological cancer leads to strong feelings of fear and dread in most people. Intense depression and cancer and confusion complicate the picture. There is frequently a difficulty in locating a cause, uncertainty about the prognosis, side effects associated with treatment, and long-term impact of the disease upon one's future and the lives of family and friends. Fears of a painful and undignified death are also common. Patients have concerns about fertility, sexual function, and self-image. Feelings of guilt with past sexual experiences and the contraceptive pill can lead to self-blame and guilt. While most doctors believe the patient should be told that they have cancer, frequently the patients remain inadequately informed which aggravates the situation.

What are the impacts of obstetrical losses on women?

Bereavement and pregnancy loss: Pregnancy loss includes miscarriage (loss of pregnancy before 20 weeks' gestation), stillbirth (baby born dead after 20 weeks' gestation), and neonatal death (death occurring within 28 days of birth). Grief is a common and natural reaction following loss of a baby at any stage. Although there are huge individual differences in the way people deal with loss or bereavement, there is a pattern to the grieving process which typically occurs in three stages:

1. There is an initial reaction of numbness and denial.
2. A second stage of full grief reaction associated with feelings of sadness, anger, guilt, self-reproach, withdrawal, and reduced contact with others
3. In the third phase of recovery, life is gradually adapted and rebuilt to accommodate the changes needed in response to the loss.

The time of this process varies greatly depending on the relationship with the deceased, previous experience of loss, ability to cope, social support, cultural factors, and the circumstances surrounding the death.

Miscarriage: Miscarriage or spontaneous problem is not an uncommon occurrence. About 20% of pregnancies end in miscarriage before 20 weeks. The health workers often assume that during the first trimester, a woman is unlikely to have become attached to the baby. However, many women do think of the fetus as a real person and seeing the baby on ultrasound scan can reinforce this feeling.

In a study, women appreciated doctors who discussed their distress and grief and were generally angry to be told that it was only an early pregnancy and that they should try again. In general, the women tended to view their miscarriage as a serious loss, while from the doctor's point of view it was a common clinical problem.

Abortion following fetal anomaly: In the current practice of obstetrics and gynecology, with the availability of sophisticated screening and diagnostic techniques, the number of terminations of pregnancies for fetal anomalies has arisen. The majority of these pregnancies are wanted pregnancies. They are usually terminated in the second trimester which requires induction of labor, which can be very distressing. Women often have feelings of guilt at having to take the decision of ending the baby's life. An additional problem is the anxiety about whether the abnormality will recur in future pregnancies.

Stillbirth, perinatal death, and neonatal death, in the first week of life: Some decades ago, studies found that parents often have grief reactions which were disregarded earlier and they were encouraged to forget about it and have another baby. Sensitive handling at the time of loss includes allowing the couple to hold the baby, have a photograph or some other memento (e.g., a lock of hair), and a funeral. In developed countries, voluntary services are now available to improve health care for couples who have lost a baby.

Anger may well be expressed within the family, toward friends, or against the hospital. Feelings of guilt and self-blame are frequently observed in the clinical scene. Those who have had emotional or psychiatric problems in the past often diminish a person's capacity to bear the loss. Loss of a twin or multiple births can complicate the grief process. There can be long-term implications of unresolved grief which can include persistent denial of the loss, excessive and long-lasting self-blame, grief, and depression.

■ COUNSELING PROCESS

What is counseling?

A definition of counseling includes most interactions between healthcare and voluntary workers and women and couples seeking help as well as settings in which counseling is arranged on a more formal basis. *The term counselor is reserved for those employed professionally and who have a recognized training.*

There are three levels of counseling, namely health worker, voluntary helper, and professional counselor. The appropriate choice will depend on the skills, expertise, role of the healthcare worker, and the needs and expectations of the person seeking help. *Nevertheless, good communication skills, the basis of all counseling, are desirable in all settings and, if practiced, yield benefits for all concerned.* Some individuals seem better than others at communicating, but these are skills that can be learnt.

What are the various types of healthcare worker/counselor and patient relationships?

Three types of healthcare worker/counselor–patient relationships have been described in counseling which vary according to the patient's feeling of autonomy and level of participation.

Activity–passivity relationship: Here, the doctor is in charge and the patient is passive, does not participate, and is expected to accept decisions that are made. This may be appropriate in certain emergency situations but is counterproductive when the aim is to understand the patient's problem.

Guidance–cooperation relationship: In this setting, the patient is offered some autonomy and participates more, but the terms of the relationship and the agenda for discussion are laid down by the doctor/helper. This model is *appropriate (for example) when patients are extremely ill*. However, the patient is unable to express her concerns and opinions, and this is a negative outcome for the relationship.

Mutual participation relationship: This is usually the most desirable relationship for health worker–patient interactions. Here it is assumed that both participants interact actively and exercise personal responsibility for the content of the interaction and its outcome. The patient's views, expectations, and opinions help to maintain this cooperative relationship.

There is an array of counseling models and psychological theories. However, many people develop their own counseling style. What is described here is the *problem management approach*.

Describe the fundamental attitudes crucial for good communication.

The crucial attitudes for good communication include *empathy, respect, and genuineness*.

Empathy refers to the attempt by the healthcare worker to enter the private world of the other person and to perceive the other's point of view accurately. The healthcare worker tries to be sensitive to the patient's understandings, feelings, and experiences and attempts to communicate this awareness to the woman or her partner. The task is to reach a fairly accurate view of the other person's model (or cognitive representation) of their problem. You may not agree with their beliefs or theories, but the process of attempting to clarify the person's thoughts and feelings can make them feel valued and thus provides the groundwork for discussion of different ways of looking at their problems.

Respect means valuing and accepting the person for themselves. This involves not judging people or assuming a superior role but taking care to listen. The knowledge, experiences, and views of the person are appreciated, taken seriously, and given equal importance when compared with expert. If treated with respect, people are more likely to feel responsible for their health and related decisions. They actively get involved in their treatment which not only increases their self-esteem but also helps in healing disturbed emotions.

Genuineness suggests a number of qualities including honesty and integrity in relation to the person seeking help. Being genuine means being truly interested in helping someone and is conveyed to the person by attention and listening and by maintaining confidentiality.

These fundamental attitudes have some overlap and how they are communicated. They help to build a relationship of trust; thus, they are more effective in solving their own problems. It is emphasized that these qualities are often discussed within the context of formal or professional counseling. However, these can be achieved by healthcare workers and should be attempted while meeting with patients.

What are the stages of counseling?
There are three stages of counseling:
1. *Clarifying the problem*: The problem is explored and clarified as well as the person's internal representation (or models) of it.
2. *Setting goals*: A common understanding of the problem is reached and goals are agreed upon and set.
3. *Problem solving*: Changes are implemented using a problem-solving approach. The impact of change is then evaluated and fed back to inform the initial understanding of the problem. The patient should feel free to explore her problems and not feel obliged to present only one side of her story. By careful attention to her words, tone of voice, and behavior, the helper is more likely to understand and empathize. Besides ascertaining facts about events and symptoms, it is important to gain impression about her current thoughts, feelings, and behavior.

Cognitive behavioral therapy: This is usually done by a professional counselor and is not covered in this chapter.

Clarification of the problem: It is a method of helping people to understand the internal representation of themselves and their problems. The patients are encouraged to challenge unhelpful assumptions in their thoughts and to look at the effects of these thoughts upon their feelings and behavior. Besides examining women's cognitive construction of her problems and events, it is important not to overlook the real social difficulties that many people face and help them to find effective ways of tackling these difficulties.

Setting goals: Based on the understandings reached in stage 1, the changes needed to find reasonable solutions are considered. The helper's role is primarily to encourage the person to devise goals that can be implemented to achieve the desired effects. The healthcare workers formulate and suggest clear, specific goals that are realistic and attainable. A woman might be helped to prioritize and carefully think through the change process and what this would involve. This might include visualizing the effect of change on her life and anticipating any difficulties that might arise or act as barriers to success.

Making the changes: Having decided on the goals, the next stage deals with how they can best be achieved, putting plans into action and evaluating progress. It can be liberating for people to "brainstorm" ways of achieving goals, that is, thinking of as many ways as possible and putting forward their own ideas, however silly they might seem. They feel supported in this process and can enhance a person's confidence. The next step is to look at each option in turn, assessing the relative benefits and costs of each strategy.

Making changes can include planning changes in lifestyle, such as taking more exercise or increasing leisure time as well as attempting to alter the way a person copes with distress, e.g., by discussing problems rather than bottling up feelings. Changing can also include thinking about things from a different perspective. Once the best available plan is reached, it may be the case of trying one option first knowing that an alternative plan is available. The person is given support and encouragement and may also be offered training in specific skills, e.g., in assertiveness, to achieve that goal. Progress is assessed regularly and if necessary, changes may be made to the plan. Therefore, evaluation is not the last step—it is an ongoing process. It is hoped that the woman seeking help will be able to put her learnt problem-solving skills, e.g., in assertiveness, to achieve the goal. At this stage, it is important to emphasize that there is considerable flexibility in the methods of counseling available to the healthcare worker to affect the change.

The approached mentioned above is a brief summary of looking at problems which can concern emotions and health or past or future events. The only criterion for helping is that the individual thinks that there is a problem and wishes to be helped.

What are the important points in setting initial contact with patient?
The health worker should ensure the following:
- Privacy must be ensured.
- Free from interruptions, e.g., telephone calls
- Comfortable room so that the patient is at ease
- Chairs to be suitably positioned, preferably at right angles between health worker and patient so that they do not directly face each other. A large desk can serve as a barrier in communication.
- Plan the amount of time to be spent with patient
- Facility to perform physical examination. A chaperone must be present.
- The health worker should know what the patient expects from the meeting.

The health worker should pay full attention to the patient so that she should not feel ignored. *Active listening* means involving oneself in what the woman is saying and trying to understand her problem. Inattention, particularly when a person feels weak, can be experienced as very painful. Concentrating on the patient can help you to be sensitive to their verbal and nonverbal communications, and the assurance that they are being listened to gives them encouragement to talk.

The *health worker's nonverbal cues*, e.g., posture, unnecessary movements, facial expression, eye contact, synchrony in conversations, indicate to the patient how much attention they are receiving. Active listening to a patient is a complex and active process which involves making sense of the person's verbal and nonverbal communications. The health worker is constantly looking for underlying meanings and searching for evidence to support his known thoughts in trying to understand the person being counseled.

Given the complexity of this process, it is important not to hurry through the process. A hasty discussion may convey negative feelings, e.g., inattention, to the patient. It can be helpful to the patient by saying, "I am interested in how you see the problem."

Communication about patients is often distorted by labels such as "menopausal", "hysterical", or "hypochondriac". Such labels imply negativity and should be avoided. The health worker should be aware of his own prejudices and biases and he should approach each person with an open mind.

What are the guidelines for dealing with a person who is distressed?
There are many and varied situations and problems that lead to distress. The following general guidelines are useful when dealing with a distressed person:
- Private place to talk.
- Give a person time to cry.
- Empathize and offer support.
- Give full attention to the person.
- Resist the urge to act and give advice.
- Let the person talk in their own time and follow the lead.
- Gradually explore their feelings and reasons for distress and give time to recover.

- Give the person time and, if necessary, a place to recover, and discuss what happens next.

For example, in a gynecological clinic, a person may feel distressed in case of a fetal anomaly and has been advised a therapeutic abortion. The health worker should not appear lacking in concern by saying that the problem of abortion for fetal anomalies is quite common in practice and she can try for another pregnancy. Such a comment is reassuring for the gynecologist but not for the patient as it may increase a patient's feeling of sadness and regret. The patient should be supported not to consider the pregnancy loss as a personal failure. Listening, empathizing, and offering support are invaluable qualities appreciated by patients in stressful situations. In many cases, all the health worker should do is to sit with the person/relative and listen and let the person vent her feelings.

What are the important tips when dealing with a person/relative who is angry?

When you are used to being in a caring or helping role, it can be very difficult when someone you are trying to help or a relative becomes angry. The following guidelines are helpful:

- Listen carefully to the angered person and attempt to understand what has happened to cause her anger.
- Give sufficient time to express her feelings.
- If the person's anger is in response to a loss or a diagnosis, try not to take it personally.
- Be honest and apologize if you have made a mistake and make efforts to ensure that it does not happen again.
- No matter how rejected or deficient you feel, you should not respond with anger or be defensive. Instead, acknowledge the other person's anger, empathize, and take it seriously.
- *If you feel you are becoming angry*, there are a few things you can do. Take a deep breath and try to relax. Do not rush in and argue back. Remember that you are there to make sense of the situation, whether you are at fault or not. Be polite and make it clear that you will give serious thought to what has been said and would like to arrange another time for further discussion. Control of temper is indeed a valuable quality in defining personality.

How should information and support be provided?

The following guidelines are useful:
- Start by finding out what the person already knows. Explore their views of the problem, their expectations, their fears, and their current knowledge.
- Try to be clear and comprehensive. Avoid using jargon or complex terminology.
- Do not give too much information. It should be simple, concise, and to the point. Start by finding out what the person already knows. Understand their views.
- Group pieces of information together in categories, such as condition, treatment, prognosis, and how to cope.
- In addition to providing verbal information, it may be explained in written leaflets and diagrams.
- Inform the person that that you are there to answer their questions.
- Involve relatives to assist those with learning difficulties and interpreters for those who do not speak the language used.
- Repeat the information given and find out if it is understood.

What guidelines should be followed while giving bad news?

All healthcare workers have to convey bad news at some time, and this is never an easy task. Having to tell someone that they have cancer, their baby has died, or they cannot have children is certainly difficult for all concerned. The following guidelines are helpful:

Be prepared
- The health worker or counselor should handle the situation with sympathy and warmth and give clear information, with enough time for tears and further questions.
- Give the woman or couple enough time.
- If the bad news is not broken in the appropriate manner, the recipient shall experience unnecessary distress; conversely if it is managed well, the person is likely to trust the healthcare system and feel supported.
- The person giving the news should know the woman or couple and have the necessary knowledge.
- If the woman has a partner, friend, or relative, then they should be included if the patient wishes.
- Plan what are the main things you should say.

Giving the news
- The patient and relative should be explained the purpose of the meeting.
- Explore the woman's expectations and knowledge about the situation; subsequently, the information should be given.
- Listen to the patient carefully and try to be relaxed. Do not hurry and try to match the woman's mood.
- Convey the news simply and clearly without jargon; technical terms should be explained.
- For a start, the test result or diagnosis should be given.
- Give the woman and partner time to absorb the news.
- Strong emotional reactions are to be expected; these are considered normal; try not to stop them. Handling distress has been discussed earlier.
- Be empathic and enquire about feelings if they are not expressed.
- Be honest and answer questions that are asked.
- Be supportive by listening and acknowledging distress.

Ending the interview
- Let the woman/couple know how much time you have left.
- Summarize the information and its implications.
- Arrange an early follow-up appointment so that further questions and concerns can be answered.
- Communicate what you have told the patient in clinical notes.

How do you counsel before investigation or minor operations?

The aim is to inform the patient before the intervention takes place in written or verbal form. The following points are useful:
- The name and purpose of the intervention
- When and where it will take place and its duration
- Who will perform the operation or the intervention
- Whether preparation prior to the intervention is necessary, e.g., drinking of water prior to ultrasound
- What will happen during the procedure
- What the woman might expect to feel
- How should she cope with any discomfort
- Explain any side effects or consequences (e.g., some bleeding after dilatation and curettage).

Principles of Counseling in Obstetrics and Gynecology

- When will the results be available and give appointment for subsequent discussion and further treatment

How do you help people to make informed choices?
- Help the woman feel confident that she has a choice to opt for a treatment/test or not.
- What are the choices and their likely results and possible side effects
- Provide sources of information—research, help groups, books, and leaflets.
- The helper should be aware of his own biases.

Processing the information about options
- Think and talk over the options and the implications of their outcome in this particular case.
- Discuss advantages and disadvantages of each option and how she feels about each option.
- Do the interest of others conflict with those of the patient? The views of relatives and friends are often sought when making difficult decisions.
- Address the woman's concern about the outcome if she does not follow the advice she has been given.

Making a choice
- There is frequently a balance to be struck between two or more options—which is the best.
- Expect mixed feeling in difficult decisions.
- The patient should be allowed to make a decision after rational consideration and may ask for more time to think, if the decision evokes strong conflicting feelings.
- If a health worker does not know the answer to a particular question, he should be honest and refer the patient to someone who has more expertise, e.g., genetic counselor, menopause clinic, oncologist or for a second opinion.

What counseling should be given before surgery?
- It is now established that preoperative anxiety is associated with postoperative anxiety, as well as postoperative pain and recovery.
- The patient should be fully informed before the procedure chronologically, with the main symptoms summarized, but this is not always systemically carried out. Leaflets are very useful as is a diagram of the operation. The necessity about catheters, dressings, and drains should be explained.
- Information about the ward, e.g., doctor's rounds, visiting hours for attendants, toilets, nurse's office
- Expected experience and recovery. Inform about the necessity of resting, when she can lift objects, drive a car, resume sexual activity, and follow-up appointments. It is useful to inform about symptoms and signs that may occur which would require medical attention.
- Ways about coping should include discussions of methods of controlling pain, ways of getting out of bed, mobilization, and related issues.
- Necessity about physiotherapy may be explained wherever required.
- It is best to have a key worker, e.g., a resident doctor or a nurse, who can develop a closer relationship with a patient and who can be in a better position to discuss concerns and provide information.

How are pregnant women given support before, during, and after childbirth?
- Antenatal classes are a standard provision in most developed countries, and they have been found useful.
- They provide information about pregnancy, self-care, and physical changes.

- Information about labor and childbirth, especially signs, stages, and the physical process
- Methods of pain relief and information about medical and surgical interventions
- Breathing and pelvic floor exercises to carry out before and during labor
- Group discussions and questions
- A visit to the labor and maternity wards
- Information about early days after birth
- Abdominal and pelvic floor exercises in the postnatal period
- Breast and bottle feeding
- Returning home and caring for the baby

Pregnancy loss
- Helping grieved people involves creating trust, by being genuine and respectful, and act like a partner to the patient instead of being an expert.
- Give the patient an active listening and time to talk about their concerns and follow their lead.
- Allow patients to express their distress freely by active listening, demonstrating empathy, and accept that their reactions are normal.
- Help them to explore what has happened and the implications in their own time.

The information commonly needed is as follows:
- Practical information about what has happened, why it has happened, and what may happen next
- Information about arrangements concerning registration of the deaths, funerals, burials, and cremations
- Information about common emotional reactions—that these are intense but normal, permissible, and part of the grief process.
- Information needed to enable choices to be made. Most people will be unaware about choices and options, so care is required in presenting possibilities in a sensitive manner.

■ SUMMARY

There is a growing body of information attesting to the benefits resulting from good communication and counseling in obstetrics and gynecology as well as many other healthcare sections. Further training can help you developing your communicating and counseling skills. Supervision and support are essential for healthcare workers and all others at varying levels of experience. Clarify your position in your organization and ask for resources you need.

Normal Values of Investigations Related to Obstetrics and Gynecology

CHAPTER 33

Samta Gupta

OBSTETRICS

Blood Chemistry Normal Values

	Nonpregnant adult	First trimester	Second trimester	Third trimester
Liver function tests				
Alanine aminotransferase (ALT) U/L	7–41	3–30	2–33	2–25
Aspartate aminotransferase (AST) U/L	12–38	2–23	3–33	4–32
Alkaline phosphatase (U/L)	33–96	17–88	25–126	38–229
Bilirubin total (mg/dL)	0.3–1.3	0.1–0.4	0.1–0.8	0.1–1.1
Bilirubin unconjugated (mg/dL)	0.2–0.9	0.1–0.5	0.1–0.4	0.1–0.5
Bilirubin conjugated (mg/dL)	0.1–0.4	0–0.1	0–0.1	0–0.1
Bile acids (µ/L)	0.3–4.8	0–4.9	0–9.1	0–11.3
Gamma-glutamyl transpeptidase (U/L)	9–58	2–23	4–22	3–36
Lactate dehydrogenase (U/L)	115–221	78–433	80–447	82–524
Protein total (g/dL)	6.7–8.6	6.2–7.6	5.7–6.9	5.7–6.7
Albumin (g/dL)	4.1–5.3	3.1–5.1	2.6–4.5	2.3–4.2
Creatinine (mg/dL)	0.5–0.9	0.4–0.7	0.4–0.8	0.4–0.9
Urea nitrogen (mg/dL)	7–20	7–12	3–13	3–11
Uric acid (mg/dL)	2.5–7.6	2.0–4.2	2.4–4.9	3.1–6.3
Sodium (mEq/L)	136–146	133–148	129–148	130–148
Potassium (mEq/L)	3.5–5.0	3.6–5.0	3.3–5.0	3.3–5.1
Magnesium (mEq/L)	1.5–2.3	1.6–2.2	1.5–2.2	1.1–2.2
Chloride (mEq/L)	102–109	101–105	97–109	97–109
Calcium total (mg/dL)	8.7–10.2	8.8–10.6	8.2–9.0	8.2–9.7
Lipase (U/L)	3–43	21–76	26–100	41–112
Amylase (U/L)	20–96	24–83	16–73	15–81

Normal Values of Investigations Related to Obstetrics and Gynecology

■ HEMATOLOGY

	Nonpregnant adult	First trimester	Second trimester	Third trimester
Hemoglobin (g/dL)	12–15.8	11.6–13.9	9.7–14.8	9.5–15.0
Hematocrit %	35.4–44.4	31.0–41.0	30–39.0	28–40.0
Red blood cell count ($\times 10^6/mm^3$)	4.0–5.2	3.42–4.55	2.81–4.49	2.71–4.43
Red cell distribution width %	<14.5	12.5–14.1	13.4–13.6	12.7–15.3
White blood cell count ($\times 10^3/mm^3$)	3.5–9.1	5.7–13.6	5.6–14.8	5.9–16.9
Platelet count ($\times 10^9$/L)	1.65–4.15	1.74–3.91	1.55–4.09	1.46–4.29
Mean corpuscular hemoglobin (MCH) (pg/cell)	27–32	30–32	30–33	29–32
Mean corpuscular volume (MCV) ($\times 1\ m^3$)	79–93	81–96	82–97	81–99
Total iron-binding capacity (µg/dL)	251–406	278–403		359–609
Ferritin (ng/mL)	10–150	6–130	2–230	0–116
Iron (µg/dL)	41–141	72–143	44–178	30–193
Transferrin saturation %	22–46		18–92	9–98
Folate (ng/mL)	5.4–18	2.6–15	0.8–24	1.4–20.7

Coagulation Parameters

	Nonpregnant adult	First trimester	Second trimester	Third trimester
Prothrombin time (s)	12.7–15.4	9.7–13.5	9.5–13.4	9.6–12.9
Activated partial thromboplastin time (s)	26.3–39.4	23–38.9	22.9–38.1	22.6–35
International normalized ratio (INR)	0.9–1.04	0.86–1.08	0.83–1.02	0.80–1.09
Fibrinogen (mg/dL)	233–496	244–510	291–538	301–696
D-Dimer (µ/mL)	0.22–0.74	0.05–0.95	0.32–1.29	0.13–0.17

Renal Functions

	Nonpregnant adult	First trimester	Second trimester	Third trimester
Renal plasma flow (mL/min)	492–696	696–985	612–1170	595–945
Glomerular filtration rate (GFR) (mL/min)	106–132	131–166	135–170	117–182
24-hour protein excretion (mg/24 hr)	<150	19–141	47–186	46–185
24-hour albumin excretion (mg/24 hr)	<30	5–15	4–18	3–22
24-hour creatinine clearance (mL/min)	91–130	69–140	55–136	50–166
24-hour calcium excretion (mmol/24 hr)	<7.5	1.6–5.2	0.3–6.9	0.8–4.2
24-hour potassium excretion (mmol/24 hr)	25–100	17–33	10–38	11–35
24-hour sodium excretion (mmol/24 hr)	100–260	53–215	34–213	37–149
Thyroid-stimulating hormone (TSH) (µmol/L)	0.34–4.25	0.60–3.40	0.37–3.60	0.38–4.04
Thyroxine-free T4 (ng/dL)	0.8–1.7	0.8–1.2	0.6–1.0	0.5–0.8
Vitamin D 25-hydroxy (ng/mL)	14–80	18–27	10–22	10–18
Vitamin B_{12} (pg/mL)	279–996	118–438	130–656	99–526

Blood Gas

	Nonpregnant	First trimester	Second trimester	Third trimester
Bicarbonate (mEq/L)	22–26	Not reported	Not reported	16–22
PCO_2 (mm Hg)	38–42	Not reported	Not reported	25–33
PO_2 (mm Hg)	90–100	93–100	90–98	92–107
pH	7.38–7.42 (arterial)	7.36–7.52 (venous)	7.40–7.52 (venous)	7.41–7.53 (venous) 7.39–7.45 (arterial)

Normal Values of Investigations Related to Obstetrics and Gynecology

GYNECOLOGY HORMONES

	Conventional units	SI units
Follicle-stimulating hormone (FSH) (reproductive years)	5–20 mIU/mL	5–20 mIU/mL
Luteinizing hormone (LH) (reproductive years)	5–20 mIU/mL	5–20 mIU/mL
Estradiol	20–400 pg/mL	70–1500 pmol/L
Estrone	30–200 pg/mL	110–740 pmol/L
Progesterone • Follicular • Secretory	<3 ng/mL 5–30 ng/mL	<9.5 nmol/L 16–95 nmol/L
17-Hydroxyprogesterone	100–300 ng/mL	3–9 nmol/L
Testosterone total	20–80 ng/dL	0.7–2.8 nmol/L
Testosterone free	100–200 pg/dL	35–700 pmol/L
Dehydroepiandrosterone sulfate (DHEAS)	80–350 µg/dL	2.2–9.5 µmol/L
Androstenedione	60–300 ng/dL	2.1–10.5 nmol/L
Prolactin	1–20 ng/mL	44.4–888 pmol/L
Insulin fasting	5–20 µU/mL	35–145 pmol/L
Growth hormone	<10 ng/mL	<10 µg/mL
Adrenocorticotropic hormone (ACTH) 6.00 AM	10–80 pg/mL	2.2–17.6 pmol/L
Cortisol 8.00 AM	5–25 µg/dL	140–690 nmol/L
11-Deoxycortisol	0.05–0.25 µg/dL	1.5–7.3 nmol/L
Blood glucose fasting	70–110 mg/dL	4–6 mmol/L
Thyroid-stimulating hormone (TSH)	0.4–4.5 µU/ml	0.4–4.5 mU/L
Thyroxine (free T4)	0.8–2.3 ng/dL	10–30 nmol/L
Triiodothyronine (T3, total)	80–220 ng/dL	1.2–3.4 nmol/L
Triiodothyronine (T3, free)	0.13–0.55 ng/dL	2.0–8.5 nmol/L

Lipids

	Conventional units	SI units
Cholesterol Low-density lipoprotein (LDL) cholesterol High-density lipoprotein (HDL) cholesterol	<200 mg/dL 60–130 mg/dL 30–70 mg/dL mg/dL	<5.2 mmol/L 1.6–3.4 mmol/L 0.8–1.8 mmol/L
Triglycerides	40–250 mg/dL	0.5–2.8 mmol/L

SUGGESTED READING

1. Cunningham F, Leveno KJ, Dashe JS, Hoffman BL, Spong CY, Casey BM. William's Obstetrics, 26th edition. New York: McGraw Hill; 2022.
2. Fritz MA, Speroff L. Clinical Gynecologic Endocrinology and Infertility, 8th edition. Philadelphia: Lippincott Williams & Wilkins; 2011.

CHAPTER 34

Classification in Obstetrics and Gynecology

Priyanka Mathe, Neha Kumar

■ GYNECOLOGY

Pelvic Organ Prolapse

Possible ranges of six site-specific pelvic organ prolapse quantitative examination measurements are given in **Table 1**.

Stages of Pelvic Organ Prolapse

The stages of pelvic organ prolapse are illustrated in **Table 2**.

TABLE 1: Possible ranges of six site-specific pelvic organ prolapse quantitative examination measurements.

Points	Description	Range
Aa	Anterior wall 3 cm from hymen	−3 to +3 cm
Ba	Most dependent portion of rest of anterior wall	−3 cm to + total vaginal length (TVL)
C	Cervix or vaginal cuff	±TVL
D	Posterior fornix (if no prior hysterectomy)	±TVL or omitted
Ap	Posterior wall 3 cm from hymen	−3 to +3 cm

TABLE 2: Stages of pelvic organ prolapse.

Stage	Feature
Stage 0	No prolapse is demonstrated
Stage I	The most distal portion of the prolapse is >1 cm above the level of the hymen
Stage II	The most distal portion of the prolapse is <1 cm proximal or distal to the plane of the hymen
Stage III	The most distal portion of the prolapse is <1 cm below the plane of the hymen but no further than 2 cm less than the TVL
Stage IV	Nearly complete eversion of the vagina. The most distal portion of the prolapse protrudes to >+(TVL − 2 cm)

Endometriosis

American Society for Reproductive Medicine
Revised Classification of Endometriosis (Table 3)

Patient's name _____ Date _____

Stage I (minimal): 1–5
Laparoscopy_____
Laparotomy _____
Photography _____

Stage II (mild): 6–15
Recommended treatment _____

Stage III (moderate): 16–40

Stage IV (severe): More than 40
Total _____ Prognosis _____

Cervical Score

Cervical score is a score to assess the quality of cervical mucous in infertility cases. It was developed by Moghissi et al. (1977). Cervical mucous is collected by aspirating

TABLE 3: Revised classification of endometriosis.

	Endometriosis	<1 cm	1–3 cm	>3 cm
Peritoneum	Superficial	1	2	4
	Deep	2	4	6
Ovary	R—superficial	1	2	4
	Deep	4	16	20
	L—superficial	1	2	4
	Deep	4	16	20
Posterior cul-de-sac obliteration		Partial	Complete	
		4	40	
Adhesions		<1/3 enclosure	1/3–2/3 enclosure	>2/3 enclosure
Ovary	R—flimsy	1	2	4
	Dense	4	8	16
	L—flimsy	1	2	4
	Dense	4	8	16
Tube	R—flimsy	1	2	4
	Dense	4*	8*	16
	L—flimsy	1	2	4
	Dense	4*	8*	16

*If the fimbriated end of the fallopian tube is completely enclosed, change the point assignment to 16.
Staging: Stage I (minimal): 1–5; stage II (mild): 6–15; stage III (moderate): 16–40; stage IV (severe): >40.
Source: Revised American Society for Reproductive Medicine classification of endometriosis: 1996. Fertil Steril. 1997;67(5):817-21.

it with a pipette or tuberculin syringe in the preovulatory period, and five properties of cervical mucous are studied. Each is given 0–3 score, 3 representing the optimum changes, and total score is calculated.

Amount
0 = 0
1 = 0.1 mL
2 = 0.2 mL
3 = 0.3 mL or more

Ferning
0 = No crystallization
1 = Atypical pattern
2 = Primary and secondary stems
3 = Tertiary and quarterly stems

Spinnbarkeit
0 = 1 cm
1 = 1–4 cm
2 = 5–8 cm
3 = 9 cm

Viscosity
0 = Thick, highly viscous
1 = Intermediate viscosity
2 = Mildly viscous
3 = Normal

Cellularity
0 = 11 cells/high-power field (HPF)
1 = 6–11 cells/HPF
2 = 1–5 cells/HPF
3 = 0 cells/HPF

Total score
>10 = Normal
5–10 = Unfavorable
<5 = Hostile

Modified Vaginal Health Index

Modified vaginal health index is used for comparative evaluation of vaginal health after hormone replacement therapy (HRT) in menopausal women **(Table 4)**.

Preoperative Score (Under Anesthesia) for Assessment of Feasibility of Nondescent Vaginal Hysterectomy

The preoperative score (under anesthesia) for assessment of feasibility of nondescent vaginal hysterectomy is given in **Table 5**.

Lasmar Submucous Myoma Classification—STEPW Classification (2005)

It is a preoperative classification of submucous myomas for evaluating the viability and

TABLE 4: Modified vaginal health index.

pH	>6.5	5–6.5	<5
Moisture/consistency of fluid	No moisture	Minimal/superficial layer of scanty thin white mucus	Normal moisture
Rugosity	None	Minimal	Good
Elasticity	Poor	Fair	Excellent
Length of vagina	<4 cm	4–6 cm	>6 cm
Thickness of vagina	Papery thin	Thin	Normal
Epithelial integrity	Petechiae	Petechiae after scraping	Normal, no petechiae
Vascularity	Minimal	Fair	Good

TABLE 5: Preoperative score (under anesthesia) for assessment of feasibility of nondescent vaginal hysterectomy.

Score	0	1	2
Size of uterus	<8 weeks	8–10 weeks	>10 weeks
Mobility of uterus	Good	Fair	Poor
Intertuberous distance	> 4 knuckles	4 knuckles	< 4 knuckles
Subpubic angle	>90°	90°	<90°
Digital examination of vagina	Three finger loose	Three finger tight	Three finger tight
Mobility of vaginal mucosa	Good	Fair	Poor
Fornix depth	>One finger crease	One finger crease	<One finger crease
Descent with vulsellum	>1°	1°	<1°
Surgeon's experience	>10 years	5–10 years	<5 years
History of previous surgery	Nil	One	>One

the degree of difficulty of hysteroscopic myomectomy (**Table 6**).

European Society of Human Reproduction and Embryology/ European Society for Gynecological Endoscopy Classification

Female Genital Tract Anomalies

The female genital tract anomalies are described in **Table 7**.

Classification System for Abnormal Uterine Bleeding (PALM-COEIN)

The classification system for abnormal uterine bleeding (PALM-COEIN) is given in **Table 8**.

The subclassification system of leiomyoma is given in **Table 9**.

Classification of Radical Hysterectomies

The classification of radical hysterectomies is illustrated in **Table 10**.

TABLE 6: Submucous myoma classification.

	Size (cm)	Penetration	Extension of the base	Topography	Lateral wall
0	≤2	0	≤1/3	Lower	+1
1	>2 to 5	≤50%	>1/3–2/3	Middle	
2	>5	>50%	>2/3	Upper	

Score	Group	Suggested treatment
0–4	I	Low complexity hysteroscopic myomectomy
5–6	II	Complex hysteroscopic myomectomy; consider preparing with GnRH analog and/or two-step surgery
7–9	III	Recommend an alternative nonhysteroscopic technique

Source: Lasmar RB, Barrozo PRM, Dias R, Oliveira MA. Submucous myomas: A new presurgical classification to evaluate the viability of hysteroscopic surgical treatment. J Minim Invasive Gynecol. 2005;12(4):308-11.

TABLE 7: ESHRE/ESGE classification of female genital tract anomalies.

	Uterine anomaly		Cervical/vaginal anomaly	
	Main class	Subclass	Coexistent class	
U0	Normal uterus		C0	Normal cervix
U1	Dysmorphic uterus	• T-shaped • Infantilis • Others	C1 C2 C3 C4	Septate cervix Double "normal" cervix Unilateral cervical aplasia Cervical aplasia
U2	Septate uterus	• Partial • Complete		

Contd...

Contd...

	Uterine anomaly		Cervical/vaginal anomaly	
	Main class	Subclass	Coexistent class	
U3	Bicorporeal uterus	• Partial • Complete • Bicorporeal septate	V0 V1 V2 V3 V4	Normal vagina Longitudinal nonobstructing vaginal septum Longitudinal obstructing vaginal septum Transverse vaginal septum and/or imperforate hymen Vaginal aplasia
U4	Hemi-uterus	• With rudimentary cavity (communicating or not horn) • Without rudimentary cavity (horn without cavity/no horn)		
U5	Aplastic	• With rudimentary cavity (bi or unilateral horn) • Without rudimentary cavity (bi or unilateral uterine remnants/aplasia)		
U6	Unclassified malformations			
U			C	V

(ESGE: European Society for Gynecological Endoscopy; ESHRE: European Society of Human Reproduction and Embryology).
Source: Grimbizis GF, Gordts S, Di Spiezio Sardo A, Brucker S, De Angelis C, Gergolet M, et al. The ESHRE/ESGE consensus on the classification of female genital tract congenital anomalies. Hum Reprod. 2013;28(8):2032-44.

TABLE 8: Classification system for abnormal uterine bleeding (PALM-COEIN).

PALM	COEIN
Polyp	Coagulopathy
Adenomyosis	Ovulatory dysfunction
Leiomyoma (subclassification given in **Table 9**)	Endometrial
Submucous	Iatrogenic
Others	Not otherwise classified
Malignancy and hyperplasia	

OBSTETRICS

Classification of Obstetric Anal Sphincter Injuries

The classification of obstetric anal sphincter injuries is described in **Table 11**.

Robson Classification for Cesarean Section

The classification of cesarean section is given in **Table 12**.

TABLE 9: Leiomyoma subclassification system.

SM—submucous	0	Pedunculated intracavitary
	1	<50% intramural
	2	>50% intramural
O—other	3	Contacts endometrium; 100% intramural
	4	Intramural
	5	Subserous ≥ 50% intramural
	6	Subserous <50% intramural
	7	Subserous pedunculated
	8	Other (specify, e.g., cervical, parasitic)
Hybrid leiomyomas (impact both endometrium and serosa)		Two numbers are listed separated by a hyphen. By convention, the first refers to the relationship with the endometrium while the second refers to the relationship to the serosa. One example is here
	2–5	Submucous and subserous, each with less than half the diameter in the endometrial and peritoneal cavities, respectively

Source: Munro MG, Critchley HO, Broder MS, Fraser IS, FIGO Working Group on Menstrual Disorders. FIGO classification system (PALM-COEIN) for causes of abnormal uterine bleeding in nongravid women of reproductive age. Int J Gynaecol Obstet. 2011;113(1):3-13.

Classification of Urgency of Cesarean Section

The classification of urgency of cesarean section is given in **Table 13**.

Biophysical Profile

The biophysical profile is given in **Table 14**.

Bishop Scoring System Used for Assessment of Induction of Labor

The Bishop scoring system used for assessment of induction of labor is highlighted in **Table 15**.

Apgar Score (Table 16)

Apgar score is used to assess neonatal oxygen status at birth. It is calculated at 1 and 5 minutes after the birth of the baby. 1 minute score indicates need for immediate resuscitation of newborn, while 5 minutes score correlates well with long-term neurological sequelae.

Sher's Grading of Abruptio Placentae (According to Severity)

Sher's grading of abruptio placentae (according to severity) is shown in **Table 17**.

Zatuchni–Andros Score (Table 18)

Zatuchni–Andros score is a prognostic scoring system to decide the mode of delivery in breech presentation.

Westin Scoring System for Selecting Mode of Delivery in Breech (Table 19)

If all the parameters of pelvis are included, a score of 12 is safe for vaginal delivery.

TABLE 10: Classification of radical hysterectomies.

Piver–Rutledge–Smith		Querleu and Morrow	
Class I	Extrafascial hysterectomy • Identification of ureter through transparency and avoiding the ureteric injury by running them outside the operator field without dissection • The uterine artery is sectioned and ligated laterally • Uterosacral and cardinal ligaments are not removed • No vaginal portion is excised	Type A	Extrafascial hysterectomy • Identification and palpation of ureters without the dissection of the ureteral layer • The uterine arteries, uterosacral ligaments and cardinal ligaments are resected as close as possible to the uterus • Removal of vaginal portion as small as possible (<10 mm)
Class II	Modified radical hysterectomy (Wertheim) • Ureters are dissected in the paracervical region but are not resected in the pubovesical ligament • Uterine arteries are sectioned medially to the ureter • Uterosacral ligaments are excised midway from the sacral insertion • Resection of the cardinal ligaments up to the medial half • Removal of the upper third of the vagina • Pelvic lymphadenectomy	Type B — B1	• Ureters are deperitonized and rolled to the lateral side • Partial resection of the uterosacral and vesicouterine ligaments • Section of paracervical tissue at the ureteral tunnel level • At least 10 mm of vagina are measured from the cervix or the tumor • Without removal of lateral paracervical lymph nodes
		B2	• Ureters are deperitonized and rolled to the lateral side • Partial resection of the uterosacral and vesicouterine ligaments • Section of paracervical tissue at ureteral tunnel level • At least 10 mm of vagina are measured from the cervix or the tumor • Removal of lateral para cervical lymph nodes
Class III	Classical radical hysterectomy (Meigs) • Complete dissection of the ureters up till the pubovesical ligaments • Uterine arteries are cut at the origin • Uterosacral ligaments are excised at their sacral insertion	Type C — C1	• Ureters are fully mobilized • Sectioning of uterosacral ligaments at the level of rectum • Sectioning of vesicouterine ligaments at the level of bladder • Complete resection of paracervical tissue

Contd...

Contd...

Piver–Rutledge–Smith		Querleu and Morrow	
	• 15–20 mm from the vaginal resected toward the cervix or tumor and corresponding paracolpos • With preservation of autonomic nerves		
		C2	• Ureters are fully mobilized • Sectioning of uterosacral ligaments at the level of rectum • Sectioning of vesicouterine ligaments at the level of bladder • Complete resection of paracervical tissue • 15–20 mm from the vaginal resected toward the cervix or tumor and corresponding paracolpos • Without preservation of autonomic nerves
		Type D	
		D1	• Full resection of the paracervical tissue up to the pelvic bone together with the hypogastric vessels exposing the sciatic nerve roots • Ureters fully ambulant
		D2	• Full resection of the paracervical tissue up to the pelvic bone together with the hypogastric vessels exposing the sciatic nerve roots • Ureters fully ambulant • Resection of muscles and adjacent fascia
Class IV	More radical dissection • Complete dissection of the ureters from the pubovesical ligament • Umbilical vesical artery is sacrificed • Removal of third-fourth of upper vagina		
Class V	It is more radical than the previous class with addition of: • Excision of portion of ureter or bladder which is invaded and then the reimplantation of the ureter into the bladder		

Source: Marin F, Plesca M, Bordea CI, Moga MA, Blidaru A. Types of radical hysterectomies: From Thoma Ionescu and Wertheim to present day. J Med Life. 2014;7(2):172-6.

TABLE 11: Classification of obstetric anal sphincter injuries.

First degree	Injury to perineal skin only
Second degree	Injury to perineum involving perineal muscles but not involving the anal sphincter
Third degree • 3a • 3b • 3c	Injury to perineum involving the anal sphincter complex • <50% of EAS thickness torn • >50% of EAS thickness torn • Both EAS and IAS torn
Fourth degree	Injury to perineum involving the anal sphincter complex (EAS and IAS) and anal epithelium

(EAS: external anal sphincter; IAS: internal anal sphincter).
Source: Society of Obstetricians and Gynecologists of Canada (SOGC). (2015). Clinical Practice Guidelines. [online] Available from www.sogc.org/clinical-practice-guidelines. [Last accessed May, 2024].

TABLE 12: Robson classification.

Robson group	Clinical characteristics
1	Nulliparous, single cephalic, ≥37 weeks, spontaneous labor
2	Nulliparous, single cephalic, ≥37 weeks, induced labor or CS before labor
2a	Labor induced
2b	Prelabor CS
3	Multiparous without previous CS, single, cephalic, ≥37 weeks, spontaneous labor
4	Multiparous without previous CS, single, cephalic, ≥37 weeks, induced labor or CS before labor
4a	Labor induced
4b	Prelabor CS
5 5.1 5.2	Multiparous with previous CS, single, cephalic, ≥37 weeks With one previous CS With two or more CSs
6	All nulliparous breeches
7	All multiparous breeches (including previous CS)
8	All multiple pregnancies (including previous CS)
9	All transverse or oblique lies (including previous CS)
10	All preterm single cephalic, <37 weeks (including previous CS)

(CS: cesarean section)
Source: World Health Organization. The Robson Classification Implementation Manual.

TABLE 13: Classification of urgency of cesarean section.

Category	Definition	Urgency
1	Immediate threat to life of woman or fetus	
		Maternal or fetal compromise
2	No immediate threat to life of woman or fetus	
3	Requires early delivery	
		No maternal or fetal compromise
4	At a time to suit the woman and maternity services	

Source: Royal College of Obstetricians and Gynecologists (RCOG). (2010). Classification of Urgency of Cesarean Section—a Continuum of Risk (Good Practice No. 11). [online] Available from www.rcog.org.uk/en/guidelines-research-services/guidelines/good-practice-11/.

TABLE 14: Biophysical profile.

Component	Score 2	Score 0
Nonstress test	Two accelerations of 15 beats/min, 15 seconds in 20–40 minutes	Zero or one acceleration in 20–40 minutes
Fetal breathing	One episode of rhythmic breathing lasting 30 seconds within 30 minutes	<30 seconds of breathing in 30 minutes
Fetal movement	Three discrete body or limb movements within 30 minutes	<3 discrete movements
Fetal tone	One episode of extension of a fetal extremity with return to flexion, or opening or closing of hand within 30 minutes	No movements or no extension/flexion
Fluid volume	Single vertical pocket >2 cm	Largest single vertical pocket <2 cm

TABLE 15: Bishop scoring system used for assessment of induction of labor.

	Factor				
Score	Dilatation (cm)	*Effacement (%)	Station (−3 to +3)	Cervical consistency	Cervical position
0	Closed	0–30	−3	Firm	Posterior
1	1–2	40–50	−2	Medium	Midposition
2	3–4	60–70	−1, 0	Soft	Anterior
3	5	80	+1, +2	–	–

*In Modified Bishop's preinduction cervical scoring system, effacement has been replaced by cervical length in cm, with scores as follows: 0 for >3 cm, 1 for >2 cm, 2 for >1 cm, 3 for >0 cm.

TABLE 16: Apgar score.

	Score		
Signs	0	1	2
Heart rate	Absent	Slow	Over 100
Respiratory effort	Absent	Slow, irregular	Good, crying
Muscle tone	Limp (flaccid)	Some flexion of limbs	Active motion
Response to catheter in nostril (reflex and irritability)	No response	Grimace	Cough
Color	Pale	Body pink, extremities blue	Pink

Classification in Obstetrics and Gynecology

TABLE 17: Sher's grading of abruptio placentae (according to severity).

Grade I (retrospective)	*Not recognized clinically before delivery:* Small retroplacental hematoma discovered on maternal surface of placenta after delivery, no APH
Grade II	Mild vaginal bleeding, uterine tenderness and tetany, no fetal distress, no maternal shock
Grade III	Severe vaginal bleeding, uterine tenderness and tetany, fetal distress then death, maternal shock, according to DIC
IIIa	Without DIC
IIIb	With DIC

(APH: antepartum hemorrhage; DIC: disseminated intravascular coagulation).

TABLE 18: Zatuchni–Andros score.

	Score		
Factor	0	1	2
Parity	Primigravida	Multipara	–
Gestational age	39 weeks or more	38 weeks	37 weeks or less
Previous breech >2.5	None	One	Two or more
Estimated fetal weight (kg)	>3.5 kg	3–3.5 kg	<2 kg
Cervical dilatation (cm)	Less than 3	3	4 or more
Station of breech	–3 and above	–2	–1 or lower
Total score = 11			

Note: 3 or less: Low somatic cell score (LSCS); 5–11: Vaginal delivery; 4: Reassess in labor.

TABLE 19: Westin scoring system for selecting mode of delivery in breech.

	Score		
Parameters	0	1	2
Inlet, anteroposterior diameter	<11.5	11.5–12	>12
Inlet, transverse diameter	<12.5	12.5–13	>13
Outlet, anteroposterior diameter	<10.5	10.5–1	>11
Outlet, interspinous diameter	<10	10–10.5	>10.5
Intertuberous diameter	<10	10–11	>11
Sum of outlet	<32.5	32.5–33.5	>33.5
Estimated weight of fetus in grams	<1,500, >4,000	1,500–2,000 3,500–4,000	2,000–3,500
Presentation	Double footling	Complete breech, and single footling	Frank
Soft parts	Unripe cervix and rigid pelvic floor	Unripe cervix or rigid pelvic floor	Ripe cervix and relaxed pelvic floor
Previous deliveries	None	Uncomplicated breech	Uncomplicated breech
	Uncomplicated breech <2,000	2,000–3,000	>3,000
	• Uncomplicated head <3,000	Uncomplicated head <3,000	
	• Complicated delivery		

TABLE 20: Tennessee classification.

Hemolysis (any 2 or more)	• Peripheral smear with schistocytes and Burr cells • Serum bilirubin ≥1.2 mg/dL (20.52 μmol/L) • Low serum haptoglobin (≤25 mg/dL) or LDH ≥2 times the upper level of normal (based on laboratory-specific reference ranges) • Severe anemia unrelated to blood loss (severe anemia in pregnancy can be defined as hemoglobin level <8–10 g/dL, depending on the trimester)
Elevated liver enzymes	AST or ALT ≥2 times the upper level of normal (based on laboratory-specific reference ranges)
Low platelets	Platelet count <100,000 cells/μL

(ALT: alanine aminotransferase; AST: aspartate aminotransferase; LDH: lactate dehydrogenase)
Source: Ditisheim A, Sibai BM. Diagnosis and Management of HELLP Syndrome Complicated by Liver Hematoma. Clin Obstet Gynecol. 2017;60(1):190-7.

However, if any single score lies within the outlined box or, any two entries within the interrupted lines, Westin considered that low somatic cell score (LSCS) was indicated irrespective of the total score. However, a lot of the parameters in this system are based on pelvimetry other than clinical, which is not routinely done.

Diagnostic Criteria for HELLP Syndrome

Two classifications Tennessee (**Table 20**) and Mississippi (**Table 21**) are given for diagnosis of HELLP syndrome.

TABLE 21: Mississippi classification.

Class 1	Platelet count ≤50,000 cells/μL plus LDH >600 IU/L and AST or ALT ≥70 IU/L
Class 2	Platelet count >50,000 but ≤100,000 cells/μL plus LDH >600 IU/L and AST or ALT ≥70 IU/L
Class 3	Platelet count >100,000 but ≤150,000 cells/μL plus LDH >600 IU/L and AST or ALT ≥40 IU/L

Mississippi classification system is based on severity of thrombocytopenia.

CHAPTER 35

New FIGO Classification of Gynecological Cancers

Shelly Agarwal, Mayuri Ahuja

INTRODUCTION

Gynecological cancers not only are the most common cancers among women, but also constitute an important cause of mortality and morbidity. Hence, public awareness, cancer screening, staging, treatment stratification and prognostication are areas of global concern.

In India, the most common malignancy noted is that of breast cancer. As far as cervical cancer is concerned, its incidence is on a declining trend due to various preventive measures instituted, but still it is the second most common cancer among women. Important however is that many of our patients report in advanced stages which affects their prognosis and 5-year survival rate.

VULVAL CARCINOMA

Vulval carcinoma accounts to about 4% of all gynecological malignancies.

It includes cancer of labia majora, labia minora, clitoris, glands of Skene, Bartholin glands, and vestibular bulb. Among these, the most common vulval malignancy is associated with labial skin, while the least common ones are those of clitoris and vestibule glands.

The disease is commonly that of older women, usually postmenopausal. However, in recent years there has been a fall in the mean age of vulval cancers due to increase in human papillomavirus (HPV) infection worldwide.

Apart from increasing age and HPV infections, other common risk factors include smoking, skin conditions like lichen sclerosis, immunocompromised states like HIV, and various precancerous lesions of vulva.

Histological Types

Squamous cell carcinoma (SCC) is the most common histological type of vulval cancer, involving the labial skin. Two types of SCC have been observed: Keratinizing SCC and warty/basaloid SCC. Keratinizing SCC is common in older women and is likely associated with conditions like lichen sclerosis or differentiated vulval intraepithelial neoplasia. Warty/basaloid SCC is common in younger women and usually caused by persistent, highly oncogenic HPV virus.

The second most common vulval malignancy is vulval melanoma with an incidence of approximately 0.1 in 100,000 women. Melanomas have poor prognosis with a poor 5-year survival rate.

Other rare vulval tumors include:
- Basal cell carcinoma
- Verrucous carcinoma
- Adenocarcinoma related to extramammary Paget's disease
- Bartholin gland carcinoma (squamous/transitional cell carcinoma)
- Sarcomas

FIGO Staging of Vulval Cancer, 2021

International Federation of Gynaecology and Obstetrics (FIGO) vulval cancer staging,

2021, was derived from data analyses of vulval cancer patients collected from United States National Cancer Database between the years 2010 and 2017. This newer staging is simplified as compared to previous revisions and includes clinical examination, imaging and pathological examination of surgical specimen, and sentinel lymph node (SLN) biopsy **(Table 1)**.

Salient changes outlined in the revised FIGO staging 2021 are as follows:

- In the revised staging of carcinoma vulva, all nonmetastatic tumors are collectively assigned to stage I. Disease involvement of the lower urethra, vagina, and anus are assigned to stage II. Lymph node involvement is extensively substaged in stage III.
- There is a newer definition of depth of invasion. In stage I, depth of invasion serves as an important prognostic factor. In the updated classification, depth of invasion is to be measured from the basement membrane of the deepest, adjacent, dysplastic tumor-free rete peg to the deepest point of invasion. Earlier, the depth of invasion was defined as the measurement of the tumor from the epithelial–stromal junction of the adjacent-most superficial dermal papilla to the deepest point of invasion.
- Lymph node involvement should reflect that in cervical cancer staging; that is, it now includes both micro- and macrometastasis. Isolated tumor cells are not to be counted as lymph node metastasis.
- New staging allows cross-sectional imaging findings to be incorporated, just similar to that of cervical cancer staging. Although vulval cancer can be clinically visualized, still imaging plays a pivotal role in tumor extension, staging, and

TABLE 1: FIGO vulval cancer staging, 2021.

Stage	Description
Stage I	Tumor confined to vulva • *IA:* Tumor size ≤2 cm and stromal invasion ≤1 mm* • *IB:* Tumor size >2 cm and stromal invasion >1 mm
Stage II	Tumor of any size with extension to lower one third of vagina, lower one third of urethra, lower one-third of anus with nodes negative
Stage III	Tumor of any size with extension to upper part of adjacent perineal structures OR with any number of nonfixed, nonulcerated lymph nodes • *IIIA:* Tumor of any size with extension to upper one-third of vagina, upper one third of urethra, bladder mucosa, rectal mucosa OR with regional lymph nodes metastasis ≤5 mm • *IIIB:* Regional lymph nodes[†] metastasis >5 mm • *IIIC:* Regional lymph nodes[†] metastasis with extracapsular spread
Stage IV	Tumor of any size fixed to the bone OR fixed OR ulcerated regional lymph node[†] metastases or distant metastases • *IVA:* Disease fixed to pelvic bone OR fixed OR ulcerated regional lymph node[†] metastases • *IVB:* Distant metastases.

*Depth of invasion is to be measured from the basement membrane of the deepest, adjacent dysplastic tumor free rete peg to the deepest point of invasion.
†Regional lymph nodes include inguinal and femoral lymph nodes which are the first draining lymph nodes.

subsequent management guidelines. MRI is the imaging of choice to assess vulval anatomy. CT and PET-CT are commonly used to evaluate nodal and extranodal spread or distant metastases. It is not just important to send the specimen with correct orientation to the pathologist, but

also full cross section of each lymph node should be included.
- With increased association of HPV with vulval cancer and increasing incidence of the same, documentation of HPV status is recommended. It can be assessed by HPV molecular testing or by p16 block-type reactivity.
- This staging can be incorporated into all types of vulval cancers, other than melanoma.

Conclusion

The updated FIGO classification of vulval cancers, 2021 is a reliable, data-analyzed and validated classification of vulval cancers which is formulated from the data collected from the United States National Cancer Database over a period of 7 years (2010–2017). It is appropriate to use for staging and management of all types of vulval cancers, other than melanoma.

■ VAGINAL CARCINOMA

Primary vaginal cancer is a rare entity and constitutes only 1–2% of all female genital tract malignancies and only 10% of all vaginal malignant neoplasm. As majority of the vaginal neoplasms are metastatic, it is important to differentiate between primary and secondary vaginal neoplasms. Primary vaginal neoplasm is defined as the vaginal cancer where there is no clinical or histological evidence suggestive of any cervical or vulval cancer or prior history of these cancers within 5 years.

It is more common in elderly and postmenopausal women, though the incidence is increasing in younger women due to increase in persistent HPV infections. But in younger women, it is imperative to rule out cervical cancer as both are etiologically linked.

The most common site of vaginal cancer is the vaginal apex, usually involving the posterior wall. The spread is direct, lymphatic, and hematogenous. The tumor in upper vagina usually drains into the pelvic group of lymph nodes, while that in lower vagina drains to inguinal and femoral lymph nodes.

The histologic types include squamous carcinoma (90%) and adenocarcinoma (9–10%). Lymphomas, sarcomas, and melanomas are extremely rare. Diagnosis is confirmed by biopsy of the suspicious lesion.

FIGO Staging of Vaginal Cancer

Vaginal cancer is primarily clinically staged. FIGO update on vaginal cancer in 2021 puts forth the role of imaging in staging of vaginal cancers. It recommends that imaging should be used to better define tumor volume and extension of disease, wherever possible **(Table 2)**.

TABLE 2: FIGO staging of vaginal cancer.

Stage	Description
Stage I	Cancer limited to vaginal wall
Stage II	Cancer has spread to paravaginal tissues but has not extended to pelvic walls
Stage III	Cancer has spread up to the pelvic side walls: • Cancer has extended to pelvic wall and/or causing hydronephrosis or nonfunctioning kidney • Pelvic or inguinal lymph node metastasis
Stage IV	• Cancer has extended beyond true pelvis and/or has involved the mucosa of the bladder or rectum • Bullous edema as such does not permit a case to be allotted in stage IV • *IVA:* Tumor invades the bladder and/or rectal mucosa and/or direct extension beyond true pelvis • *IVB:* Spread to distant organs

Among the imaging techniques available, MRI plays a key role in determining tumor size and soft-tissue involvement due to its superior soft-tissue resolution, whereas PET-CT is most sensitive in detecting nodal disease or a recurrent disease.

- FIGO stage I is limited to vaginal wall. Its size can be smaller than 2 cm (T1a) or larger than 2 cm (T1b) according to TNM staging.
- FIGO stage 2 is when cancer has spread to paravaginal tissues but has not extended to pelvic walls. Again, according to TNM, it can be T2a (if size is <2 cm) or T2b (if size is >2 cm).
- FIGO stage III is when cancer has spread up to the pelvic side walls stage T3 in TNM classification. If lymph nodes are involved it is N1, according to TNM stage.
- FIGO stage IV is when cancer has extended beyond true pelvis and/or has involved the mucosa of the bladder or rectum. This is equivalent to T4 of TNM classification.

Conclusion

FIGO update on vaginal cancer in 2021 highlights the importance of imaging in adjunct to clinical staging for primary vaginal cancers, as clinical assessment at times can be challenging. This can then guide in individualized treatment with better prognostication and patient survival.

■ ENDOMETRIAL CARCINOMA

Endometrial cancer is primarily a disease of postmenopausal woman, usually occurring in the sixth and seventh decades of life.

In recent years, there has been an increase in the incidence of cancer endometrium. In western countries, the ratio of endometrial to cervical cancer is becoming almost 1:1, whereas in developing countries, cancer endometrium is reported as the third most common gynecological malignancy. In India, the incidence of endometrial to cervical cancer still remains low, the ratio ranging between 1:8 and 1:15.

This rising incidence could be both real and apparent. It can be attributed to various reasons such as increase in life expectancy, rising obesity, higher chances of diabetes and hypertension as the age advances, and even the use of menopause hormonal therapy in older women.

Classification of Endometrial Cancer

Based on biological and histological behavior, endometrial carcinoma can be broadly classified into two types: Type 1 and Type 2 **(Table 3)**.

TABLE 3: Classification of endometrial cancer.

Features	Type 1	Type 2
Age	Perimenopause	Postmenopause
Risk factor	*Occurs in*: • Nullipara • Obese • Unopposed estrogen	*Occurs in*: • Multipara • Nonobese • Nonestrogen dependent
Endometrial hyperplasia	Present	Absent
Histology and grading	Grade 1 and 2 endometrioid	Grade 3 endometrioid serous/clear
Her2/neu and p53 over expression	No	Yes
PTEN and *KRAS* mutations	Yes	No
Prognosis	Favorable	Not favorable

Cancer body uterus can be of various histological types. These histological varieties can prognosticate the survival of patients. The World Health Organization (WHO) (2014) has classified them as follows:
- *Endometrioid adenocarcinoma:*
  - Variant with squamous differentiation
  - Villo-glandular variant
  - Secretory variant
  - *Ciliated variant:* It is the most common microscopic type and accounts to about 80% of all cases and have a favorable prognosis.
- Serous carcinoma (5–10%)
- Clear cell adenocarcinoma (<5%)
- Mucinous adenocarcinoma (1–2%)
- SCC
- Mixed cell carcinoma
- *Undifferentiated carcinoma:*
  - Monomorphic type
  - Dedifferentiated type
- *Neuroendocrine tumors:*
  - Carcinoid tumors, well differentiated
  - Small cell, poorly differentiated
  - Large cell, poorly differentiated

Among these, majority of cancer endometrium (80%) are of endometrioid type and have favorable prognosis. Serous carcinomas, clear cell carcinomas, and grade 3 endometrioid carcinomas are aggressive tumors and have poor prognosis.

Molecular Typing

The Cancer Genome Atlas by the National Cancer Institute has proposed the molecular subtypes in cancer endometrium. These prognosticate the patient and help in planning therapy and have been incorporated in the updated molecular FIGO classification of endometrial carcinoma, 2023.

Current recommendations are to do a complete molecular typing (POLEmut, p53, MMRd, NSMP) in a biopsy or hysterectomy specimen. The details have been outlined below.

FIGO Staging of Carcinoma Endometrium

FIGO staging has recently been updated in 2023 since its previous publication in 2009. This updated 2023 classification considers both the pathology of tumor and molecular findings, as both are of prognostic value **(Table 4)**.
- *Important points to note are:* Surgical staging is important in cancer endometrium.

Type of surgery?
In early endometrial cancer, standard surgery is total hysterectomy with bilateral salpingo-oophorectomy with SLN biopsy with or without infracolic omentectomy.

Route of surgery?
Minimally invasive route (robotic/laparoscopic) is the preferred approach for early stages.

Sentinel lymph node biopsy or systematic lymph node dissection?
Sentinel lymph node biopsy is now an alternative to systemic lymphadenectomy as a part of surgical staging.

Role of infracolic omentectomy?
Infracolic omentectomy is reserved for specific subtypes like serous and undifferentiated carcinoma and carcinosarcoma. This is because the chance of omental micrometastasis is high in these conditions.
- The recent updated staging lays emphasis on the grade and histological type of tumor.

Low-grade endometrioid tumors (grades 1 and 2) are considered nonaggressive histological types, whereas high-grade endometrioid tumors (grade 3), serous, clear

Stage	Description
Stage I	Confined to uterine corpus and ovary • *IA:* Disease limited to endometrium OR nonaggressive histological type, i.e., low-grade: endometrioid type with invasion of less than half of Myometrium with no or focal lymphovascular space involvement (LVSI) OR good prognosis disease • *IA1:* Nonaggressive tumor limited to an endometrial polyp or confined to endometrium • *IA2:* Nonaggressive tumor involving less than half of myometrium with no or focal LVSI • *IA3:* Low-grade endometrioid carcinoma limited to uterus and ovary
Stage II	Invasion of cervical stroma with no extrauterine involvement or with substantial LVSI or aggressive histological type with myometrial invasion: • *IIA:* Invasion of cervical stroma with nonaggressive histological type • *IIB:* Substantial LVSI with nonaggressive histological type • *IIC:* Aggressive histological type with myometrial invasion

Stage III	Local and/or regional spread of tumor of any histologic subtype:
	• *IIIA:* Invasion of uterine serosa, adnexa, or both, by direct extension or metastasis
	• *IIIA1:* Spread to ovary or fallopian tube (other than criterion of stage IA3)
	• *IIIA2:* Involvement of uterine subserosa or spread to uterine serosa
	• *IIIB:* Metastasis or direct spread to vagina and/or to the parametria or pelvic peritoneum
	• *IIIB1:* Metastasis or direct spread to vagina and /or to the parametria
	• *IIIB2:* Metastasis or direct spread to pelvic peritoneum
	• *IIIC:* Metastasis to pelvic or para-aortic lymph nodes or both
	• *IIIC1:* Metastasis to pelvic lymph nodes.
	   – *IIIC1i:* Micrometastasis
	   – *IIIC1ii:* Macrometastasis
	• *IIIC2:* Metastasis to para-aortic lymph nodes up to renal vessels, with or without metastasis to pelvic lymph nodes
	   – *IIIC2i:* Micrometastasis
	   – *IIIC2ii:* Macrometastasis

Stage IV	Spread to bladder mucosa and/or intestinal mucosa and/or distant metastasis: • *IVA:* Spread to bladder mucosa and/or intestinal/bowel mucosa • *IVB:* Abdominal peritoneal metastasis beyond the pelvis • *IVC:* Distant metastasis, including metastasis to extra or intra-abdominal lymph nodes above the renal vessels, lungs, liver, brain, and/or brain

TABLE 4: FIGO staging of endometrial cancer, 2023.

cell, undifferentiated, mixed, mesonephric-like, gastrointestinal mucinous-type carcinomas and carcinosarcomas all are aggressive tumors. Grading of tumor is dependent on the proportion of solid component: Grade 1 (5 or less), grade 2 (6–50%), and grade 3 (>50%). For high-risk endometrioid tumors, molecular staging is found to be extremely beneficial for risk stratification, prognostication, and treatment guidance and should be done.

Stage I

This stage now includes tumors limited to endometrial polyps or disease confined to the uterus or low-grade endometrioid endometrial cancer limited to uterus and ovary, without LVSI. The rationale behind the same is that they all have good prognosis. There is sufficient evidence which suggests that low-grade endometrioid carcinomas limited to uterus and ovary have good

prognosis and do not require any adjuvant therapy. However, it is very important to distinguish between tumors which will fall into stage IA1 and tumors into stage IIIA1. FIGO clearly states that the tumor should be classified into stage IA1 only if it meets the following criteria:
- Only unilateral ovarian involvement without capsule invasion/rupture
- Not more than 50% of myometrial invasion
- Involvement of extensive/substantial LVSI, which means less than five vessels are involved
  (To note: Extensive/substantial LVSI is when five or more vessels are involved)
- Absence of any additional metastasis

Stage II

Marked change has been observed in stage II. It takes into consideration histology and grade of the tumor, along with its extent. LVSI has emerged as an important and strong indicator for staging and prognosticating the disease.

Stage III

- Revised staging of stage III enables prognostication and treatment decision-making.
- Subclassification of stage IIIA into stages IIIA1 and A2 reflects the tumor behavior.
- Stage IIIB1 involves direct spread to vagina and/or to parametria. This is equivalent to previously classified stage IIIB.
- Stage IIIB2 indicates involvement of pelvic peritoneum which was previously in stage IV. This change guides in decision-making in terms of whether a surgical or nonsurgical method should be chosen as a first-line treatment modality for patients with advanced stage disease.
- Another mention is the terms micro-metastasis and macrometastasis to lymph nodes in stage IIIC. Macrometastasis is defined when tumor cells are >2 mm; micrometastasis refers as tumor cells are 0.2–2 mm or >200 cells, and isolated tumor cells are ≤0.2 or ≤200 cells. This substaging reflects better prognosis in patients who have micrometastasis as compared to those who have macro-metastasis.

Stage IV

- There is addition of an extra substage IVB which suggests extraperitoneal metastasis.
- Peritoneal metastasis which does not spread beyond pelvic brim is now classified as stage IIIB2.

FIGO Staging with Molecular Classification

- Molecular classification in FIGO staging is written by letter "m".
- FIGO states that addition of molecular subtype to staging will improve prognostication. Therefore, complete molecular classification (p53, POLEmut, MMRd, NSMP) should be added wherever feasible.
- This molecular classification can be done on biopsy specimen itself. Thereafter, repeat subtyping is not required on hysterectomy specimen.
- POLEmut typing is associated with good prognosis.
- MMRd and NSMP are associated with intermediate prognosis.
- p53 is associated with poor prognosis.
- In case molecular classification reveals POLEmut or p53 in stages I and II, then FIGO stage is modified in early stage of disease. On the other hand, if molecular subtyping is suggestive of MMRd and NSMP, they do not modify the staging in early stage of disease. So, in case there

Stage designation	Molecular findings in stages I and II after surgical staging
Stage IAm$_{POLEmut}$	POLEmut endometrial carcinoma limited to uterine corpus or with cervical extension, regardless of the degree of LVSI or histological type
Stage IICm$_{p53abn}$	p53abn endometrial carcinoma limited to uterine corpus with any degree of myometrial invasion, with or without cervical invasion, regardless of the degree of LVSI or histological type

TABLE 5: FIGO staging with molecular classification.

is a POLEmut mutation in a patient with endometrial carcinoma, either limited to uterine corpus or with cervical extension, regardless of the degree of LVSI or histological type, it will be classified as stage IAm$_{POLEmut}$. On the other hand, if there is a *p53* mutation, endometrial cancer is limited to uterine corpus with any degree of myometrial invasion, with or without cervical invasion, regardless of the degree of LVSI or histological type, then the staging is upstaged to stage IICm$_{p53abn}$.

- FIGO surgical stages III and IV are not modified by molecular classification; however, molecular classification should still be recorded **(Table 5)**.

Conclusion

The purpose of this revised FIGO endometrial cancer is to incorporate the essential research evidence to prognosticate and to decide treatment modality.

■ CERVICAL CANCER

Cervical cancer is the fourth most common cancer for women across the world. It is still the leading cause of cancer-related death in low-income countries. In the year 2020, cervical cancer burden was estimated to be 6,04,100 new cases globally, with 3,41,831 deaths attributed to it.

In India, it is the second most common cancer amongst women. Major risk factors include HPV infection with high-risk oncogenic strain, early marriage, multiple pregnancies, genital hygiene, poor nutritional status, smoking, and unsafe sexual practices like multiple sexual partners.

Since cervical cancer is largely preventable, the WHO has proposed cervical cancer elimination program, by 2030. It outlines three key steps:

1. 90% of girls fully vaccinated with the HPV vaccine by 15 years of age
2. 70% of women should be screened for cervical cancer
3. 90% of women identified with cervical disease should receive treatment

Five-year survival rate for a cancer patient depends upon appropriate management guidelines, which in turn are dependent upon staging of the disease and various prognostic factors. Earlier, the staging done for cancer cervix was only clinical staging. However recently, in 2018, FIGO has updated its cervical cancer staging which hereby not only includes clinical staging but also lays emphasis on cross sectional imaging and pathology.

Updated FIGO Staging of Cervical Cancer, 2018

FIGO has updated the cervical cancer staging in 2018. The basic rationale to bring about this update is to optimize stage-based treatment and to prognosticate the disease according to its stage and substage **(Table 6)**.

CHANGES IN FIGO CLASSIFICATION

- In stage IA, only depth of lesion is taken into consideration. The width of lesion

TABLE 6: Updated FIGO staging of cervical cancer, 2018.

Stage	FIGO 2009	FIGO 2018
Stage I	*IA:* ≤5 mm depth and ≤7 mm wide • *IA1:* ≤3 mm depth • *IA2:* >3 mm and not >5 mm depth *IB:* >5 mm depth • *IB1:* ≤4 cm maximum diameter • *IB2:* >4 cm maximum diameter	*IA:* ≤5 mm depth • *IA1:* <3 mm depth • *IA2:* >3 and ≤5 mm *IB:* >5 mm depth • *IB1:* ≤2 cm maximum diameter • *IB2:* >2 and ≤4 cm • *IB3:* >4 cm maximum diameter
Stage II	Beyond the uterus but not involving lower one-third of vagina or pelvic side walls *IIA:* Upper two-thirds of vagina • *IIA1:* Upper two-third of vagina and tumor size ≤4 cm in maximum diameter • *IIA2:* Upper two-third of vagina and tumor size >4 cm in maximum diameter *IIB:* Parametrial invasion	Beyond the uterus but not involving lower one-third of vagina or pelvic side walls *IIA:* Upper two-thirds of vagina • *IIA1:* Upper two-third of vagina and tumor size ≤4 cm in maximum diameter • *IIA2:* Upper two-third of vagina and tumor size >4 cm in maximum diameter *IIB:* Parametrial invasion
Stage III	Lower vagina, pelvic sidewalls, and ureters *IIIA:* Lower one of vagina *IIIB:* Pelvic side walls	Lower vagina, pelvic sidewalls, ureters, and lymph nodes. *IIIA:* Lower one-third of vagina *IIIB:* Pelvic side walls *IIIC:* Pelvic and para-aortic lymph node involvement • *IIIC1:* Pelvic lymph node involvement • *IIIC2:* Para-aortic lymph node involvement
Stage IV	Adjacent and distant organ metastasis • *IVA:* Rectal or bladder involvement • *IVB:* Distant organ outside pelvis	Adjacent and distant organ metastasis • *IVA:* Rectal or bladder involvement • *IVB:* Distant organ outside pelvis

has been removed. This is to reduce potential artifact error.
- Substaging for stage IB has changed to IB1, IB2, and IB3. This new substaging provides guide to management. For example, in patients with FIGO stage IB1 (2018) who require fertility sparing, trachelectomy can be offered, whereas FIGO stage IB2 (2018) tumors are usually not eligible for the same. Evidence also suggests that there is a two-fold increased survival rate for patients with stage B1 as compared with stage B2.
- There has been no change in stage II and stages IIIA and IIIB between 2009 and 2018 FIGO staging of cervical cancer, but a new substage has been added in stage III, that is, stage IIIC3. This substage indicates pelvic and para-aortic involvement. There is sufficient data which suggests that lymph node involvement has prognostic implications and is associated with a decreased 5-year survival rate and increased chances of recurrence. In other words, lymph node involvement will upstage the disease.
- Cross sectional imaging has been included in the recent classification. Its role has been utilized in identifying tumor size as well as suspected lymphadenopathy. A meta-analysis compared the diagnostic performance of FDG PET/CT, MRI, and

CT for nodal involvement. It reported that FDG PET/CT had sensitivity of 82% and specificity of 95%, CT had sensitivity of 50% and specificity of 92% and MRI had sensitivity of 56% and specificity of 91%, respectively. To summarize, FDG PET/CT has the best overall diagnostic performance for depicting nodal disease and pelvic and para-aortic lymph node involvement. The size of the lymph node is one of the main criteria used to identify lymph node involvement. It has been documented that a lymph node of size >8 mm in short axis and those which have a rounded, spiculated, or lobulated contour and have similar signal intensity to that of primary cervical tumor are suspicious on MRI and CT and fall into stage IIIC1 or IIIC2.

Conclusion

Updated FIGO classification of cervical cancer, 2018 aims at improving prognostication, thereby revisiting the treatment options with improved patient outcomes.

■ OVARIAN CARCINOMA

In 2014, FIGO Committee for Gynecologic Oncology revised the staging of ovarian cancer, incorporating ovarian, fallopian, and peritoneal cancer into the same classification. The reason behind this change is largely evidence based. It was observed that as large as 80% of tumors which were initially classified as high-grade serous carcinomas (HGSC) of the ovary or peritoneum probably had their origin from the fimbrial end of the fallopian tube. Thus, cancers of ovary and fallopian tube and peritoneal cancers should be considered collectively. Since majority of these are HGSC, they can be referred to as "serous carcinoma". It is however suggested that the primary site (ovary, fallopian tube, or peritoneum) should be designated, wherever possible and where it is not possible, it should be listed as "undesignated".

Primary Site

Ovarian epithelial tumors can either originate from Mullerian inclusions developed below the ovarian surface or within endometriotic tissue in the ovary. Histologically, ovarian neoplasm can be low-grade serous carcinomas, mucinous tumors, low-grade endometrioid carcinomas, clear cell carcinomas, seromucinous tumors, and others (Brenner, undifferentiated, and mixed epithelial tumors).

Fallopian tube carcinomas arise in the distal fallopian tube and the majority of these are high-grade serous carcinomas. Serous tubal intraepithelial carcinoma (STIC) lesions are the precursors of high-grade serous tumors which have been found in tubal epithelium.

The peritoneum is the most common site for metastasis of ovarian and fallopian tube cancers. So, after excluding tubal or ovarian site of origin, malignancies that appear to arise primarily on the peritoneum are considered as primary peritoneal malignancies. These peritoneal tumors are thought to arise in endosalpingiosis.

Types I and II Epithelial Ovarian Cancer

According to the tissue from where epithelial ovarian cancer (EOC) originate, they are classified as types 1 and type 2 **(Table 7)**.

FIGO Classification of Ovarian Cancer

The updated FIGO staging system combines the classification for ovarian, fallopian tube, and peritoneum cancer **(Table 8)**.

The salient features of the revised FIGO classification of ovarian cancer are:
- Staging should be based on findings mainly after surgical exploration. Imaging

helps to identify intra-abdominal spread, but still staging is primarily surgical.
- Stage IC is divided into three substages: IC1—surgical spill, IC2—capsule ruptured before surgery or on ovarian or fallopian tube surface, and IC3—when malignant cells in the ascites or peritoneal washing
- Stage IIC has been eliminated.
- Revision of the stage IIIC which is based on spread to retroperitoneal lymph nodes

TABLE 7: Types of epithelial ovarian cancer.

Type 1	Type 2
Arise from Müllerian inclusion or surface epithelium of ovary	Arise from the fimbrial end of fallopian tube or peritoneum
Slow-growing tumors, usually evolving from low-grade precursor lesion	High-grade tumors which are rapidly progressing
Less common than type 2	More common than type 1
Not associated with *BRCA1* and *p53* mutations	Associated with *BRCA1* and *p53* mutations

TABLE 8: Updated FIGO staging system of ovarian cancer.

Stage	Description

Stage I	Tumor confined to ovaries or fallopian tube:
	• *IA:* Tumor limited to one ovary (capsule intact) or fallopian tube surface; no malignant cells in the ascites or peritoneal washing
	• *IB:* Tumor limited to both ovaries (capsule intact) or fallopian tubes; no malignant cells in the ascites or peritoneal washing
	• *IC:* Tumor limited to one or both ovaries or tumor fallopian tube with any of the following:
	  – *IC1:* Surgical spill
	  – *IC2:* Capsule ruptured before surgery or on ovarian or fallopian tube surface
	  – *IC3:* Malignant cells in the ascites or peritoneal washing

Stage II	Tumor involves one or both ovaries or fallopian tubes with pelvic extension (below pelvic brim) or peritoneal cancer • *IIA:* Extension and/or implants on uterus and/or fallopian tubes/or ovaries • *IIB:* Extension to other pelvic intraperitoneal tissues

Stage III	Tumor involves one or both ovaries or fallopian tube, or peritoneal cancer, with cytologically or histologically confirmed spread to the peritoneum outside the pelvis and/or metastasis to the retroperitoneal lymph nodes
	IIIA1: Positive retroperitoneal lymph nodes only (cytologically or histologically proven)
	  – *IIIA1(i):* Metastasis <10 mm in greatest dimension
	  – *IIIA1(ii):* Metastasis >10 mm in greatest dimension
	• *IIIA2:* Microscopic extrapelvic (above the pelvic brim) peritoneal involvement with or without positive retroperitoneal lymph node metastasis
	• *IIIB:* Macroscopic peritoneal metastases beyond the pelvis up to 2 cm in greatest dimension with or without metastasis to the retroperitoneal lymph nodes
	• *IIIC:* Macroscopic peritoneal metastasis beyond the pelvis > 2 cm in greatest dimension with or without metastasis to the retroperitoneal lymph nodes (includes extension of tumor to capsule of liver and spleen without parenchymal involvement of either organ)

Stage IV	Distant metastasis excluding peritoneal metastasis: • *IVA:* Pleural effusion with positive cytology • *IVB:* Parenchymal metastasis and metastasis to extra-abdominal organs (including inguinal lymph nodes and lymph nodes outside of the abdominal cavity)

alone and subsequent substaging as it significantly changes the survival
- Retroperitoneal lymph nodes involvement must be biopsy proven.
- Stage IVB includes involvement of inguinal lymph nodes.
- Extension of tumor to omentum, spleen, and liver should be differentiated from isolated parenchymal spleen or liver metastasis
- Histological type of tumor should be recorded as it is an important prognostication factor.

SUGGESTED READING

1. Adams TS, Rogers LJ, Cuello MA. Cancer of the vagina: 2021 update. Int J Gynecol Obstet. 2021;155(Suppl. 1):19-27.
2. Adhikari P, Vietje P, Mount S. Premalignant and malignant lesions of the vagina. Diagn Histopathol. 2016;23:28-34.
3. Berek JS, Friedlander M, Hacker NF (Eds). Epithelial ovarian, fallopian tube, and peritoneal cancer. In: Berek and Hacker's Gynecologic Oncology, 7th edition. Philadelphia: Wolters Kluwer Health; 2020.
4. Berek JS, Matias-Guiu X, Creutzberg C, Fotopoulou C, Gaffney D, Kehoe E, et al. FIGO staging of endometrial cancer: 2023. Int J Gynecol Obstet. 2023;162:383-94.
5. Choi HJ, Ju W, Myung SK, Kim Y. Diagnostic performance of computer tomography, magnetic resonance imaging, and positron emission tomography or positron emission tomography/computer tomography for detection of metastatic lymph nodes in patients with cervical cancer: meta-analysis. Cancer Sci. 2010;101(6):1471-9.
6. Hellman K, Silfversward C, Nilsson B, Hellstrom AC, Frankendal B, Pettersson F. Primary carcinoma of the vagina: factors influencing the age at diagnosis. The Radiumhemmet series 1956–96. Int J Gynecol Cancer. 2004;14:491-501.
7. Jhingran A. Updates in the treatment of vaginal cancer. Int J Gynecol Cancer. 2022; 32(3):344-51.
8. Jonathan B, Malte R, Sean K, Lalit K, Michael F. Cancer of the ovary, fallopian tube, and peritoneum:2021 update. Int J Gynecol Obstet. 2021;155:61-85.
9. Kang YJ, Smith M, Barlow E, Coffey K, Hacker N, Canfell K. Vulvar cancer in high-income countries: increasing burden of disease. Int J Cancer. 2017;141:2174-86.
10. Konar H, Dutta DC. Genital malignancy. In: DC Dutta's Textbook of Gynecology. New Delhi: Jaypee Brothers Medical Publishers; 2020. p. 297.
11. Mehrotra R, Yadav K. Cervical Cancer: Formulation and Implementation of Govt of India Guidelines for Screening and Management. Indian J Gynecol Oncol. 2022;20(1):4.
12. Olawaiye AB, Cotler J, Cuello MA, Bhatla N, Okamoto A, Wilailak S, et al. FIGO staging for carcinoma of the vulva: 2021 revision. Int J Gynecol Obstet. 2021;155:43-7.
13. Olawaiye AB, Cuello MA, Rogers LJ. Cancer of the vulva: 2021 update. Int J Gynecol Obstet. 2021;155(Suppl 1):7-18.
14. Prat J. FIGO Committee on Gynecologic Oncology. Staging classification for the ovary, fallopian tube and peritoneum. Int J Gynecol Obstet. 2014;124:1-5.
15. Ruan J, Zhang Y, Ren H. Meta-analysis of PET/CT detect lymph nodes metastases of cervical cancer. Open Med (Wars). 2018;13(1):436-42.
16. Salib MY, Russell JHB, Stewart VR, Sudderuddin SA, Barwick TD, Rockall AG, et al. 2018 FIGO Staging Classification for Cervical Cancer. RadioGraphics. 2020; 40(6):1807-22.
17. Siegel RL, Miller KD, Jemal A. Cancer statistics, 2020. CA Cancer J Clin. 2020;70:7-30.
18. Tewari KS, Agarwal A, Pathak A, Ramesh A, Parikh B, Singhal M, et al. Meeting report, "First Indian national conference on cervical cancer management—expert recommendations and identification of barriers to implementation." Gynaecol Oncol Res Pract. 2018;5:5.
19. Virarkar M, Vulasala SS, Daoud T, Javadi S, Lall C, Bhosale P. Vulvar Cancer: 2021 Revised FIGO Staging System and the Role of Imaging. Cancers (Basel). 2022;14(9):2264.

Index

Page numbers followed by *b* refer to box, *f* refer to figure, *fc* refer to flowchart, and *t* refer to table.

A

Abdomen 173
  acute 263
  fetal 292
  maternal 77
  pain 254, 288, 290
  right lower 288
Abdominal cavity 167, 174
Abdominal circumference 302, 402
Abdominal compartment syndrome 422
Abdominal examination 13, 52
Abdominal exercises 454
Abdominal hysterectomy 151
Abdominal incision
  advantages of 198*t*
  disadvantages of 198*t*
  types of 195
Abdominal Koch's 198
Abdominal palpation 81
Abdominal radical trachelectomy 273
Abdominal surgeries 166
Abdominal wall 167, 172-174, 191
  anatomy 194
    of anterior 194
  blood supply of anterior 196*t*
  preparation of 150
  vessel injury, manage 177
  with breathing, mobility of 14
Abdominal wound closure 213
Abdominopelvic masses, causes of 14
Abnormal uterine bleeding 12, 151, 179, 222, 252, 255, 256, 339, 396
  acute 252
  causes of 252, 256, 257
  chronic 252
  classification for 462, 463*t*
  medical management of nonstructural 255
  polyp category of 254
Abortion 6, 104, 366, 442
  following fetal anomaly 447
  incomplete 151
  septic 261
  therapeutic 330
Abortus 400
  hydropic degeneration of 233
  karyotype of 231
Abruptio placenta 111, 228, 240, 401
Absolute fetal contraindications 90
Absolute maternal contraindications 90
Abstinence 346
Accidental bladder injury, diagnosis of 162
Acetaminophen 411
Acidosis 37
Acoustic stimulation 41, 99
Acquired immunodeficiency syndrome 369
Acromegaly 326, 426
Acyclovir 345
Adenocarcinoma 274, 471
  component 274
Adenomyosis 12, 249, 253, 258, 323, 398
  made, diagnosis of 254
Adequate amniotic fluid 32
Adhesions 290, 212
  filmy 285
  risk of 177*t*
Adhesives, topical 210, 212, 212*f*
Adjuvant radiotherapy, postoperative 270
Admission
  date of 393
  test, role of 53
Adnexal mass 290
Adrenal hyperplasia, congenital 294
Adrenal insufficiency 426
Adrenocorticotropic hormone stimulation test 220
Advanced assisted reproductive technology 428
Advanced cardiac life support 123, 413, 414
  algorithm of 413*fc*
Advanced-stage disease, treatment for 267
Advisory Committee on Immunization Practices 19
Agonist protocol 433
Air
  bubbles 284
  embolism 185
  replaces fluid 126*f*
Airway 121, 414
  and breathing 123
  protect 113
Alanine aminotransferase 470
Alcohol-related illnesses 427
Alfentanil 408
Alloimmune 106
Allylestrenol 323
Alpha-fetoprotein 223, 266
Altruistic surrogacy 429
Ambu bag
  with reservoir 131*f*
  without reservoir 131*f*
Ambulatory analgesia 408
Amendments 374
Amenorrhea 234, 267, 353, 365
  primary 394
  secondary 394
  traumatica 183
Amniocentesis 100, 103-105, 228
  hazards of 104
  indications for 103
Amniotic fluid 98, 225
  embolism 113, 412
  microscopic examination of 225
  presence of 298
  volume 32
Amnisure test 225
Amoxicillin 344, 346, 347
Ampicillin 338, 343, 346
Ampullary pregnancy ruptures 241
Anal sphincter, internal 467
Analgesia 411
Anaphylaxis 114
Anastrozole 294

Anatomical pelvic axis 46
Androgen excess society 294
Android 47
Androstenedione 219
Anejaculation 430
Anemia 230, 234, 245, 318, 341, 402
    mild 230
    moderate 230
    refractory 231
    severe 230
    types of 230
Anencephaly 67, 227, 237, 237f, 238, 301
    develop 237
    diagnoses of 237
Anesthesia 185, 189
    depth of 174
    epidural 97, 406
    general 152, 406
    local 104
Anesthetic complications 176, 412
Anesthetic techniques 406, 407
Aneuploidy 3
    preimplantation genetic testing for 101
    screening 23
Angiotensin receptor blockers 423
Angiotensin-converting enzyme inhibitors 423
Anisotropy index 215
Anomaly 237, 405
Anovulatory infertility 328
Antagonist protocol 433
Anteflexion 15
Antenatal anti-D prophylaxis 7
Antenatal risk factors 128t
Antenatal scans 76
Antenatal sonogram 290, 292
Antenatal sonographic scan 293
Antenatal visit
    number of 2
    second 2
    third 2
Antepartum 8, 342
    period 341
Antepartum fetal surveillance
    initiation of 29
    normal 29
    techniques 29
    tests 33
Antepartum fetal test 29
    indications for 29, 29b
    management of abnormal 33

Anterior abdominal wall 174
    anatomy 199f
    muscles 194f
Anthropoid 47, 79
Antiandrogenic effects, pills with 358
Antiandrogens 326, 336
Antianxiety agents 337
Antiarrhythmic therapy 125
Antibiotic
    prophylaxis 66, 185
    role of 185
    therapy 427
Anticardiolipin antibodies 232, 401
Anticoagulant use, indications of 316
Anticoagulation 343
    therapy 175
Anticonvulsant therapy, principles of 314
Anti-D
    administration 98
    immunoglobulin 6
    prophylaxis 236
Antidepressants, tricyclic 326
Antidiuretic hormone 424
Antiestrogenic action 362
Antifibrinolytic agents 258
Antifungal preparations 339
Antihypertensives 311
Antimicrobial agent 203
Anti-Müllerian hormone 219, 220
Antioxidants, use of 432
Antiphospholipid
    antibody syndrome 316, 401
    syndrome 232
Antiprogesterone 255
Antiprogestins 337
Antiretroviral therapy
    highly active 105
    triple-drug 343
Aortic compression, external 116
Aortic dissection 412
Apgar score 96, 464, 468t
Aplastic 463
Aqueous crystalline penicillin 346
Arm
    delivery of posterior 109
    extraction, posterior 110f
    movement for releasing 74f
Aromatase inhibitors 259, 294
Arterial disease, peripheral 198
Arterial perfusion, twin-reversed 245

Artery 196
Asherman's syndrome 163, 180, 183, 285, 325, 340
    management of 183, 285
Aspartate aminotransferase 470
Aspermia 396
Asphyxia 77
    perinatal 126
Aspirator, preparation of 170
Assisted breech delivery 69, 70
Assisted delivery, failure of 91
Assisted reproductive technology 324, 396, 428
    and surrogacy 428
    banks 434
    clinic 434
    and banks, registration of 434
Assisted vaginal birth 95
    risk of 89
Assisted vaginal delivery 86, 124
Asthenospermia 396
Atherosclerosis 250
Atosiban 318, 341
Atrial fibrillation 35, 316
Atrial thrombus, left 316
Atropine 31, 35
Automated external defibrillator 122, 413
Auvard speculum 165f
Ayre's spatula 168, 168f
Azithromycin 343, 346
Azoospermia 382, 396, 429
    nonobstructive 430
    obstructive 430

B

Backward flip 98
Bacterial vaginosis 338
Bacteriuria, asymptomatic 6, 402
Bad obstetric history 400
Bag-and-mask ventilation 128, 135
Balfour retractor 167, 167f
Bandl's ring 240
Barium enema 224
Barr bodies 168
Bartholin gland 471
    carcinoma 471
Basal body temperature method 351
Basal cell carcinoma 471
Basal-bolus regimen 312

Index

Basic life support 121, 413
  steps of 122
Beck's sign 82
Bed rest 411
Benzathine penicillin 346
Bereavement 446
Beta-agonist 317
Beta-human chorionic
      gonadotropin 24,
      233, 266
Betamethasone phosphate 321
Bicarbonate 424
Binovular twin 244
Biochemical hyperandrogenism
      219
Biophysical profile 468*t*
  components of 32
  modified 33
Biopsy 221
Biopsychosocial model 438
Biparietal diameter 302
Bipolar cautery instruments 189
Bipolar electrosurgical resection
      system 182
Bird's modification 93*f*
Birth
  asphyxia 80, 91
  companion 54
  corpora conduplicata 84, 85
  defects, types of 405
  preparation for 127, 129
Bisacromial diameter 69
Bishop scoring system 468*t*
Bitrochanteric diameter 69
Bladder
  injury 163
  neck and clitoris, level of 171
  separation of 151
  sound 162, 162*f*
  wall 290
Blake's uterine curette 151
Blastocyst 101
Blastomere
  analysis 101
  single 101
Bleeding 289
  amount of 11
  cause of 116
  irregular 353
  on oral pills, manage
      breakthrough 358
  per vaginum 299
  postmenopausal 179, 252
  postprocedural 105
Bleomycin 277

Blood
  chemistry normal values 455
  gas 457
  oxygen saturation,
      peripheral 118
  transfusion, indications for
      340, 341*b*
Blood loss
  minimal 194, 197
  reduction of 353
  replace 419
Blood pressure 51, 112, 118
  control 112
  improvement in 421
Blood sugar 228, 229
  fasting 230
  random 240
Blood urea 240
  nitrogen 415
Bloodborne viral infections,
      screening for 105
B-Lynch suture 117
Body
  habitus 194
  potassium, total 422
Body mass index 7, 176, 359, 431
  effect of 176
  elevated 294
  high 176
  low 176
Bogota bag 213
Bone
  injuries 77
  marrow aspiration 231
  shortened long 27
Bonney clamp 157*f*
Bonney myomectomy clamp 157
Bowel dysfunction 256
Bowel injury 176
  management of 176
  risk of 176
Bowel perforation 292
Bradycardia 35, 105, 409
Brainstorm 449
Braun–Stadler episiotomy
      scissors 154, 155*f*
Braxton hicks version 99
BRCA-2 genes 265
Breast
  cancer 265, 360
  disease 361
  examination 9, 13
  malignancy, history of 265
  tenderness 357

Breastfeeding 366
Breathing 111, 414
Breech
  aftercoming head of 90
  complete 67
  deliver aftercoming head of 72
  extraction 69
  fetuses, preterm 76
  in labor, management of 69
  infant 77
  irregular 75
  mode of delivery in 464, 469*t*
  vaginal delivery 76
Breech delivery 71, 77, 78
  during 73
  spontaneous 69
Breech presentation 67, 76, 77
  antenatal management of 68
  diagnosed 68
  etiology of 67
  management of 69
  varieties of 67
Bregma 48
Breisky–Navratil
      retractor 166, 166*f*
Brenner tumors 264
Bromocriptine 326
Brow posterior position 83*f*
Brow presentation, etiology of 82
Bullous edema 473
Bupivacaine 260
Burns–Marshall
  method 70
  technique 71*f*
Busch episiotomy scissors 155*f*
Busch scissors 154
Butoconazole 339
Buttock
  arrest of 73*t*
  at brim, arrest of 72*t*
  management of arrest of 72
  pain 217

C

Cabergoline 259, 326
  contraindications of 327
Caffeine 411
Calcium 337
  channel blockers 317
Caldwell–Moloy classification 46
Calendar method 351
Camper's fascia 276
Cancellous bone 82

Cancer
　antigen 125 223
　endometrium, incidence of 474
　screening 471
Cannula 172, 173f
　insert 170
　large-bore 111
Cannulation sheaths 179
Caput succedaneum 404
Carbamazepine 314
Carbetocin 118
Carbon dioxide 173, 181, 184
Carboprost 116
Carcinoembryonic antigen 223
Carcinoma cervix 168, 270, 271
　primary management of 271
　risk factors for 271
　staging of 271
　treatment of 273
Carcinoma endometrium 268, 269, 475
　staging of 268
　treatment of 269
Carcinoma ovary, history of 265
Carcinosarcoma 270
Cardiac arrest 120, 121, 412
　cause of 124, 412
　role of fetal assessment during 124
Cardiac contractility 426
Cardiac disease 113, 316, 412
　severe 175
Cardiac output 420, 421
　maintain 415
Cardinal ligaments 272
Cardiopulmonary resuscitation 120, 122, 412, 413
Cardiotocograph machine 34f
Cardiotocographic monitoring 84
Cardiotocography 31, 39t, 40
　management of
　　abnormal 39
　　nonreassuring 39
　trace
　　recordkeeping of 40
　　speed of 35
　use of 34
Cardiovascular disease
　multiple risk factors for 354
　risk 220
Cardiovascular evaluation 326
Cardiovascular system 426
Carnitine 432

Catheter, type of 432
Cefotaxime 338, 343
Cefotetan 338
Cefoxitin 338
Ceftizoxime 338
Ceftriaxone 338, 344, 346
Cell
　carcinoma, mixed 475
　large 475
　obtained 101, 104
Cell-free DNA screening test, disadvantages of 3
Centchroman 348, 361, 361f
　binds 361
Central nervous system 20, 291
Central neuraxial analgesia 406
Central precocious puberty 394
Central venous pressure 415
Cephalexin 346
Cephalhematoma 91, 94, 404
Cephalic application 87, 88
Cephalic curve 86
Cephalic version, techniques for external 98
Cephalocele 227, 238
Cephalopelvic disproportion 55, 75, 239
Cephalosporin 346
Cephalotribe 156f
Cerclage 293
Cerebellar diameter 229
Cerebral artery
　Doppler, normal middle 307f
　middle 229, 307
Cerebral hemispheres 237
Cerebral hypoxia 111
Cerebroplacental ratio 402
Cerebrospinal fluid 75, 237, 291
Cerebrovascular accidents 366, 369
Cerebrovascular stroke 360
Cervical
　canal 161, 163, 168
　cap 348, 356f
　carcinoma 224, 271f
　dilatation 51, 57
　dilation 42
　dilators, types of 151
　ectopic pregnancy, diagnose 242
　examination 37
　index 293
　injury 161

　intraepithelial neoplasia 353, 359
　laceration 185, 293
　leiomyomas 157
　malignancy 442
　os, internal 304
　perforation 161
　position 468
　score 459
　screening 442
　secretions 225
　spine 76
　stenosis 102
　tears 152
　tumor, primary 480
Cervical cancer 180, 273, 274, 471, 478
　cytological screening for 168
　incidence of 271
　screening 442
　staging of 472, 478, 479t
　treatment of early-stage 271
Cervical consistency 468
　index 226
Cervical fibroid 256, 257f
　large 198
Cervical incompetence 227, 232, 293f
　causes of 293
　treatment of 293
Cervical length 303
　and dilatation 226
Cervical punch biopsy 442
　forceps 168, 169f
Cervicitis, severe 102
Cervix 149, 153, 157, 161, 165, 272, 360
　dilated 99
　incomplete dilatation of 75
　lymphatic drainage of 274
　preparation of 235
　technique of dilating 152
Cesarean delivery 80, 91, 247, 260
Cesarean hysterectomy 239, 443
Cesarean scar implantation 242
Cesarean section 76, 80, 96, 163, 463, 467
　classification of urgency of 464, 467t
　role of forceps during 91
Chemical sterilization 177
Chemotherapy, role of 277
Cherney's incision 198
Chest compressions 123, 129, 131

Index

Chhaya 361
Chiari–Frommel syndrome 326
Chickenpox 345
Chignon 93
Childbirth
    experience of 443
    natural 407
    process, monitoring
        during 411
Chimerism 402
Chlamydia 434
    trachomatis 344
Chlorpheniramine 343
Chlorpromazine 326
Cholinesterase inhibitors 406
Chorioamnionitis 102, 261, 343
Choriocarcinoma 233, 234, 266
Chorionic plate 247
Chorionic villus 106
    biopsy 100, 101
    degeneration of 233
    sampling 25, 102
Chorionicity 303
    determine 245
Choroid plexus cysts 28
Chromopertubation test 175
Chromosomal aberrations 101
Chromosomal abnormality 100
Chromosomal analysis 104
Chvostek sign 426
Ciliated variant 475
Cimetidine 326, 330
Circumflex iliac vessels 177
Circumvallate placenta 247
Cirrhosis, mild 369
Clamps, types of 157
Classical radical
    hysterectomy 250
Clavicle 84
Clavulanic acid 347
Clear cell
    adenocarcinoma 475
    tumors 264
Cleidotomy 111
Clindamycin 338, 341, 344, 347
Clinicohysteroscopic scoring
    system 285
Clinodactyly 28
Clitoris 471
Clomiphene 322
    citrate 294, 322, 431
    failure 395
    mechanism of action of 321
    resistance 395

Clonidine 406, 410
Cloning 405
Cloquet's node 276
Clotrimazole 339
Coagulation parameters 456
Coagulation profile 240
Coagulogram 226
Coagulopathy 249, 252, 253
Coccyx, tip of 46
Cochrane metanalysis 94
Codeine 411
Coein 397, 463
Coenzyme Q 432
Coercion, allegation of 380
Coexistent class 462, 463
Cognitive behavioral
    therapy 337, 449
Cognitive factors 439
Coitus 326
    interruptus 348, 351
Collin's knife 184, 184f
Collin's loop 184, 184f
Colloid 115, 416, 418t
    advantages of 416, 418t
    composition of 416
    disadvantages of 416, 418t
    osmotic pressure 418
    solutions 419
Colpomicroscopy 165
Colporrhexis 241
Colposcopy 165, 224, 442
Combined contraceptive
    patch 351, 363f
    vaginal ring 351
Combined estrogen and
    progestogen 331
Combined injectable
    contraceptives 351
Combined low-dose pills 348
Combined oral contraceptive pills
    180, 327, 351, 358, 359,
    359t, 362
    contraindications of 358
Combined oral pill 356
Combined pill 348, 363, 367
    cardiovascular side
        effects of 360
    side effects of 360
Community health center 372
Compartment syndrome 422
Complete blood count 113,
    117, 266
Compressed air 177
Compression methods 116

Conception, products of 236
Condom
    female 348, 351, 356f
    male 348, 351
Cone biopsy 442
Congestive dysmenorrhea 397
Conjugated equine
    estrogen 325, 340
Conray 281
Consent 377, 380
Contact hysteroscopy 182
Continuous positive airway
    pressure 137
Contraception 348, 350
    different methods for 348
    failure 372
    safe 237
    temporary 348
Contraceptive
    barrier 348
    device 352
    effectiveness 351t
    male 367
    preparations 358
Contraceptive combined pills 360
    effect of 360
Contraceptive implants 366t
    types of 365
Contraceptive method 186,
    362-365
    categories for 348
Contraction stress test 29, 30
Controlled cord traction 65f, 310
    steps of 65
Conventional units 458
Convulsions, control 111
Coombs test 231
Copper intrauterine contraceptive
    devices 352
Copper-bearing intrauterine
    device 354
    insertion 354
Copper-T 261, 351
    380a 352
Cord
    entanglement 37
    insertion site 308
    prolapse, incidence of 77
Cordocentesis 100, 105
    complications of 105
    indications for 105
Corkscrew fashion 109
Cornual block, bilateral 284f
Cornual spasm 285

Corticosteroids, role of 321
Cosmetic results 203
Counseling 337, 438, 447
    biopsychosocial model of 438
    principles of 438
    process 447
    stages of 449
    steps of good 349
Counselor, types of 447
COVID-19 vaccination 22
Cranioclast 156*f*
Craniotomy 155
C-reactive protein 55, 225
Crochet, use of 156
Crown-rump length 300
Cryopreservation, role of 430
Crystalloid 416
    advantages of 115, 416, 418*t*
    disadvantages of 416, 418*t*
    fluids 417
    infusion 422
    replacement solutions,
        composition of 417*t*
    solutions 416
CT scan 280
Cu-7 352
Culdocentesis 222
Cumulus-oocyte complex pills,
    extended-use of 362
Curettage 224, 442
Curve of Carus 46*f*
Curved blades 163
Cusco's speculum 164, 164*f*
Cushing syndrome 331
Cut 200 352
Cut 380A 352, 352*f*
Cu-T insertion 337
Cyclooxygenase inhibitors 255
Cyproterone acetate 330, 336, 360
Cyst 262
    arachnoid 238
    cavity 262
    follicular 288
    sonolucent 291
    suburethral 162
    torsion of 263
    treatment of 262
Cystadenoma 263
Cystic adnexal mass 264
Cystic anechoic spaces 254
Cystic fibrosis 101
Cystic hygroma 24, 101
Cystic lesion, large 290
Cystic mass 289

Cystic teratoma, mature 261
Cystitis 251
Cystoscopy 223
Cytological smear 168
Cytomegalovirus 238
    infection 5
Cytoreductive surgery,
    primary 267
da Vinci Xi surgical system 188

D

Dalteparin 316
Danazol 259, 322, 328, 339, 340
Danazol-loaded intrauterine
    device 323
Danger signs 118
Deaver's retractor 166*f*
Decapitation saw 155*f*
Deep transverse arrest 79, 80
Deep vein thrombosis 316,
    347, 369
    treatment of 316
Defibrillation 123, 414
Deficiency, chronic 427
Deflexed head 75
Degenerations, types of 258
Dehydration, laboratory signs
    of 415
Dehydroepiandrosterone 433
    sulfate 219
Deliver vaginally 82
Delivery
    and care, preparation
        of 128, 131*t*
    preterm 258, 261
Dense adhesions 285
Depot medroxyprogesterone
    acetate 339, 348, 365
Depression 186
    symptoms of moderate-to-
        severe 445
Depressive disorder 369
Dermoid cyst 261, 262, 262*f*, 264,
    286, 295
    asymptomatic 286
    calcification in 286*f*
    diagnosis of 262
    laparoscopic removal of 262
    twisted 263*f*
Dermoid mesh 286
Dermoid plug 262, 286
Desogestrel 323, 360
Destructive operations,
    instruments for 155

Detrusor overactivity 399
Dexamethasone 343
    sodium phosphate 321
Dextran 70 184
Diabetes mellitus 1, 359, 353, 427
    uncomplicated 369
Diagnostic aids 242, 262
Diagnostic tests, candidates
    for 23
Diagonal conjugate 45*f*
Dialysis 427
Diamniotic twin pregnancies 246
Diaphragm 121, 348, 356*f*
Diaphragmatic hernia 175
Diarrhea, secretory 427
Dichorionic pregnancy,
    uncomplicated 246
Diencephalon 301
Dienogest 323, 337
Dihydrotestosterone 329
Dilatation 224, 442
Dinoprostone suppositories 315
Diphtheria, reduced 6
Direct occipitoposterior
    position 80
Discharge of patient, date of 393
Discordant growth 245
Disseminated intravascular
    coagulation 469
Distended veins 14
Distension media 181, 184, 185
Doctor–patient relationships 442
Dolichopellic pelvis 79
Donor
    egg 428
    eligibility criteria for 434
    semen 428
    tests done for 434
Dopamine
    agonist 337
    inhibitory effect of 326
    metabolism 253
Doppler principle 305
Doppler ultrasound 306
    Principle of 305
Double application technique 89
Double bleb sign 300
Double decidual sign 299
Down's syndrome 23, 405
    history of 100
Doxycycline 338
Doyen's retractor 153, 153*f*
Drospirenone 330, 360, 363

Drug
  abusers 21
  antiangiogenic 323
  antiarrhythmic 427
  antiepileptic 314
  antithyroid 320
  oxytocic 65
  parasympatholytic 31
  sympathomimetic 31
  tocolytic 97
  toxicity 113
Ductus venosus
  Doppler 27, 308
  waveform 306
    components of 306
Duhrssen's incision 75, 76
Dura mater 411
Dural punctures, number of 411
Dydrogesterone 323, 324, 337
  oral 324
Dynamic passive leg raising test 421
Dyslipidemia 354
Dysmenorrhea 12, 290, 397
  primary 13, 397
  reduction of 353
  secondary 13, 397
  symptoms of 254
  triple 13
  types of 13
Dyspareunia 202, 290, 398
  symptoms of 254
Dysuria 276

E

Early amniocentesis, disadvantages of 103
Early diastolic notching 308
Early obstetric warning score, modified 121
Early pregnancy 103
  failure 300
Early term neonate 399
Echocardiography 420
Echogenic bowel 27
Echogenic intracardiac focus 27
Echogenicity septum, intermediate 282
Eclampsia 37, 87, 111, 113, 311, 400, 427
  drill, algorithm for 113
  magnesium for 427
Ectocervix 168
Ectodermal dysphasia 106

Ectopic gestation specimen 241
Ectopic pregnancy 6, 222, 241, 242, 242f, 243, 244, 301
  prevention of 361
Ectopic production 326
Ectopic tubal gestation 241f
Edema 9, 82f
Edwards lifesciences 420
Edwards syndrome 23
Ehlers–Danlos syndrome 106
Eisenmenger's syndrome 316
Elective subtotal hysterectomy, advantages of 250
Electrocardiogram 117
Electrolyte 415, 422, 427
  imbalance 114
Embryo 432, 436
  donation 429
  evaluation of 301
Embryonal carcinomas 266
Embryotomy scissors, uses of 156
Emergency contraception 337, 348, 355, 399
  pill 348, 367
Emergency laparoscopy, indications of 288
Emergency medical services, activation of 122
Emotional problems 441
Emotional stress 326
Empathy 448
Encephalocele 292, 293f
End occlusion expiratory test 421
Endo-bag, use of 263
Endocervical curettage 224
Endocervix 168
Endocrinal screening test 218
Endodermal sinus tumor 266, 267
Endometrial ablation 182
  methods of 256
Endometrial aspiration 254
Endometrial biopsy 224, 254
  curette, types of 160
  premenstrual 218
Endometrial cancer 268, 270, 478
  advanced-stage 270
  classification of 474, 474t
  risk factors for 269
  staging of 476t
  types of 268
Endometrial carcinoma 224, 268, 268f, 474
  diagnosis of 151
  early stage 269
  high-risk 269

Endometrial contractility 257
Endometrial hyperplasia 249, 254, 474
  treatment of 255
  with atypia 255
  without atypia 255
Endometrial injury 432
Endometrial polyp 249f, 284
Endometrial resection 183f
Endometrial sampling 222
Endometrial tissue 223
  sampling 224
Endometrial tuberculosis, diagnosis of 151
Endometrioid adenocarcinoma 475
Endometrioid tumors 264
  low-grade 475
Endometrioma 262, 290, 290f
Endometriosis 258, 289, 290, 331, 336, 353, 397, 459, 460
  locations of 290
  newer therapies for 322
  revised classification of 459, 460t
Endometritis 161
Endometrium 161, 183, 358
  maturation of 358
Endoscopy 172
Endotracheal intubation, indications of 128
Endotracheal tube 121, 136
Endo-wrist instruments 188, 189, 191
Enoxaparin 316
EnSeal tissue sealing 178
Entry dyspareunia 398
Enzyme-linked immunosorbent assay 221
Epidermolysis
  atrophica gravis 106
  atrophica inversa 106
  bullosa 106
Epididymal sperm aspiration, percutaneous 430
Epidural analgesia 37, 55, 89
  patient-controlled 89, 406
Epigastric artery, superficial 197
Epigastric vessels 177
Epilation 336
Epilepsy 369
Epinephrine 260
Episiotomy 71, 201, 346
  advantages of median and mediolateral 202, 201t

complications of 202
disadvantages of median and
　　mediolateral 201t, 202
evidence regarding 64
role of 71, 89
scissors, type of 154
Epithelial carcinoma, types of 264
Epithelial integrity 461
Epithelial ovarian cancer 480
genetic risk for 265
types of 481t
Epithelial ovarian tumor 264
malignant 265
Equipment, list of 130t
Erythema, vestibular 398
Erythrocytes 105
Erythromycin 344
ethylsuccinate 344
Escherichia coli 113
Estradiol valerate 325
Estrogen 258, 326, 336, 357, 432
agonist 322
hormones 357t
on uterus, antagonizes effect
　　of 255
pills with very low-dose 357
preparations 325
therapy 255
Estrogen-producing ovarian
　　tumors 269
Ethinylestradiol 325, 337
Ethosuximide 315
Ethylene oxide gas 177
Ethynodiol diacetate 323
Eugenic 371
Excessive ventriculomegaly 292
Executive magistrate 436
Exercise 337
Exfoliated cells 168
Exogenous
doses of 433
estrogen 269
Extended head 75
External beam radiation
　　therapy 277
External cephalic version 68,
　　96-98
contraindications of 96
External iliac
artery 173
nodal regions 277
Extracellular
fluid 181, 422
volume 424
water 424

Extrachorial placenta 247
Extrafascial hysterectomy,
　　simple 272
Extrauterine 13
intrauterine device,
　　management of 261
Extremity compartment
　　syndrome 422
Eyes 82, 83

F

Face 48
Face presentation 81
diagnostic points for 81
etiology of 81, 81b
Facial nerve palsy 91
Failed resuscitation, causes of 127
Fallopian tube 154, 290, 298
carcinomas 480
classification of 264
parts of 280
patent 281
rupture of 242
Fallot tetralogy 238
False labor 50
pains 50, 50t
Familial hypocalciuric
　　hypercalcemia 426
Familial monogenic disease 101
Family planning 378
indemnity scheme 382
Far-far suture placement
　　204, 208f
Fascia 197
lata 276
Fat 197
Fat-fluid level 286
Fatigue 186
Favorable fetal attitude 68
Fecundity 395
Female genital tract
anomalies 462
classification of 462t
Female sterilization 351, 379
categories for 369t
contraindications for 369
failure of 370
causes of 370
Femoral length 302
Femoral nerve 276
Femur 72
length 304
Fentanyl 408
Ferric carboxymaltose 319

Fertility awareness-based
　　methods 348
Fertility rate 399
Fertility-reducing factors,
　　history of 243
Fertility-sparing treatment,
　　role of 271
Fetal acidosis 80
Fetal aneuploidy 27
Fetal anomaly 67
Fetal ascites 292f
causes of 292
Fetal biometry 302
standard 303f
Fetal blood
sample 41, 42
use of 106
Fetal body 69
Fetal bradycardia 105
causes of 31
development of 409
Fetal breathing movements 32
Fetal buttocks 67
Fetal cardiac activity 236
Fetal cerebral oxygenation 42
Fetal circulation 305
Fetal cochlear 40
Fetal complications 91, 94
Fetal contraindications,
　　relative 90
Fetal death 111
causes of 32
Fetal descent 63
assessment of 53f
Fetal echocardiogram 342
Fetal electrocardiogram 403
Fetal fibroblast 104
Fetal fibronectin 225
Fetal goiter 320
Fetal growth restriction 105,
　　401, 402
Fetal hazards 104
Fetal head 108
assessing descent of 52f
descent of 50
in breech delivery, causes for
　　arrest of 74
in vaginal breech delivery,
　　causes for arrest of 74
Fetal heart
deceleration 36f-38f
tracing 31f
Fetal heart rate 31, 32, 35, 76, 112,
　　113, 412

Index

bradycardia 31
changes 97
decelerations of 35
monitoring 54
Fetal hydrocephalus 291, 291f
Fetal hypothyroidism 320
Fetal hypoxia 37
Fetal imaging 305
Fetal indications 87
Fetal infection, risk of 6
Fetal injuries 77
Fetal karyotype 229, 235
Fetal kidney biopsy 106
Fetal lie 51, 305
Fetal liver biopsy, indications for 106
Fetal loss, risk of 102
Fetal lower jaw 156
Fetal malformation 372
Fetal membranes 247
Fetal monitoring 29
Fetal movement 32, 304
Fetal muscle biopsy, indications for 106
Fetal nasal bone 26
Fetal position 51
Fetal presentation 51, 51t, 305
Fetal pulse oximetry 403
Fetal renal abnormalities 301
Fetal scalp electrode, application of 37
Fetal skin biopsy, indications for 106
Fetal skull 44, 48, 48f
  diameters of 49, 49t
  sutures of 48, 49f
Fetal surveillance 227
Fetal tachycardia 31
Fetal tissue biopsy 100, 106
Fetal tone 32
Fetal urinary
  ascites 292
  tract, rupture of 292
Fetal weight, estimated 402
Fetogram 228
Fetopelvic disproportion 68, 72, 73
Fetoplacental circulation 305
Fetoplacental contribution 50
Fetus 237, 242f
  chest 110
  dead 81, 83
  live 85
  normal 299

part of 51
preterm 41, 93
Fibers, interlacing 215f
Fibrin glue 212
Fibroid 180, 257, 258, 268f, 287, 331
  beneficial effects on 353
  complications of 258
  larger 182
  location of 287
  medical management of 327
  red degeneration of 258
  smaller 260
  surgical management of 259
  symptoms of 256
  types of 287
  vaporizing 182
Final suture placement 204
Finasteride 329, 336
Finger, middle 53
First antenatal visit 2
First-generation techniques 182
First-trimester
  aneuploidy screening 23
  masses 301
  pregnancy termination 151
  scan 298, 302
  screening 23
    test 23
  ultrasound markers 26
Fistula
  rectovaginal 149
  vesicovaginal 149, 223, 251
Fixed groin lymph nodes 279
Flexion, maintain 71
Fluconazole 339
Fluid 415, 418
  administration 415, 420
    complications of 422
    purpose of 415
  challenge
    quantity of 422
    test 421
  expansion 420
  incidence of 181
  increased 411
  loss 416, 418
    evaluation of 415
  media 181
  movement of 419
  oral 54
  overload 181, 182
  redistributed 419
  replacement 114, 419

requirement 419, 419t
responsiveness 420
  significance of 421
status, advanced assessment of 420
therapy, perioperative 416
Fluorescence in situ hybridization 104
Fluorouracil 332
Fluoxetine 326
Flutamide 329
Foam tab 348
Focal lesions 161
Foley's catheter 163, 163f, 177, 232
  in situ 282, 283
  indications of 163
Folic acid 7
  preconceptionally 238
  supplementation 7
Folinic acid 344
Follicle matures 336
Follicle-stimulating hormone 358
Follicular phase 180
Fontanelle 48f, 49, 83
Forbes–Albright syndrome 326
Forceps 80, 86
  Adson's 159
  Allis 153, 153f
  application of 87
  applied 89
  Armytage 152
  artery 159, 159f
  babcock 154f
  Barnes–Neville 88
  Barton's 91, 91f
  bipolar 178f
  Dartigues 163, 164, 164f
  failed 91
  fenestrated 189
    bipolar 190f
  green armytage 153f
  Heigh-Ferguson 88
  Kelly's 171
    placental 170, 171f
  Kielland's 86, 87, 88f, 89
  long-curved 87
  low 87
  midpelvic 87
  Milne–Murray 88
  obstetric 86
  outlet 86
  ovum 151f
  phantom application of 88

Piper's 72, 74, 88f, 90
placenta 170, 171
Shirodkar's 163, 163f, 164
short-curved 87
Simpson–Braun 88f
smooth nontoothed 158
sponge holding 150
Tischler–Kevorkian 168
toothed 159
traction 88
trial 91
types of 87, 88f
Wrigley 88f
  outlet 86f
Forceps application 87
  classification of 86
  contraindications for 90
  indications of 87
Forceps delivery 91, 92, 94
  after 92
  complications of 91
Forceps-assisted
  deliveries 89
  vaginal birth 95
Foreign body 180
Forensic evidence 15
Fothergill's operation 151
Fothergill's surgery 160
Free androgen index 219
Free-floating head 52
Frequent cycles, causes of 12
Fresh frozen plasma 117
Fundal fibroids 239
Fundal grip 68
Fundal height 9
Fusion, types of 245

G

Galactorrhea, causes of 325
Gallbladder 359
  disease 353
Gamete
  donation 428
  intrafallopian tube transfer 396, 429
Gas embolism 185, 200
Gastric access 426
Gastrointestinal causes 13
Gastrointestinal changes 121
Gastrointestinal symptoms 265
Gastrointestinal tract 211, 424
Gastroschisis 238
Gelatin-thrombin matrix 260

Genetic
  disorders, specific 101
  myopathies 106
  sonogram 28
  syndromes 245
  tests 104
Genital herpes
  active 102
  pregnancy with 345
  recurrent 345
Genital lesions, recurrent 345
Genital malignancy 360, 361
Genital tract, trauma of 117
Genital tuberculosis 221
Genitalia, external 14
Genitourinary causes 13
Gentamicin 338, 343, 347
Genuine stress incontinence 399
Genuineness 448
Germ cell tumor 267
Gestation 318
Gestational age 4, 98
  small for 401
Gestational diabetes mellitus 229, 312, 313
Gestational hypertension 310, 400
Gestational sac 243
  normal 235
  visualization of 299
Gestational trophoblastic disease 233, 320
  classification of 233
  diagnosis of 237
Gestodene 323
Gestrinone 323, 328, 337
Gibson incision, modified 198
Glanzmann thrombasthenia 319, 320
Glibenclamide 313
Glucocorticoids 330
Glutaraldehyde 154
  solution 177
Glyburide 313
Glycine 184
Goal-directed therapy 419, 420
Golf-club appearance 221
Gonadotropin 294, 432
  recombinant 328
  therapeutic uses of 328
  therapy 431
Gonadotropin-dependent precocious puberty 394
Gonadotropin-releasing hormone 183, 255, 322, 433

  agonists 322, 327, 331
  analogs 327, 337
  antagonists 259, 327
  release of 358
Gonorrhea 346
Gore-Tex meshes 215
Goserelin 331, 339
Graft in prolapse surgery, indications of 217
Granulosa cell tumor 267, 268f
Graspers 179
Graves disease 320, 321
Gravid uterus 308
  manual left uterine displacement for 412f
Gravida 4
Groin traction 72
Growth hormone 432
Gynecoid 47
  pelvis 52
Gynecologic
  causes 13
  consultation 442
  examination 13
  oncology 480
  surgery 191
Gynecological cancer 446, 471
  classification of 471
Gynecological indications 160, 163
Gynecological malignancy 474
Gynecology
  hormones 458
  investigations in 218
  specimens 249

H

Haas rule 241
Hair
  loss 186
  removal, physical measures for 336
  tufts of 262
Halban's disease 253
Haloperidol 326
Hand washing 128
Hanging drop
  method 174
  test 200
Hank dilator 152
Harmonic scalpel 177
Hartmann's solution 419
Hasson's technique 176, 201
Head, molding of 49

Index

Headache 186, 410
Healing 334
Health care workers 21
Health worker 452
   nonverbal cues 450
Healthcare
   professional 127
   worker 451
   types of 447
Heaney clamps 157, 158
Heaney retractor 166f
Heart
   disease, pregnancy with 87, 226, 342
   failure 426
   rate 54, 134, 137
Hegar cervical dilators 152f
Hegar dilator 151
HELLP syndrome 231, 401, 470
   diagnosis of 470
Hematinic deficiency 341
Hematology 456
Hematuria 240
Hemi-uterus 463
Hemochromatosis 319
Hemodilution resulting 422
Hemodynamic monitoring 420
Hemoglobin 117, 234, 240
Hemogram, complete 222, 226
Hemolysis 401, 470
Hemophilia screen 222
Hemorrhage 100, 105, 113, 152, 176, 184, 185
   acute 341
   antepartum 34, 96, 228, 247, 401, 469
   cerebral 111
   fetomaternal 97, 104, 310
   intracranial 77, 91, 113
   severe 99, 100
Hemosiderosis 319
Hemostasis 203
   system 178
Hemostatic reanimation 116
Heparin 316, 347
   unfractionated 316, 347
Hepatitis 21
   B 42, 105
      immunoglobulin 21
      virus 430
   B vaccine 21
      dose of 21
   C 42
      virus 430
   D 42
   E 42

Hepatocellular carcinoma, malignant 361
Hernial orifices 14
Herpes zoster infection
   reactivation of 20
   risks of 20
Heterosexual puberty 394
Heywood Smith's ovum forceps 151
Hirsutism 220, 336, 395
   pharmacologic therapy for 329
   treatment of 329
Hormonal contraception 367
Hormonal contraceptive 348
   method 364
   oral 348
Hormonal makeup 441
Hormonal treatment 336
Hormone assays 430
Hormone replacement therapy 222
   short-term 325
Hormone therapy 337
   role of 270
Human arm and wrist 189
Human chorionic gonadotropin 3, 23, 289, 405, 429
Human immunodeficiency virus 42, 343, 353, 369, 430
Human menopausal gonadotropin 328, 428
Human papillomavirus 5, 271, 275, 332, 442
   immunization 338
   vaccine 22
Human plasma 6
Humanitarian ground 372
Husband's semen analysis 218
Hybrid leiomyoma group 287
Hydatidiform mole 189f, 233, 233f, 236, 289
Hydralazine 112, 311
Hydrocephalus 238, 238f, 239, 290, 291
   antenatally 238
   fetus 239
   incidence of 238
Hydrocephaly 67
Hydrogen peroxide gas plasma 177
Hydrometrocolpos 292
Hydronephrosis 237
Hydrosalpinx 283
   bilateral 283f

Hydroureteronephrosis, bilateral 287f
Hydroxyprogesterone caproate 325
Hyperandrogenemia 294
Hyperbilirubinemia 8
Hypercalcemia 426
   causes of 425
   signs of 426
   symptoms of 426
Hypercarbia 176
Hyperemesis gravidarum 400
Hyperextended head in breech, causes of 75
Hyperkalemia 120, 423
   signs of 423
   symptoms of 423
   treatment measures for 424
Hypernatremia 415, 425
   causes of 425fc
Hyperplasia 12, 252, 253
Hyperprolactinemia 220, 294, 325, 336
Hypersensitivity 319
Hyperstimulation 403
Hypertension 1, 34, 359, 366
   chronic 231, 310, 400, 401
   control 113
   pregnancy with 231
   pregnancy-induced 359
   severe 34
   uncontrolled 327
Hyperthyroidism 320, 321
Hypnosis 99
Hypocalcemia 426
   acute 426
   causes of 426
   signs of 426
   symptoms of 426
Hypogastric artery 173
Hypoglycemic agents, oral 312, 313
Hypogonadotropic hypogonadism state 327
Hypokalemia 120, 422, 423
Hypomagnesemia 427
   symptoms of 427
   treatment of 427
Hyponatremia 113, 424, 425
   asymptomatic 425
   etiology of 424fc
Hypotension, management of 421
Hypotensive resuscitative approach 115

Hypothalamic-pituitary stalk
    damage 326
Hypothermia 113, 120
Hypothyroidism 321, 369
Hypotonic distension media 181
Hypotonic fluids 181
Hypoventilation 176
Hypovolemia 113, 120
    signs of 416*t*
Hypovolemic shock 251
Hypoxemia 121
Hypoxia 42, 113, 120
    resultant 126
Hysterectomy 100, 153, 175, 191,
        249, 249*f*, 261
    clamps 157, 158*f*
    class of 270
    complications of 251
    performed, type of 249
    subtotal 250
    total 241, 249, 249*f*, 250
    types of 250
Hysterical personalities 446
Hysteromat 181
Hysterosalpingogram 186, 280,
        282, 282*f*, 284, 285
    complications of 280
    indications for 280
    normal 280*f*
Hysterosalpingography 431
Hysteroscope 179
Hysteroscopic ablative
        techniques 182
Hysteroscopic findings 285
Hysteroscopic myomectomy 182
Hysteroscopic procedures 185
Hysteroscopic resection 183
Hysteroscopic sterilization 180
Hysteroscopic surgery 184, 286
    type of 181
Hysteroscopy 172, 179,
        180, 185, 186, 282
    complications of 184, 185*t*
    contraindications of 180
    diagnostic 179, 186
    incidence of 185*t*
    indications for 179
    risk factors of 185*t*
    role of 183, 184

I

IA1 disease 273
Ibuprofen 346
Iceberg sign, tip of 286

Iliac
    artery, branches of
        internal 275
    crest 195
    spine, anterosuperior 197
    vessels, common 274
Imiquimod 333
Immobilization 354, 426
Immunization 17
    active 18
    passive 18, 20
Immunoglobulin G 18
Immunosuppressive therapy 354
Implanon 366
Implanon NXT 365, 366*f*
    contraindications for 367
Implantation failure,
        recurrent 430
In vitro fertilization 301, 396,
        428, 432
    indications for 429
    metformin treatment
        during 432
    procedure of 428
Inactive capsular polysaccharide
        vaccine 22
Incision
    number of 178
    selection of 194
    type of 194
Incisional hernia 177
Incontinentia pigmenti 106
Index finger 149
Indian Contract Act 377
Indian Council of Medical
        Research 340
Indian Penal Code 379
Indocyanine 270
Infant death 399
Infant mortality rate 399
Infection 184
    chances of 204
    prevention 130*fc*
Inferior epigastric
    artery 196, 198
    vessels 197
Infertile couple 428, 431
    eligibility criteria for 434
    evaluation of 430
Infertility 151, 179, 395
    causes immense mental
        exhaustion 428
    investigations 444
    primary 218

treatment 444
unexplained 335, 434
Inflammatory bowel disease 318
Inflammatory illness, chronic 318
Inflating pneumoperitoneum 190
Influenza
    vaccination 19
    vaccine 17, 18
        inactivated 20
Informed consent, types of 377
Informed written consent 378
Infracolic omentectomy 475
    role of 475
    staging 269
Infrequent cycles, causes of 12
Inguinal femoral
        lymphadenectomy 278
Inguinal ligament 195
Inherited thrombophilia 231
Inhibits deoxynucleic acid 331
In-hospital maternal cardiac
        arrest algorithm 122*fc*
Instrument 149
    parts of 149
Instrumental delivery 86
Insulin 312
    intermediate-acting 313
    long-acting 313
    rapid-acting 313
    short-acting 313
Insurance coverage 434, 436
Integrated test 25
    types of 25
Intensive care unit 19
Intercourse, unprotected 355
Intermenstrual bleeding 252
    causes of 12
Intermittent auscultation 33, 34
Internal iliac
    artery ligation 100
    nodal regions 277
Internal podalic version 99
    contraindications of 99
    indications of 99
International normalized
        ratio 317
Intersex 394
Interstitial cystitis 399
Intestinal surgeries 201
Intra-abdominal
    injury 77
    pressure 173, 174, 190,
        200, 213
Intracellular compartment 416
Intracellular fluids 422

Intracytoplasmic sperm injection 396, 428, 429
Intradecidual sign 299
Intramuscular methotrexate administration, methods of 332t
Intrapartum 8, 343
    fetal surveillance, methods of 33
    period 341
    risk factors 128, 128t
    situation, methods of revalidation in 40
Intraperitoneal bleeding 236
Intraperitoneal hemorrhage, severe 361
Intrauterine 13
    death 227
    fluid pressure 52
    growth restriction 228, 247
    infection 151, 292
    insemination 396, 428
    pressure 182
    progesterone 339, 340
Intrauterine adhesions
    classification of 183, 184t
    extent of 184
Intrauterine contraceptive device 337, 348, 350, 351, 353, 355
    contradictions for 353
    insertion 377
    postpartum insertion of 355
Intrauterine device 102, 239, 260, 261f, 351
    in situ 261
    insertion, contraindications for 353t
    transmigrated 175
Intrauterine fetal 246
    death 75, 81, 246
Intrauterine pregnancy 243
    normal 299
Intravascular volume status 420
Intravenous 117
    fluid 346, 416
        administration of 415
    oxytocin 30
    pyelogram 271
    pyelography 223
Intubate baby 128
Invasive mole 233
Ipsilateral port position 201

Iron
    deficiency anemia 340, 341t
    dextran 318
    parenteral 318
    sucrose 318
    supplementation 7
Iron-sorbitol-citrate complex 318
Irregular cycles 4, 5
Irregular periods 186, 441
Irregular shedding 253
Irregular spotting 365
Ischemic heart disease 366
Ischial spines, level of 52
Ischial tuberosities 11
Isolated tumor cells 477
Isotonic fluids 181
Isotonic media 182
Isoxsuprine 31
Isthmic fibrosis 285
Isthmus 164

J

Joel-Cohn's skin incision 197
Judicial magistrate 435, 436

K

Karman cannula 169
Karyotypic abnormalities 291
Kelly's plication 163
Keyes punch biopsy forceps 169, 169f
Khanna's sling operation 153
Kidney
    disease 369
    function test 113, 117, 223
Kielland's forceps application, methods of 89
Kielland's rotational forceps 95
Kleihauer-Betke
    stain 105
    test 228
Kocher's clamp 157, 158, 158f
Kristeller pressure 76
Kustner's incision 198

L

Labetalol 311
Labia majora 275
    cancer of 471
Labia minora 471
    anterior 276, 277

Labia, separating 86
Labial skin 471
Labor 343
    abnormal 57
    active phase of 54, 60f
    analgesia, protocol for 408
    care 60
        guide 57, 62f, 63, 63t
    diagnosis 57
    during 54, 78, 84, 239
    dysfunctional 404
    first stage of normal 54
    induction of 315, 404, 464, 468t
    initiation of 50
    mechanism of 61, 69, 81, 83, 84
    normal 50, 52, 57
    partograph depicting normal 59f
    pregnancy with preterm 340
    preterm 226, 238, 321, 402
    role of augmentation of 76
    stages of 51
    threatened preterm 402
    tolerate stress of 76
    version during 99
    walking epidurals during 408
Lactate dehydrogenase 470
Lactated Ringer's solution 417
Lactational amenorrhea method 348, 351
Lahey's right-angled hemostat 159, 159f
Lambda 48
Lamivudine 338
Lamotrigine 315
Langenbeck retractor 165f
Laparoscope 172f
Laparoscopic guidance 184
Laparoscopic instruments 177
Laparoscopic myomectomy 260
Laparoscopic needle holder 178f
Laparoscopic ovarian drilling 294
Laparoscopic scissors 178f
Laparoscopic surgery 172, 192, 193
    single-incision 178
Laparoscopic tooth 178f
Laparoscopic tubal clipping 432
Laparoscopic-assisted vaginal hysterectomy 175, 249
Laparoscopy 172, 176
    advantages of 175
    complications of 176

contraindications for 175
indications for 175
open 176, 177, 201
role of 290
scars 177
Laparotomy 288
advantages of 175
incisions 196*f*
pads 417
staging 266
Laryngeal mask airway 121
Lasmar submucous myoma
classification 461
Last menstrual period 1
Latent syphilis of unknown 346
Leech-Wilkinson
cannula 161, 161*f*
Lee-Huang point 173, 200
Left sacrum
anterior 403
posterior 403
Left upper quadrant 200
insertion technique 176
Legal abortion services 371
Leiomyoma 12, 249, 253
diagnose 258
effects of 258
medical management of 258
multiple 256*f*
subclassification
system 257*t*, 464*t*
Lemon sign 291
Leopold's fourth maneuver 10
Leopold's third maneuver 10
Letrozole 259, 294, 322, 335, 431
resistant cases 335
Leuprolide 331
acetate depot 339
Levetiracetam 314
Levobupivacaine 410
Levofloxacin 346
Levonorgestrel 337, 351, 360
intrauterine device 323
Levonorgestrel-releasing
intrauterine
devices 348
system 327, 339
Levothyroxine therapy 321
Life span 352, 366
Lifestyle
change in 445
modification 337
Ligament hematoma 241
Ligasure 178, 178*f*
Lignocaine 169

Linen fibers 204
Lipids 458
Lipoprotein
cholesterol, high-density 294
low-density 220
Liquid chromatography, high-
performance 231
Listening, active 450
Live and non-live vaccines 18*b*
Live ectopic pregnancy 243
Live vaccines 18
Live-attenuated influenza
vaccine 19
Liver
dullness, obliteration of 174
enzyme, elevated 401, 470
function test 113, 117, 230, 455
transplantation 327
tumors 369
Lobe, succenturiate 247*f*
Loop electrosurgical excision
procedure 271, 293
Lovset's maneuver 70, 73, 74*f*
Löwenstein-Jensen medium 221
Lower segment cesarean
section 8, 69, 72, 73
Lower uterine
cavity 171
segment 152
Low-estrogen levels 253
Low-molecular-weight
heparin 316, 347
L-shaped blades 164
Lumbar vertebra, sacralization
of 79
Lupron overlap protocol 433
Lupus anticoagulant 232, 401
Luteal phase defect 395
investigations for 232*b*
Luteinizing hormone 218, 220,
322, 358
Lymph node 274, 472, 477
dissection, systematic 475
drainage, primary 274
metastases, incidence of 276
negative 277
para-aortic 270, 274, 480
retroperitoneal 482
secondary 274
staging 269
Lymphadenopathy, generalized 9
Lymphatic metastasis 271
Lymphovascular space 274
invasion 272
Lysol 154

M

Mackenrodt's ligament 271
Macro-adenomas 336
Macrometastasis 472, 477
Magic bullet 433
Magnesium 337, 427
blood levels of 312
sulfate 311, 318, 341
regimens of 311
toxicity 112*t*
therapy 427
toxicity 412
Maingot's clamp 157, 158
Mala N 357*f*
Malabsorption syndrome 318
Malaria 344
complicated 344
severe 344
uncomplicated 344
Malformation 314, 372, 405
Malignancy 12, 253
Malmstrom 92
Malpresentation 403
Maltese-cross appearance 221
Mammalian bite 22
Maneuvers 108
internal 109
postural 99
Mannitol 181
Manual left uterine
displacement 120
Manual vacuum
aspirator 170, 170*f*
Marital status, change of 372
Mask, correct position of 134*f*
Master-slave systems 187
Maternal blood 100
Maternal body mass index 91
Maternal cardiac arrest 124
causes of 120
Maternal coagulopathy 102
Maternal collapse 121
causes for 113
sudden 113
Maternal complications 91,
94, 238
Maternal death 111
causes of 241
Maternal epilepsy 37
Maternal hazards 104
Maternal hypoxia 37
Maternal immunization 17
Maternal kyphosis 83
Maternal mortality

rate 412
ratio 400
Maternal pelvis 44, 86
  type of 79
Maternal resuscitation 120, 124
Maternal serum alpha
  fetoprotein 227
Maternal supine hypotension 37
Matthew Duncan method 64
Mauriceau-Smellie-Veit
  maneuver 70
  method, modified 71*f*
  technique 71
Maylard and Cherney's
  incision 197
Mayo's scissors 159*f*
McDonald procedure 293
McRoberts maneuver 108, 109*f*
Mean arterial pressure 182
Mean sac diameter 299
Measles, mumps, and rubella 5
  indications for 20
  vaccine 20
Medical eligibility
  categories 349, 349*f*
Medical management,
  indications of 243
Medical oophorectomy 337
Medical record-cum-checklist 383
Medical termination in molar
  pregnancy, role of 235
Medical termination of pregnancy
  150, 315, 368, 371-373,
  378, 380
  act 371
  indications for 372
  method of 393
  records 380
Medications, role of 135
Mediolateral episiotomy 201
Medroxyprogesterone acetate
  337, 360
Mefenamic acid 339
Megestrol acetate 337
Meglumine diatrizoate 281
Membrane
  artificial rupture of 96
  prelabor rupture of 55
  premature rupture of 76, 225,
    258, 402
  preterm
    prelabor rupture of 341
    premature rupture of 402
  ruptured 96

Membranous placenta 247
Menadiol sodium phosphate 343
Menarche 441
Meningomyelocele 67
Menometrorrhagia 270
Menopausal females 429
Menopausal problems 445
Menopausal symptoms,
  prevention of 250
Menopause
  attained premature 429
  hormone therapy for 340
  natural 340
  transition 253
Menorrhagia, control of 327
Menstrual bleeding
  causes of heavy 12
  frequent 252
  heavy 12, 252, 397
  infrequent 252
  prolonged 252
  shortened 252
Menstrual changes 441
Menstrual cycle 280, 361
Menstrual history 1
Menstrual pattern 285
Menstruation
  frequent 397
  infrequent 397
  painful 12
Mentally sound 374
Menticoglou maneuver 109
Mesh 203, 214
  complications of 217
  ideal 215
  natural 214
  prolene 215*f*
  types of 214*t*
Metabolic abnormalities 294
Metabolic acidosis 176
  progressive 415
Metabolic disorders,
  history of 101
Metabolic syndrome 398
Metal cup 92
Metallic ventouse cup 92*f*
Metformin 313, 336
Methergine 116
  contraindications of 310
Methimazole 320, 321
Methotrexate 100, 243, 331
  role of 331
Methyldopa 311, 326
Methylene blue 223
  dye 164

Methylergometrine 411
Metoclopramide 326
Metronidazole 338, 343, 344, 347
Metroplasty 180, 282
Metropolitan magistrate 435, 436
Metzenbaum scissors 159, 159*f*
Miconazole 339
Microdose flare protocol 433
Microhysteroscope 179
Microinvasive disease 271
Microinvasive squamous
  carcinoma 276
Microinvasive vulvar cancer 278
Micrometastasis 472, 477
Microsurgical epididymal sperm
  aspiration 430
Midpelvis, level of 75
Midtrimester fetal ultrasound
  scan, role of 302
Mifepristone 255, 259,
  328, 330, 331, 340
Migraine 353
Minimally invasive
  surgery 199, 269
  role of 269
Mini-pill 348, 357
Mirena 337, 352, 353*f*
Miscarriage 366, 447
  recurrent 324
  threatened 324
Miscellaneous causes 426
Misoprostol 260, 315
Misses combined oral
  contraceptives 362
Mississippi 470
  classification 470*t*
Miya hook 169*f*
Mobius syndrome 315
Molar pregnancy 234-236
  complete 235
  diagnose 235
  high-risk 236
  partial 233
  risk of 236
Molar tissue 234
Molding 404
Mole
  complete 233, 234, 234*t*, 236
  partial 233, 234, 234*t*, 236
Molecular classification 477, 478*t*
Monoamniotic monochorionic
  twins 244
Monochorionic pregnancy,
  complications of 245

Monogenic disorders, preimplantation genetic testing for 101
Monopolar cautery instruments 189
Monopolar scissors 190f
Monozygotic multiple gestation 245
Monthly reporting form 374
Morphine 408
Morphology, poor 396
Moschcowitz culdoplasty 153, 164
Mothering skills 445
Mother-to-child transmission, risk of 105
Motion, expanded range of 192
Moxibustion 99
Mucinous
　adenocarcinoma 475
　cystadenocarcinoma 290
　cystadenoma 263, 264
　ovarian cystadenoma 264
　tumors 263, 264
Mucus plugging 284
Mueller-Hillis maneuver 47
Müllerian agenesis 222
Müllerian anomalies 180
　congenital 293
Müllerian duct 282
Müllerian inclusions 480, 481
Multiload 250 352, 352f
Multiload 375 352
Multiload Cu 250 352
Multiload Cu 375 352
Multipara 4, 63
Multiple gestation 67, 306
Muscle
　and skin, blood supply to 195
　injury 424
Myelomeningocele 238
Myocardial infarction 360, 412
Myoinositol 331
　role of 331
Myoma 156
　screw 156f
Myomectomy 154, 183, 191
　abdominal 156
　procedure 157
Myometrial cells 259
Myometrial invasion 269
　degree of 478
Myometrial penetration, depth of 182

Myometrium
　damage of 239
　layer of 243

N

Nadroparin 316
Naegele's formula 4
Nafarelin 331, 339
Nasal bone 302f
　hypoplasia 26
National Family Health Survey 350
National Neonatology Forum 127
Natural behavioral family planning methods 348
Near-infrared spectroscopy 42
Near-near suture placement 204, 208f
Necrotic tissue 214
Needle 203
　affect, type of 210
　bevel orientation 411
　driver 190f
　holder 167f
　Miya hook, type of 168
　placement of 174
　tip design 411
　types of 211, 211t
Neisseria gonorrhoeae 102
Neoadjuvant chemotherapy 267
　before surgery, role of 273
Neonatal death 447
Neonatal endotracheal intubation 124
Neonatal hypothermia 66
Neonatal intensive care unit 80, 321
Neonatal intubation, steps of 131, 134fc
Neonatal medications 136t
Neonatal resuscitation 126, 128, 135, 136t
　components of 127
　during maternal cardiac arrest, role of 124
　sequential steps for 127, 129t
Neonatal Resuscitation Program 127, 135, 137fc
Neonatal tetanus 19
　control areas 19
　elimination 19
Neonate
　full-term 399
　preterm 400

Neoplastic diseases 426
Neostigmine 410
Nephrosis, congenital 106
Nerve
　injuries 77, 91
　supply 195
Nestorone 366
Neural tube defect 227, 237
　previous history of 227
Neuraxial analgesia 410
　recent advances in 410
Neuroendocrine tumors 475
Neurologic injury, permanent 109
Neurological signs 425
Neurological symptoms 425
Neuromuscular function 422
Neuromuscular irritability, increased 427
Neurosyphilis 346
Newborn baby 66
Nifedipine 311, 341
Nipple stimulation 30
Nitric oxide donors 318
Nitrofurantoin 346
Nitroglycerin 311, 318
Nitrous oxide 407
Nonabsorbable sutures 203, 204, 206t
　indications of 209
Nonfunctional fluid 126
Nonhormonal pill derived 367
Noninvasive prenatal screening test 3
　advantages of 3
Noninvasive prenatal test 25, 100
Non-nucleoside reverse transcriptase inhibitors 359
Nonpharmacological methods 407
Nonpneumatic anti-shock garment 116
Nonpregnant patients 227
Nonreactive nonstress test 30
Nonsteroidal anti-inflammatory drugs 254, 322, 336, 423
Nonstress test 29-31
　basic principle of 30
　normal 32
Nonstructural systemic causes 12
Nontooth graspers 178f
Norethisterone 339, 360
　acetate 323
　enanthate 365

Index

Norethynodrel 323
Norplant 366
Nortestosterone derivatives 323
Nose 82
No-touch technique 170
Novak's and Pipelle's biopsy curette 160
Novak's endometrial biopsy curette 160f, 161
NovaSure 182
Nuchal fold 27
Nuchal translucency 3, 24, 24f, 302f
Nulliparas
   with epidural 63
   without epidural 63
Nulliparous state 290
Nutrition, tolerating enteral 426
Nuvaring 364f
Nylon 206
Nystatin 339

O

Obesity 398
Oblique muscle
   external 195
   internal 195
Oblique serrations, advantage of 158
Observe systemic circulation 421
Obstetric
   anal sphincter injuries 95
      classification of 463, 467t
   cholestasis 343
   complications 96
   conjugate 45
   drills 108
   examination 9
   grips 10
   history taking 1
   indications 150, 160, 163
   investigations in 225
   losses 446
   outlet, diameters of 46, 46f
   pelvic axis 46
   problems 1
   procedures 6, 96
   specimens 233
   surgeries 407
Obstructed labor 57, 61f
   signs of 99
Obstructive abnormality 13
Occiput anterior, right 403

Occlusion techniques 368
Oculocutaneous albinism 106
Odon device 95
Office hysteroscopy 185
Oligoasthenoteratozoospermia 396
Oligohydramnios 33, 104
Oligomenorrhea 353
Oligospermia, severe 396
Omega-3 fatty acid 337
Omphalocele 238
Oncogenic strain, high-risk 478
Only progestogen 348
Oocyte
   donation 429
   in vitro maturation of 396
Oophorectomy 244, 263
Operation theater 379
Operative hysteroscopic procedures 185
Operative hysteroscopy 180
Operative instruments 179
Operator's forearm 77
Opiates 326
Opioids 407
   parenteral 55
Opportunistic salpingectomy 251
Oral combined contraceptives 362
   use of 362
Oral contraceptive pills 258, 265, 339
   mechanism of action of 358
   use of 359t
Oral hypoglycemic agents, role of 312
Orbital ridges 83
Organ formation, clinical significance of 299
Original Mauriceau-Smellie-Veit method 71f
Ormeloxifene 255
Orodental hygiene 9
Orthostatic hypotension 423
Osteomyelitis, risk of 198
Osteoporosis 250
Ovarian artery 275
   ligation 117
Ovarian cancer 480
   advanced-stage 267
   classification of 480
   development of 290
   early stage disease of 266
   signs of 265

   staging system of 481t
   symptoms of 265
Ovarian cyst 198
   rupture 292
   simple 288
Ovarian cystectomy 262
   laparotomy for 153
Ovarian cysts, functional 361
Ovarian dermoid cyst 297
Ovarian epithelial tumors 480
Ovarian function, history of abnormal 265
Ovarian hyperstimulation syndrome 322, 395, 432
Ovarian insufficiency, premature 340, 395
Ovarian malignancy 223, 265
   development of 265
   role of tumor markers in 266
Ovarian mass 287f, 301
   benign 263
Ovarian stimulation
   controlled 428
   protocols 432
Ovarian tissue 262
Ovarian tube, classification of 264
Ovarian tumor
   benign 263
   common 290
   malignant 264, 290, 290f
Ovary 264f, 268f, 272
   advantages of retaining 250
   bilateral 234
   dysgerminoma of 267f
   mucinous cystadenoma of 263f
   serous cystadenoma of 263f, 264, 288f
   surface epithelium of 481
Ovary-containing hair, dermoid cyst of 261
Overactive bladder syndrome 399
Ovulation induction 335, 429, 431
   methods of 294
Ovulatory dysfunction 252, 253
Ovulatory function, testing 430
Oxygen 413
   saturations 111, 342
   supplemental 123
   therapy 423, 427
Oxytocic infusions 235
Oxytocin 116, 238, 310
   agonist 118
   titration technique 310

P

P53 mutation 477, 478
Paget's disease
    extramammary 471
    of bone 426
Pain relief 54
    methods of 454
Painful bladder syndrome 399
Palm 397, 463
Palmer's point 173, 176
Palpation 14
Pap's smear, guidelines for 273
Papillary serous
            cystadenocarcinoma
            264f
Para-aortic lymphadenectomy 268
Paracervical block 409
    adverse effects of 409
    contraindications of 409
Paracervix 250, 251
Paracetamol 347
Parametrium 270
    dorsal 251
    lateral 251
Parasympathetic blockers 35
Parental karyotype 231
Paresthesia 197
Parity denote 4
Partogram 404
Partograph 55, 56f, 57, 63, 63t
Parvovirus B19 infection 5
Patau syndrome 23
Patellar reflex 112
Pathological retraction ring 85
Patient cart 188
    components of 189f
Patient's bladder 14
Pawlik's grip 10
Peak coagulant action 320
Pelvic
    application 87
    assessment 11, 52
    brim 44, 44f, 52
        bony landmarks of 44
    causes 12
    cavity 46
    curve 86
    dimension 45
    examination 14
    exenteration 273
        role of 273
    floor exercises 454
    grip 68
    infection, active 180
    inflammation 258
    lymph nodes, enlarged 250
    lymphadenectomy 268, 271
    nodes 278
    plane, narrow 45
    pressure 256
    radiation 277
    status of 270
    surgery 251
Pelvic inflammatory disease 182,
            301, 353, 354, 369
    management of acute 338
    prevention of 361
Pelvic inlet 52
    diameters of 44, 45f
    level of 75
Pelvic masses 14
    large 200
Pelvic organ prolapse 216, 399,
            459, 459t
    stages of 459, 459t
Pelvic outlet 108
    level of 74
Pelvic pain 446
    causes of
        acute 13
        chronic 13
    chronic 180, 398
Pelvis 294f, 296f
    anatomical variation of 46
    cavity of 46
    central 273
    contracted 96
    flat 47
    forepart of 79
    inclination of 44
    left side of 89
    movement of 409
    on pelvic assessment,
            normal 52
    true 261
    types of 47, 47f, 79
Penicillin 343
Pentazocine 408
Per speculum examination 15
Per vaginum examination 15
Peri cervical tourniquet 260
Perimortem cesarean
    delivery 120, 122, 124
    section 114
        role of 114
Perinatal death 447
Perinatal mortality 96
    rate 399
Perineal compresses 64
Perineal lacerations, severe 80
Perineal trauma 64
    anterior 64
Perineum stretches 80
Peripheral Health Centers 55
Peritoneal cavity 197
Peritoneal metastasis 477
Peritoneum 195, 480
Peritonitis, generalized 175
Periumbilical adhesions 177, 200
Persistent trophoblastic
            disease 234, 236
Personnel protective
            equipment 122
Pethidine 407
Pfannenstiel incision 197
Phenytoin 314
Physical disabilities 372
Pill 348
    amenorrhea 358
    beneficial side effects of 361
    contraceptive 357t
    male 348
    mechanism of action of 357
    multiphasic 348
    newer 357
    oral 358
    postcoital 358
    progesterone-only 357
    side effects of 361
    standard dose 348
    very low-dose 348
Pinard's maneuver 72, 73f
Pipelle's biopsy curette 161
Pistol-style handle 169
Pituitary prolactin
            hypersecretion 326
Piver-Rutledge-Smith
            classification 250,
            465, 466
Pivot point 94f
Placenta 102, 229, 247, 305
    abnormality 247
    abruption 6, 37
    accreta 247, 248, 304
        diagnosis of 248
    alkaline phosphatase 223
    alpha-microglobulin-1,
            measurement of 225
    and cord 228
    and membranes 100
    cornual-fundal implantation
            of 67

develop, normal 247
diffusa 247
increta 99
insertion, level of 105
lacunae 248
manual removal of 99, 100
method for removal of 310
percreta 99, 247
previa 6, 67, 228, 258, 401
retained 99
separation of 64
   signs of 64
site trophoblastic tumor 233
succenturiate 247
technique of manual removal
   of 100
type of 247
Plasma protein, Pregnancy
   with 24
Plasmalyte® 419
Plasmodium
   falciparum malaria 344
   vivax malaria 344
Plastic spatula 168
Platelet 117
   count 111, 401
Platypelloid 47
Pneumococcus 113
Pneumoperitoneum 172, 173, 176
Podalic pole 67
Podalic version, risks of
   internal 99
Polar body biopsy 101
Polycystic ovarian
   disease 219, 232, 336
   morphology 219, 220
   syndrome 175, 219, 219*fc*, 258,
      294, 322, 331, 336, 395
         diagnosis of 219*t*
Polycystic ovary 294, 294*f*
   diagnosis of 294
Polydioxanone 205, 207
Polyembryoma 266, 267
Polyester fiber uncoated 206
Polyglactin 205
Polyglecaprone 205
Polyhydramnios 238
   causes of 237
Polymerase chain reaction 106
Polyp 12, 180, 249
Polypropylene 206
Poor prognostic factors 270, 274
Popliteal fossa, abduction of 73*f*

Port
   creation of 189
   placement 199*f*
   primary 173
   secondary 173
Portio vaginalis 162
Port-site herniation, incidence
   of 177
Postablation sterilization
   syndrome 185
Post-abortion 354, 362
   contraception 393
Post-arrest care 125
Post-cesarean section 354
Postcoital contraception 331
Postdatism 403
Postdural puncture headache
   410, 411
   treatment of 411
Posthysterectomy vault
   prolapse 168
Postmenopausal woman 255
Postnatal depression 445
   causes of 445
Postpartum 8, 343, 347, 354, 362,
   366
   blues 404, 445
   breastfeeding 362
   endometritis 343
   nonbreastfeeding 362
   period 341
   woman 354, 362
Postpartum hemorrhage 51, 99,
   114, 117, 118, 238, 315,
   319, 404
   bundles for 118*fc*, 119
   management of 114, 117*fc*
      algorithm for 119
   prevention of 310
Postspinal headache 410
Post-term neonate 400
Potassium 422
   removal 424
   shift 424
   sparing diuretics 423
   therapy 423
      contraindications of 423
Pouch of Douglas 242, 290
   free fluid in 301
PPIUCD 355
Prague maneuver 77
Pratt dilators 152
Prazosin 311
Precocious puberty 394

Preconceptional counseling 314
Pre-eclampsia 34, 245, 400, 401
   severe 87
Pregnancy 181, 341
   coma during 111
   complications of 401
   duration of 393
   during 78, 84, 341
   high-risk 34
   intrahepatic cholestasis of 319
   late 103
   loss 446
   low-risk 34
   monochorionic 245
   multifetal 303
   multiple 85, 96, 240, 244, 247,
      304, 311
   prolonged 403
   registered 2
   safety during 313, 328
   teenage 1
   test, urine for 222
   triplet 246
   uncomplicated 298
   vaccines in 17, 17*b*
Pregnant woman 21
   normal 8
Preimplantation genetic
   diagnosis 101
      indications for 101
   screening 101
   testing 101
Premenopausal women 180
Premenstrual syndrome 337, 397,
   444, 445
Premenstrual tension 444
Prenatal diagnostic
   techniques 100
   indications of 100
Primaquine 345
Primary health center 372
Primigravida 69
Primrose oil 337
Prior breech delivery 67
Private health facility 373
Proctoscopy 224
Progesterone 258, 324, 337, 360
   administration of 432
   continuous 255
   derivatives 323
   doses of micronized 325
   hormones 357*t*
   micronized 324
   natural micronized 323

stereoisomers of 323
supplementation 324, 325
   candidates for 324
Progesterone-only pills 357
Progestin 258, 322, 331, 336, 358, 360, 360t, 365
   impregnated intrauterine device 255
Progestin-only contraceptive 365f
   mechanism of action of 364
Progestogen 323, 357
   newer 348
Progestogen-only
   contraceptives 364, 365t
   injectables 351, 365
   pills 348, 351
      contraindications of 366t
Prolactinoma 326
Prophylactic antibiotics 92, 354
Prophylactic chemotherapy, role of 236
Prophylactic medication 337
Prophylaxis 316, 341
Propylthiouracil 320
Prostaglandin
   side effects of 331
   synthetase inhibitors 318
Prostodin 65
Pruritus 276
Psammomatous calcification 264
Pseudosinusoidal pattern 39
Psychosis, postpartum 405
Puberty 394
Pubic arch 71
Pubic symphysis 53, 189, 198
Pudendal block 70
Pudendal nerve block 409, 410f
   analgesia 45
Puerperal fever 404
Puerperal sepsis 346
Pulmonary artery catheter 420
Pulmonary disease 175
Pulmonary edema 111, 422
   subsequent 181
Pulmonary embolism 369
Pulmonary hypertension, primary 316
Pulmonary thromboembolism 412
Pulsatility index 402
Pulse 112
   pressure variation, high 421
   rate 9, 118
Pulseless electrical activity 413
Pulsion medical systems 420

Pyelectasis 27
Pyramidalis 194
Pyrimethamine 344

Q

Quadruple test 24
Querleu-Morrow classification 250, 251t

R

Radiation therapy, role of 227
Radical hysterectomy 251t, 272, 274
   classification of 462, 465t
   modified 272
   types of 251, 271, 272t
Radical trachelectomy 399
Radical vulvectomy 276
   modified 279
Radiofrequency coagulates endometrium 182
Raloxifene 331
Randall's endometrial biopsy curette 160
Ranitidine 326
Reactive nonstress test 30
Reactive vibroacoustic stimulation test 41
Recombinant follicle-stimulating hormone 428
Rectal administration 424
Rectal examination 15
Rectus abdominis 194, 195
Rectus muscle 173, 195, 198
Recurrent pregnancy loss 231, 324, 400, 430
Red blood cells 6, 419
Red rubber catheter 157
Re-entry incisions 198
Registration, application for 435
Relaxation techniques 337
Remifentanil 408, 410
Renal agenesis 301
Renal failure 427
   chronic 326
Renal function 457
   monitoring 427
   test 220
Renal system 423
Replace sensible fluid losses 415
Reproductive changes, biopsychosocial model of 439fc

Reproductive cycle 444
Reproductive performance 285
Reproductive problems, chronic 446
Reserpine 326
Residual disease 267
Respiratory changes 121
Respiratory distress syndrome, acute 422
Respiratory failure 126
Respiratory rate 112, 118
Restricted fluid administration strategies 419
Resuscitation 114, 127
Retractors 165
Retrograde ejaculation 430
Retroperitoneal dissection 159
Reviparin 316
Rhesus
   alloimmunization 6
   D 117
   isoimmunization 6
Rh-negative mother 310
Rhombencephalon 301
Rhythm method 351
Ribs 84
Richardson's retractor 166, 166f
Rigby retractor 167f
Ringer lactate 346
Rising hematocrit 415
RISUG 368
Ritodrine 31, 35
Robotic cannula 189
Robotic gynecological surgery 190f
Robotic instruments 192
Robotic port 190
Robotic surgery 187, 189, 191, 192
   history of 187
   over laparoscopic surgery
      advantages of 192
      disadvantages of 192
   systems, types of 187
Robotic systems 192
Robotic trocar 189, 190f
Robson classification 463, 467t
Rokitansky nodule 262
Rokitansky protuberance 262
Rollerball endometrial ablation 183f
Romberg's sign 408
Ropivacaine 410
Rosette type 221
Rotate fetal 110

RU 486 330
Rubella infection 5
Rubin's maneuver 110f
Rubin's test 161
Rudimentary horn 283
Rugosity 461
Rule of 30 119
Rupture uterus 99, 239, 239f, 241
    danger of 99
    differential diagnosis of 240
    during labor, causes of 240
    during pregnancy, causes of 239
    management of 240
    repair of 240
Ruptured rudimentary horn 242f

S

Sacral nerve roots, lower 409
Sacrococcygeal teratoma 67
Sacrocolpopexy 191
Sacrosciatic notch 11
Sacrum 79
    anterior, right 403
    posterior, right 403
Safe abortion services 371
Safe ambulation 408
Safest distension media 182
Salbutamol 35
Saline
    infusion sonohysterography 223
    instillation sonography 163
Salivary estriol 226
Salpingectomy 244
Salpingogram 280
Salpingo-oophorectomy, bilateral 249f, 250
Sarcomas 274, 471
Sawtooth pattern 305
Scalp 212
    stimulation test 403
    trauma 93
Scanty periods, causes of 12
Scanzoni maneuver 89
Scar
    endometriosis 202
    rupture, incidence of 241
Schial spines 11
Schuchardt incision 202
Scissors 179
    types of 159

Scoliosis 238
Screen-negative test result 25
Screen-positive test result 26
Seasonale, pack of 362
Second stage of labor 38, 61, 63, 64
    managed 64
Second trimester 455-457
    aneuploidy screening 23
    scan 298
    ultrasound in 27
Second-generation techniques 182
Security index 215
Sedlis criteria 274
Seeking behavior 441
Seizures, control 113
Selective estrogen receptor modulator 321
Selective growth restriction 245
Self-inflating bag 128, 133
    and mask 131f
Self-retaining Rigby retractor 167
Semen analysis, reference for 218t
Sensations, loss of 276
Sensitive manner 454
Sentinel lymph node 270, 472
    biopsy 269, 475
Sepsis 113
Septate, differentiate 282
Septum, rectovaginal 290
Seroma 276
Serous
    carcinoma 475, 480
    cystadenomas 264
    tubal intraepithelial carcinoma 251, 480
    tumors 264, 290, 480
        sonographic appearance of 290
Sertoli-Leydig cell tumor 268
Serum
    anti-müllerian hormone 429
    beta-human chorionic gonadotropin 222
    bilirubin 231
    chloride 419
    electrolytes 226, 240
    follicle-stimulating hormone 218, 220
    glutamate pyruvate transaminase 230
    integrated test 25

    iron 230
    luteinizing hormone 220
    potassium 422
    pregnancy test 234
    progesterone 222, 242
    prolactin 219, 220, 223
    quadruple 3
    testosterone 220
    thyroid-stimulating hormone 220
Sex cord-stromal tumor 266, 267
Sex predilection 237
Sex variation 238
Sexual assault 15, 337
    care 15
Sexual partners, multiple 21
Sexually transmitted
    disease 271
    infections 353
Shanks facing downward 157
Sher's grading of abruptio placentae 464, 469t
Shirodkar's procedure 293
Shirodkar's sling procedure 153
Shirodkar's test 152, 162
Shock
    index 119
    postoperative 157
Shoulder 83
    palpating anterior 10
    presentation 85
Shoulder dystocia 108, 109, 404
    complications of 109b
    management of 108fc
Sickle cell
    disease 369
    test 231
Silastic cup 92, 92f
    advantages of 92
Silicon material 128
Sim's anterior vaginal wall retractor 150
Sim's speculum 149, 149f
Simpson's perforator 155, 155f
Sinusoidal fetal heart 38f
Sinusoidal pattern 38
    causes of 38
Sjögren-Larsen syndrome 106
Skin 197
    abdominal 195
    edges 203
    incision 171
    patch, continuous-release 325

Skull
  depressed fracture of 91
  fractures 77
Small cell 475
  keratinizing 274
  neuroendocrine 272
Smear made 168
Smith–Lemli–Opitz syndrome 24
Soaked lap 417
Social supportive network,
    lack of 445
Sodium 281
  ferric gluconate complex 318
Soft-tissue 165
  obstruction 91
Solvent dimethyl sulfoxide 368
Sonogram 288*f*
Sounding uterus, method of 162
Specimens 249, 256, 261
Sperm 428
Spermicidal substances 348
Sphincter 467
Spina bifida 237, 238
Spinal anesthesia 97, 406
Spiramycin 344
Spironolactone 329, 336
Spleen 482
Split-mix regimen 312
Sponge holder 150*f*
Squamous cell carcinoma
    273, 471
  of cervix 274
Stainless steel wire 206
Star-gazing fetus 75
Status epilepticus 112
Stem cells 405
STEPW classification 461
Sterile package 209
Sterilization 368, 378, 442
  eligibility criteria for 368
  female 351, 379
  male 351
  procedure 379
    for female 368, 368*t*
  surgery, success of 382
Steroidal contraceptives 348
Steroids
  antenatal 340, 342
  long-acting 411
Stillbirth 399, 447
  rate 399
Stimulation cycles, mild 428
Stomach empty 176
Stool 231

Stress
  incontinence 399
  reduction 337
  volumes 421
Stroke volume 421
Stromal invasion, depth of 277
Struma ovarii tumor 262
Styrene maleic anhydride 368
Subchorionic fibrin 245
Subclinical hypothyroidism,
    management of 321
Subcutaneous fat 195
Subgaleal hemorrhage, risk of 93
Submucosal fibroid 183*f*, 256,
    257*f*, 258, 260
  symptomatic 260
Submucosal group 287
Submucous myoma
    classification 462*t*
Subserosal fibroid 256, 257*f*
Subumbilical placement 199
Subumbilical trocar 200
Sudden maternal collapse,
    management of 115*fc*
Sufentanil 408, 410
Sulbactam 338
Sulfadiazine 344
Sulfamethoxazole 346
Sulfonylureas 313
Sumatriptan 411
Superfecundation 245, 402
Supracervical hysterectomy 249
Suprapubic
  laterally 173
  midline 173
  pressure 109, 110*f*
Supraumbilical placement 200
Surgeon console 188, 188*f*
Surgeon fatigue, reduced 192
Surgery
  duration of 182
  major 443
  type of 197, 475
Surgical fluid loss 417
Surgical gut 205
Surgical incision, type of 201
Surgical needle 210
  parts of 210, 210*f*
Surgical procedures, perform 172
Surgical silk 206
Surgical sperm extraction
    procedures 430
Surrogacy 429
  clinics 435

  Rules 435, 436
  woman opt for 435
Surrogacy (Regulation) Rules 435
Surrogate mother, safeguard
    rights of 435
Survival rate 412
Suture 203, 209
  absorbable 203, 204, 205*t*
  absorbed 209
  antimicrobial-coated 210
  body react to 209
  buried 204
  compression 117
  deep 204
  determined, size of 210
  line
    primary 204
    secondary 208
  mattress 204
  monofilament 203, 209
  multifilament 209
  purse-string 204
  retention 208
  selection, principles of 203
  skin 203
  subcuticular 204
  tensile strength of 207*t*, 210
  tension 208
  types of 204, 208
Symphysiotomy 111
Symphysis 228
  fundal height 2
  pubis 44, 90, 108
Syndrome of inappropriate
    antidiuretic hormone
    secretion 424
Synechiolysis 180
Synthetic meshes 214
  classification of 214
Synthetic polymer 203
Synthetic progesterone 323
Synthetic tension-free vaginal
    tape obturator 171*f*
Syntometrine 116
Syphilis 346, 434
Syringe
  barrel test 174
  test 200
Systemic causes 12
Systemic disorders 326
Systemic lupus erythematosus
    353, 366

T

Tachycardia 35
  supraventricular 35
  ventricular 427
Tachysystole 403
Tactile feedback, lack of 192
Tamponade 120
Tapering 339
Technology, dependency on 192
Teflon 172
Telencephalon 301
Telescope
  sheath 179
  types of 172
Tennessee classification 470t
Tension pneumothorax 120
Tentorium cerebelli 77
  tears of 91
Teratogenic effects 330
Teratomas, immature 267
Terbutaline 31, 35, 317
Termination of pregnancy 315, 385, 442
  date of 393
  surgical 236
Testicular sperm
  aspiration 430
  extraction 429
Testosterone
  derivatives 323
  total 219
Tetanic uterine contraction 118, 311
Tetanus
  diphtheria, and pertussis vaccination 19
  immunization 6
  immunoglobulin, single dose of 18
  prophylaxis 18
  toxoid 6, 17, 338
Thalassemia 369
Theca lutein cyst 234, 289f
Theophylline 411
Therapeutic applications 330
Thermal balloon ablation 182, 256
Thiazide diuretic induce 426
Third stage of labor 65, 310
  active management of 65, 310
Third-trimester 455-457
  scan 298
  ultrasound scan, role of 304

Thorax, rotate 73
Three-swab test 223
Thrombin 114
Thrombocytopenia 106
Thromboembolism 120
Thrombophilia
  acquired 232
  screening 231
Thromboprophylaxis 347
Thumb 149
Thyroid 13
  disorders 294
  dysfunction 254
  examination 9
  function test 222
  storm 235
Tinidazole 338
Tissue
  adhesives 212
  forceps 158, 159f
    types of 158
  perfusion 415
  retrieval specimens 191
  trauma 419t
  degree of 419
Tocolysis 340, 342
  role of 317, 342
  unless for 97
Tocolytic 96, 317
Topical imiquimod cream, use of 333
Topography 462
Total hysterectomy, indication of 249, 250
Toxicity
  signs of 312t
  symptoms of 312t
  treatment of 312
Toxins 120
Toxoids 18
Toxoplasmosis 292, 344
Tracheoesophageal fistula 238
Traditional robotic gynecologic surgeries 190
Tramadol 407
Tranexamic acid 255, 327, 339
Transabdominal chorionic villus sampling
  advantages of 102
  disadvantages of 102
Transcervical chorionic villus sampling

  advantages of 102
  disadvantages of 102
Transcutaneous electrical nerve stimulation 407
Transhysteroscopic myolysis 183
Transient hyperthyroidism, used for 320
Transitional cell carcinoma 471
Transvaginal approach 409
Transvaginal sonography 222, 228, 237
Transvaginal ultrasound 288, 293, 304
Transverse abdominis 195
  aponeurosis 195
Transverse axis 164
Transverse lie 83, 85
  etiology of 83
  incidence of 83
Trauma 104, 120, 240
Trendelenburg's position 173, 175, 189
Treponema pallidum 434
Trichomonas vaginalis 338
Tricuspid valve Doppler 27
Trimethoprim 346
Triplet delivery, placenta of 244f
Trocar 172, 173f
  insertion
    primary 176
    secondary 176
  introduce 174
  placement, primary 200
  secondary 173
  sleeve 172
Trophoblast cells 101
Trophoblastic tissue 243
Trousseau sign 426
True labor 50
  pains 50, 50t
Tubal cannulation 180, 184
Tubal embryo transfer 429
Tubal ligation 351, 393
Tubal obstruction, proximal 284
Tubal occlusion, causes of 284
Tubal ostia 179
Tubal ostium 180f, 285
Tubal patency
  assessment of 431
  tests 218
Tubal recanalization 191
Tubal spasm 284, 285
  occur 284

Tuberculosis
  abdominal 201
  rule out 218
Tubes, bilateral 268
Tubo-ovarian mass 262
Tubular cavity 285
Tubular instrument 160, 161
Tumor 85, 157, 269
  carcinoid 475
  cells, massive lysis of 424
  epithelial 264
  histological type of 482
  histopathologic 269
  intracranial 292
  malignant 235
  marker 223
    CA-125, role of 265
    CA-19-9 264
  primary 278
  slow-growing 481
  types of 274
  urgical excision of
      primary 279
Turner syndrome 340
Twin 246
  both 245
  conjoint 244f, 245
  delivery, placenta of 244f
  diagnose discordant 246
  dizygotic 244, 245, 402
  fraternal 244
  monoamniotic 247
  monozygotic 402
  pregnancy 235, 246
    complications of 245
  reversed arterial perfusion
      sequence 245
  surviving 246
  syndrome, vanishing 245
  types of 244
  uniovular 244, 245
Twin-peak sign 246
Twin-to-twin transfusion
    syndrome 245, 246
Typhoid vaccine 22

U

Ulipristal acetate 259, 327,
    337, 340
Ultrasonography 287, 298
  diagnoses on 237
  indications for 298
Ultrasound 407
  depth 407

during pregnancy,
    contraindications for
    doing 299
Umbilical artery 105, 229,
    300, 402
  flow 305
  role of 33
Umbilical blood sampling,
    percutaneous 105
Umbilical cord 100, 136f, 155, 305
  assessment 303
  formation of 300
  insertion 307
  knots 37
  placental site of 308
  scissors 155, 155f
Umbilical hernia, history of 200
Umbilical vein 106, 305, 308
Uniform tensile strength 209
Ureter 272
  abdominal part of 275
Ureteric branch 275
Urethra 223
  distal 277
  underneath 171
Urethral diverticulum 162
Urge incontinence 399
Urgency 398
Urinary bladder 272
Urinary frequency 265
Urinary incontinence 398
Urinary ketones 230
Urinary osmolality 415
Urinary retention 251
Urinary sodium 415
Urinary specific gravity 415
Urinary stress incontinence 277
Urinary tract
  infection 5, 6, 175, 276, 345
  injury 111
Urine 223, 226, 229, 231
  albumin 111
  examination 230
  output 112, 421
  pregnancy test, persistent
      positive 234
Urografin 281
Ursodeoxycholic acid 319, 343
Uterine 275
  anomaly 67, 462, 463
    congenital 240
  balloon tamponade 116
  curette 151f, 160, 160f
  displacement, left 122, 413

fibroids 14, 369
fundus 154
hyperactivity 37
hypertonus 403
leiomyoma 183, 258
lesion 284
ligaments 290
malformations 232
massage 311f
masses 302
myoma 102
perforation 151, 152, 161, 184
relaxants 96
size 120
sound 162f
wall 65
Uterine artery 250, 308, 402
  constriction of 409
  Doppler pulsatility index 302
  embolization 100, 260
  ligation 117
  waveform 306
Uterine cavity 160, 180f, 350, 429
  distorted 285f
  size of 182
  visualization of 179
Uterine contraction 52, 89
  sudden 310
Uterine rupture 239, 240
  incidence of 241
Uterocervical length 162
Uteroplacental insufficiency 36
Uterosacral ligaments 272
Uterotonics 116
Uterotubal junction devices 348
Uterus 241, 260, 261f, 272, 275
  anteverted 15
  bicornuate 281, 281f, 282
  bicorporeal 463
  complete evacuation of 170
  congenital malformation of 96
  craniocaudally, parts of 298
  fibroid 256, 258, 287f, 339
  filling defect in 283f
  fundus of 9
  intact 272
  packing 150
  portion of 283
  pregnant 160
  retroverted 15, 162
  scar 97
  septate 67, 282
  subseptate 83
  tonicity of 117

Index

unicornuate 67, 282f
with cervix, specimen of 249
Uterus-holding forceps,
types of 163

V

Vacuum cup, bird's modification of 92
Vacuum-assisted birth 94
Vagina 64, 110, 149, 161, 165, 212, 277
    cuff of 270
    cut edges of 153
    length of 461
    posterior wall of 149
    preparation of 150
    thickness of 461
Vaginal anomaly 462, 463
Vaginal bleeding 236, 240
Vaginal breech delivery 78
Vaginal canal 186
Vaginal cancer 271, 473
    primary 473
    staging of 473t
Vaginal carcinoma 473
Vaginal delivery 68, 124, 345, 407
    normal 346
    operative 95
    planned 78
    spontaneous 82
Vaginal estrogenic creams 325
Vaginal examination 15, 52, 53f, 68, 442
Vaginal fornix 171
    posterior 168
Vaginal health index, modified 461, 461t
Vaginal hysterectomy 151, 153, 162
Vaginal incision 171
Vaginal margin 272
Vaginal mesh systems 216f
Vaginal myomectomy 156
Vaginal radical trachelectomy 273
Vaginal replacement 110
Vaginal secretions 225
Vaginal speculum 186
    self-retaining 165
Vaginal sponge 356f
Vaginal surgery 166, 168
Vaginal wall 149
    posterior 165
    retractor, anterior 150f

Vaginismus 398
Vaginoscopy 223
Valproic acid 314
Varicella
    infection 20
    virus vaccine 20
    zoster immunoglobulins 20
Vas deferens, congenital bilateral absence of 430
Vasa previa 304, 401
Vascular disease 353
Vasectomy 351
Vasopressin, use of 260, 332
Vasovagal reaction 185
Vault granulation 252
Vena cava
    collapsibility index 421
    inferior 229
Venous intravasation 281f
Venous return 420
Venous system 421
Venous thromboembolism 360
    management of 347
Ventilation, positive-pressure 126, 128, 129, 134-137
Ventilatory problems 176
Ventouse 92, 92f
    cups, types of 92
    over forceps, advantages of 93
Ventouse application 80, 93
    complications of 94
    contraindications for 93
    indications for 93
Ventral parametrium 251
Ventricular fibrillation 427
Ventriculomegaly 27
Verapamil 326
Verbal consent 377
Veress needle 172, 173, 173f, 176
    correct placements of 200
    double-click sound of 200
    insertion 199
Verrucous carcinoma 471
Versapoint 182
Vertex 48
Vertical abdominal incisions, types of 195
Vesicovaginal repair 163
Vessel injury 176
    major 177
    primary 177
Vestibular bulb 471

Vibroacoustic stimulation 41
    test 40, 41, 403
Video laparoscopy 200
Villo-glandular variant 475
Virilization 395
Virtual hysteroscopy 185
Visceral injury 176
Vision cart 188
    components of 189f
Visual field test 221
Vitamin
    B_6 337
    E 337
Vomiting 245
Vulva
    carcinoma 275, 276
    precancerous lesions of 471
    preparation of 150
    protection 333
Vulval cancer 276, 277, 471
    classification of 473
    development of 275
    histological type of 471
    incidence of 275
    prognostic factors for 277
    spread 276
    treatment of 277, 278
    types of 276
Vulval carcinoma 275f, 471
Vulval intraepithelial neoplasia 471
Vulval lesion 276
Vulval malignancy 224, 471
Vulval melanoma 471
Vulvar dystrophie 275
Vulvar intraepithelial neoplasia 275
Vulvar pain syndrome 398
Vulvectomy, simple 276
Vulvodynia 398
Vulvovaginal candidiasis 339

W

Warfarin 316, 347
Water birth method 411
Weakness 426
Wedge biopsy 276
Weight fluctuations 186
Weight gain 7, 7t
Weight reduction 336
Wertheim's clamp 164f
Wertheim's hysterectomy 163, 164, 250

Index

Wertheim's smears 168
Wertheim's vaginal clamp 164
Westin scoring system 464, 469*t*
Wheel aligns contraceptive
    methods 349
Woods corkscrew maneuver
    109, 110*f*
Wound
    closure, options for 210
    dehiscence 197, 199
    edges 165
    kind of 210
    therapy, negative pressure 213
Writ petition 372

Writing prescription, principles
    for 334
Written consent 377

X

Xiphisternum 197
Xiphoid process 195
X-ray 280
    skull 221

Y

Yolk sac 299
    tumors 266

YS joins, wall of 300
Yuzpe regimen 337

Z

Zatuchni-Andros score 69,
    464, 469*t*
Zavanelli maneuver 110
Zidovudine 338
Ziehl–Neelsen staining 221
Zoster vaccine 20
Zuspan regimen 112, 312
Zygote intrafallopian
    transfer 396